TARGET

NEET PG

2019

(Review of NEET PG 2019 – Model Questions with Solved Explanatory Answers)

Dr. KANTAMANI BALA TEJA, MS ENT, Mch
Head and Neck Oncosurgery, Senior Resident

Dr. T. ARUN BABU
MD Pediatrics (JIPMER), DAA (CMC Vellore), MBA (HM)
Fellow in Neonatal Perinatal Medicine (Canada)
Associate Professor and Head, Department of Pediatrics
All India Institute of Medical Sciences (AIIMS)
Mangalagiri – 522 503
Website: www.drarunbabu.in

Peepee Publishers and Distributors (P) Ltd.®

TARGET NEET PG 2019

Published by
Pawaninder P. Vij and Anupam Vij

Peepee Publishers and Distributors (P) Ltd.
Head Office: 160, Shakti Vihar, Pitam Pura, Delhi-110 034 (India)

Correspondence Address:
7/31, First Floor, Ansari Road, Daryaganj
New Delhi-110 002 (India)
Ph: 41512412, 23246245, 9811156083
e-mail: peepee160@yahoo.co.in
e-mail: peepee160@gmail.com
www.peepeepub.com
join us on facebook.com/pp.publishers

First Edition: 2019

ISBN: 978-81-8445-272-3

DEDICATION

Dr. Teja: To my Parents and Family along with my Teachers

Dr. Arun Babu: To my Parents, Teachers, my wife Dr. Sharmila, my kids Akshaya and Akash

DISCLAIMER

PREFACE

The NEET PG exam is the single largest medical entrance exam in India, which decides the fate of thousands of budding medicos. As we all know, the exam conducting team, the pattern of exam and MCQs asked keep changing every year. It is extremely important for a PG aspirant to be aware of these changes in examination pattern and recent trends about questions being asked in various subjects to outshine their competitors. Most of these exams have direct repeats and favourite topic repeats all the time, which plays a crucial role in deciding your rank. On reviewing the most recent NEET PG exam pattern which is there for last 2 years (single session/ same paper pattern), it is very obvious there are only few books available in the market specifically targeting this recent pattern exam.

This book was written with the sole purpose of guiding aspirants to crack the recent NEET PG. This book includes collection of model MCQs from the most recent 2019 exam. The important advantage of this book is that the students will be aware of the recent trends in questions asked and can strategize their preparations accordingly. This book will give PG aspirants the cutting edge required to excel in these exams.

We have put in tremendous effort to make sure that all the questions discussed in the book are accurate. Questions solved using references from standard textbooks/articles and a detailed background theory has been included. Book also contains numerous tables and illustrations, which will help in easy understanding and long-term retention. MCQs have been solved by a team of well-qualified and experienced subject experts from various reputed institutes of India. ***For controversial questions, every attempt has been made to trace the source textbook or article and solve the questions.*** Every subject MCQs have references, Tables, Magical points, Illustrations and Flowcharts for the better understanding and authenticity. Highlighted points are essential for answering repeat questions in forthcoming exams.

We would like to express our sincere gratitude to all the contributors, for their hard work and commitment, which has led to this high quality content. We wish to thank our publishers, Mr. Pawaninder Pal Vij and Mr. Anupam Vij, the Directors of Peepee Publishers and Distributors (P) Ltd, for their support and special interest on this project. We would also like to thank our publishing team for their relentless efforts in releasing this book in a short notice. We are deeply indebted to students for their overwhelming support, feedback and critical appraisal on our previous projects. We are looking forward to hear your feedback on this book and are fully committed in bringing out better editions in the future. "Our happiness lies in your success" and the only path for success is "Persistence" and "Hard work". Have faith in yourselves, your parents and Almighty God. All the best!

Kantamani Bala Teja

T. Arun Babu

ACKNOWLEDGEMENTS

Mr. Thirunavukkarasu D, Government School English Lecturer (Retd), Puducherry.
Mrs. Sampurnam, Principal (Retd), SSVHSS, Puducherry.
Mr. Vijayan D, Cash Officer (Retd), SBI, Puducherry.
Mrs. Sagoundala, Under Secretary (Retd), Government of Puducherry.
Mr. Srinivasan@Babu, PWD, Puducherry.
Mr. Dhinesh Shankar, MCA, RS Solutions, Chennai.
Mr. Rajkumar, System Engineer, Apple, CA, USA.
Mr. Kantamani Bhanu Teja, Veterinary Assistant Surgeon, Tanuku.
Mr. Kantamani Veera Raghavulu, Chief Engineer, Andhra Sugars Limited, Tanuku.

Write to Us:
Any observations, suggestions, criticisms are welcome. Write to the author at ***babuarun.t@gmail.com***

Errata
Please visit: ***www.drarunbabu.in*** & ***www.peepeepub.com***

Follow Author in Facebook: ***www.facebook.com/targetjipmer/***and ***www.facebook.com/targetneetpg/***
Dr Arun Babu's Pediatrics Discussion group

CONTRIBUTORS

Dr. Kantamani Bala Teja, MS ENT, Mch
Head and Neck Oncosurgery Senior Resident
(Chief Editor)

Dr. Arun Babu T, MD Pediatrics (JIPMER), DAA (CMC), Fellow NPM (Canada)
Associate Professor and Head, Department of Pediatrics
All India Institute of Medical Sciences (AIIMS)
Mangalagiri – 522 503
(Chief Editor)

Dr. Mugunthan N, MS Anatomy, DNB, PhD, MBA
Professor of Anatomy
Sree Mookambika Institute of Medical Sciences
Kulasekaram, Kanyakumari District, Tamil Nadu – 629161
(Anatomy)

Dr. Jean Fredrick, MD Physiology
Assistant Professor, Department of Physiology
Mahatma Gandhi Medical College and Research Institute
Puducherry
(Physiology)

Dr. Usha Sachidananda Adiga, MD PhD
Professor, Department of Biochemistry
KS Hegde Medical Academy, NITTE–DU
Mangalore, Karnataka – 575018
(Biochemistry)

Dr. Arundhathi S, MD Pathology
Associate Professor, Department of Pathology
All India Institute of Medical Sciences (AIIMS)
Mangalagiri – 522 503
(Pathology)

Dr. Archana Voleti, MSc.PhD
Assistant Professor, Department of Microbiology
Gayathri Vidya Parishad
Visakhapatnam – 530048
(Microbiology)

Dr. Bharath Kumar VD, MD Pharmacology
Assistant Professor, Department of Pharmacology
BGS Global Institute of Medical Sciences
Bangalore, Karnataka
(Pharmacology)

Dr. Yatiraj Singi, MD Forensic Medicine
Professor, Department of Forensic Medicine
Sree Mookambika Institute of Medical Sciences
Kulasekaram, Kanyakumari District
Tamil Nadu – 629161
(FMT)

Dr. Prakash Mathiyalagen, MD PSM (AFMC)
Assistant Professor, Department of Preventive and Social Medicine
Indira Gandhi Medical College and Research Institute (IGMC and RI)
Puducherry – 605009
(PSM)

Dr. Rajesh Vepuri, MS–ENT, Fellow in Rhinoplasty (Jaipur), Fellow in Rhinology (Australia), Fellow in Anterior Skull Base (Malaysia)
Assistant Professor, Department of ENT
Katuri Medical College, Guntur – 540019
(ENT)

Dr. Srikanta Kumar Padhy, MD Ophthalmology (AIIMS, New Delhi)
Fellow Retina and Vitreous
LV Prasad Eye Institute, New Delhi
(Ophthalmology)

Dr. Soumya Sathyan, MD General Medicine
Senior Resident
MES Medical College, Perintalmanna
(Medicine)

Dr. Deepthi Ala, MD General Medicine
Assistant Professor
Katuri Medical College
Guntur – 540019
(Medicine)

Dr. Rakesh Chintala, DM–Endocrinology
Senior Resident
Vijayawada
(Medicine)

Dr. Ram Prakash Gurram, MS, Mch–Gastrosurgery
Senior Resident
JIPMER
Puducherry
(Surgery)

Dr. Sharmila, MS OBG (JIPMER)
Assistant Professor, Department of Obstetrics and Gynecology
Indira Gandhi Medical College and Research Institute (IGMC and RI)
Puducherry – 605009
(OG)

Dr. Dinesh Kumar, MD Pediatrics
Assistant Professor, Department of Pediatrics
Indira Gandhi Medical College and Research Institute (IGMC and RI)
Puducherry – 605009
(Pediatrics)

Dr. Mukul Mohindra, MS Ortho, DNB, MNAMS, Dip. SICOT (Belgium)
Fellow National Board (Arthroscopy and Sports Medicine)
Sports Injury Center, Safdarjung Hospital and VMM College
New Delhi
(Orthopedics)

Dr. Prabhakaran N, MD Dermatology (JIPMER), DNB
Assistant Professor, Department of Dermatology
All India Institute of Medical Sciences (AIIMS), Mangalagiri
(Dermatology)

Dr. Kethireddi S Divya, MD, DVL
Assistant Professor, Department of Dermatology
Gayathri Vidya Parishad and Medical College
Visakhapatnam – 530048
(Dermatology)

Dr. Sangeeta Dhanger, DA, DNB, MNAMS
Assistant Professor, Department of Anesthesiology
Indira Gandhi Medical College and Research Institute
(IGMC and RI)
Puducherry – 605009
(Anesthesia)

Dr. Prudhvinath Reddy A, MD, DNB, Fellow in Body Imaging
Assistant Professor, Department of Radiodiagnosis
AIIMS, Mangalagiri
(Radiology)

Dr. Challa SV Krishna Vasan, MD Psychiatry
Resident, Department of Psychiatry
Andhra Medical College
Visakhapatnam – 530017
(Psychiatry)

EXPERT REVIEWERS

Dr. Chidanand KJC, MS Ortho
Assistant Professor, Department of Orthopedics
Sanjay Gandhi Institute of Trauma and Orthopedics
Bangalore, Karnataka
(Orthopedics)

Dr. Madhusudhan NS, MD Microbiology
Assistant Professor, Department of Microbiology
Indira Gandhi Medical College and Research Institute
(IGMC and RI)
Puducherry – 605009
(Microbiology)

EDITORIAL ASSISTANCE

Gaurang Narayan, MBBS Student
Indira Gandhi Medical College and Research Institute
(IGMC and RI)
Puducherry – 605009

Padmapriya, MD Pathology
Resident, Department of Pathology
Andhra Medical College
Visakhapatnam – 605009

CONTENTS

Chapter 1

ANATOMY

1. Movement at the following joint permits a person to look towards the right or left:

A. Atlantoaxial B. Atlanto-occipital

C. C2-C3 D. C3-C4

Key:

- *Atlanto-occipital (between skull and C1) joint permit nodding of head (indicating approval–YES)*
- *Atlantoaxial joint permits the head to be turned from side to side (indicating disapproval–NO)*

CRANIOVERTEBRAL JOINTS (SYNOVIAL JOINTS)

- **Atlanto-occipital**
- **Atlantoaxial**

- ***Both are synovial joints.***
- Provide relatively wide range of motion compared with other joints of vertebral column.
- Atlanto-occipital joint allows one to nod head up and down (Flexion and Extension).
- ***Atlantoaxial joint is a pivot joint that permits one to rotate head from side to side, as if to indicate "no".***
- Axis (C2) is point of articulation where head turns on neck, providing an "axis of rotation".

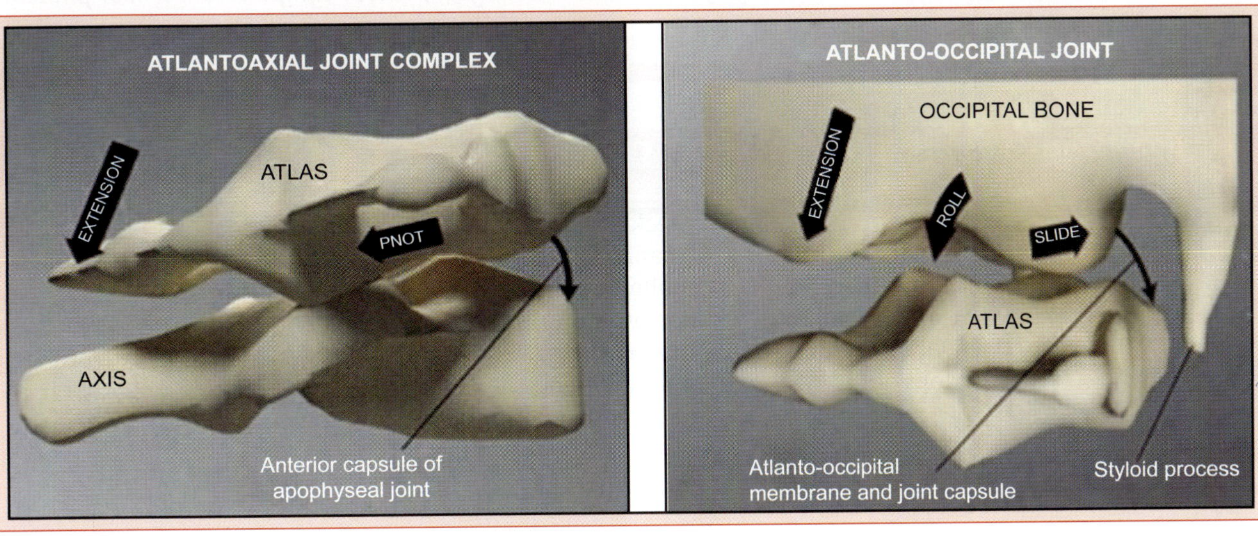

Contd.

Contd.

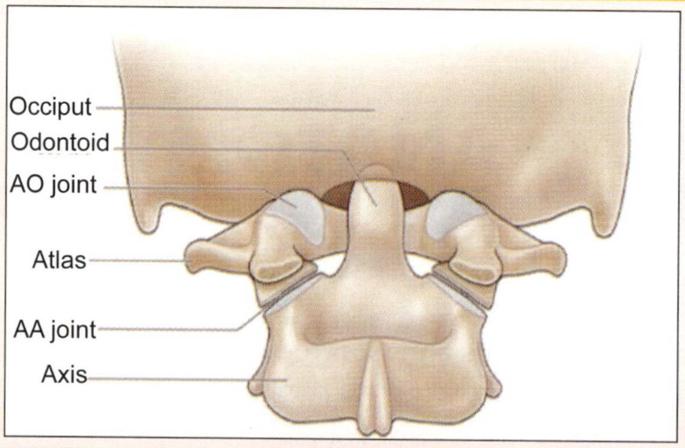

Clinical Importance

- Jefferson fracture–Burst fracture atlas (C1) often caused by blow to top of the head.
- "Hangman" fracture is a pedicle fracture of the axis.

Ref: Netter's Clinical Anatomy 2nd Edition Page 43, Gray's 41st Edition Page 737, Snell Clinical Anatomy Page 26

Ans: (A) Atlantoaxial

2. Which of the following muscle is derived from 1st pharyngeal arch?

A. Stylopharyngeus
B. Stapedius
C. Anterior belly of digastric
D. Posterior belly of digastric

Key:

Anterior belly of digastrics is a muscle derivative of first pharyngeal arch

- Stylopharyngeus is the only muscle derived from the 3rd pharyngeal arch.
- Stapedius is a muscle of 2nd arch
  - *Muscles of the hyoid arch or 2nd pharyngeal arch are the stapedius, stylohyoid, posterior belly of the digastric, auricular, and muscles of facial expression.*
- **Anterior Belly of Digastric is a muscle of 1st pharyngeal arch**
  - ***Musculature of the first pharyngeal arch includes the muscles of mastication (temporalis, masseter, medial and lateral pterygoids), anterior belly of digastric, mylohoyoid, tensor tympani and tensor palatini.***

Arch	Cranial nerve	Muscles	Cartilages/bones	Cleft/pouch derivatives	Aortic arch remnant
1	V	Muscles of mastication, anterior belly of digastric, tensor veli palatini, tensor tympani, mylohyoid	Meckel's cartilage (mandible, malleus, incus, sphenomandibular ligament), maxilla, palatine bone, squamous temporal bone	**Cleft:** External acoustic meatus **Pouch:** Middle ear cavity, Eustachian tube, mastoid air cells	Maxillary artery

Contd.

Contd.

2	VII	Muscles of facial expression, stylohyoid, stapedius, posterior belly of digastric	Reichert's cartilage (stapes, styloid process, stylohyoid ligament, lesser horn of hyoid bone)	**Pouch:** Palatine tonsils	Stapedial and hyoid arteries
3	IX	Stylopharyngeus	Greater horn and inferior body of hyoid bone	**Pouch:** Inferior parathyroid glands, thymus	Common and internal carotid arteries
4	X (Pharyngeal, superior laryngeal)	Pharyngeal and palatal muscles (except stylopharyngeus, TVP), cricothyroid	Thyroid cartilage	**Pouch:** Superior parathyroid glands, ultimobranchial body	Arch of aorta, right subclavian artery
6	X (Recurrent laryngeal)	All intrinsic muscles of larynx except cricothyroid	Cricoid cartilage, arytenoids, corniculate and cuneiform cartilages	None	Ductus arteriosus, pulmonary arteries

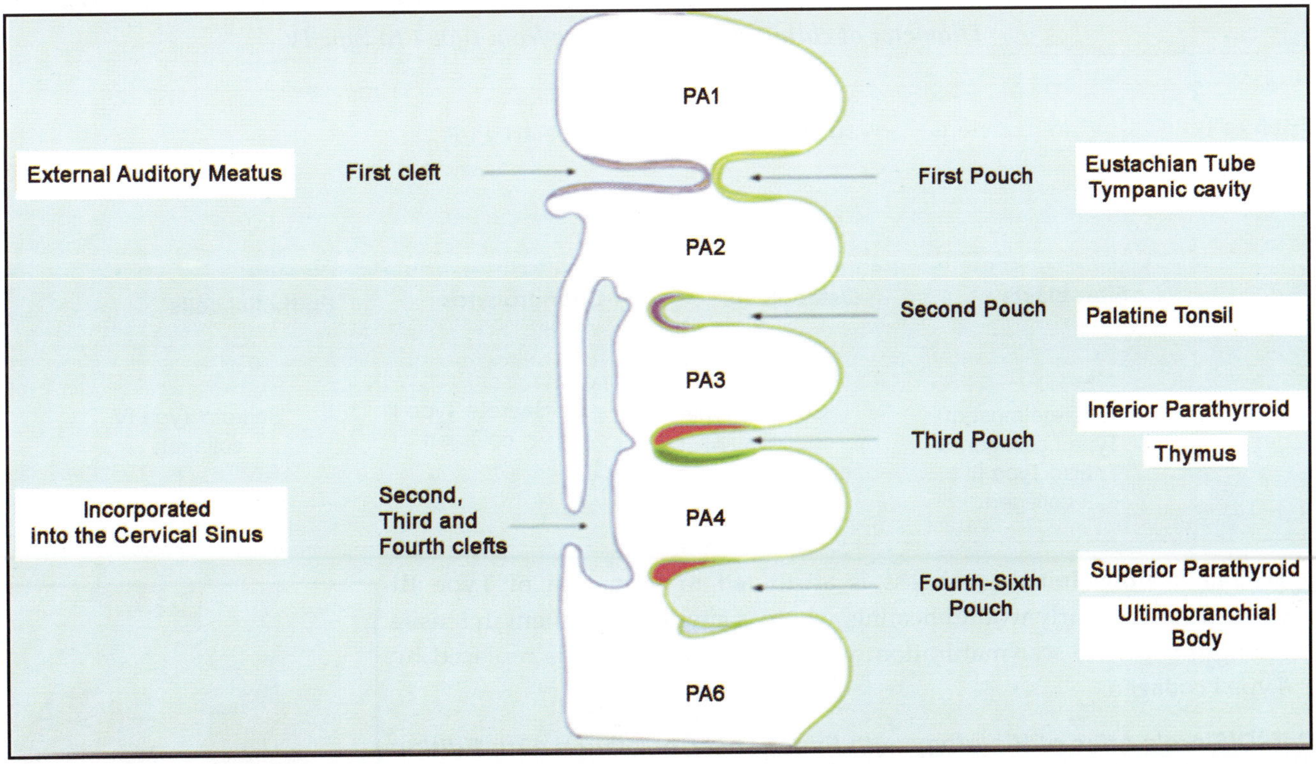

Ref: Langman's Medical Embryology 12th Edition Page 264, Gray's Anatomy 40th Edition Page 597, Keith Moore 9th Edition Page 165, Keith Moore 9th Edition Page 165

Ans: (C) Anterior belly of digastric

3. Type of collagen that is maximum in skin is:

A. Type I B. Type II C. Type III D. Type IV

Key:

Type I collagen–Most common connective tissue fibres found in the dermis of the skin

Collagen	
Type I	• 90% of body collagen • Very strong • Offers great resistance to tensile strength • Present in fibrocartilage, bones, tendons, ligament, fasciae, dermis of skin and capsules of organs
Type II	• Provides support to • Resist pressure • Present in hyaline and elastic cartilages
Type III	• Delicate • Support cells of Lymph nodes, spleen and bone marrow
Type IV	• Found in the basal lamina of basement membrane
Diameter of collagen fibres decrease from type I to type IV	

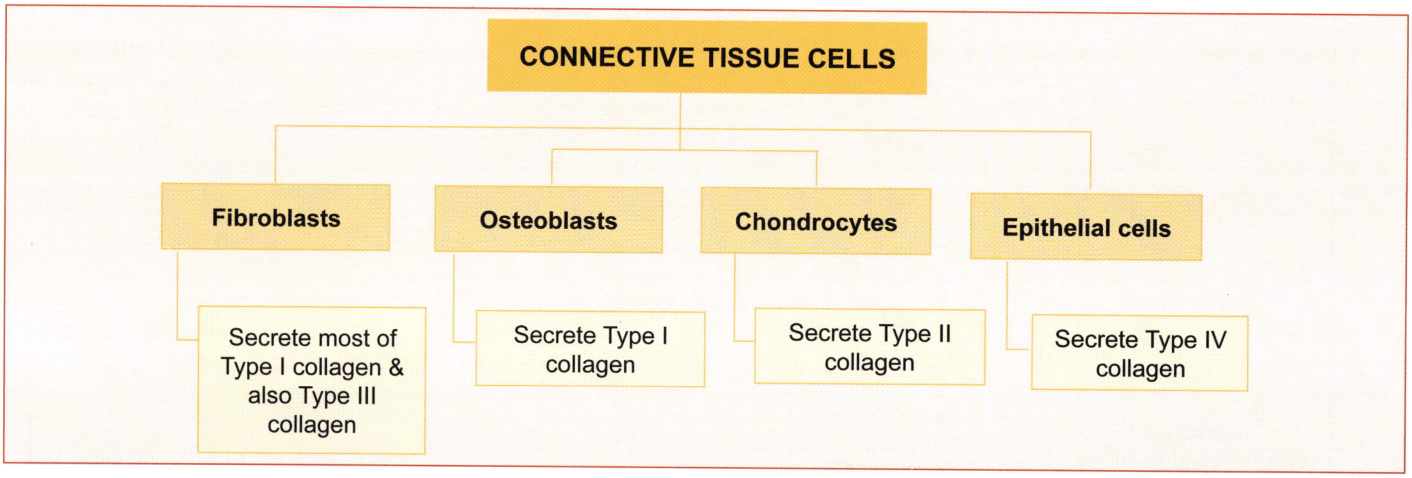

- ***Wound healing:*** Initial weakness is attributed to formation of Type III collagen during early wound healing, whereas later improvement in tensile strength is due to scar maturation, when Type III collagen is replaced by Type I collagen.

Ref: DiFiore's Atlas of Histology with Functional Correlation 13th Edition Page 76, Bloom and Fawcett's Concise Histology 2nd Edition Page 65, Harper 30th Edition Page 628

Ans: (A) Type I

4. Nerve that supplies below marked structure is:

A. Median nerve
B. Ulnar nerve
C. Posterior interosseous nerve
D. Anterior interosseous nerve

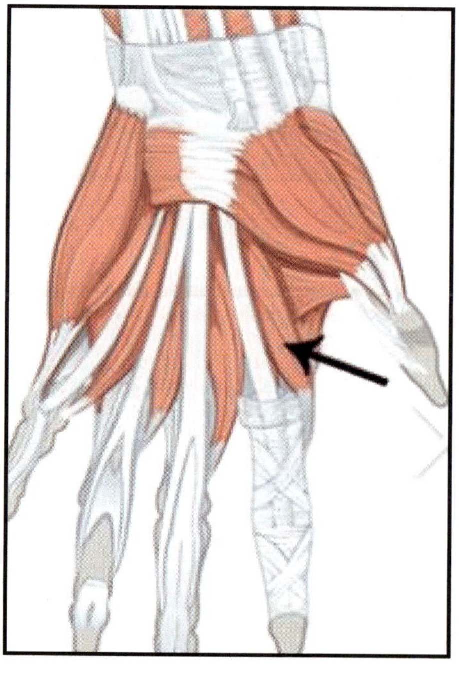

Key:

Picture depicted shows marked structure with pointed arrow–1st Lumbrical.
Distal to carpal tunnel median nerve supplies thenar muscles and 1st and 2nd lumbricals.

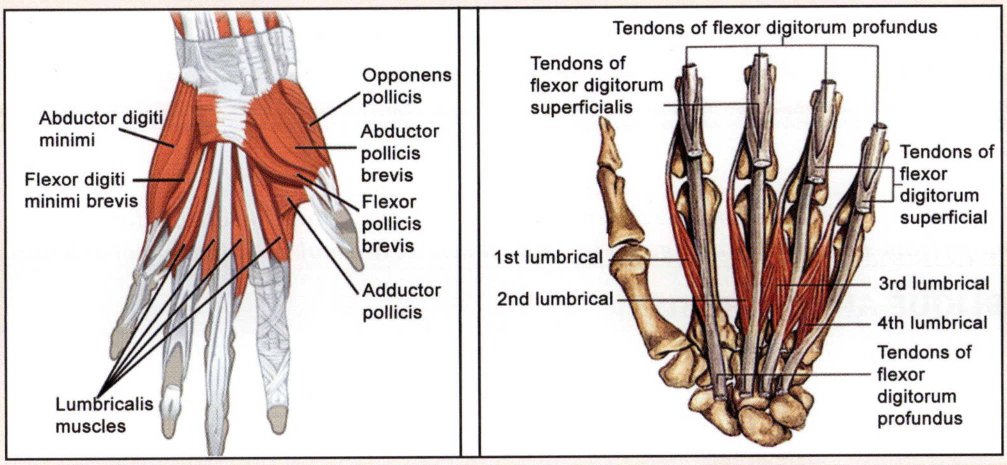

- Lumbricals are 4 small fasciculi that arise from flexor digitorum profundus tendons.
- Lumbricals 1 and 2 arise from lateral two tendons and lumbricals 3 and 4 arise from medial three tendons of Flexor digitorum profundus respectively.
- Lumbricals flex the fingers at Metacarpophalangeal joints and extend Interphalangeal joints.

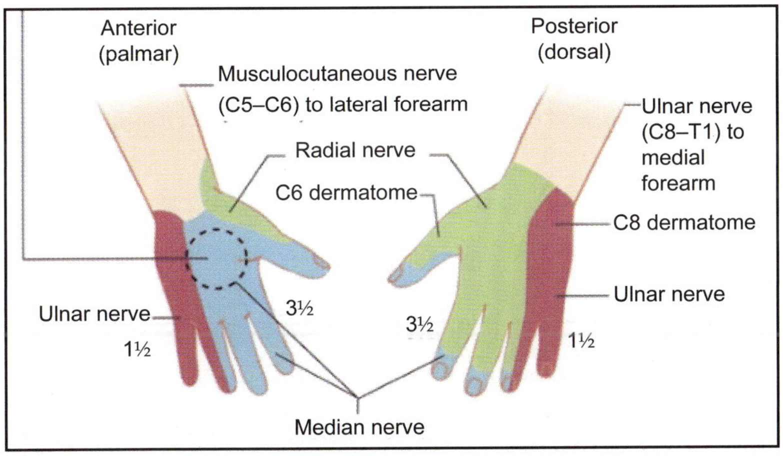

1st and 2nd Lumbricals	Unipinnate	Median Nerve
3rd and 4th Lumbricals	Bipinnate	Ulnar Nerve

Nerve	Motor Supply	Sensory Supply
Median	Thenar muscles–Abductor pollicis brevis, Flexor pollicis brevis, Opponens pollicis and Lumbricals of index and middle fingers	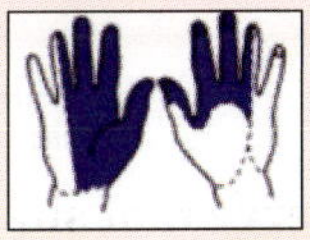
Ulnar	Flexor carpi ulnaris, Flexors of distal phalanx of ring and little fingers, All intrinsic hand muscles except thenar muscles	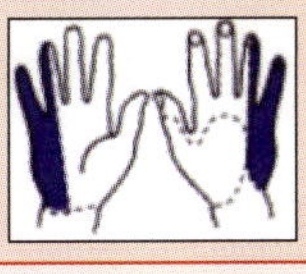
Radial	Triceps, Brachioradialis, Supinator, All extensors of wrist, thumb and fingers	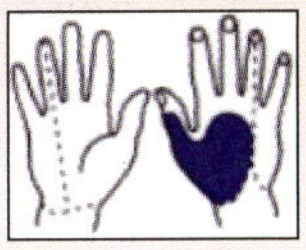

Ref: Keith L Moore Clinically Oriented Anatomy 5th Edition Page 835, Netter's Clinical Anatomy 2nd Edition Page 331, Gray's Anatomy 40th Edition Page 886

Ans: (A) Median nerve

5. **All of the following are extensions of External Oblique Aponeurosis except:**
   A. Lacunar ligament
   B. Pectinate ligament
   C. Linea semilunaris
   D. Inguinal ligament

Key:

Linea semilunaris is semilunar line/spigelian line. Curved tendinous insertion found on both sides of rectus muscle extending from 9th costal cartilage tip to pubic tubercle. It is not an extension of external oblique aponeurosis

EXTERNAL OBLIQUE APONEUROSIS

- **External oblique aponeurosis presents these extensions mainly.**
- ***Inguinal Ligament:*** Thickened lower border of the aponeurosis of the external oblique.
  - Attached laterally to the anterior superior iliac spine, medially, to pubic tubercle.
- ***Lacunar ligament:*** Apex is formed by the pubic tubercle and its concave base forms the medial boundary of femoral ring.
- ***Pectineal ligament:*** Attached to the pecten pubis upto to ilio-pubic eminence.

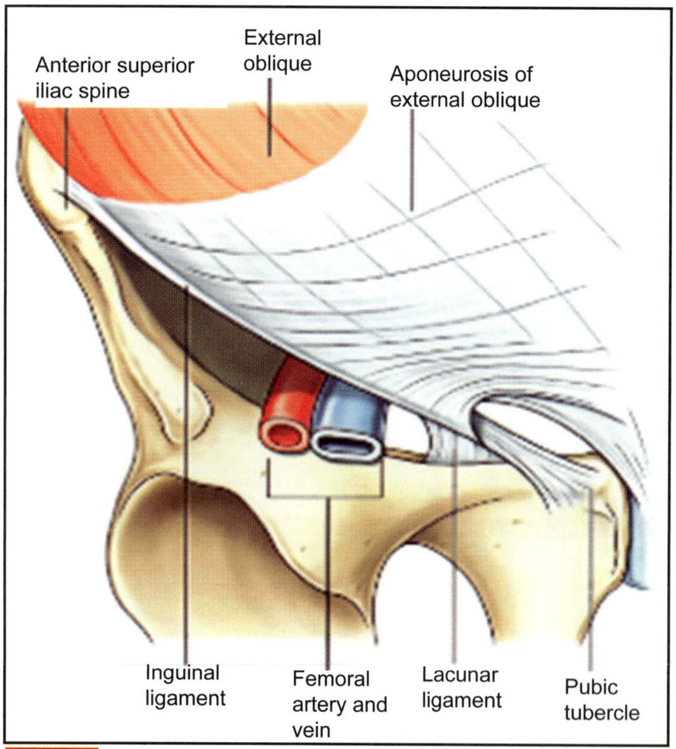

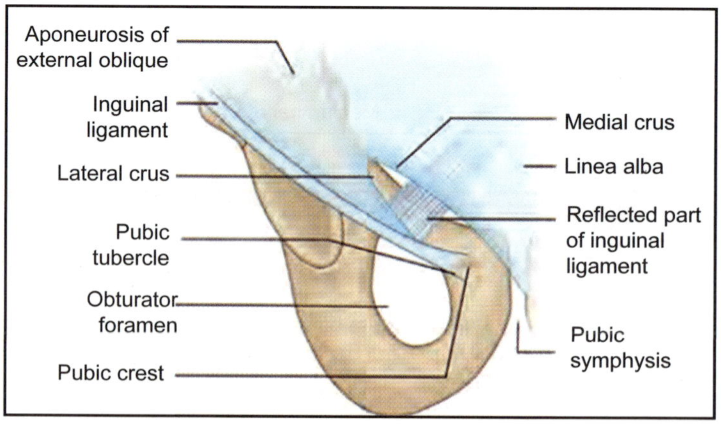

Linea Semilunaris

- Curved fibrous line extending from pubic tubercle to tip of the 9th costal cartilage.
- Forms lateral margin of rectus sheath.

Contd.

Contd.

- Anterior rami of lower six thoracic nerves enter the rectus sheath after passing across this line between the aponeurosis of internal oblique and transversus muscles.
- Surgical incision of anterior abdominal wall along linea semilunaris may produce segmental paralyisis of recuts abdominis muscle due to injury of lower thoracic nerves.

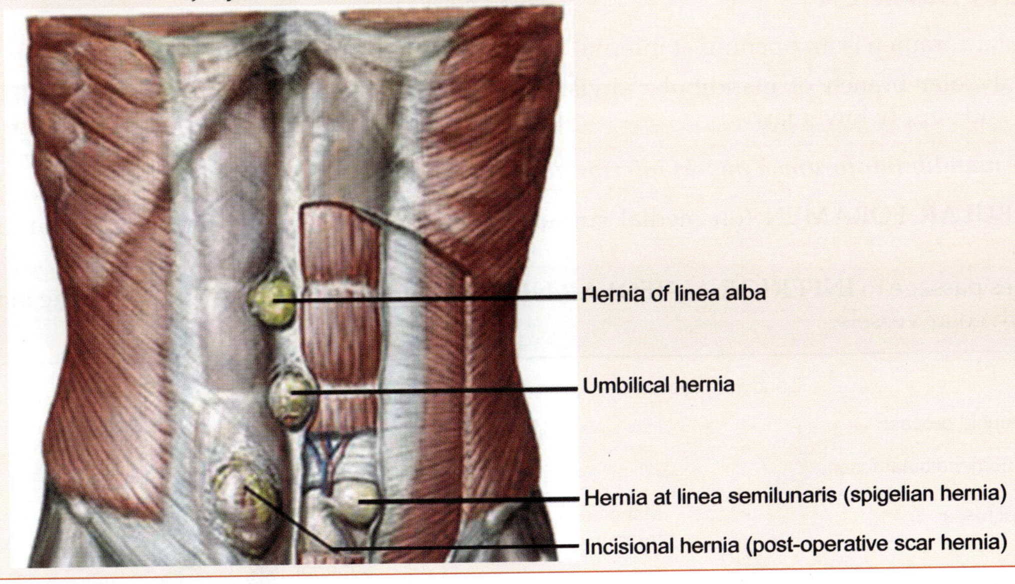

Ref: A K Dutta 9th Edition Page 121, Gray's Anatomy 41st Edition Page 1079, Inderbir Singh, 6th Edition, Chapter 14 Page 165, Vishram Singh 2nd Edition Page 54

Ans: (C) Linea semilunaris

6. **Identify structure that passes through below marked structure:**

A. Maxillary nerve
B. Inferior alveolar nerve
C. Lingual nerve
D. Chordatympani nerve

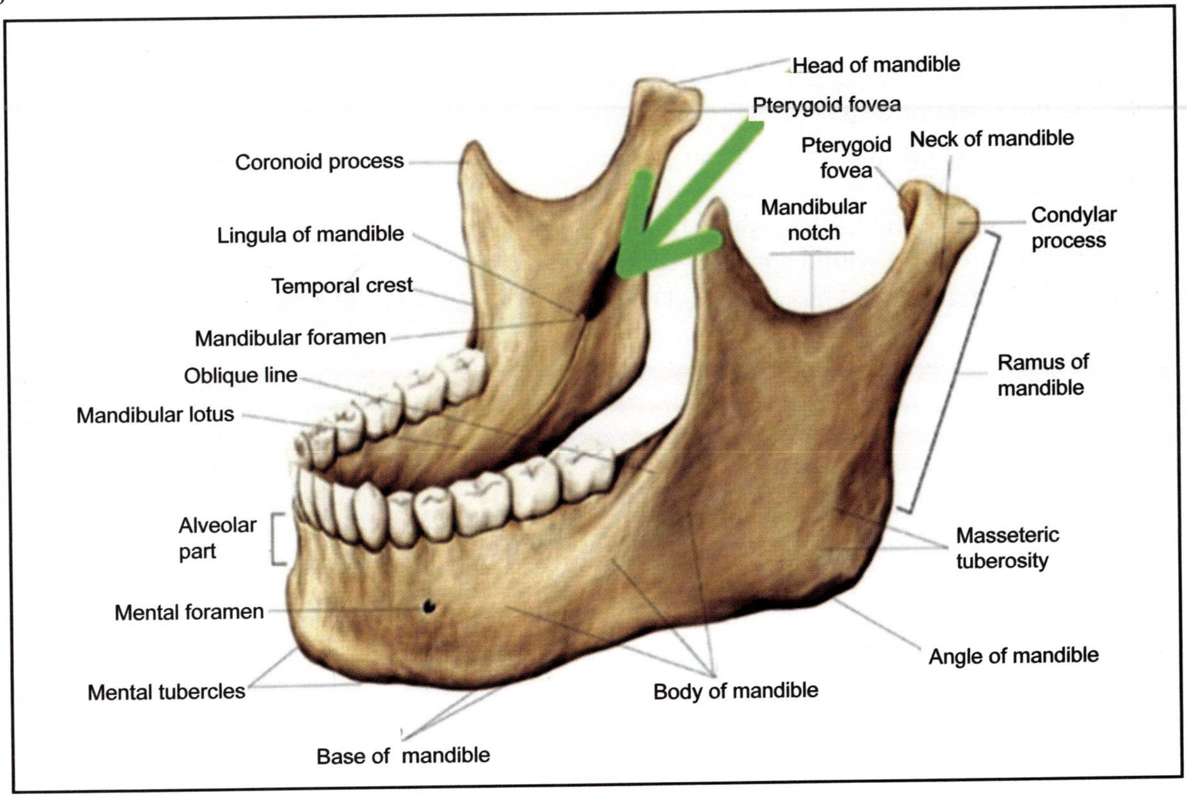

Key:

Picture depicts opening in inner aspect of ramus of mandible–MANDIBULAR FORAMEN

MANDIBULAR FORAMEN

- Mandibular foramen is an opening at internal aspect of ramus of mandible.
- Inferior alveolar branch of mandibular division of trigeminal nerve along with inferior alveolar vessels enter foramen and supply lower jaw.

Through the mandibular foramen passes inferior alveolar neurovascular bundle to gain access to mandibular canal.

- **MANDIBULAR FORAMEN** (on medial surface of ramus) leads into mandibular canal and opens as mental foramen.
- It provides passage to **INFERIOR ALVEOLAR NERVE** (branch of posterior division of the mandibular nerve) and inferior alveolar vessels.

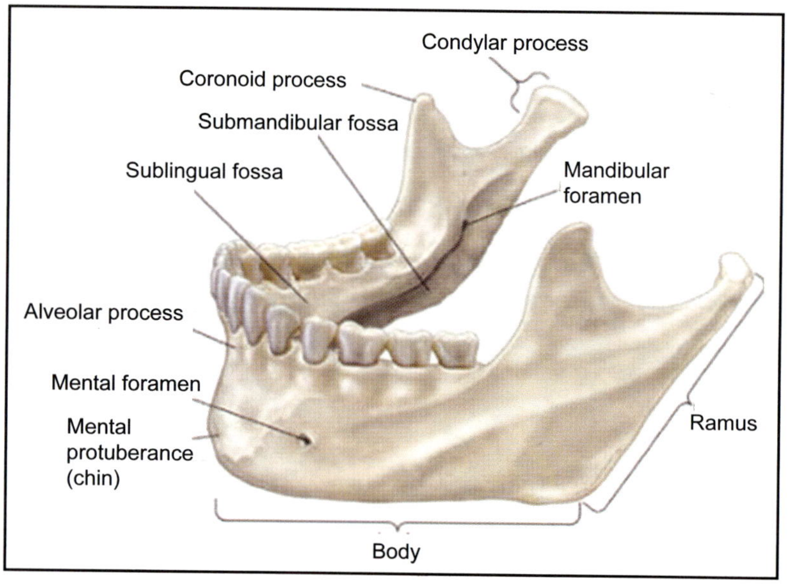

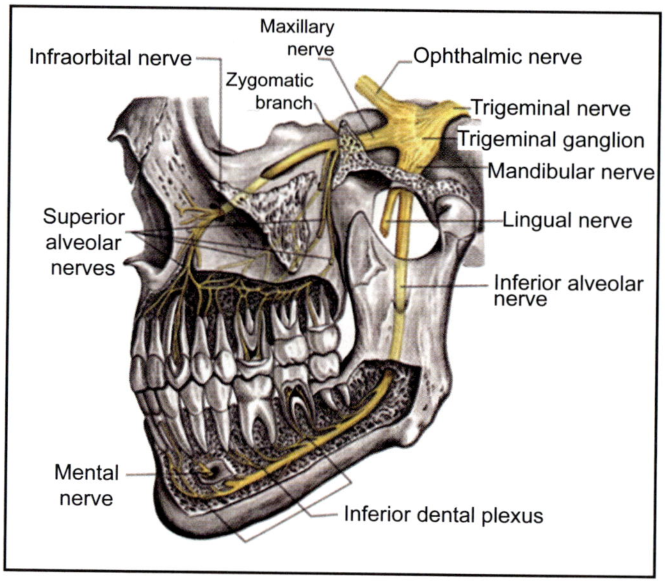

- Maxillary division of trigeminal nerve is wholly sensory. Leaves the skull via the foramen rotundum, which leads directly into the posterior wall of pterygopalatine fossa.
- Three main sensory branches arising from posterior division of the mandibular nerve are auriculotemporal, lingual and inferior alveolar nerves.
- Inferior alveolar nerve divides into mental nerve that leaves the mandible through the mental foramen and incisive nerve that remains within bone and supplies anterior teeth.
- Lingual nerve in infratemporal fossa is joined by Chordatympani branch of 7th nerve.

Nerve	Foramen
Maxillary nerve	Foramen rotundum
Inferior alveolar nerve	Mundibular foramen
Chordatympani nerve	***Canal of Hughier*** Exits cranium through **Petrotympanic fissure** and internal acoustic meatus Enters petrotympanic fissure to continue to infratemporal fossa
Lingual nerve	Close to submandibular duct

Ref: Gray's Anatomy 41st Edition Page 538, Grants Atlas 13th Edition Page 626, Snell's Clinical Anatomy Page 236

Ans: (B) Inferior alveolar nerve

7. **Uvula vesicae is seen in:**

A. Median lobe of prostate
B. Lateral lobe of prostate
C. Posterior lobe of prostate
D. Anterior lobe of prostate

Key:

Uvula vesicae is a small rounded elevation just behind urethral orifice at apex of trigone. Raised by median lobe of prostate gland and becomes prominent in BPH leads to urine stagnation

Small elevation in mucous membrane immediately above and behind internal urethral orifice

PROSTATE

- **Anterior Lobe**
  - *Isthmus (Lies in front of urethra and devoid of glandular substance)*
- **Middle (Median) Lobe**
  - *Lies between urethra and ejaculatory ducts (Prone to BPH obstructing internal urethral orifice)*
- **Posterior Lobe**
  - *Lies behind urethra and below ejaculatory duct Contains glandular tissue and prone to carcinomatous transformation*
- **Lateral Lobes**
  - *Situated on either side of urethra and form main mass of gland*

Median Lobe of Prostate

- Wedge shaped.
- Apex directed below towards colliculus seminalis.
- Base forms ***uvula vesicae*** at apex of trigonusm vesicae.
- Apex of the trigonum vesicae is formed by internal urethral orifice.
- In male rounded elevation uvula vesicae projects upwards behind urethral orifice and is formed by median lobe of prostate.
- Uvula lies within so called sphincter vesicae.
- Uvula vesicae may be enlarged in old age due to enlargement of prostate, and acts as a ball-valve to obstruct outflow of urine.
- ***During BPH Uvula vesicae is also enlarged.***

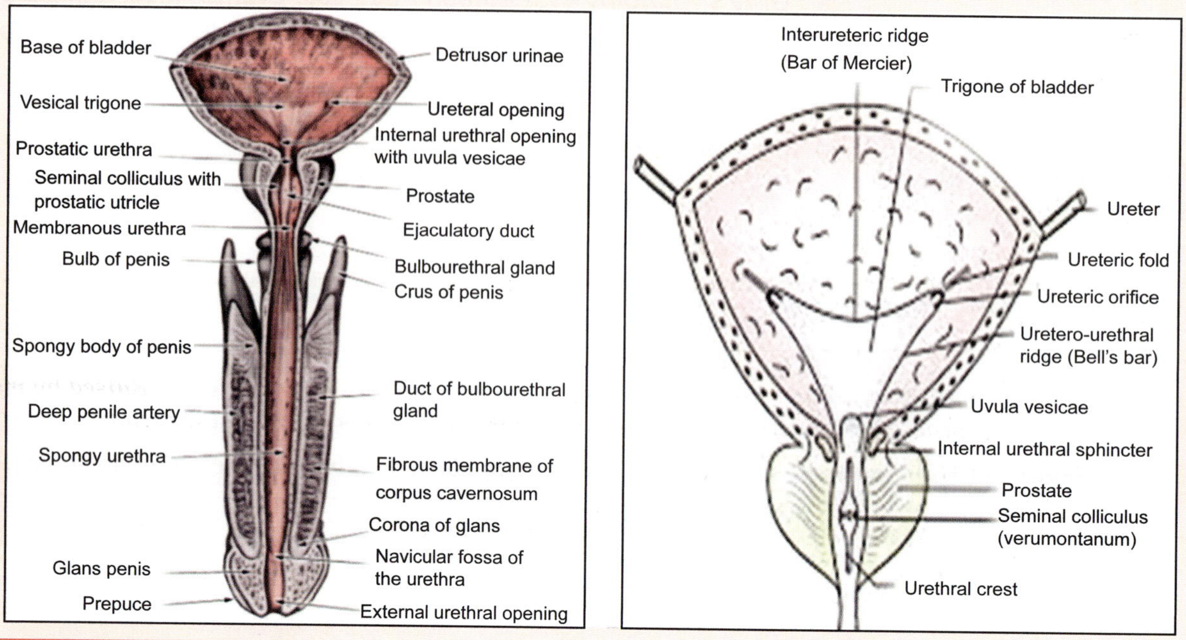

Ref: A.K.Dutta, Essentials of Human Anatomy 9th Edition Page 342, Gray's Anatomy 40th Edition Page 1249, BDC, 6th Edition Page 400, Snell Clinical Anatomy Page 375

Ans: (A) Median lobe of prostate

8. **Identify structure marked below:**
   A. Commissural fibers
   B. Projection fibers
   C. Long association fibers
   D. Short association fibers

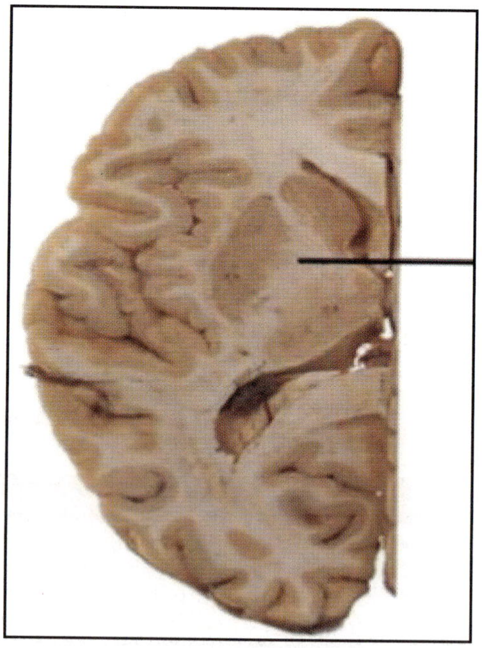

Key:

Projection fibers pass from brainstem to entire cerebral cortex between large nuclear masses of grey matter within cerebral hemisphere

- When a considerable number of fibers pass from a mass of grey matter in one part of brain to another mass of grey matter in another part of the brain or spinal cord, these are referred to as ***projection fibers***.

Corticofugal fibers go away from cortex (cortical efferents) to centres in other parts of CNS.
Corticopetal fibers, which come to the cerebral cortex from the other centres in the CNS.

- Fibers interconnecting different areas of the cerebral cortex or of the cerebellar cortex are called ***Association fibers***.
- Fibers connecting identical areas of 2 halves of brain are called ***Commissural fibers***.

WHITE MATTER OF CEREBRAL HEMISPHERE
(Composed of myelinated nerve fibers)

- **Commissural fibers**
  - **Connect corresponding regions of 2 hemispheres** (Corpus callosum, Anterior commissure, Posterior commissure, Fornix, Habenular commissure)
- **Association fibers**
  - Essentially connect cortical regions within same hemisphere & may be divided into short & long groups
    - **Short association fibers:** Lie immediately beneath the cortex and connect adjacent gyri; these fibers run transversely to the long axis of the sulci
    - **Long association fibers:** Uncinate fasciculus, cingulum, superior longitudinal fasciculus, inferior longitudinal fasciculus, fronto-occipital fasciculus
- **Projection fibers**
  - Connects cortex to subcortical areas– Internal capsule & Fornix

Association Fibers	Commissural Fibers	Projection fibers
Superior longitudinal fasciculus	Corpus callosum	Internal capsule
Inferior longitudinal fasciculus	Anterior commissure	Corona radiata
Cingulum	Posterior commissure	Tracts
Uncinate fasciculus	Habenular commissure	
	Hippocampal commissure	

- Projection fibers interconnect hippocampus and mammillary body.
- Commissural fibers interconnect two hippocampi.
- Association fibers connect the hippocampus to cingulate gyrus of same side.

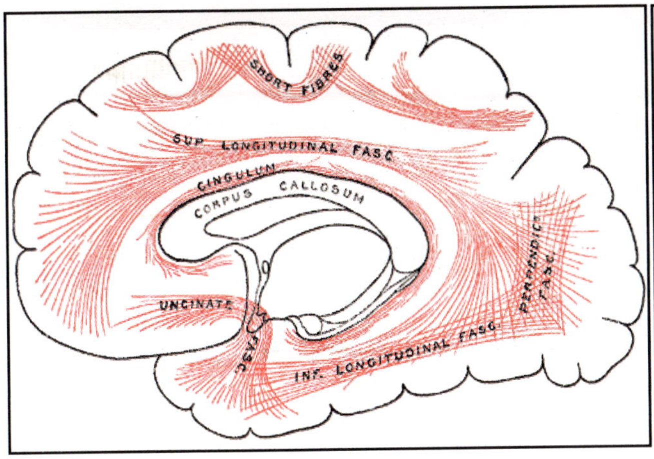

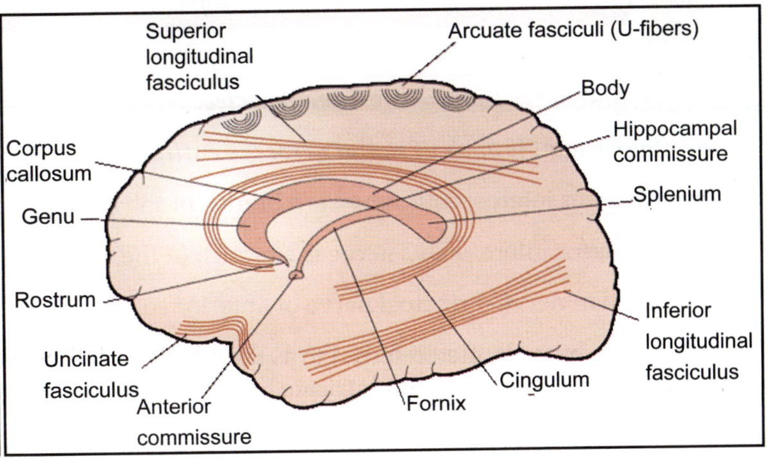

Ref: Snell Clinical Neuroanatomy 7th Edition Page 266, Vishram Singh 2nd Edition Page 395, Inderbir Singh 6th Edition Page 420, BDC 5th Edition Page 400, Gray's 41st Edition Page 394

Ans: (B) Projection fibers

9. Area marked below is supplied by which of the following nerve?

A. Radial nerve
B. Ulnar nerve
C. Posterior interosseus nerve
D. Median nerve

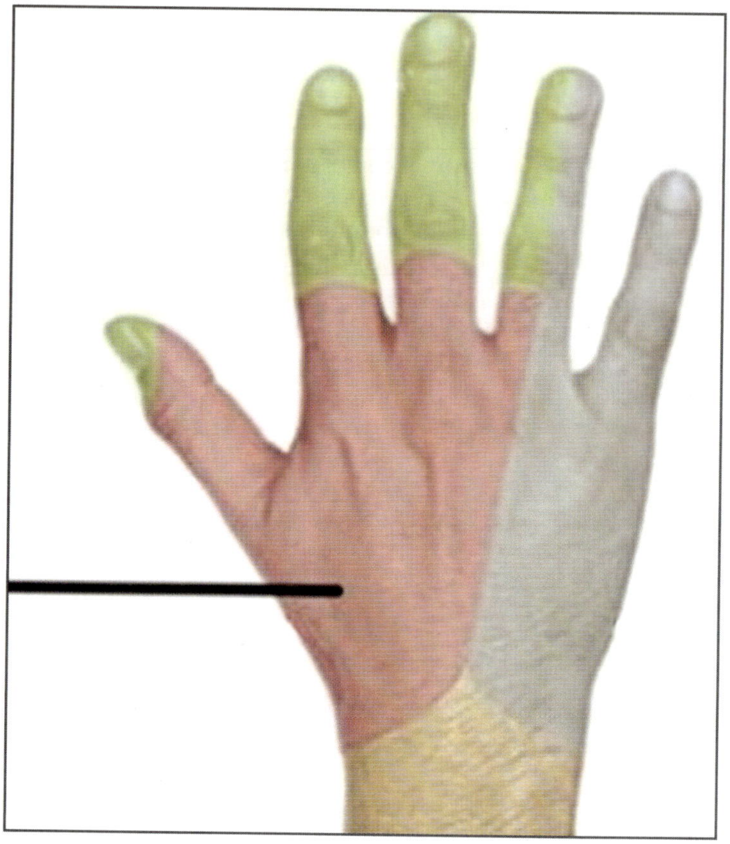

Key:

Picture depicts area corresponding to lateral three and half digits which is supplied by superficial branch of radial nerve (sensory branch)
Superficial branch of radial nerve provides cutaneous innervation to lateral 2/3rd of dorsum of hand and dorsum of index finger, middle finger and lateral ½ of ring finger over proximal and middle phalanx

- ***Radial nerve supplies no hand muscles.***
- ***Superficial branch of radial nerves is entirely sensory.***
- Anterior interosseous nerve is a branch of the median nerve.
- Posterior interosseous nerve is a branch of the radial nerve.
- Median nerve–Principal nerve of anterior compartment of forearm.
- Ulnar nerve is often referred to as the nerve of fine movements because it innervates most of the intrinsic muscles that are concerned with intricate hand movements.

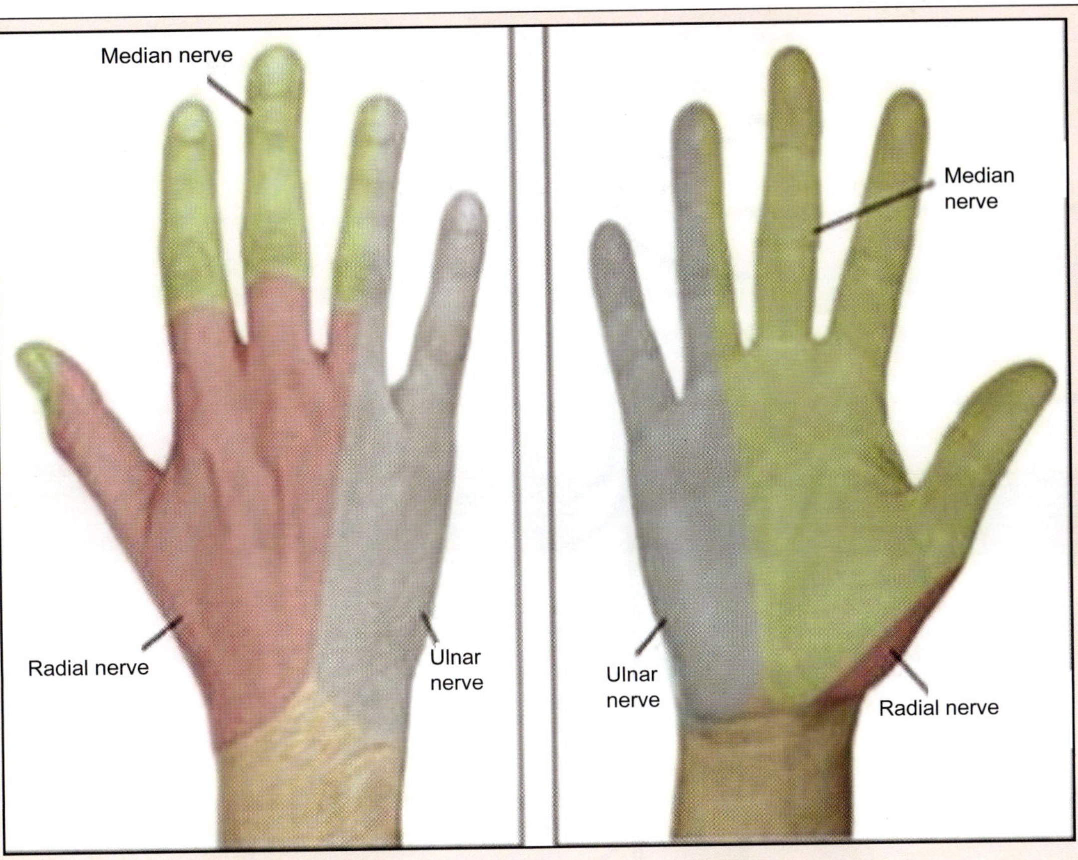
Median nerve
Radial nerve
Ulnar nerve
Median nerve
Ulnar nerve
Radial nerve

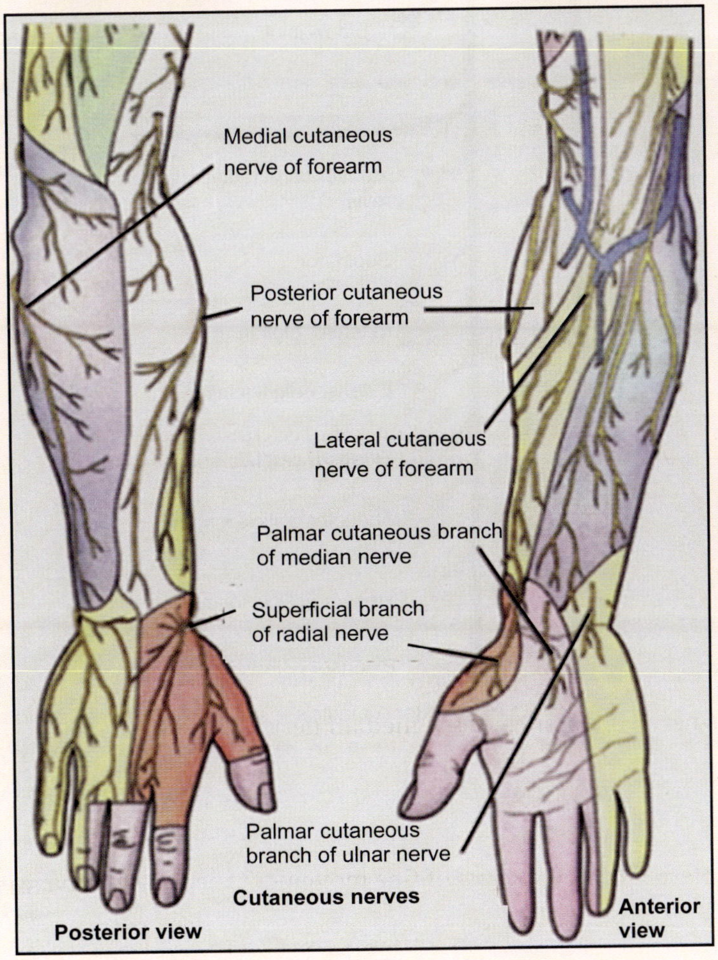
Medial cutaneous nerve of forearm
Posterior cutaneous nerve of forearm
Lateral cutaneous nerve of forearm
Palmar cutaneous branch of median nerve
Superficial branch of radial nerve
Palmar cutaneous branch of ulnar nerve
Cutaneous nerves
Posterior view
Anterior view

RADIAL NERVE

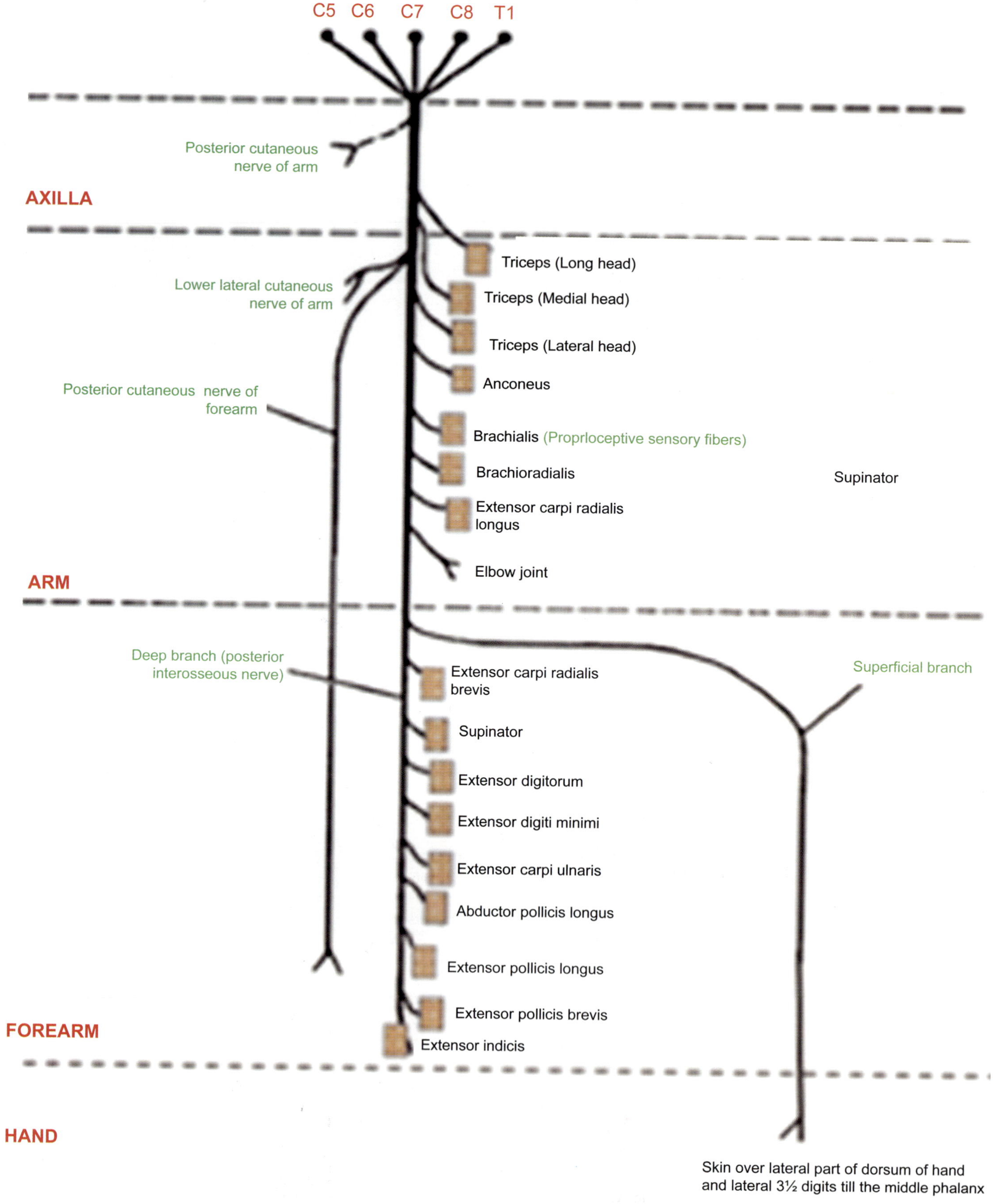

MEDIAN NERVE

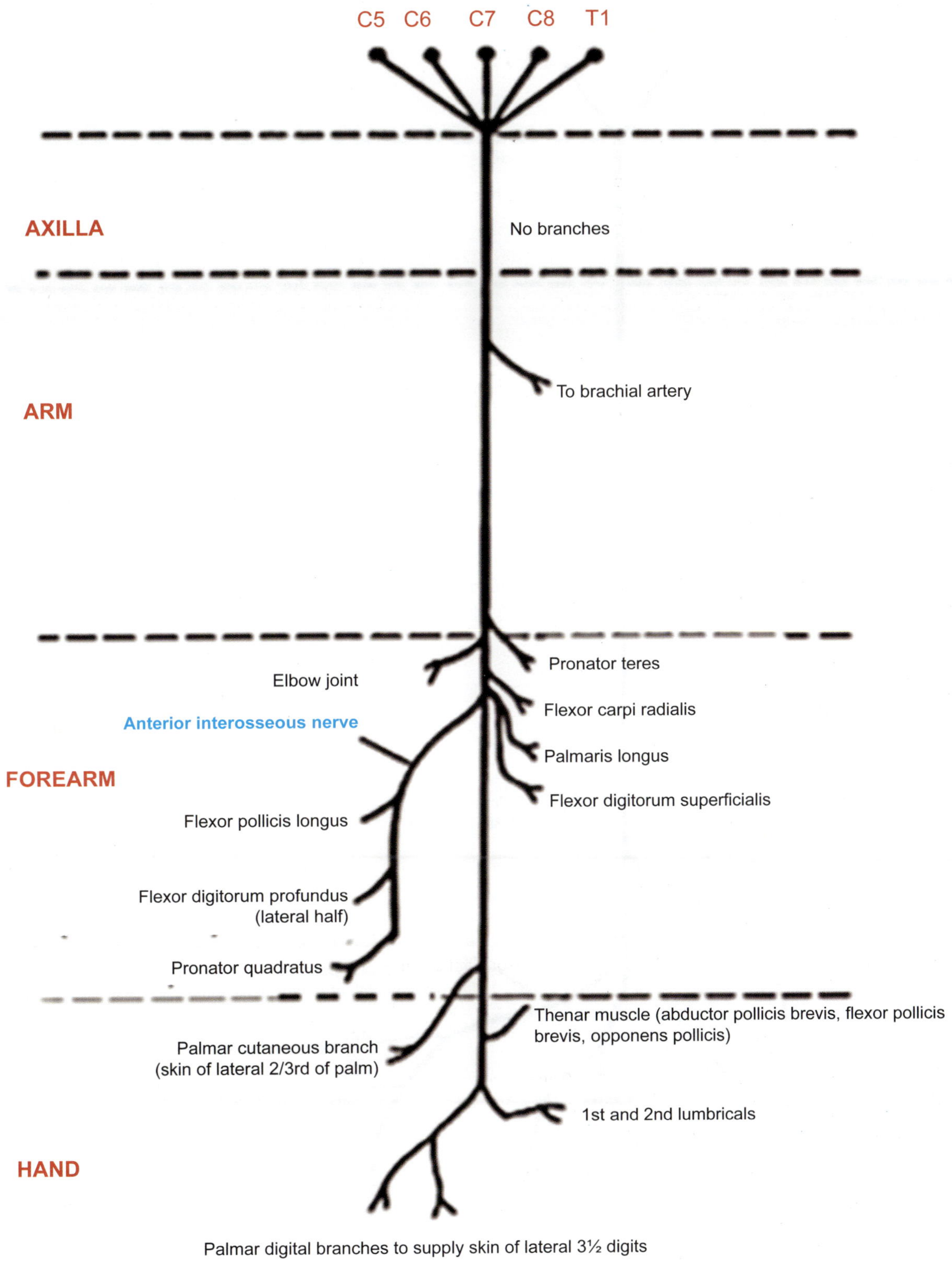

ULNAR NERVE

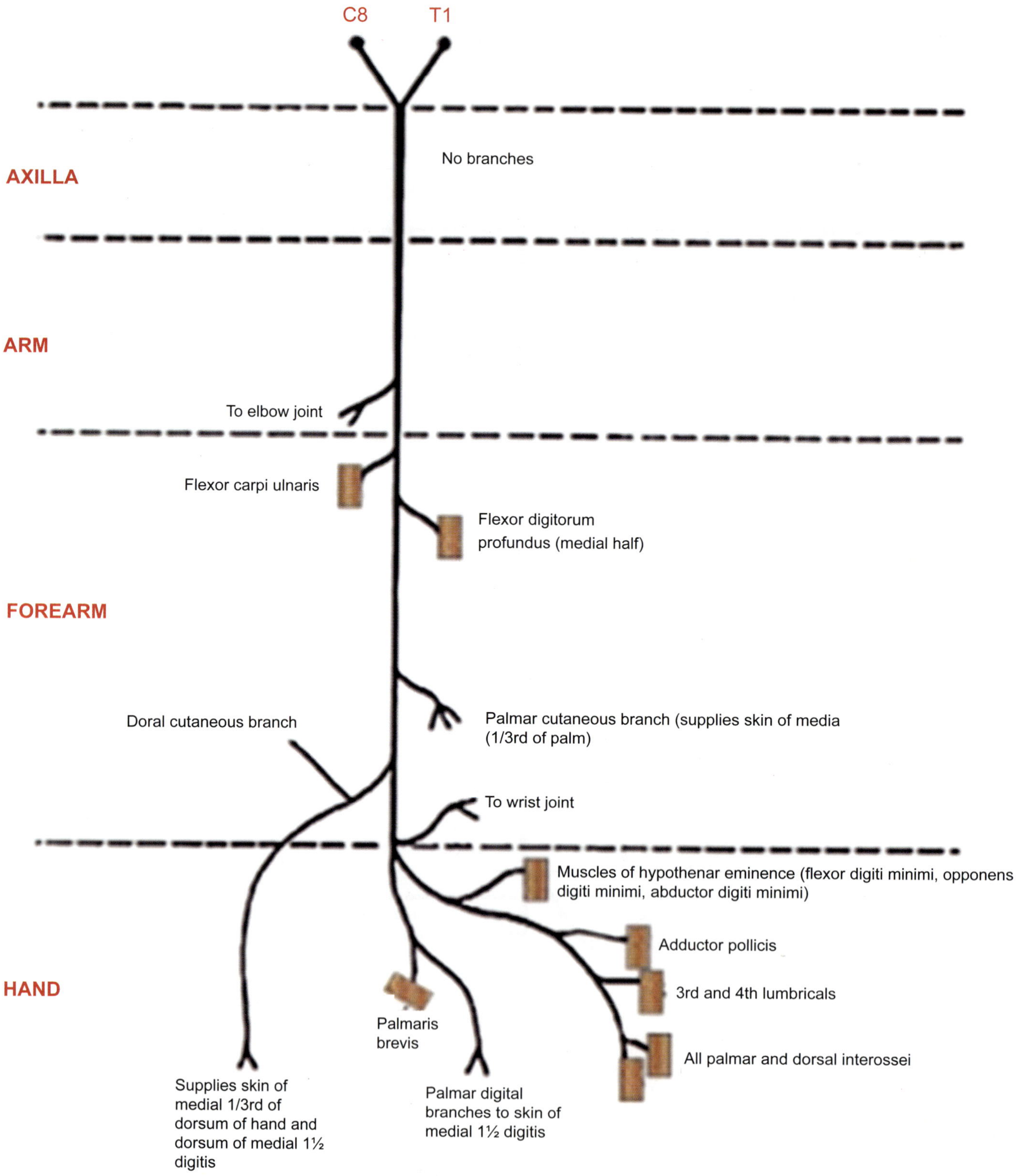
C8
T1
AXILLA
No branches
ARM
To elbow joint
Flexor carpi ulnaris
Flexor digitorum profundus (medial half)
FOREARM
Doral cutaneous branch
Palmar cutaneous branch (supplies skin of media (1/3rd of palm)
To wrist joint
Muscles of hypothenar eminence (flexor digiti minimi, opponens digiti minimi, abductor digiti minimi)
Adductor pollicis
3rd and 4th lumbricals
HAND
Palmaris brevis
All palmar and dorsal interossei
Supplies skin of medial 1/3rd of dorsum of hand and dorsum of medial 1½ digitis
Palmar digital branches to skin of medial 1½ digitis

Ref: Keith Moore 9th Edition Page 838, Gray 41st Edition Page 893, Grants Atlas, 13th Edition, Page 490

Ans: (A) Radial nerve

10. Identify the marked structure in the figure:

A. Fornix
B. Pineal gland
C. Pituitary gland
D. Insula

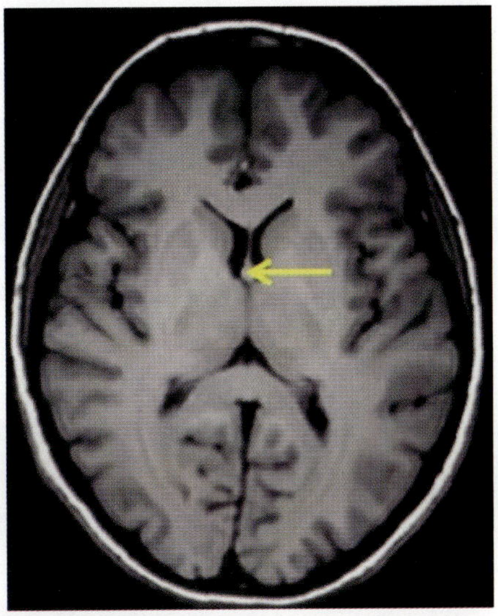

Key:

Picture depicts C-shaped bundle of nerve fibers in brain known as Fornix

Fornix

- ***Fornix is C-shaped bundle of nerve fibers in brain that acts as major output tract of hippocampus.*** (Part of the limbic system)
- Also carries afferent fibers to hippocampus from structures in diencephalon and basal forebrain.
- Fibers of fornix arise from pyramidal cells of hippocampus.

Parts of Fornix

- Crura–Seen at splenium of corpus callous at level of superior colliculus.
- Commissure–Connects crura.
- Body–Provides one of the major path through which hippocampus communicates with each other.
- Columns (Anterior pillars)–Dive into hypothalamus (Mammillary bodies).

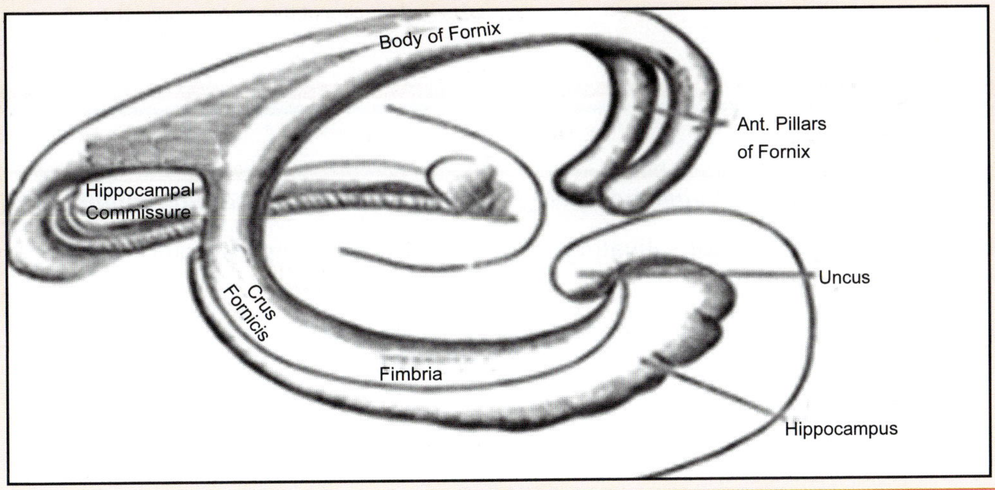

EXTRA EDGE

- Cortical region of limbic system consists of limbic lobe and hippocampal formation.
- ***Most important function of hippocampus formation is retention of information in short-term memory and its transfer into long-term memory.***
- Majority of fibers of fornix are projection fibers, some of the fibers are commissural fibers and association fibers.
- ***Septum pellucidum and anterior column of fornix form medial wall of anterior horn of lateral ventricles.***

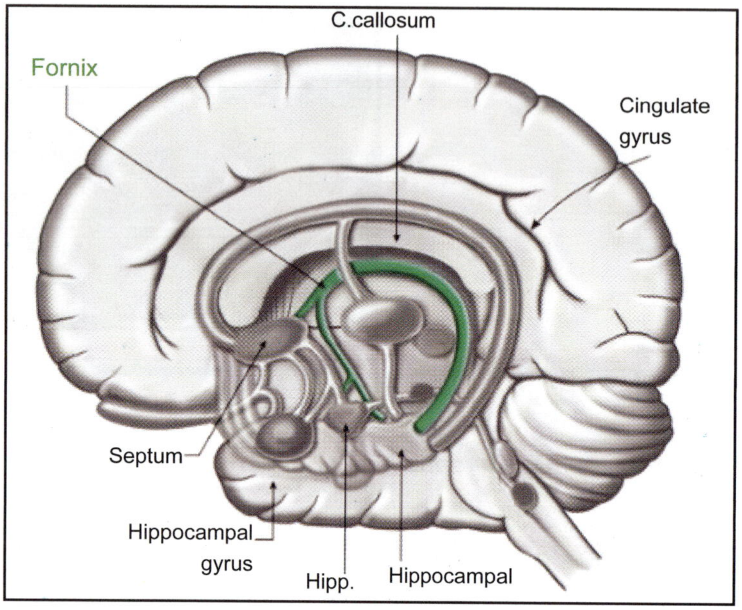

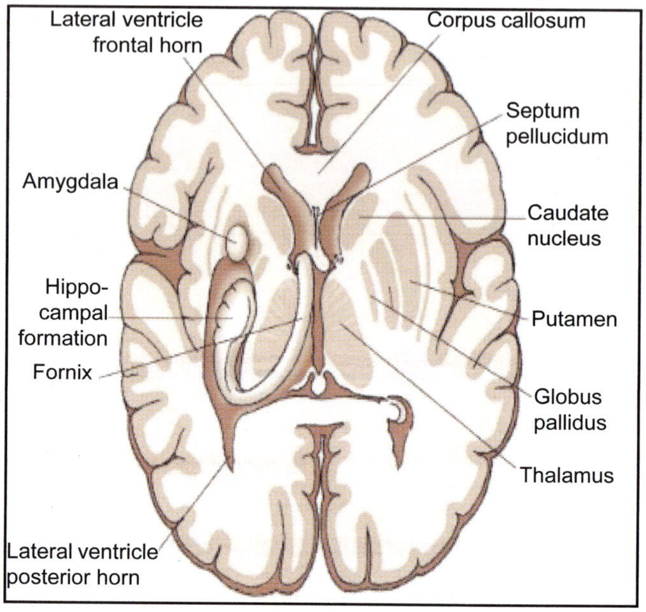

Ref: Gray 41st Edition Page 385,
Snell's Clinical Neuroanatomy 7th Edition Page 446,
GP Pal Illustrated Textbook of Neuroanatomy 1st Edition Page 293

Ans: (A) Fornix

11. Which of the following nerve carries Parasympathetic supply of Submandibular gland?

A. Glossopharyngeal

B. Facial nerve

C. Inferior alveolar nerve

D. Auriculotemporal nerve

Key:

Parasympathetic supply of Submandibular gland occurs through Chordatympani branch of 7th nerve

- **Parasympathetic supply:** Superior salivatory nucleus → Chordatympani branch of 7th nerve → Submandibular ganglion→Submandibular gland.
- **Sympathetic supply:** Postganglionic fibers via superior cervical ganglion.

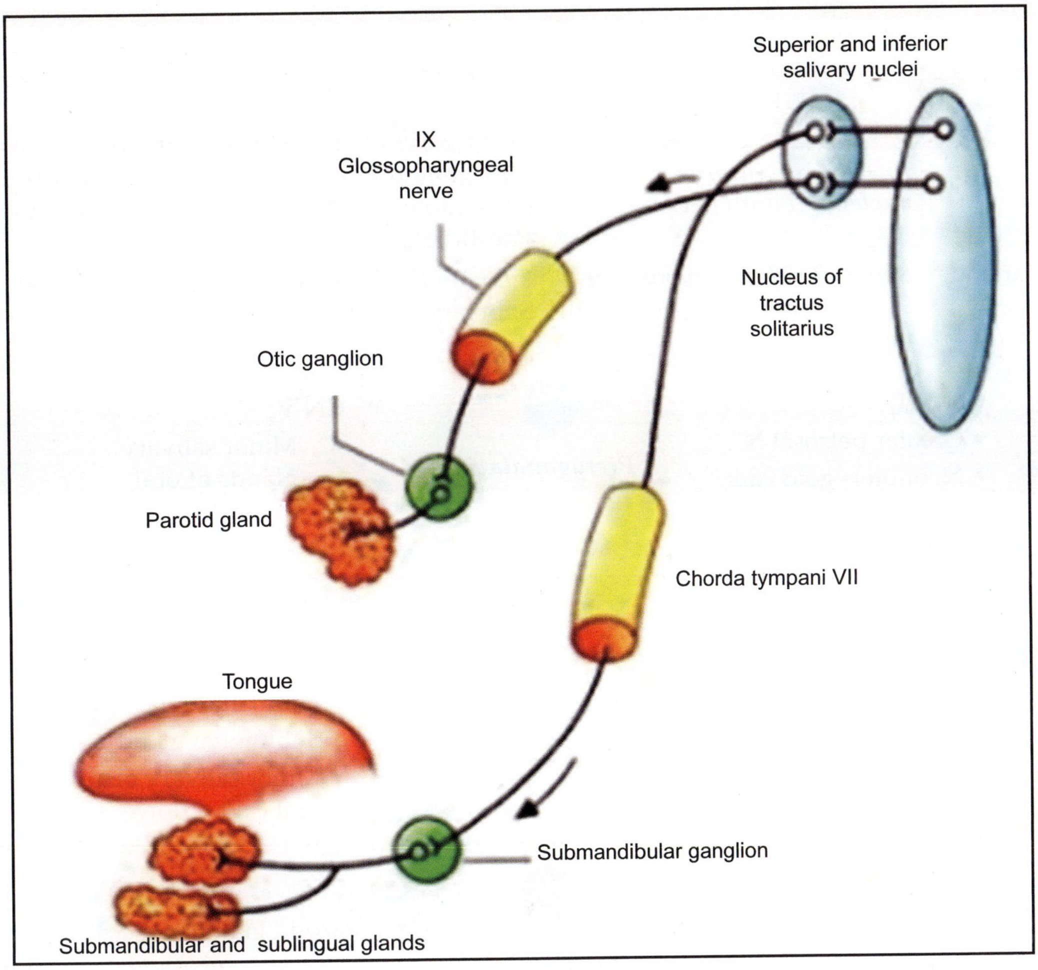
Superior and inferior salivary nuclei
IX Glossopharyngeal nerve
Nucleus of tractus solitarius
Otic ganglion
Parotid gland
Chorda tympani VII
Tongue
Submandibular ganglion
Submandibular and sublingual glands

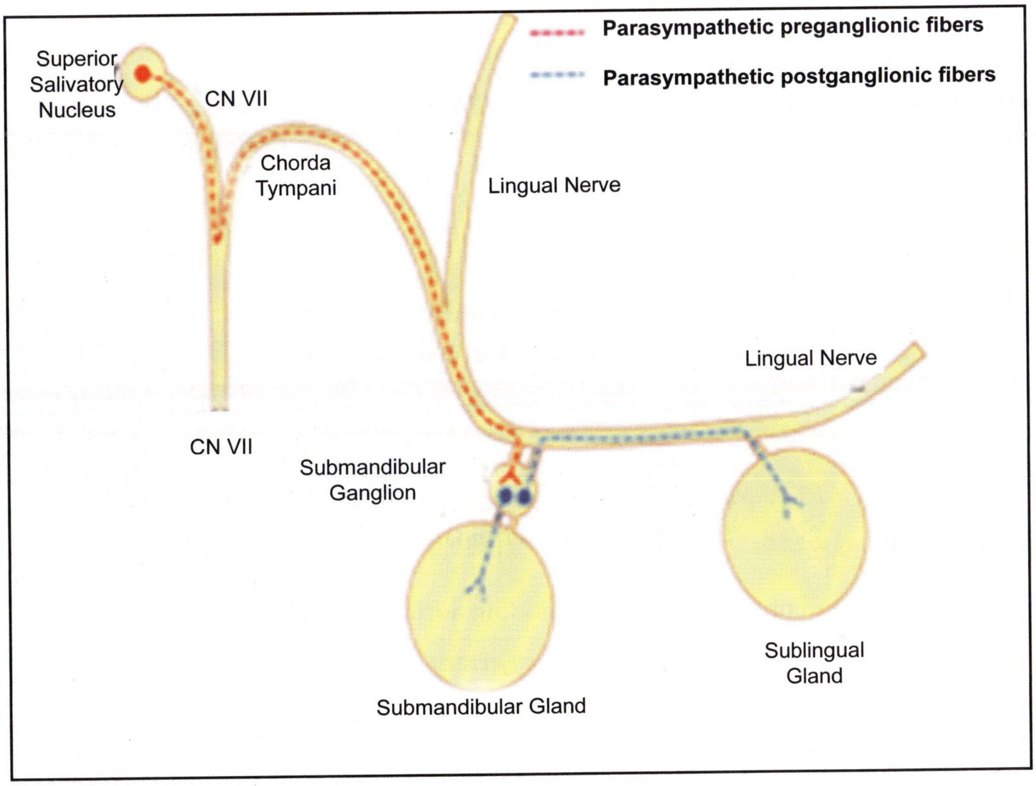
Parasympathetic preganglionic fibers
Parasympathetic postganglionic fibers
Superior Salivatory Nucleus
CN VII
Chorda Tympani
Lingual Nerve
Lingual Nerve
CN VII
Submandibular Ganglion
Sublingual Gland
Submandibular Gland

Gland	Parasympathetic		Sympathetic
	Preganglionic	Postganglionic	
Parotid	*Inferior salivatory nucleus*→Ninth nerve	*Otic ganglion*→ Auriculotemporal nerve→ Parotid gland	Postganglionic fibers via superior cervical ganglion
Submandibular and Sublingual	*Superior salivatory nucleus*→ Chordatympani branch of 7th nerve	*Submandibular ganglion*→ Submandibular gland	Postganglionic fibers via superior cervical ganglion

CN VII → *Pterygopalatine* → **CN V_2**

- Greater petrosal N.
- N. of pterygoid canal

CN V_2:
- Minor salivary glands of oral cavity (upper ½)

CN VII → *Submandibular* → **CN V_3**

- Chorda tympani n.
- Lingual br. of V_3

CN V_3:
- Submandibular gland
- Sublingual gland
- Minor salivary glands of oral cavity (lower ½)

CN IX → *Otic* → **CN V_3**

- Tympanic n.
- Lesser petrosal n.

CN V_3:
- Parotid gland

Parasympathetic innervations of salivary glands

Ref: Gray's 41st Edition Page 528, Grant Atlas 13th Edition Page 350, Snell Clinical Anatomy Page 22, Bailey and Love 27th Edition Page 795

Ans: (B) Facial nerve

12. Right coronary artery arises from:

A. Coronary sinus
B. Left aortic sinus
C. Right aortic sinus
D. Posterior aortic sinus

Key:

RCA arises from anterior aortic sinus (Right aortic sinus)
LCA arises from left posterior aortic sinus

- Coronary arteries are first and only branches of ascending aorta.

Mouth of right coronary artery is in the right aortic sinus

- Mouth of left coronary artery is in left aortic sinus and no artery arises from the posterior aortic (non-coronary) sinus.
- Coronary sinus is a wide venous channel that runs from left to right in the posterior part of the coronary groove *(Main vein of heart).*

Right posterior aortic sinus is known as Non-coronary sinus.

AORTA

- ⇩ **Right coronary artery**
  - ⇩ **Posterior interventricular artery** ⇩ **Ventricular wall**
  - ⇩ **Marginal artery** ⇩ **Walls of right atrium and right ventricle**
- ⇩ **Left coronary artery**
  - ⇩ **Circumflex artery** ⇩ **Walls of left atrium and left ventricle**
  - ⇩ **Anterior interventricular artery** ⇩ **Ventricular walls**

⇩ **Cardiac veins**

⇩ **Coronary sinus**

⇩ **Right atrium**

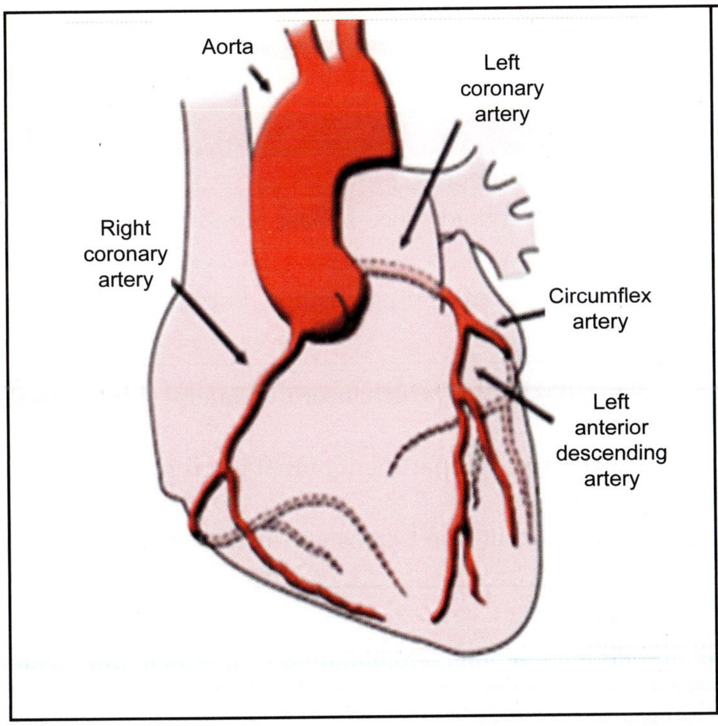

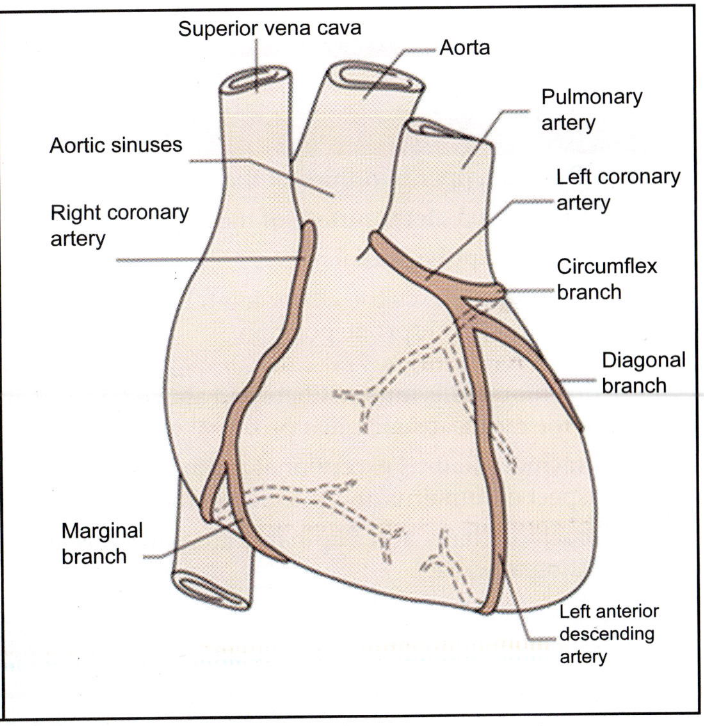

Ref: Keith Moore Clinical Anatomy 5th Edition Page 158, Gray's Anatomy 41st Edition Page 1017, Vishram Singh 2nd Edition Page 274, Inderbir Singh 6th Edition Page 93

Ans: (C) Right aortic sinus

13. Identify the marked muscle in the diagram.

A. Brachioradialis
B. Extensor carpi radialis longus
C. Flexor carpi radialis
D. Extensor carpi ulnaris

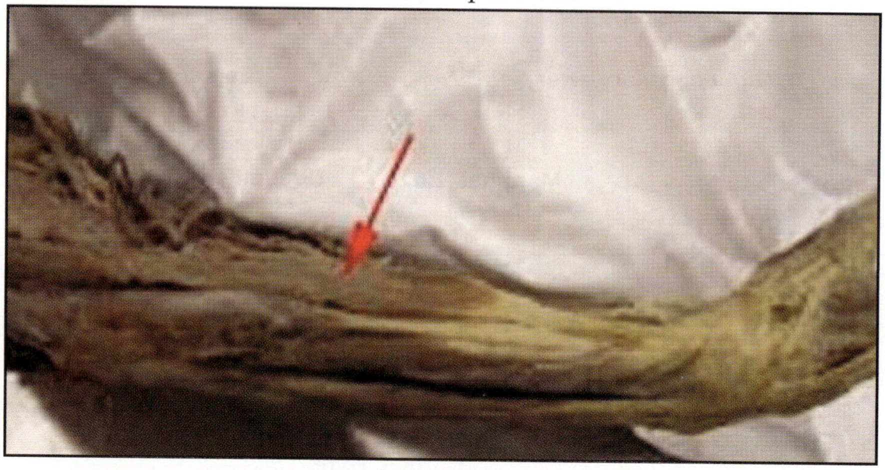

Key:

Depicted Picture shows Brachioradialis muscle
Brachioradialis–Most superficial muscle along radial side of forearm and forms lateral border of cubital fossa

Brachioradialis

- **Origin:** Upper two-third of the lateral supracondylar ridge of the humerus.
- **Insertion:** Lateral surface of the distal end of radius just above the styloid process (Base of radial styloid process).
- **Nerve supply:** Radial nerve.
- **Function:** Flexes the elbow joint, Pronates the supinated forearm to midprone position, Supinates the pronated forearm to midprone position.

- Brachioradialis muscle fibers end above mid-forearm level in a flat tendon which inserts on lateral side of distal end of the radius, usually just proximal to its styloid process.
- Brachioradialis is exceptional among muscles of posterior (extensor) compartment in that it has rotated to anterior aspect of humerus and thus flexes forearm at elbow.
- Brachioradialis and Supinator are only muscles of compartment that don't cross and therefore are incapable of acting at wrist.

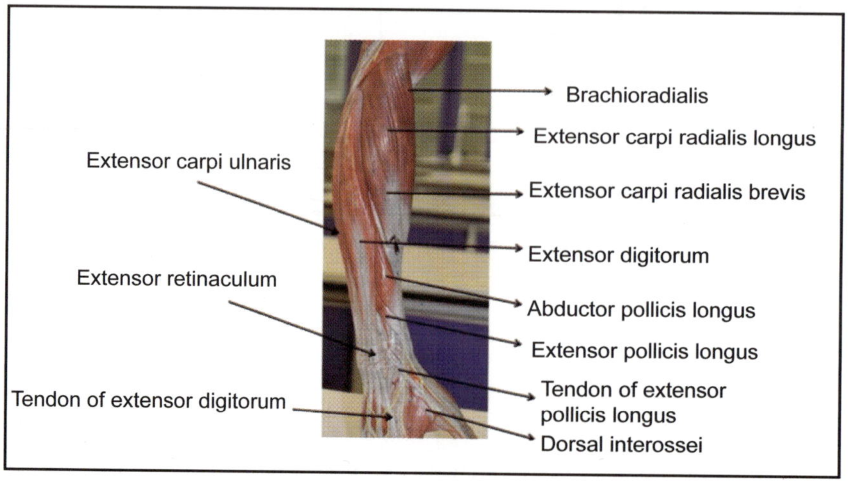

Muscle	Origin	Insertion	Nerve	Action
Brachioradialis	Lateral supracondylar ridge of humerus	Base of radial styloid process	Radial	Flexes the elbow joint, pronates supinated forearm to midprone position and Supinates pronated forearm to midprone position
Extensor carpi radialis longus	Lateral supracondylar ridge of humerus	Dorsum of base of 2nd metacarpal	Radial	Acting with extensor carpi ulnaris extends wrist Acting with flexor carpi radialis abducts wrist
Extensor carpi radialis brevis	Lateral epicondyle of humerus	Posterior base of 3rd metacarpal	Radial (Posterior interosseous nerve)	Acting with extensor carpi ulnaris extends wrist Acting with flexor carpi radialis abducts wrist
Extensor digitorum	Lateral epicondyle of humerus	Extensor expansion, Base of medial and distal phalanges	Radial (Posterior interosseous nerve)	Extends medial four digits. Can also extend wrist
Extensor digiti minimi	Common extensor tendon and interosseous membrane	Extensor expansion, Base of medial and distal phalanges	Radial (Posterior interosseous nerve)	Extends little finger. Helps in extension of wrist
Extensor carpi ulnaris	Lateral epicondyle and posterior surface of ulna	Base of 5th metacarpal	Radial (Posterior interosseous nerve)	Acting with extensor carpi radialis it extends wrist, Acting with flexor carpi ulnaris it adducts wrist

Ref: Gray's Anatomy 40th Edition Page 848, Keith Moore Clinically Oriented Anatomy 5th Edition, Page 807, Vishram Singh 2nd Edition Page 118, Inderbir Singh 6th Edition Page 191

Ans: (A) Brachioradialis

14. Dermatome for below marked structure is:

A. T3
B. T4
C. T10
D. T9

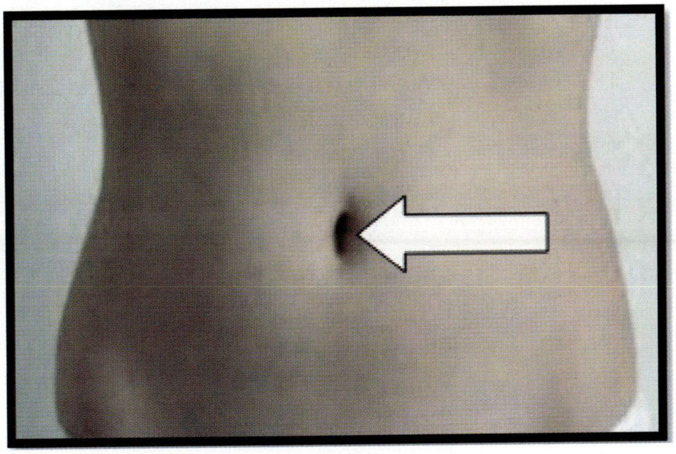

Key:

Dermatome for Umbilicus is T10

Dermatomes	
C1	Top of head
C2	Face
C3	Lateral neck
C4	Lower neck and Top of shoulder
C5	Shoulder to base of thumb outside of arm
C6	Front of shoulder, down arm into thumb and back of hand
C7	Back of shoulder, down back of arm into back of hand
C8	Little finger and wrist
T1	Inside elbow down into wrist
T10	Umbilicus
L1	Back and over trochanter
L2	Back and anterior thigh to knee
L3	Back, upper buttocks, anterior thigh and knee, inner lower leg
L4	Inner buttocks, outer thigh inside of leg and dorsum of foot and big toe
L5	Buttock, back side of thigh, lateral leg, dorsum of foot, inner half of sole of foot, 2nd and 3rd toes
S1 and S2	Buttock, posterior thigh to knee
S3	Groin and inner thigh to knee

Students just memorize below tables

Level	Supply
C2	Occiput
C3	Thyroid cartilage
C4	Suprasternal notch
C5	Infraclavicular fossa
C6	Thumb
C7	Index finger
C8	Little finger
T4	Nipple line
T10	Umbilicus
L1	Inguinal ligament
L2 and L3	Medial thigh
L4	Medial foot
L5	Web space between big toe and 2nd toe
S1	Lateral foot
S2-4	Perineal area

Spinal Level	Myotomes
C5	Elbow Flexors
C6	Wrist Extensors
C7	Elbow Extensors
C8	Finger Extensors
T1	Intrinsic hand muscles
L2	Hip Flexors
L3	Knee Extensors
L4	Ankle dorsiflexors
L5	Long toe extensors
S1	Ankle plantar flexors

Level	Corresponding Structure
C2-3	Mandible
C3	Hyoid bone
C4-5	Thyroid cartilage
C6	Cricoid cartilage
C7	Vertebra prominens
T3	Spine of scapula
T8	Point of IVC pierces diaphragm
T10	Xiphisternal junction
T10	Point of esophagus entering stomach
T12	Point of aorta entering abdomen
L1	End of spinal cord
L3	Subcostal plane
L3-4	Umbilicus
L4	Bifurcation of aorta
L4	Iliac crests
S2	End of dural sac

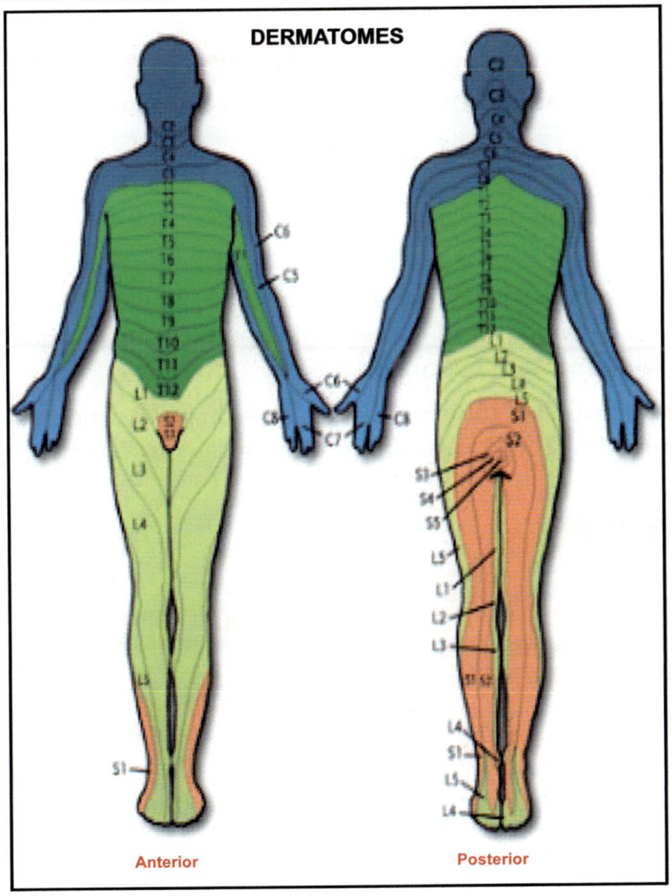

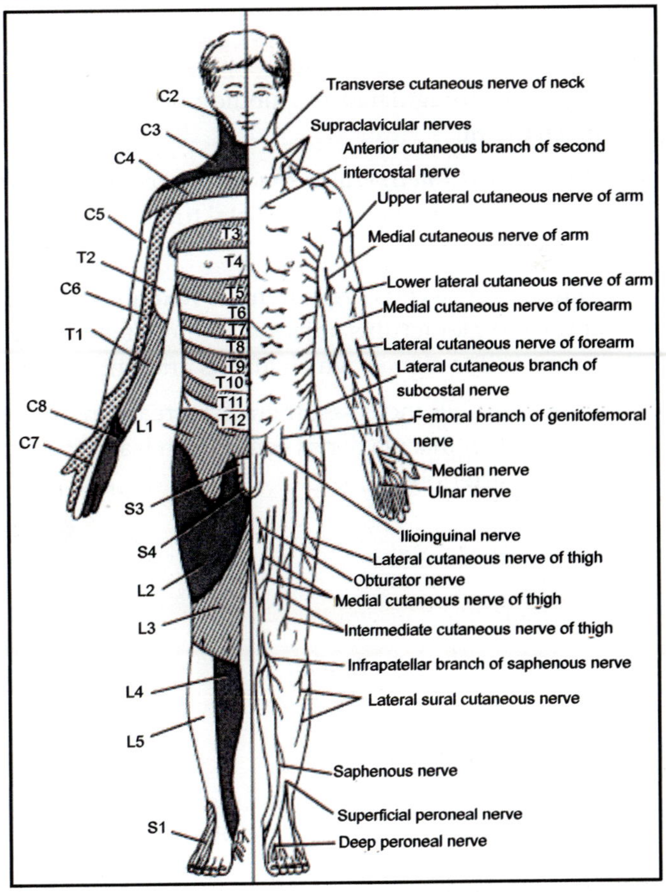

Ref: Keith L Moore Clinically Oriented Anatomy 5th Edition Page 53, Snell Clinical Anatomy Page 6, Gray 41st Edition Page 233

Ans: (C) T10

Chapter 2

PHYSIOLOGY

1. Tubuloglomerular feedback is for:

A. Controlling plasma volume

B. Maintenance of systemic BP

C. Controlling GFR

D. Controlling blood Na^+ level

Key:

Tubuloglomerular feedback controls GFR

GFR is closely matched to transport capacity of tubules by glomerulotubular feedback

Tubuloglomerular Feedback

- GFR is autoregulated by tubuloglomerular feedback mechanism which is a **NaCl concentration dependent mechanism.**
- *Rate of NaCl delivery to the distal nephron significantly influences glomerular blood flow and therefore GFR.* Rate of NaCl delivery to the distal tubule is dependent on the tubular concentration of NaCl as well as the tubular flow rate.
- **Macula densa cells** present in the **juxtaglomerular apparatus** (located at the end of the thick ascending limb and abuts the glomerulus adjacent to the afferent arteriole) senses the NaCl concentration on the tubular fluid and converts it to signals which affects afferent **arteriolar resistance** and hence affects GFR.
- When the GFR increases, there is increase in NaCl concentration of tubular fluid. This rise in NaCl concentration is sensed by macula densa cells which leads to formation of ATP and adenosine which causes vasoconstriction of afferent arteriole.

COMPONENTS

- **Signal:** *NaCl delivery to distal tubule*
- **Sensor:** *Macula densa*
- **Effector:** *Vascular smooth muscle cells within wall of afferent arteriole*

- When filtration increases, through an unclear mechanism the increased NaCl delivery to the macula densa triggers vasoconstriction of the afferent arteriole.
- Result is reduced renal blood flow (RPF) and therefore decreased GFR, which reduces delivery of NaCl to the macula densa.

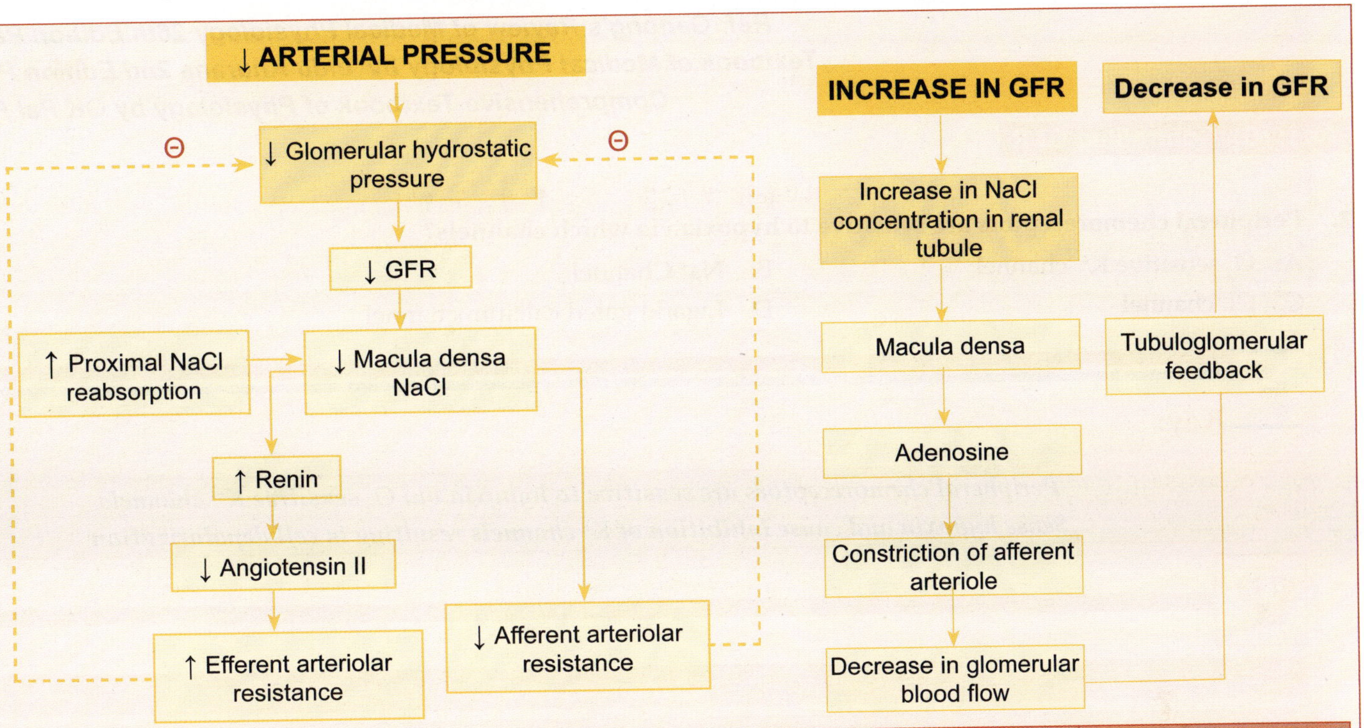

Effect	RPF	GFR	Filtration Fraction (GFR/RPF)
Constriction of afferent arteriole	↓	↓	NC
Constriction of efferent arteriole	↓	↑	↑
Increased plasma protein concentration	NC	↓	↓
Decreased plasma protein concentration	NC	↑	↑
Constriction of the ureter	NC	↓	↓

GFR, Glomerular filtration rate; NC, no change; RPF, Renal plasma flow.

- High-protein diet increases GFR by increasing Na^+ and Cl^- reabsorption, decreasing Na^+ and Cl^- delivery to macula densa, and thereby increasing GFR via tubuloglomerular feedback.

EXTRA EDGE

Hormones influencing the RBF and GFR

Hormone	Stimulus	Effect on GFR	Effect on RBF
Vasoconstrictors			
• Norepinephrine	↓ ECV	↓	↓
• Angiotensin II	↓ ECV	↓	↓
• Endothelin	↑ Stretch, ECV, angiotensin II, bradykinin, epinephrine	↓	↓
Vasodilators			
• Prostaglandins (PGI_2 and PGE_2)	↓ ECV, stretch, angiotensin II	NC	↑
• Nitric oxide (NO)	↑ Stretch ACh, histamine, bradykinin, ATP	↑	↑
• Bradykinin	Prostaglandin, ↓ ACE	↑	↑
• ANP	↑ ECV	↑	↑
• Glucocorticoids	Administration in therapeutic dose	↑	↑
• Dopamine	–	NC	↑
• Histamine	Inflammation, injury	NC	↑

NC– No change

Ref: Ganong's Review of Medical Physiology 26th Edition Page 272, Textbook of Medical Physiology by Indu Khurana 2nd Edition Page 275, Comprehensive Textbook of Physiology by GK Pal Page 681

Ans: (C) Controlling GFR

2. Peripheral chemoreceptors are sensitive to hypoxia via which channels?

A. O_2 sensitive K^+ channel
B. Na^+ Channel
C. Cl^- channel
D. Ligand gated calcium channel

Key:

Peripheral chemoreceptors are sensitive to hypoxia via O_2 sensitive K^+ channels
Sense hypoxia and cause inhibition of K^+ channels resulting in cell depolarization

Chemoreceptors

Type of chemoreceptor	Location	Stimuli that increase breathing rate
Central	Medulla	↓ pH
		↑ PCO_2
Peripheral	Carotid and aortic bodies	↓ PO_2 (if <60 mm Hg)
		↑ PCO_2
		↓ pH

At birth central chemoreceptors are active and peripheral chemoreceptors become sensitive in the weeks following birth.

Peripheral Chemoreceptors

- Carotid body located near bifurcation of aorta and aortic bodies located near arch of aorta are the peripheral chemoreceptors of respiration.
- ***Each carotid and aortic body contains Type I and Type II cells which is surrounded by sinusoidal cells.***

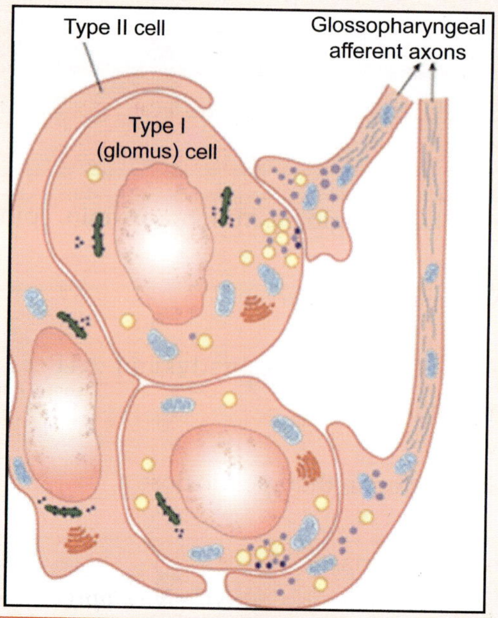

Type I Cells (Glomus Cells)
• They are closely associated with cup like ending of afferent nerve fibers.
• Resemble adrenal chromaffin cells and has dense core granules that contain catecholamines.
• On exposure to hypoxia and cyanide, they release catecholamines.
• These cells are excited by **hypoxia**.
• Dopamine is the principal neurotransmitters and act via D_2 receptors.
• Glomus cells are surrounded by 4 to 6 type I cells whose function is not known.
• Afferents from the carotid bodies ascend to the medulla via the **carotid sinus and glossopharyngeal nerves.**
• Fibers from the aortic body ascend **via Vagus nerve.**
• Increase in impulse traffic in afferent nerve fibers has been noted in hypoxia and hypercapnia
• **Conductance of O_2 sensitive K^+ channels present in Type I glomus cell is reduced during hypoxia**. This reduces the K^+ efflux, depolarizing the cell and causing Ca^{2+} influx, primarily via L-type Ca^{2+} channels. Ca^{2+} influx triggers action potentials and transmitter release, with consequent excitation of the afferent nerve endings.

Type II Cells
• Type II cells are also called **sustentacular cells**. They surround clusters of glomus cells. They are supporting cells for glomus cells as glial cells support neurons in brain.

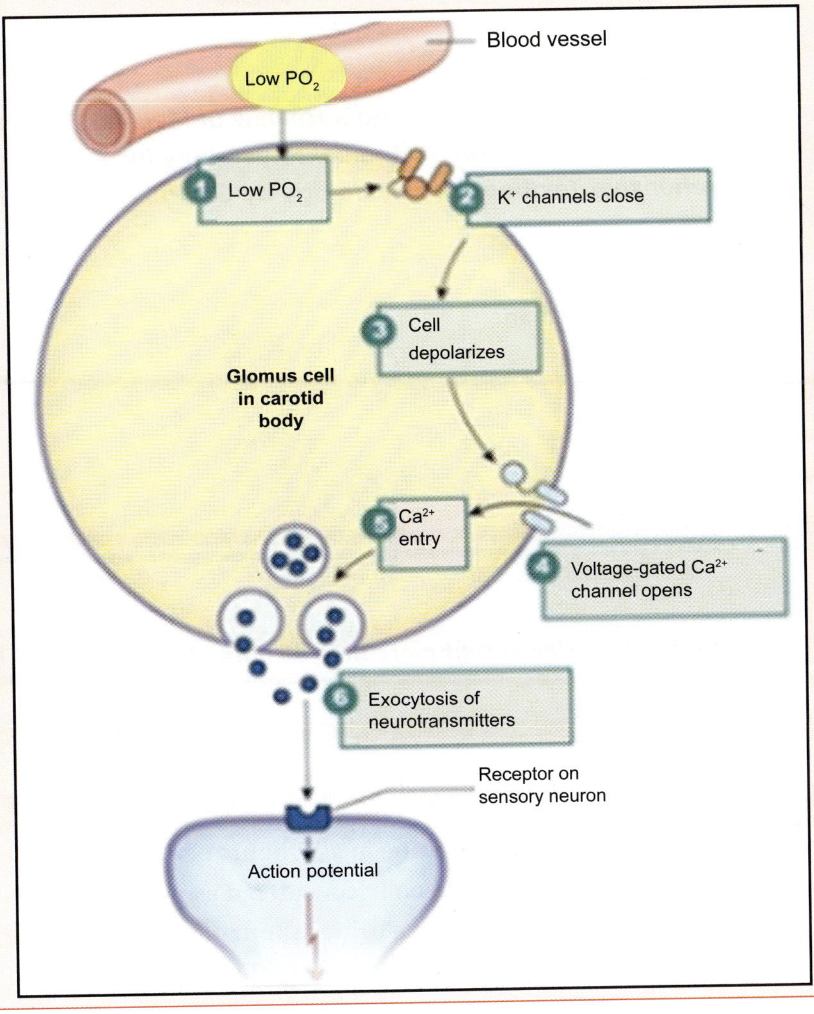

Contd.

Contd.

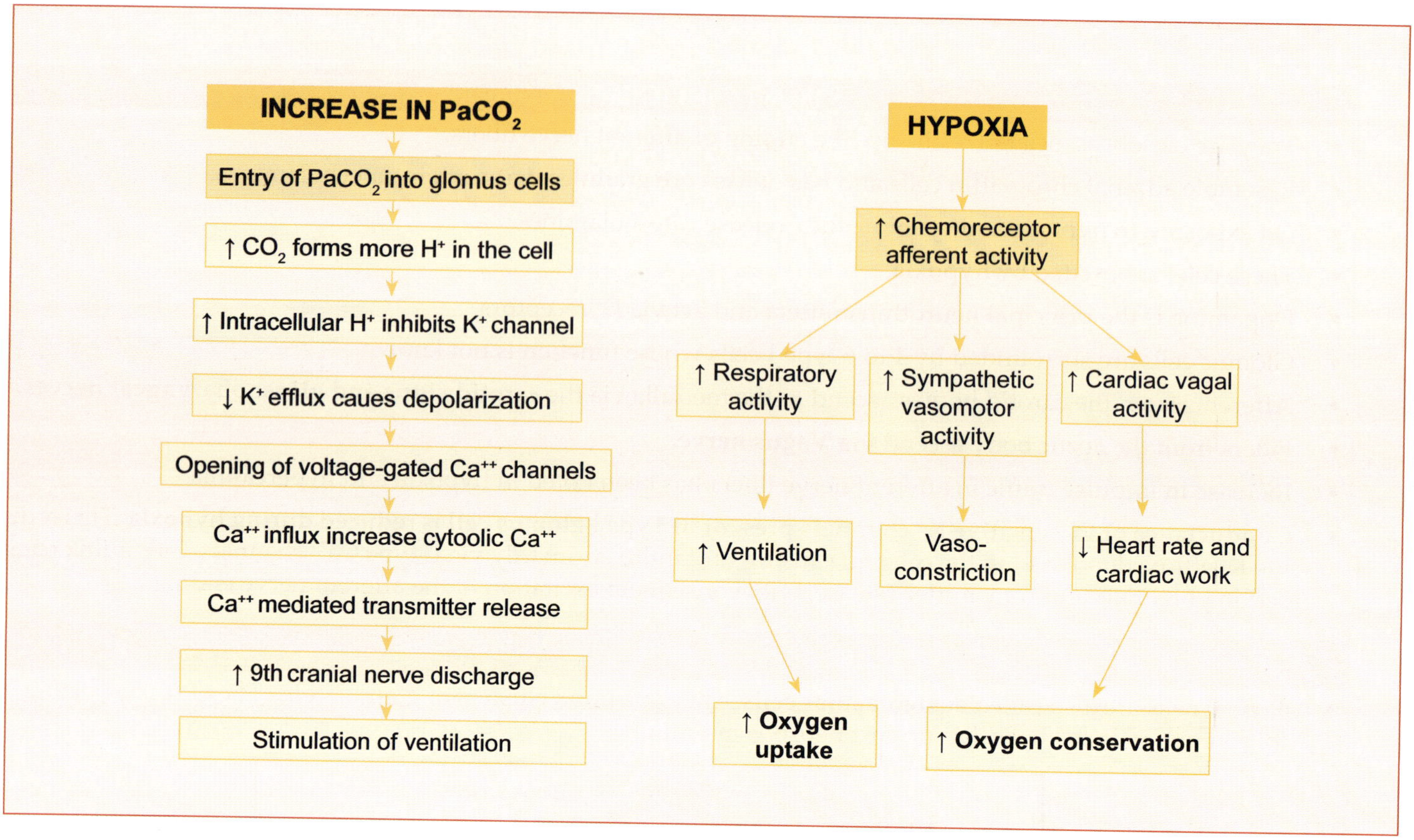

Ref: Ganong's Review of Medical Physiology 26th Edition Page 648, Textbook of Medical Physiology by Indu Khurana 2nd Edition Page 186, Comprehensive Textbook of Physiology by GK Pal Page 939, Boron 2nd Edition Page 738

Ans: (A) O_2 sensitive K^+ channel

3. Polyuria is defined as urine output more than:

A. 30 ml/kg body weight
B. 50 ml/kg body weight
C. 60 ml/kg body weight
D. 70 ml/kg body weight

Key:

Polyuria is urine output more than 30 ml/kg body weight/24 hours

Polyuria

- Polyuria is defined as an excessive excretion of urine in a 24 hours period.
- Urine output of more than **3 L/day** in adults is usually considered as polyuria.
- More accurately in children, polyuria is defined as a urine output of more than **30 ml/kg body weight/24 hours.***
- Average person excretes between **600 mosmol and 800 mosmol of solutes per day.**

Contd.

Contd.

POLYURIA (URINE OUTPUT >3 L/D)

↓

Urine Osmolality

U_{osm} < 100 mOsm/kg (Water Diuresis)
- Psychogenic polydipsia
- DI (central and nephrogenic)

→ Water Deprivation Test

U_{osm} < 100-300 mOsm/kg (Mixed Polyuria)
- Partial DI (central and nephrogenic)
- Simultaneous water and solute intake
- CKD

→ Water Deprivation Test; 24-hour urine collection

U_{osm} > 300 mOsm/kg (Solute Diuresis)
- Hyperglycemia
- Azotemia*
- High solute intake
  - Intravenous fluids
  - Enteral and parenteral nutrition
  - Exogenous supplements

→ 24-hour urine collection (estimation of osmoles)
- Urine sodium
- Urine potassium
- Urine glucose
- Urine urea nitrogen
- Other osmoles

Diabetes Insipidus

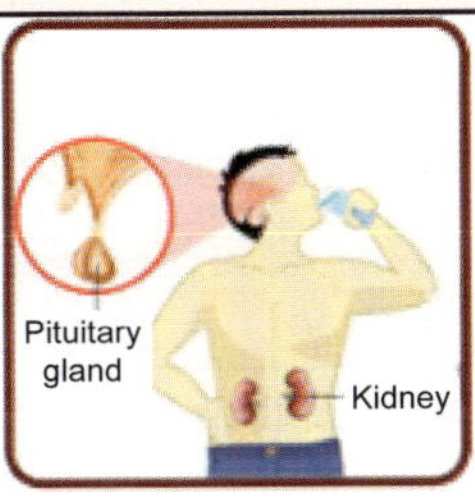

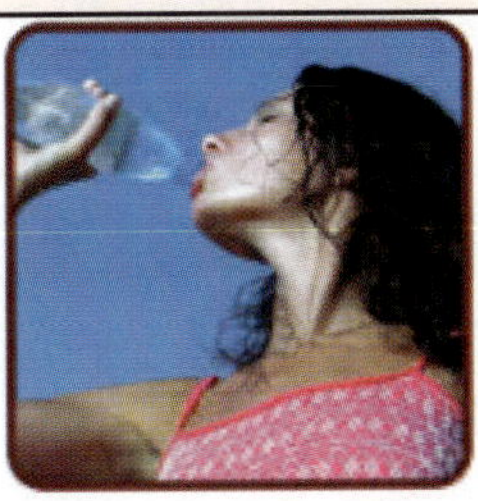

Psychogenic Polydipsia

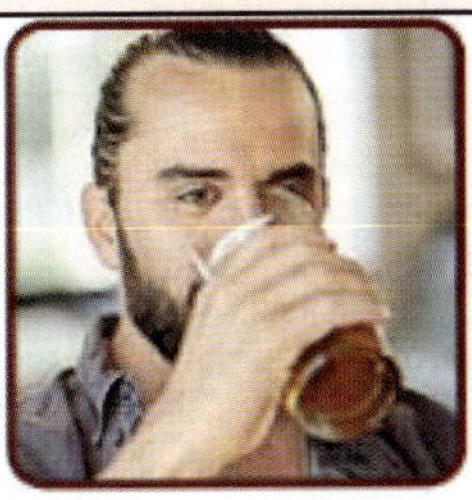

Heavy Drinking

Diuretics

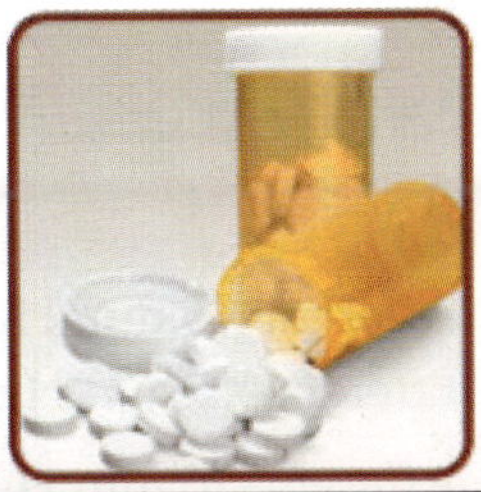

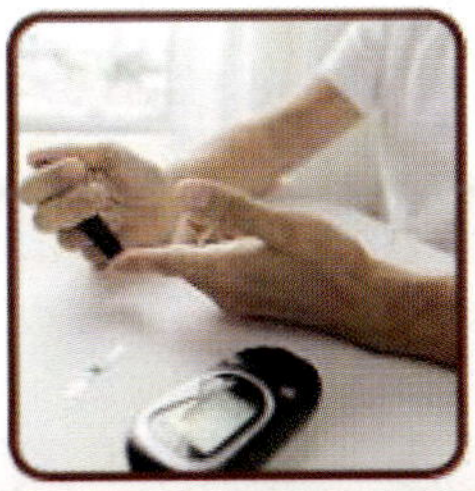

Diabetes Mellitus

Mechanism

- Excretion of non-absorbable solutes such as glucose (Solute diuresis); or
- Excretion of water usually due to defect in ADH production or renal responsiveness (Water diuresis).

- **Water Diuresis:**
  - Urine output **> 3 L/day** and **urine osmolality of < 250 mosmol/**L.
  - This occurs from **polydipsia** due to inadequate secretion of vasopressin (**central DI**) or failure to respond to vasopressin (**nephrogenic DI**).

- **Solute Diuresis:**
  - Urine output **> 3L/day** and urine osmolality **of >300 mosmol**.
  - **Poorly controlled diabetes mellitus** with **glucosuria (MC Cause)**.
  - Common iatrogenic solute diuresis occurs in **mannitol administration**, **radiocontrast** media and **high protein feedings** leads to increased **urea production** and **excretion**.

EXTRA EDGE

Oliguria
• *Urine output <300 ml/24 hrs.*
• **CAUSES:** *Dehydration, Renal failure, Hypovolemic shock, Urinary obstruction/Retention, Preeclampsia and UTI.*
Anuria
• *Urine output <50 ml/24 hrs.*
Microalbuminuria
• Low levels of proteinuria in range of 30-300 mg/day (20-200 microgram/min).

Important Values in Renal System	
Renal blood flow (RBF)	***12 L/min*** *(300-400 ml/100 gm/min*
Glomerular filtration rate (GFR)	***125 ml/min*** *(7.5 L/hr OR 180 L/day)*
Urine volume	*1-1.5 L/day*
Glomerular capillary pressure	*45-55 mm Hg*
Renal vein pressure	*4 mm Hg*
Normal plasma renin	*200 ng/10 ml*

24 hr Urinary Protein and Protein Creatinine Ratio in Different Conditions

24 hr Urinary protein (gm)	Protein/Creatinine ratio	Significance
<0.03	<2.5 (M), <3.5 (F)	Normal
0.03-0.3	3.5-15	Microalbuminuria
0.3-0.5	15-50	Dipstick +ve
>2.5	>250	Glomerular disease likely
>4	>400	Glomerular disease

Pressures in Glomerulus	
Glomerular capillary pressure	Afferent–45 mm Hg Efferent–45 mm Hg
Pressure in Bowman's capsule	Afferent–10 mm Hg Efferent–10 mm Hg
Glomerular oncotic pressure	Afferent–20 mm Hg Efferent–35 mm Hg
Net filtration pressure	15 mm Hg

Ref: Harrison 20th Edition Page 294, Ganong's Review of Medical Physiology 26th Edition Page 688, Textbook of Medical Physiology by Indu Khurana 2nd Edition Page 294, Comprehensive Textbook of Physiology by GK Pal Page 717, Axel S Mexburger, Urology at a Glance Page 23

Ans: (A) 30 ml/kg body weight

4. Antidiuretic hormone acts on collecting duct through:

A. Aquaporin 2
B. GLUT 4
C. Aquaporin 1
D. Aquaporin 3

Key:

ADH acts on collecting duct through Aquaporin 2

Vasopressin

- Secreted by Supraoptic nucleus of Hypothalamus
- **Half life**–18 min

Name	Subtype	Signaling pathway	Location	Function
V1	**V1A**	G protein coupled, Phosphatidylinositol/calcium	Vascular smooth muscle, Platelet, Hepatocytes, Myometrium	Vasoconstriction, Myocardial hypertrophy, Platelet aggregation, Glycogenolysis, Uterine contraction
V3	**V1B**	G protein coupled, Phosphatidylinositol/calcium	Anterior pituitary gland	Releases ACTH, Prolactin and Endorphins
V2	**V2**	Adenylyl cyclase/cAMP	***Basolateral membrane of collecting duct***, Vascular endothelium and Vascular smooth muscle cell	Insertion of AQP2 water channels into apical membrane, induction of AQP2 synthesis, releases Vwf and Factor VIII, Vasodilatation

Control of vasopressin secretion

Stimulating factors	Inhibiting factors
Increased ECF osmolality	Decreased ECF osmolality
Severe hypovolaemia (via angiotensin II and arterial and venous receptors)	Hypervolaemia Alcohol
Stress, including pain	
Nausea	
Exercise	
Drugs Narcotic analgesics, nicotine, some sulphonylureas, carbamazepine, vincristine	

RISE IN PLASMA OSMOLALITY (NORMAL–285 mOsm/kg)

↓

Shrinkage of osmoreceptors

↓

↑ Discharge rate of the osmoreceptors

↓

↑ Release of neurotransmitter

↓

Acts on magnocellular cells of supraoptic nucleus of hypothalamus

↓

Release of ADH

↓

Increase permeability of the membrane of collecting ducts for reabsorption of water (plasma osmolality is maintained)

↓

↓ Urinary output

Contd.

Contd.

Channel	Location
Aquaporin 1	Luminal membrane of PCT
Aquaporin 2	Luminal membrane of CD
Aquaporin 3	Basolateral membrane of CD
Aquaporin 4	Basolateral membrane of MCD

Water Reabsorption in Kidneys

- Aquaporin 1 localized in basolateral and apical membranes of proximal tubules allows water to move rapidly due to osmotic gradient created by active transport of solutes.
- ***60 – 70% of the filtered water is removed in proximal convoluted tubule.***
- **Descending limb** of the loop of Henle is permeable to water, due to the presence of **aquaporin-1** but **ascending limb** is **impermeable*** to water.
- While passing through the descending limb of loop of Henle **15%** of the filtered water is removed. Hence only **20%** of the filtered water enters **distal tubule.**
- **Distal tubule** is **relatively impermeable*** to water. Removal of solute in excess of solvent dilutes the tubular fluid in the distal tubule.
- *Vasopressin or ADH from posterior pituitary acts on collecting ducts*.*
- **ADH** increases permeability of collecting duct to water by acting on **AQP 2***.
- Aquaporins are stored in the vesicles of the principal cells.
- Vasopressin causes insertion of these vesicles into the apical membrane of these cells.
- Effect is mediated via **V2 receptor,** cAMP and **protein kinase A**.
- **10%** of water is removed from the **cortical collecting duct** in the presence of **vasopressin.**

Water Reabsorption Sites in Kidney

Site	Percentage
Proximal convoluted tubule	**60 – 70%**
Descending limb of 'Loop of Henle'	**15%**
Distal convoluted tubule	**5 –10%**
Collecting duct	**10%**

Hormone	Major Stimulus	Major Site of Action	Effect
Angiotensin II	Renin release	***Proximal tubule***	Increase NaCl and water absorption
ADH	Increase plasma osmolality	***Collecting duct***	Increase NaCl and water absorption
Aldosterone	Increase Angiotensin 2 and K^+	***Collecting duct***	Increase Nacl and water absorption
ANP and BNP	Increase ECF volume	***Collecting duct***	Decrease NaCl and water absorption
Dopamine	Increase ECF volume	***Proximal tubule***	Decrease NaCl and water absorption
PTH	Decrease calcium	***Proximal tubule***	Increase calcium and decrease phosphate reabsorption

Ref: Ganong's Review of Medical Physiology 26th Edition Page 686, Textbook of Medical Physiology by Indu Khurana 2nd Edition Page 376, Comprehensive Textbook of Physiology by GK Pal Page 476

Ans: (A) Aquaporin 2

5. **Functional residual capacity (FRC) is the volume which remains in lungs after:**

A. Full inspiration
B. Full expiration
C. Normal inspiration
D. Normal expiration

Key:

FRC– Volume of air remaining in lungs after normal tidal expiration. Therefore, it equals expiratory reserve volume plus residual volume (ERV + RV)

It is about 2500 mL in normal adult male

SIGNIFICANCE OF FRC

- It is also called as ***Equilibrium volume***–Inward elastic recoil of lung balances with outward recoil of chest wall at FRC.
- Helps in ***steady state exchange of gases*** through out respiratory cycle without any sudden change in arterial PO_2 and PCO_2 ***(Maintains stable gas tension)***.
- Decreases energy required to ***reinflate lungs*** during inspiration (Without FRC, alveoli will collapse completely at end of expiration and it requires tremendous force to reinflate them–***Prevents sudden alteration of gas tension***).
- Increases when there is air trapped within lungs–Asthma/Emphysema.
- Breath holding is possible only with FRC.
- Dilutes toxic inhaled gases.

Parameter	Definition	Volume
Tidal Volume (TV)	Amount of air that is inspired/expired during quiet breathing	**500 – 750 ml**
Inspiratory Reserve Volume (IRV)	Volume of air inspired with a maximal inspiratory effort in excess of the TV	**~ 2 L**
Expiratory Reserve Volume (ERV)	Volume of air expelled by an active expiratory effort after passive expiration	**~ 1 L**
Residual Volume (RV)	Volume of air left in lungs after maximal expiratory effort	**~ 1.3 L**
Total Lung Capacity (TLC)	TV+IRV+ERV+RV	**~ 5 L**
Vital Capacity (VC)	Maximum amount of air expired after maximum inspiration (TV+IRV+ERV)	**~ 3.5 L**
Inspiratory Capacity (IC)	Maximum amount of air inspired from the end-expiratory level (TV+IRV)	**~ 2.5 L**
Functional Residual Capacity (FRC)	Volume of the air remaining in the lungs after normal tidal expiration (ERV+RV)	**~ 2.5 L**

- All of these volumes and capacities are measured by spirometry ***(Except RV, CV, FRC and TLC–Measured by N2 washout, Helium dilution method, Body plethysmography)***
- ***Best method of estimation of volumes and capacities is Body plethysmography (See Figure on the next page)***

Change in VC with different body position	
Body position	**Decrease in VC with sitting position is baseline**
LITHOTOMY	18%
TRENDELENBERG	15%
JACK KNIFE	12.5%
SUPINE	9%

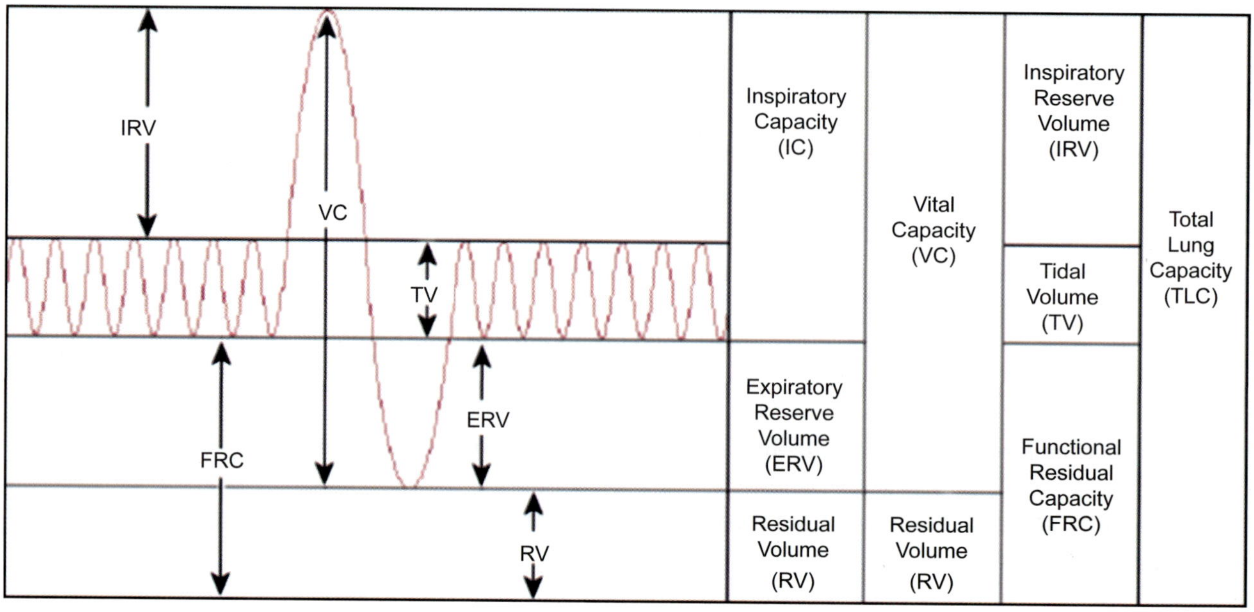

Ref: Ganong's Review of Medical Physiology 26th Edition Page 617, Textbook of Medical Physiology by Indu Khurana 2nd Edition Page 216, Comprehensive Textbook of Physiology by GK Pal Page 893

Ans: (D) Normal expiration

6. In Brown-Séquard syndrome, which of the following is lost on ipsilateral side?

A. Pain, crude touch and temperature
B. Kinesthesia and stereognosis
C. No sensory loss on ipsilateral side
D. Touch, vibration and proprioception

Key:

In Brown-Séquard syndrome there is ipsilateral loss of touch, vibration and proprioception, contralateral loss of pain and temperature along with ipsilateral weakness and spasticity

BROWN-SÉQUARD SYNDROME

- Caused due to **functional hemisection** of the spinal cord.
- **Damage to:**
  - **Dorsal column pathway**–*Ipsilateral loss of discriminative touch, vibration and proprioception* below the level (lesion in fasciculus gracilus or fasciculus cuneatus).
  - **Ventrolateral spinothalamic tract (sensory)**–*Contralateral loss of pain and temperature* sensation beginning one or two segments below the lesion.
  - **Corticospinal tract (motor) pathways**–*Ipsilateral weakness and spasticity* in certain muscle groups.

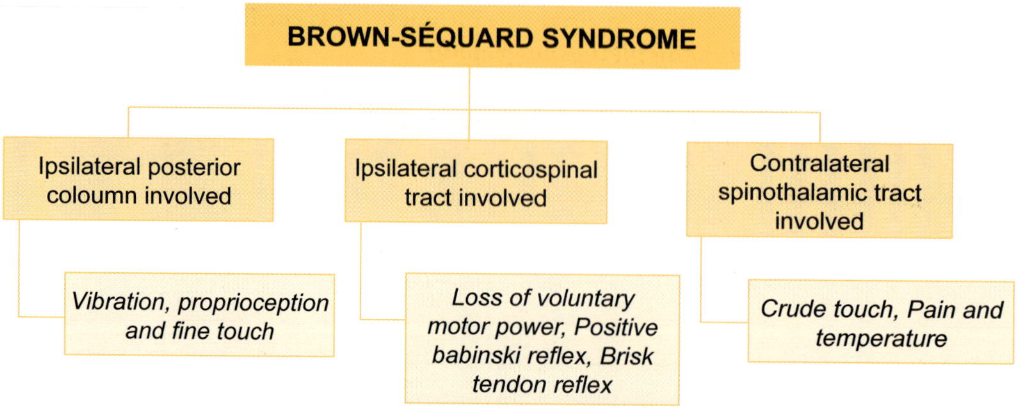

Etiology

- Spinal cord tumor, Spinal cord trauma, Degenerative disk disease and Ischemia

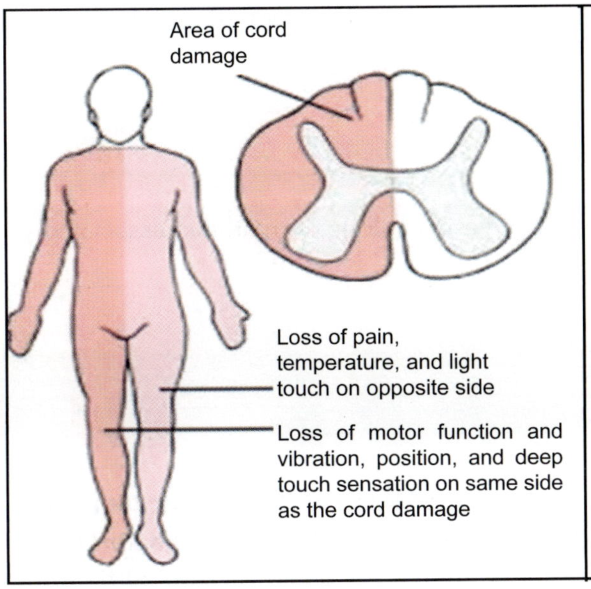

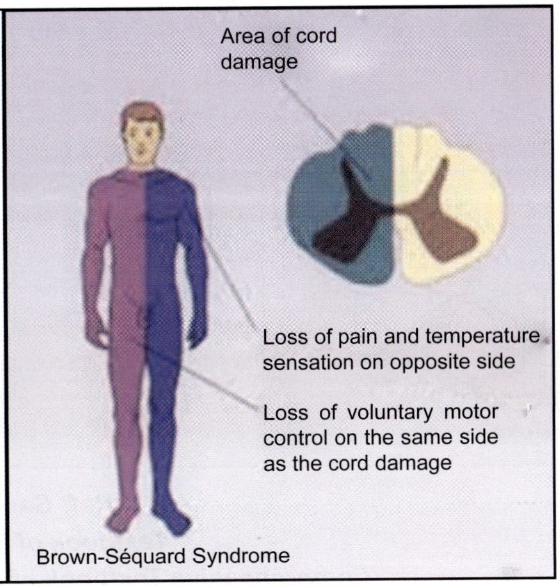

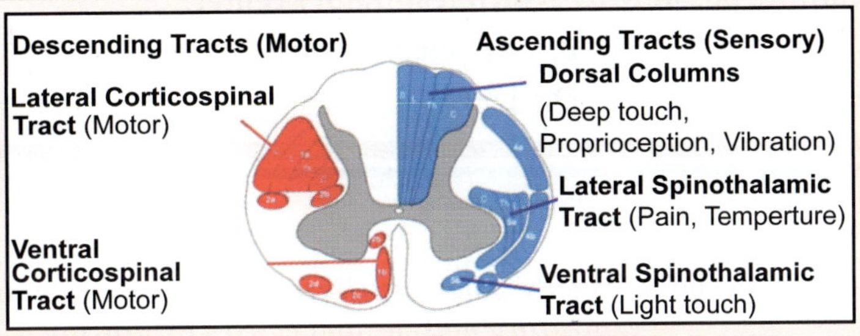

Disease	Cause	Clinical Features
Brown-Séquard syndrome 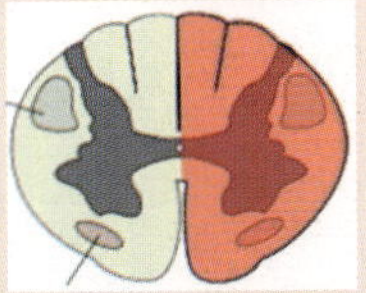	*Trauma*	I/L loss of joint position and vibratory sense (Posterior column) C/L loss of pain and temperature (Spinothalamic tract) Ipsilateral weakness below lesion (Corticospinal tract)
Syringomyelia 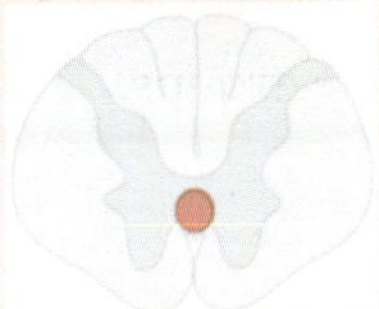	*Associated with Arnold type 1 malformations*	Dissociated sensory loss (Loss of pain and temperature with sparing of touch and vibration in neck, shoulders and upper arms) Once central cavity enlarges, long tracts are compressed→ Spasticity and weakness of legs, bladder and bowel dysfunction with Horner's syndrome
Subacute combined degeneration (SACD) 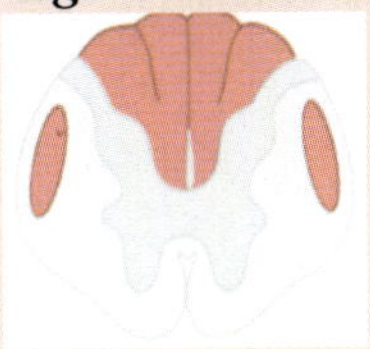	*Vitamin B_{12} deficiency*	Paresthesia of limbs, loss of vibration and position sense, Ataxia

Contd.

Contd.

Tabes Dorsalis 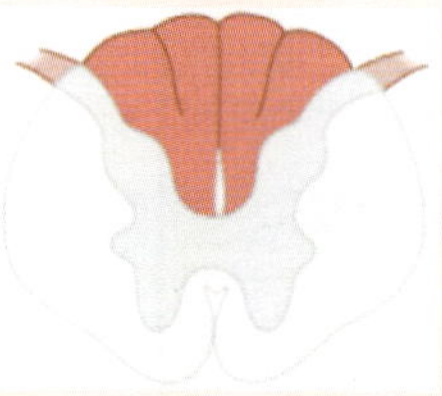	***Syphilis***	Loss of leg reflexes, Impaired position and vibration, Romberg sign, Bilateral Argyll Robertson pupil, Charcot's joint
Herpes zoster (Shingles) 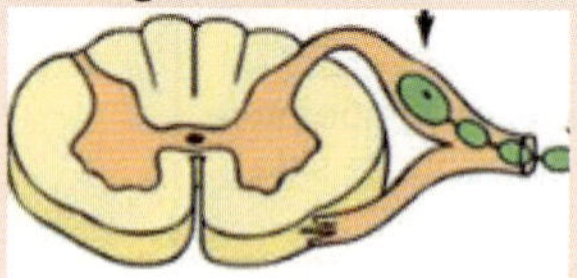	***Reactivation of latent virus in dorsal root ganglia***	Unilateral vesicles along dermatomes associated with severe pain

Ref: Ganong's Review of Medical Physiology 26th Edition Page 617, Textbook of Medical Physiology by Indu Khurana 2nd Edition Page 216, Comprehensive Textbook of Physiology by GK Pal 893, Harrison 20th Edition Page 3173

Ans: (D) Touch, vibration and proprioception

7. **During exercise rapid breathing possible by which respiratory center?**

A. Pneumotaxic center B. Apneustic center
C. VRG D. DRG

Key:

VRG stimulates expiratory muscles only when ventilation is high particularly during Exercise. Stimulate expiratory muscle and causes expiration

RESPIRATORY CENTERS

- Respiratory center is composed of several group of neurons located bilaterally in ***medulla and pons of the brainstem.***

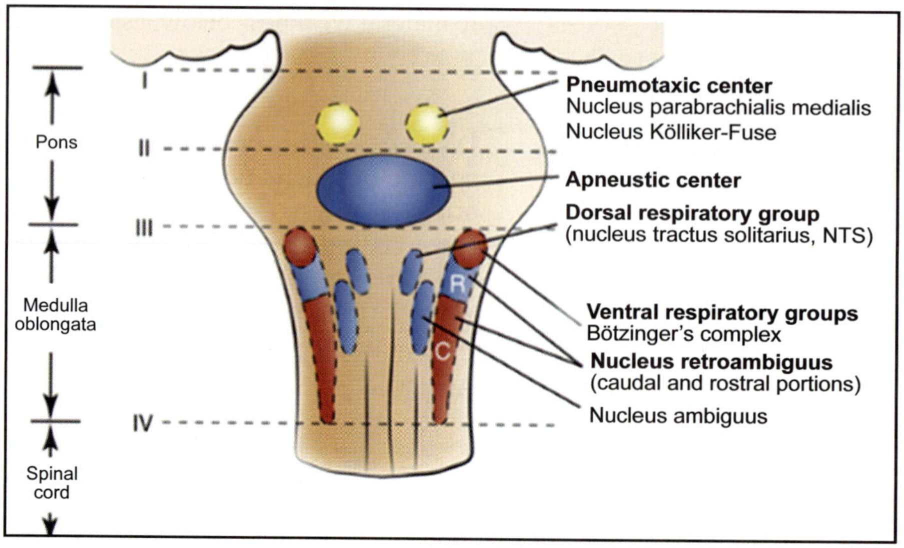

Dorsal Respiratory Group (DRG)	**Located in Nucleus Tractus Solitarius of Medulla** DRG controls inspiration and respiratory rhythm causes inspiration. Signals from these neurons to inspiratory muscles especially the diaphragm are ramp signals.
Ventral Respiratory Group (VRG)	Located in **nucleus ambiguus** and nucleus retroambiguus of medulla. Stimulate expiratory muscle and causes **expiration.** Since expiration is a passive process, stimulation from **VRG stimulates expiratory muscles only when ventilation is high.** *Ex: Exercise*
Pneumotaxic center	***Located in superior portion of pons (Nucleus Parabrachialis).*** Neurons from Pneumotaxic center project to DRG. Primary role is to control the "switch off" point of the ramp signal. **Limit the size of tidal volume** and **increases respiratory rate.**
Apneustic center	***Located in inferior portion of pons.*** Neurons project to DRG. Increase the duration of inspiratory signals and causes increase in duration of diaphragmatic contraction. ***Increase the tidal volume and reduces the respiratory rate.***

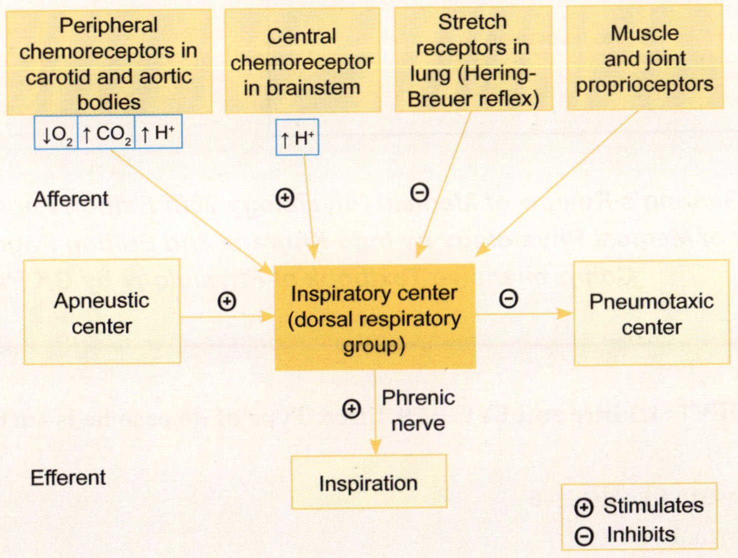

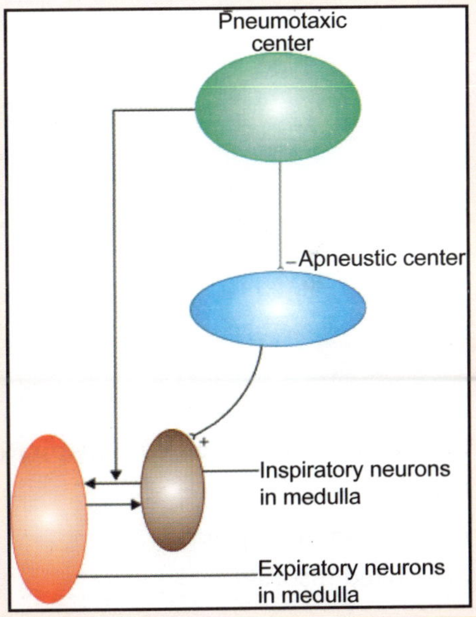

Effects of Transaction At Various Levels			
Site of Lesion	**Effect**	**Inference**	
		Vagi intact	**Vagi cut**
Above pons	Respiratory neurons of medulla and pons are intact	***Normal breathing*** Loss of voluntary control by higher centers	***Slow and Deep breathing*** (Lung stretch information via vagus)

Contd.

Contd.

Mid pons	Pneumotaxic center separated from Apneustic center	***Slow and deep breathing*** (Inhibition of apneustic center lost)	***Inspiration is markedly prolonged*** (Apneusis/Inspiratory spasm)
Pontomedullary junction	Pons and medulla are separated	***Irregular respiration*** (No regularization of rhythm by pons)	***Irregular respiration*** (No regularization of rhythm by pons)
Below medulla	–	***Stops respiration***	***Stops respiration***

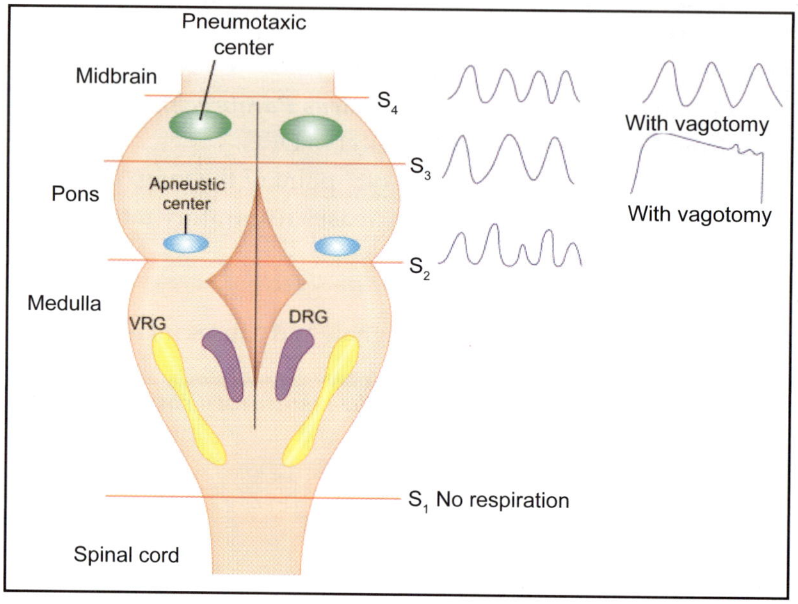

Ref: Guyton and Hall 13th Edition Page 539, Ganong's Review of Medical Physiology 26th Edition Page 647, Textbook of Medical Physiology by Indu Khurana 2nd Edition Page 242, Comprehensive Textbook of Physiology by GK Pal 934

Ans: (C) VRG

8. **In a 50-year-old patient with respiratory distress, FEV1=1.3 litre and FVC =3.9 litres. Type of disease he is suffering from:**

A. Restrictive disease
B. Obstructive disease
C. Mixed disorder
D. Normal

Key:

Reduced FEV1/FVC indicates obstructive lung disorder

ANALYTICAL SOLUTION

- *In the given question, FEV1 = 1.3 L, FVC = 3.9 L. So FEV1/FVC = 33.33%.*
- *Normally FEV1= 80% of FVC→ So FEV1/FVC= 80%.*
- *So there is reduced ratio of FEV1/FVC indicating obstructive disorder.*

Obstructive Lung Disorders (Asthma/COPD)	Restrictive Lung Disorders (Fibrosis)
• Marked decrease in FVC • Marked decrease in FEV1/FVC	• Decrease in FVC • Normal FEV1/FVC

	TLC	RV	VC	FEV1/FVC
Obstructive disease	Normal/Increased	Increased	Reduced	Reduced
***Restrictive**–Parenchymal disease*	Reduced	Reduced	Reduced	Normal/Increased
***Restrictive**–Extraparenchymal disease*	Reduced	Increased	Reduced	Variable

FEV1/FVC Ratio

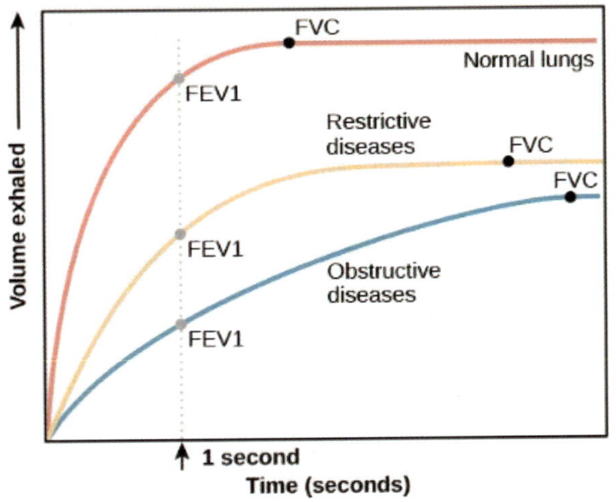

- **Forced Vital Capacity (FVC):** Volume of air forcefully expired after maximal inspiration
- **Forced Expiratory Volume (FEV1):** Volume of air that can be expired in the first second of a forced maximal expiration
  - o *FEV1–Volume of FVC expired in 1 sec of exhalation= 80% of FVC*
  - o *FEV2–Volume of FVC expired in 2 sec of exhalation= 95% of FVC*
  - o *FEV3–Volume of FVC expired in 3 sec of exhalation= 99-100% of FVC*
- **Forced expiratory flow during 25-75% of Expiration (FEF $_{25-75\%}$):** Average expiratory flow rate during middle 50% of FVC–Also called as Maximum Mild Expiratory Flow rate (MMEFR). Normal= 300 L/min
- **Minute ventilation (MV)/Pulmonary ventilation (PV):** Tidal volume × Respiratory rate = 6000 mL/min
- **Alveolar ventilation:** (TV– Dead space) × Respiratory rate= 4200 mL/min
- **Maximum volume ventilation (MVV)/Maximum Breathing capacity (MBC):**

  Largest volume of air that can be taken into and out of lungs in 1 min by maximum voluntary efforts. Normal= 100 L/min
- **Pulmonary reserve/Breathing reserve:** MVV–PV → Expressed as percentage of MVV– ***Expressed as Dyspnoeic index***

  Normal Dyspnoeic Index → more than 60-70%

Flow Volume Loop Patterns

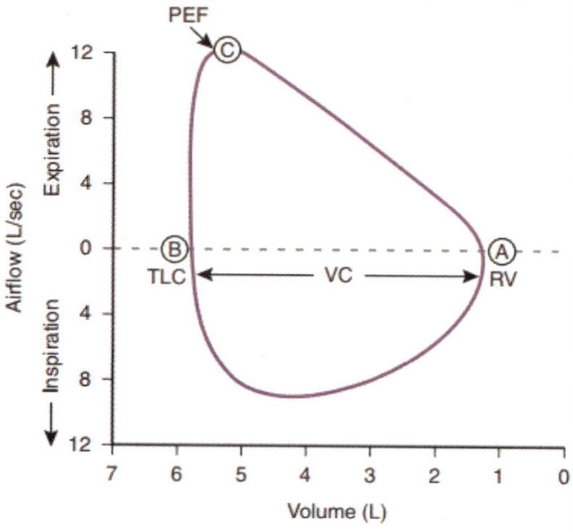

Normal flow volume loop

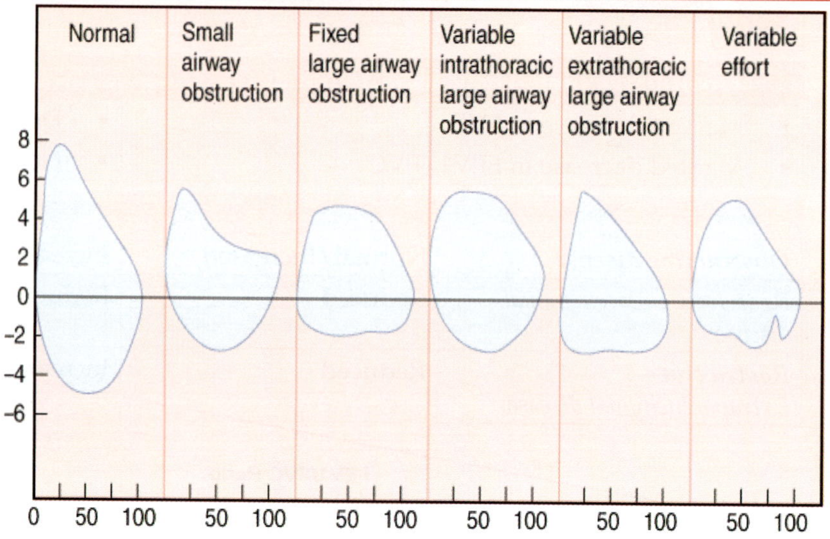

Different patterns of flow volume loop

Ref: Ganong's Review of Medical Physiology 26th Edition Page 647, Textbook of Medical Physiology by Indu Khurana 2nd Edition Page 242, Comprehensive Textbook of Physiology by GK Pal Page 904

Ans: (B) Obstructive disease

9. **Testosterone secreted from:**

A. Leydig's cell
B. Sertoli cell
C. Vas deferens
D. Epididymis

Key:

Leydig cells are steroidogenic stromal cells that synthesize and secrete testosterone

LH acts in Leydig cells to increase testosterone secretion

Leydig cells appear at 8–9 weeks. Testis starts secreting testosterone during this period. Helps in development of male sex

SYNTHESIS OF TESTOSTERONE

- Principal hormone of the testes
- Synthesized in **Leydig cells*** from **cholesterol**.
- It is also formed from **androstenedione** secreted by **adrenal cortex***
- **LH** controls secretion of **testosterone** from Leydig cells by increasing formation of cyclic adenosine monophosphate (**cAMP**) via the **G protein coupled LH receptor and Gs.**
- *Leydig cells don't contain 21 beta hydroxylase or 11 beta hydroxylase and therefore doesn't synthesize glucocorticoids/mineralocorticoids*
- Cyclic AMP increases the formation of cholesterol from cholesterol esters and conversion of cholesterol to pregnenolone via activation of protein kinase A.

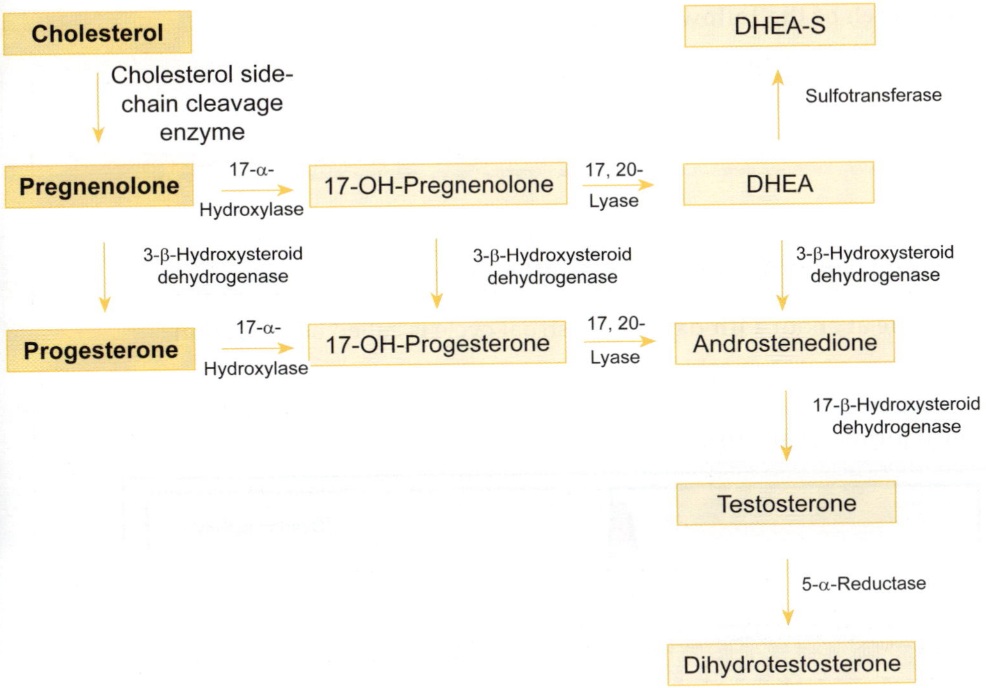

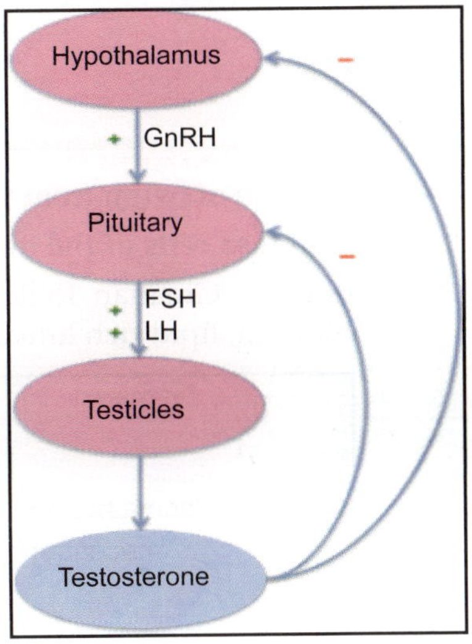

- **Normal testosterone** secretion rate in adult male is **4–9 mg/d (13.9–31.33 µmol/d).**
- **95%** of the Testosterone is bound to β **globulin (65%)** called **gonadal steroid binding globulin** (**GBG**) or **sex steroid binding globulin** and **albumin (33%).**
- **Plasma testosterone level** (free and bound) is **300–1000 ng/dL** (10.4–34.7 nmol/L) in adult men.

Functions of Testosterone

Binds to intracellular receptor forms receptor-steroid complex that binds to DNA in nucleus

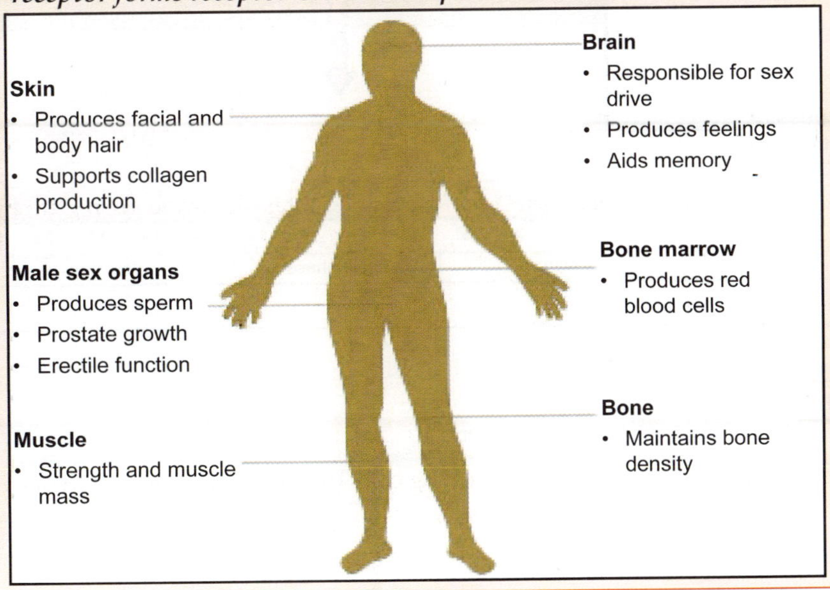

Ref: Ganong's Review of Medical Physiology 26th Edition Page 417, Textbook of Medical Physiology by Indu Khurana 2nd Edition Page 438, Comprehensive Textbook of Physiology by GK Pal Page 579

Ans: (A) Leydig's cell

10. After ovulation, corpus luteum releases which of the following hormone?

A. Progesterone
B. Estrogen
C. LH
D. Inhibin

Key:

Corpus luteum releases Progestrone after ovulation

- Extrusion of ovum from **Graffian follicle** at about **14th day** of menstrual cycle is called as **ovulation**.
- **Granulosa cells of the ovaries** are primary source of **estrogen**.
- Ruptured Graafian follicle forms **corpus hemorrhagicum** which is filled with blood. Blood is replaced with yellowish, lipid rich luteal cells which forms **corpus luteum.**

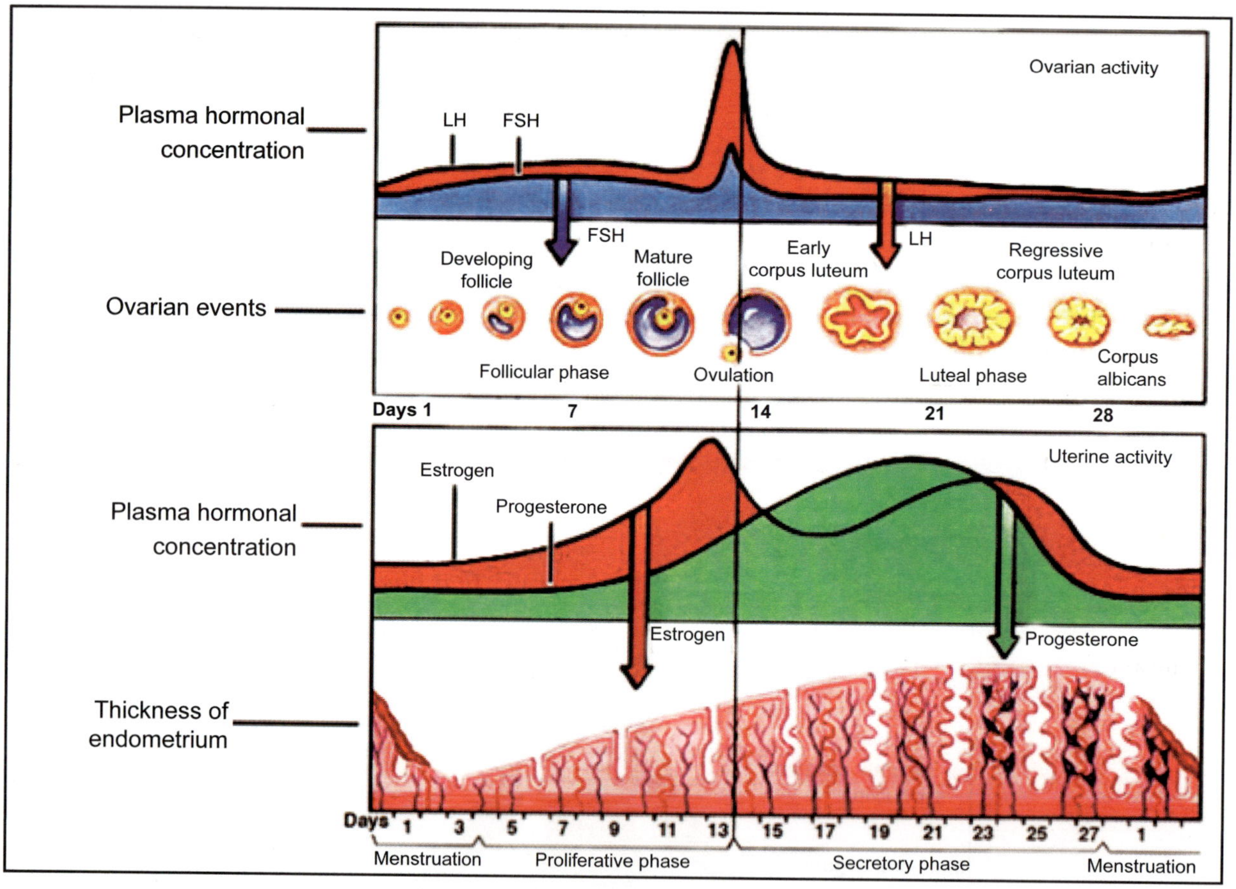

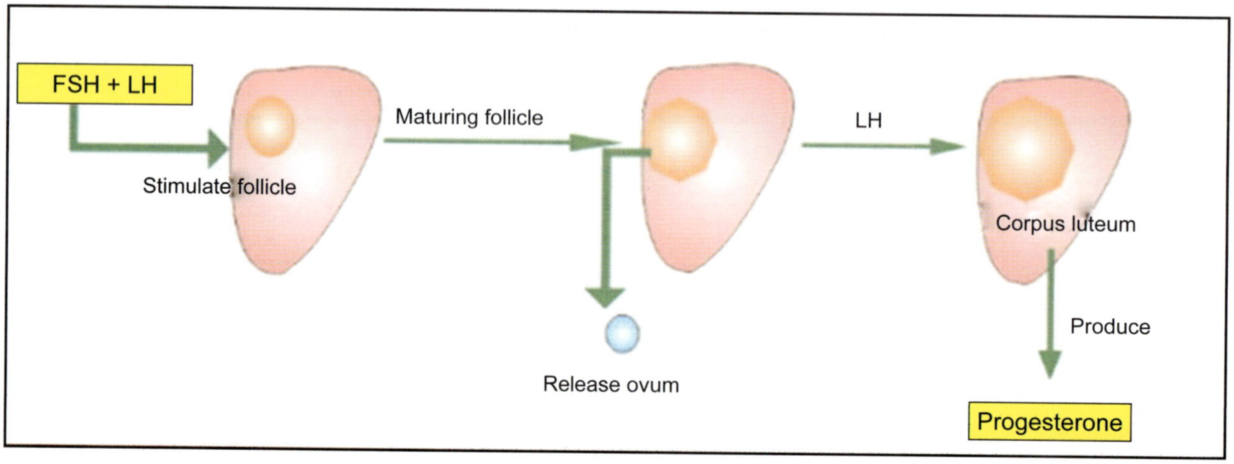

Progesterone	Estrogen
• ***Concentration is minimal in proliferative phase.*** • Starts rising following ovulation and reaches peak in 4 to 5 days after ovulation. • ***Peak is maintained till corpus luteum is active.*** • With regression of corpus luteum, progesterone concentration decreases toward end of luteal phase.	• Has **two peaks** in menstrual cycle. • ***First peak,*** which is major peak, occurs about 48 hours before ovulation and ***second peak*** (minor peak) occurs in post-midluteal phase. • With growth of ovarian follicle, estrogen concentration slowly increases in early part of follicular phase. Concentration rises rapidly from 8th day of cycle to ***reach peak about one or two days before ovulation.*** • Concentration decreases thereafter and decreases further after ovulation. • About two days after ovulation (after formation of corpus luteum), again estrogen concentration increases slowly to reach **smaller peak** that occurs just after mid secretory phase.

- This phase after formation of corpus luteum is called **luteal phase** of menstrual cycle. Luteal cells secrete **estrogen** and **progesterone** during this phase.
- Although both estrogen and progesterone are produced after ovulation, luteal phase is dominated by progesterone secretion from corpus luteum.
- During luteal phase, corpus luteum secretes large quantities of **progesterone**.
- ***Serum progesterone levels increase upto a level of 18 ng/mL.***
- There are **two peaks** of **estrogen** secretion in menstrual cycle. **First** peak is just **before ovulation** and during **mid luteal phase**.

Menstrual cycle	Follicular phase	Luteal phase
Synonym	Proliferative phase	Secretory phase
Days	1-14	14-28
Main hormone	Estrogen	Progesterone
Cervical mucus	Thin	Thick
	Viscous, Abundant mucus	Tenacious
	Penetrable to sperms	Impermeable to sperms
Vagina	Superficial cells with glycogen	Intermediate cells

Ref: Ganong's Review of Medical Physiology 26th Edition Page 393, Shaw Gynecology 16th Edition Page 43, Textbook of Human Physiology Indu Khurana Page 450, Comprehensive Textbook of Physiology by GK Pal Page 618

Ans: (A) Progesterone

11. Golgi tendon organ of skeletal muscle is responsible for maintaining:

A. Tension in the muscle
B. Length of the muscle
C. Pressure
D. Proprioception

Key:

Golgi tendon detects tension in muscle

Golgi Tendon Organ

- Golgi tendon organs are arranged in series with **extrafusal muscle fibers.**
- ***Detects tension in muscle.****
- ***3-25 muscle fibers per tendon organ.***
- **Afferents** are **group Ib afferent fibers** which terminate on **inhibitory interneurons** in the **spinal cord** which inhibits the motor neurons causing the relaxation of muscle which was originally contracted.
- **Group Ib afferents** also make **excitatory connections** with **motor neurons** that supplies **antagonistic muscles.**

Golgi Tendon Reflex

- Also called as ***disynaptic reflex or inverse stretch reflex.***
- When a muscle is stretched it leads to reflex muscle contraction.
- When stretch is stronger and tension becomes very high, contraction ceases and muscle relaxes. This relaxation in response to strong stretch is called **inverse stretch reflex.**
- Golgi tendon organ is **receptor for inverse stretch reflex.**

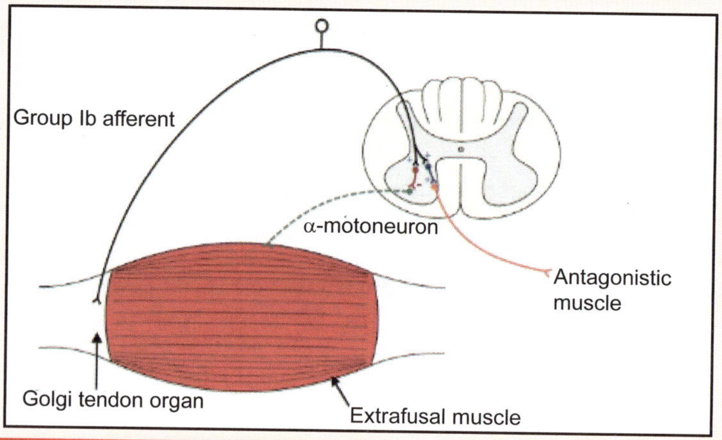

Muscle Spindles

- Distributed throughout the muscle along the extrafusal fibers.
- Each muscle spindle consists of a group of intrafusal fibers, **Group Ia and group II afferents and small myelinated efferent fibers.**
- Muscle spindle detects **static and dynamic changes** in muscle length.
- It is the sense organ for **stretch reflex or myotatic reflex.**

Characteristic	Stretch reflex/Myotactic reflex	Inverse stretch reflex/Lengthening reflex
Synonym	**Monosynaptic**	**Disynaptic**
Stimulus	Passive muscle stretch	Passive stretch and Active contraction
Receptor	Muscle spindle	Golgi tendon organ
Receptor location	Parallel to muscle fibers	Lies in series to muscle fibers
Detects	Muscle length	Muscle tension
Afferent	Ib and II endings	Ib endings
Center	Spinal cord	Spinal cord
Efferent	Alpha motor neuron	Alpha motor neuron
Mechanism	Activated Alpha motor neuron	Inhibited Alpha motor neuron
Gamma motor innervation	Innervates contractile parts of spindle	Absent

Ref: Guyton and Hall 13th Edition Page 701, Ganong's Review of Medical Physiology, 26th Edition Page 228, Textbook of Medical Physiology by Indu Khurana 2nd Edition Page 522, Comprehensive Textbook of Physiology by GK Pal Page 1052

Ans: (A) Tension in the muscle

12. Which of the following are respiratory changes that occur in old age?

A. Increase mucociliary clearance and cough
B. V/Q mismatch decreases
C. Increase chest wall compliance
D. Increased residual volume

Key:

Reduced volume of thoracic cavity and lung volumes increased residual volume is seen with aging

CHANGES IN LUNG WITH AGING

- Reduced chest wall compliance is in counter balanced by loss of elastic recoil.
- Reduced number of parenchymal elastic fibers.
- Chest wall and thoracic spine deformities lead to increase work of breathing.
- Dilatation of air spaces–SENILE EMPHYSEMA.
- ***Reduced mucociliary clearance with ciliary dysfunction.****
- ***Alveolar dead space increases with age–Affects arterial oxygen without impairing CO_2 elimination*.***
- ***Reduced volume of thoracic cavity and lung volumes.***
- ***Reduced respiratory muscle strength and impaired strength of cough.****
- *Reduced sensation of dyspnea along with diminished ventilator response to hypoxia.*
- *Most vulnerable to ventilator failure, less likely response to drugs (Airway undergoes functional changes).*

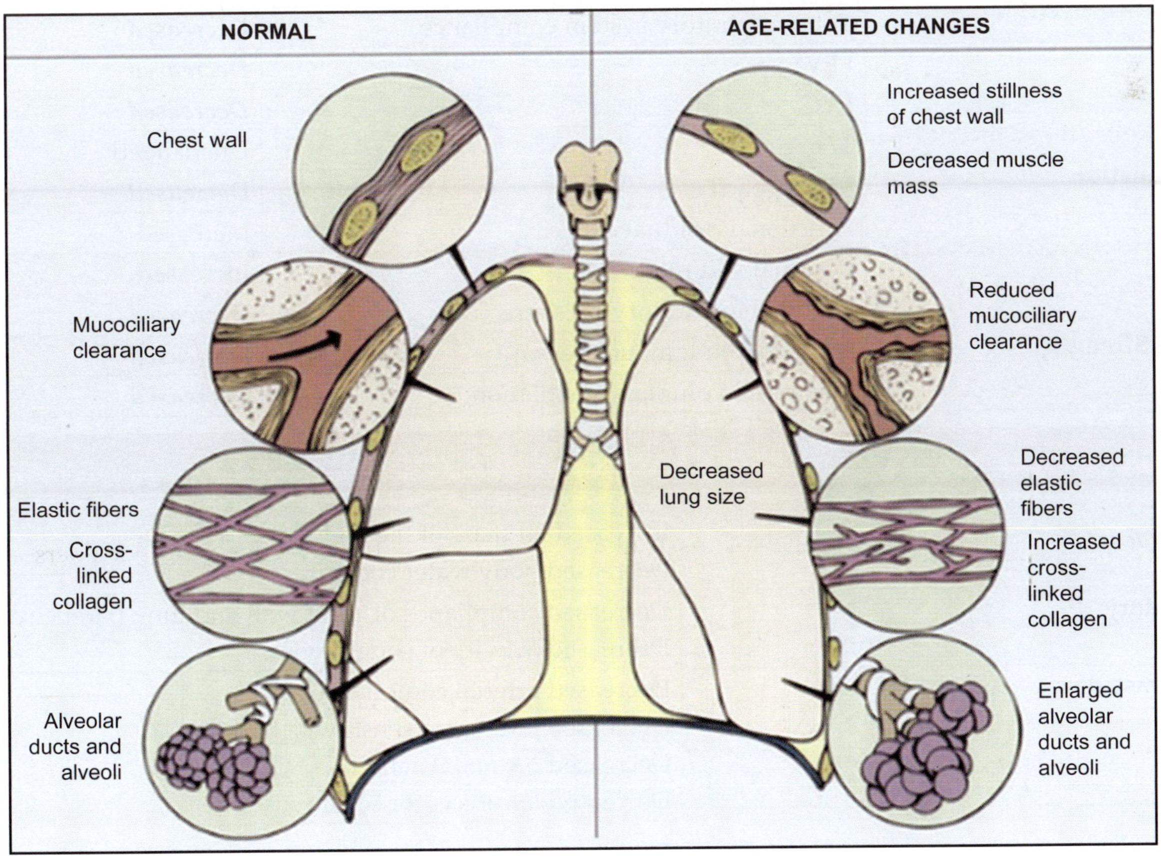

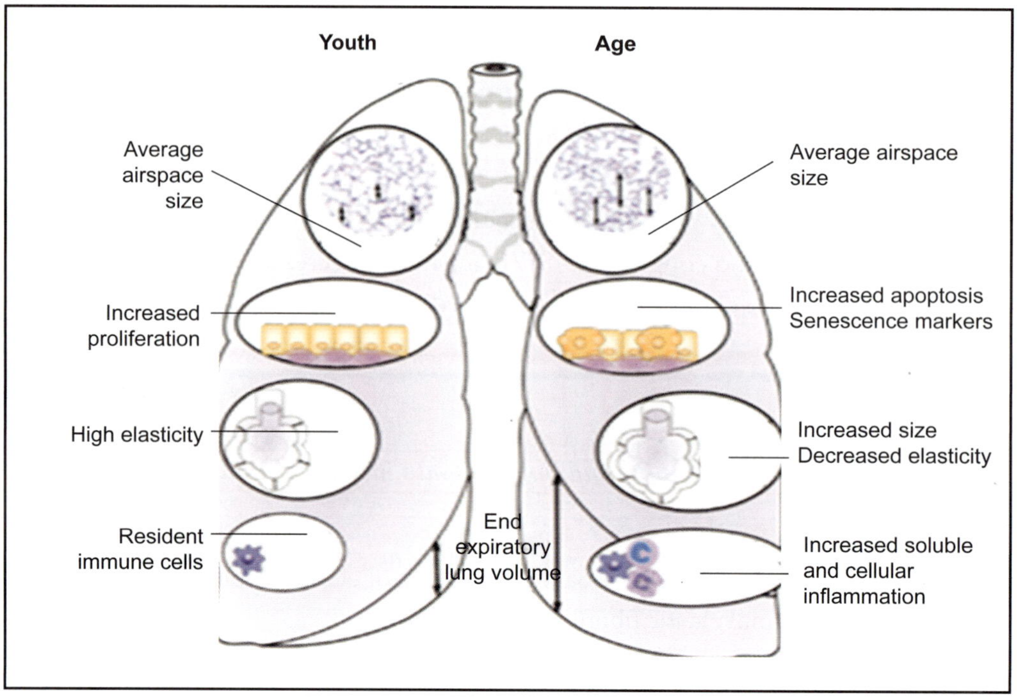

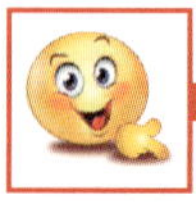

Physiological Changes of Respiratory System with Aging		
Parameter	**Change**	
Compliance	Chest wall compliance	***Decreased***
	Lung compliance	Increased to unchanged
	Total respiratory system compliance	***Decreased***
Lung function	FEV1	***Decreased***
	FVC	***Decreased***
	TLC	Unchanged
	Vital capacity	***Decreased***
	Functional residual capacity	Increased
	Residual volume	Increased
Muscle Strength	Maximal inspiratory pressure	***Decreased***
	Trans diaphragmatic pressure	***Decreased***
	Maximum voluntary ventilation	***Decreased***

Physiological Changes in Geriatric Age Group	
Organ system	**Physiological change**
General	Increased fat mass of the body Decreased body water content
Respiratory	Decreased compliance of chest wall and lung parenchyma Decreased activity of cough reflex
Cardiovascular	Decreased arterial compliance Decreased β receptor sensitivity Decreased SA nodal activity Decreased baroreceptor sensitivity

Contd.

Contd.

GI system	Decreased hepatic function Decreased gastric acidity Decreased colonic motility
Hematologic	Decreased bone marrow activity
Immune system	Decreased T cell function Increased autoantibodies
Renal	Decreased GFR Impaired capacity for urine concentration and dilution
Endocrine	Impaired insulin secretion Decreased thyroxine secretion and thyroxine clearance Increased ADH release and decreased aldosterone secretion Decreased testosterone secretion Vitamin D activation
Nervous system	General brain atrophy Decreased catecholamine secretion Decreased brain dopaminergic synthesis Decreased righting reflexes Decreased stage 4 sleep Impaired thermal regulation
Musculoskeletal	Decreased muscle mass Decreased bone density
Genitourinary	Atrophy of vaginal mucosa In males, prostate enlargement
Eyes and ears	Presbyopia Opacification of lens Decreased sound conduction

Ref: Comprehensive Textbook of Physiology by GK Pal Page 1297, Sharma, Goodwin Effect of Aging on Respiratory System Physiology and Immunology. Clin Interv Aging 2006;1(3):253-60

Ans: (D) Increased residual volume

13. Calcitonin levels are increased in:

A. Hyperthyroidism
B. Hypoparathyroidism
C. Hyperparathyroidism
D. Cushing syndrome

Key:

Calcitonin is secreted in response to rise in calcium level which is seen in hyperparathyroidism. It causes fall in calcium level

CALCITONIN

- **Calcium lowering hormone.**
- Secreted by **C cells (Parafollicular cells)** of **Thyroid.**
- Secretion of calcitonin is increased when plasma calcium **increases >9.5 mg/dL.**

Calcitonin secretion is stimulated by

- *β adrenergic agonists*
- *Dopamine*
- *Estrogens*
- *Hormones such as gastrin, CCK, glucagon and secretin*

- **Gastrin** is most potent stimulus of calcitonin and hence increased level of calcitonin is seen in **Zollinger-Ellison Syndrome** and **pernicious anemia**.

Hypercalcemia–Potent stimulus for secretion of calcitonin

⇩

Reduces calcium and phosphate level

⇩

Bones–Decrease osteoclastic activity
Kidney–Reduced calcium and phosphate reabsorption

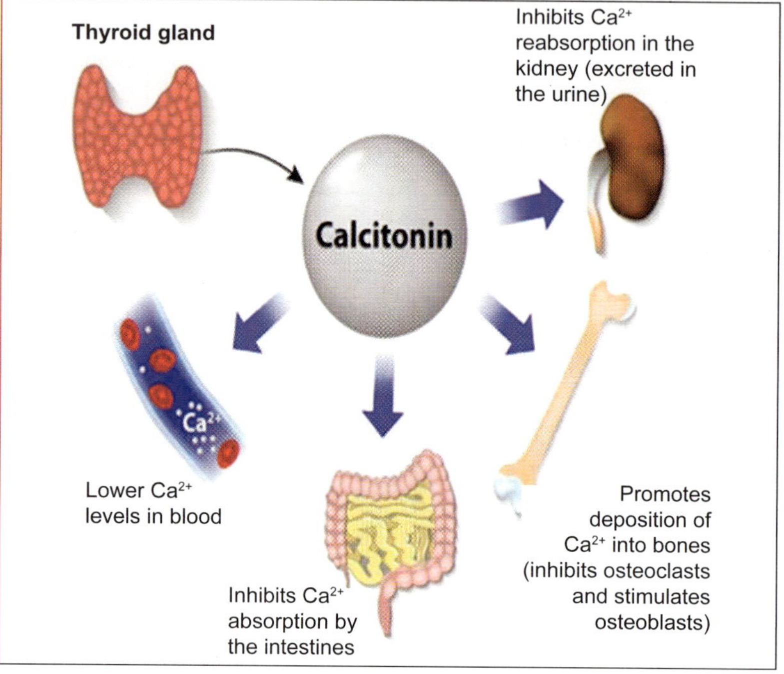

- Acts through **G Protein coupled receptors** found in **bones** and **kidneys**.
- Hypocalcemic effect of calcitonin is seen in **Hyperparathyroidism**.
- Calcitonin exerts its calcium lowering effect by **inhibiting bone resorption** and also **calcium excretion.**

	PTH	1,25-dihydroxycholecalciferol	Calcitonin
Stimulus for secretion	↓ Serum Ca^{2+}	↓ Serum Ca^{2+} ↑ PTH ↓ Serum phosphate	↑ Serum Ca^{2+}
Actions on:			
• Bone	↑ Resorption	↑ Resorption	↓Resorption
• Kidney	↓ P Reabsorption ↑ Ca^{2+} Reabsorption	↑ P reabsorption ↑ Ca^{2+} Reabsorption	– –
• Intestine	↑ Ca^{2+} Absorption	↑ Ca^{2+} Absorption	–
Overall effect on:			
• Serum Ca^{2+}	↑	↑	↓
• Serum phosphate	↓	↑	–

Version 2

Calcitonin elevated in:

A. Adrenocortical tumour
B. Zollinger-ellison syndrome
C. Cushing syndrome
D. Primary hyperaldosteronism

Calcitonin

- Hypocalcemic peptide hormone that in several mammalian species acts as an indirect antagonist to the calcemic actions of PTH.
- It is of medical significance because of its role as a tumor marker in sporadic and hereditary cases of medullary carcinoma and its medical use as an adjunctive treatment in **severe hypercalcemia and in Paget's disease of bone.**
- Hypocalcemic activity of calcitonin is accounted for primarily by inhibition of osteoclast-mediated bone resorption and secondarily by stimulation of renal calcium clearance.
- **Extrathyroidal tumors that can produce ectopic calcitonin include:**
  - Pheochromocytomas, Pancreatic NET's, Adrenocortical carcinomas
  - Gastrointestinal tract tumors, NET's of esophagus, Acute leukemia, Lung cancers.
  - Prostatic carcinomas.
  - Breast cancers, Cervical tumors.

Ref: Harrison 20th Edition Page 2923

Ans: (A) Adrenocortical tumour

Ref: Boron Medical Physiology 2nd Edition Page 1108, Guyton and Hall 13th Edition Page 1001, Ganong's Review of Medical Physiology 26th Edition Page 370, Textbook of Medical Physiology by Indu Khurana 2nd Edition Page 394, Comprehensive Textbook of Physiology by GK Pal Page 1052

Ans: (C) Hyperparathyroidism

14. Antegrade peristalsis due to:

A. Acetyl choline
B. Serotonin
C. Substance P
D. Vasoactive intestinal peptide

Key:

Antegrade peristalsis occurs due to Serotonin

PERISTALSIS

- **Peristalsis** is defined as a motor pattern of the gut organ musculature that can propel contents of gut.

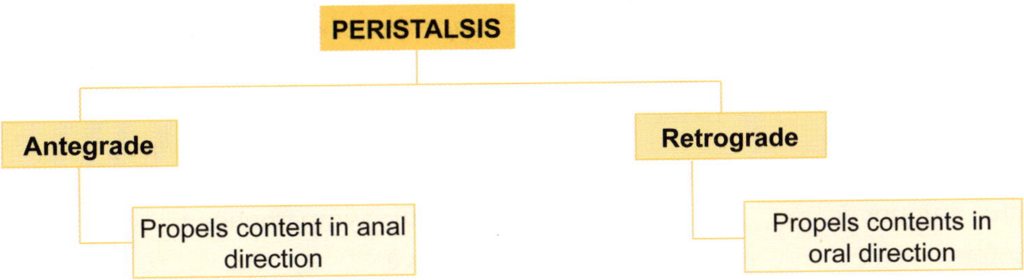

- Bolus present in the intestine stretches intestinal musculature which stimulates inhibitory neurons present in front of bolus to cause relaxation and stimulatory neurons at oral end of bolus to propel bolus in anal direction. This occurs due to myenteric plexus. This is called as ***myenteric reflex or peristaltic reflex***.
- Peristaltic reflex plus anal direction of movement of peristalsis is called ***"law of gut"***.
- Apart from nervous signals, several hormonal factors also affect peristalsis.
- ***Gastrin, CCK, insulin, motilin and serotonin*** enhances intestinal motility.
- ***Secretin and Glucagon*** inhibit small intestinal motility.
- Cholinergic neurons that are **present in antegrade direction** (cell bodies toward oral cavity and terminals toward anus) activate the neurons that secrete VIP and nitric oxide. These neurons assist in ensuing relaxation of circular muscle in the portion of the gut ahead of the stimulus.
- Cholinergic neurons that are **present in a retrograde direction** (with cell bodies toward anus and terminals toward oral cavity) activate the neurons that ***release substance P and acetylcholine.*** These neurons *stimulate circular muscle contraction*, and help in formation and progression of contractile ring behind stimulus.

- ***Impulses travelling in cephalad direction cause ascending contraction***–Mediated by Ach, Substance P and Neurokinin A.
- ***Impulses travelling in caudal direction cause descending relaxation***–Mediated by VIP, NO and PACAP.

Patterns of GI Motility

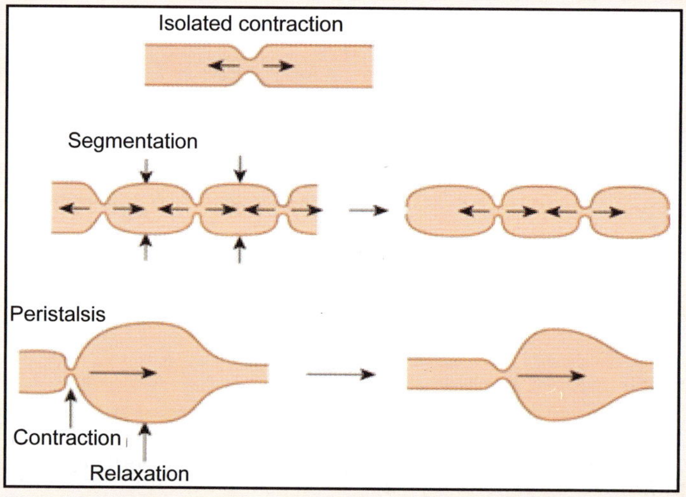

- **An *Isolated contraction*** moves contents orally and aborally.
- ***Segmentation*** mixes contents over short stretch of intestine, as indicated by time sequence from left to right. In diagram on left, vertical arrows indicate sites of subsequent contraction.
- ***Peristalsis*** involves both contraction and relaxation, and moves contents aborally.

Ref: Guyton and Hall Textbook of Medical Physiology, 13th Edition Page 813, Hamid Said Physiology of Gastrointestinal Tract Page 325, Ganong's Review of Medical Physiology 26th Edition Page 485, Textbook of Medical Physiology by Indu Khurana 2nd Edition Page 324, Comprehensive Textbook of Physiology by GK Pal Page 396

Ans: (B) Serotonin

15. Slowest conduction velocity is seen with which of the following fibers:

A. Preganglionic autonomic
B. Post ganglionic sympathetic
C. Somatic motors
D. Proprioceptive

Key:

Slowest conduction velocity is seen with post ganglionic sympathetic fibers

Erlanger and Gasser Classification of Sensory Nerve Fibers

Types of mammalian nerve fibers and its properties

Type of nerve fiber	Function	Fiber diameter (μm)	Conduction velocity (m/s)
Aα	Proprioception; somatic motor	12–20	70-120
Aβ	Touch, pressure	5–12	30–70
Aγ	Motor to muscle spindles	3–6	15–30
Aδ	Pain, temperature	2–5	12–30
B	Preganglionic autonomic	< 3	3–15
C, Dorsal root	Pain, temperature	0.4–1.2	0.5–2
C, Sympathetic	***Post ganglionic sympathetic***	***0.3–1.3***	***0.7–2.3***

Type of nerve fibers		Origin
Ia	A alpha	*Muscle spindle (Annulospiral endings)*
Ib	A alpha	*Golgi tendon organ*
II	A beta	*Muscle spindle (Flower spray endings), touch and pressure*
III	A delta	*Pain and cold receptors, Some touch receptors*
IV	C	*Pain, temperature and other receptors*

***Type A fibers**–Largest, fastest and Myelinated*
***Type C fibers**–Smallest, slowest and Non myelinated*

Ref: Ganong's Review of Medical Physiology 26th Edition Page 94, Textbook of Medical Physiology by Indu Khurana 2nd Edition Page 41, Comprehensive Textbook of Physiology by GK Pal Page 237

Ans: (B) Post ganglionic sympathetic

16. Physiological change in pregnancy include all *except*:

A. Increased cardiac output
B. Increase in total plasma protein
C. Increased GFR
D. Decreased residual volume

Key:

Total plasma proteins are reduced as a physiological change in pregnancy

Physiological Changes in Mother During Normal Pregnancy	
CVS Changes	**Respiratory Changes**
Increase in heart rate Increase in cardiac output Increase in stroke volume Increase in Femoral venous pressure Decrease in diastolic blood pressure during second trimester Decrease in Mean arterial pressure Decrease in systemic vascular resistance No change in systolic blood pressure No change in CVP and PCWP	Increase in Respiratory rate Increase in subcostal angle Increase in transverse diameter Increase in chest circumference Increased vital capacity Increased inspiratory capacity Increased tidal volume Increased minute ventilation Increased gas exchange due to increased pulmonary blood flow Decreased residual volume, FRC and ERV during second half of pregnancy Reduced chest wall compliance No change in FVC, FEV1 and PEFR and Total lung capacity
Renal Changes	**Hematological Changes**
Increase in GFR Increase in renal blood flow Presence of glycosuria and proteinuria Decreased creatinine, BUN and Uric acid	Increase in blood volume Decrease in RBC count, hemoglobin and PCV Increase in Reticulocyte count Increase in ESR Decrease in total concentration of plasma protein Increase in fibrinogen, factors VII, VIII, IX and X

Plasma proteins: *Increase in total plasma proteins and globulin with reduced plasma protein concentration, Albumin and Albumin/Globulin ratio.*

Ref: Comprehensive Textbook of Physiology by GK Pal Page 636, Textbook of Human Physiology Indu Khurana Page 456, LoMauro Aliverti Respiratory Physiology of Pregnancy: Physiology Masterclass. Breathe 2015;11(4):297-301, Williams Obstetrics 25th Edition Page 22

Ans: (B) Increase in total plasma protein

17. Bundle of Kent is:

A. Accessory pathway in WPW syndrome
B. Pathway that connects SA node and ventricular fibres
C. SA →AV connection
D. Left bundle branch

Key:

Bundle of Kent is an accessory pathway to ventricle that occurs before conduction of impulse through AV node and bundle of His and ventricles are pre-excited during sinus rhythm

It is involved in WPW syndrome

- **Bundle of Kent** is an extra electrical connection across annulus fibrosus in addition to bundle of His.
- Bundle of Kent allows electrical impulses to bypass AV node, thus avoids AV nodal delay, reaches rapidly and depolarizes area of ventricles. By pass tract can conduct in both direction retrograde (ventricle to atria) or anterograde (atria to ventricle).

- Most prominent manifestation due to bundle of Kent is pre-excitation of ventricles known as **Wolff-Parkinson-White (WPW) syndrome.**
- ***It is characterized by Supraventricular tachycardia.***
- *Wolff-Parkinson-White syndrome has familial inheritance. In these families, there is mutation in gene that codes for an **AMP-activated protein kinase.** Presumably, this kinase is normally involved in suppressing abnormal atrioventricular pathways during fetal development.*

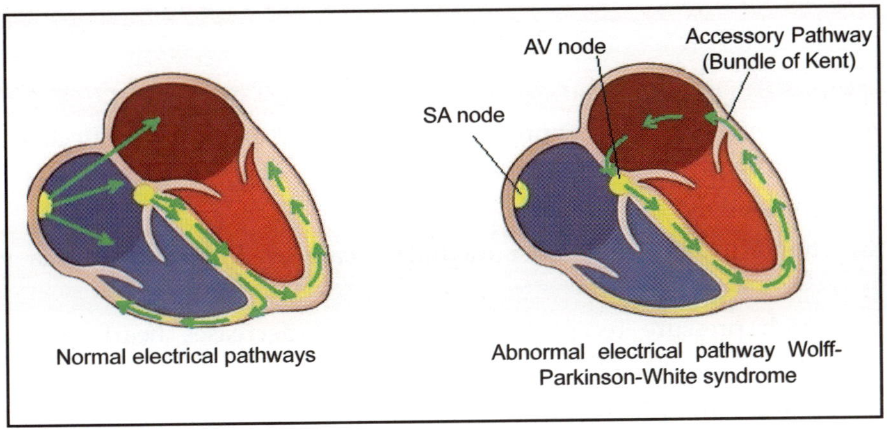

Characteristic ECG findings of WPW include:

- Wide QRS complexes
- Shortened PR interval (<0.12 sec)
- Upstroke of QRS complexes is slurred/notched called as **Delta wave*** ***(Delta wave**–Initial portion of QRS complex with slow upstroke in ECG).*

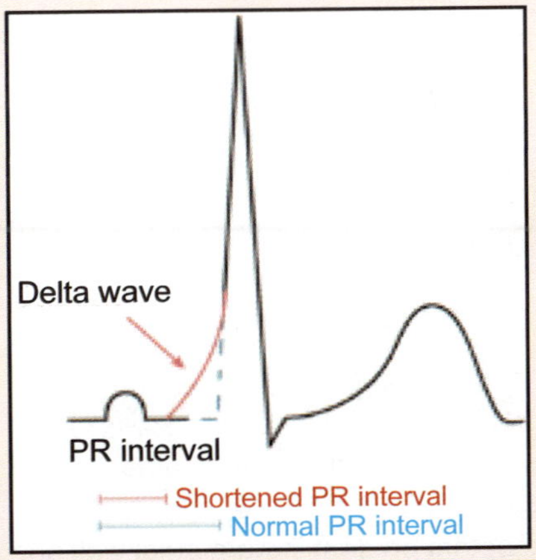

Ref: Goldberger's Clinical Electrocardiography 8th Edition Page 108, Alam LC, WPW Syndrome Presented with Ventricular Tachycardia–A Case Report. Indian Anaesthetists forum 2009 Oct 1 (Page 1-5), Harrison 20th Edition Page 1731, Ganong's Review of Medical Physiology 26th Edition Page 522, Comprehensive Textbook of Physiology by GK Pal Page 773

Ans: (A) Accessory pathway in WPW syndrome

18. Which of the following stimulates Bainbridge reflex?

A. Increased pulse pressure
B. Right atrial engorgement
C. Reduced venous return
D. Bradycardia

Key:

Bainbridge reflex is stimulated by right atrial engorgement which stimulates right atrial stretch receptors

Bainbridge reflex/Arterial stretch reflex/Volume reflex

- **B type atrial stretch receptors** are the low pressure receptors that monitor the effective circulating volume and venous return to the heart.
- **Stretch receptors are located in both left and right atria.**
- Afferent pathways travel to **NTS** and other medullary cardiovascular centers via **vagus** nerve similar to **Baroreflex**.
- Increase stretch of high pressure receptors (Baroreceptors) decreases heart rate and causes generalized vasodilation.
- **Increase stretch** of **atrial B receptors** due to **increased venous return, raises heart rate** and also decreases **sympathetic vasoconstrictor** output only to kidney.
- Net effect of Bainbridge reflex is **tachycardia** and **renal vasodilation** and hence increase in **renal blood flow and diuresis**.
- Increase in atrial stretch **decreases ADH secretion** and hence leads to **diuresis**. The afferent fibers from atrial stretch receptors that projects to NTS also projects to magnocellular neurons in the paraventricular nucleus of the hypothalamus that synthesize **antidiuretic hormone (ADH).** ADH is released through posterior pituitary into the blood.
- Stretch of atrium also causes release of Atrial Natriuretic peptide that causes water diuresis and renal sodium excretion.

- ○ ***Receptor:*** Stretch receptors in both atrial walls.
- ○ ***Afferent:*** Vagal afferent.
- ○ ***Center:*** Brainstem.
- ○ ***Efferent:*** Parasympathetic and Sympathetic.
- ○ ***Response:*** Increase in Heart rate.

↑ Vagal tone

↑ Right sided filling pressure

↓

Stretching of atria

↓

Stimulates stretch receptors present in right atrial wall and cavoatrial junction

Vagal myelinated afferent fibers	Directly stimulates SA node
↓	↓
Cardiovascular center of medulla	↑ HR
↓	
Efferents of vagus nerve	
↓	
Inhibit parasympathetic activity	
↓	
↑ HR	

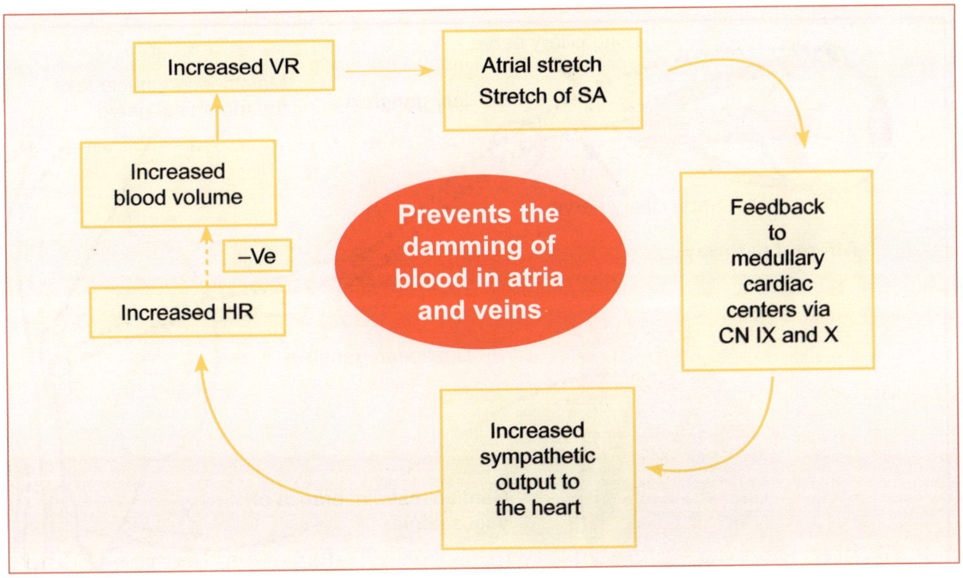

Bezold Jarisch Reflex/Cardiopulmonary Reflex

- Intracardiac injection (Serotonin, Veratridine, Capsaicin) activates this reflex.
- Afferents travel via Unmyelinated Vagal C fibers.
- **Reflex response:** *Apnea followed by rapid breathing, Hypotension and Bradycardia.*
- **Responsible for sinus bradycardia during MI.**
- Cause of Profound bradycardia and circulatory collapse after spinal anesthesia.

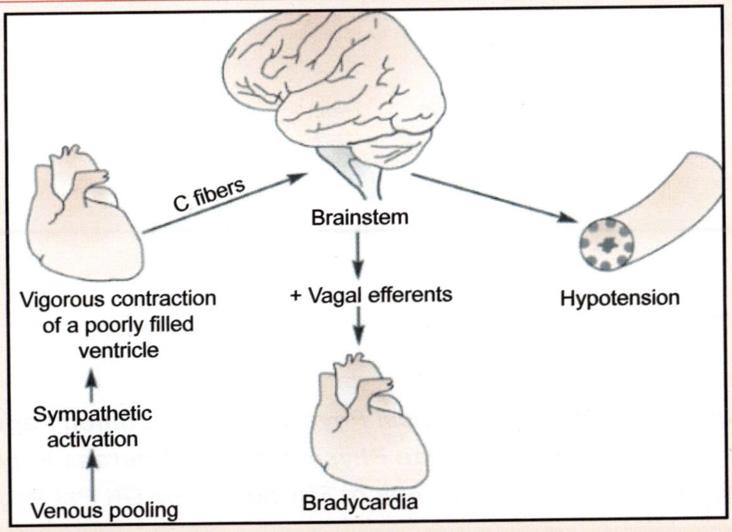

Triggering factors
↓
Stimulates cardiopulmonary chemoreceptors and mechanoreceptors of LV wall
↓
Unmyelinated vagal afferent type C fibers
↓
Inhibit medullary vasomotor center
↓
↑ Parasympathetic tone
↓
Triad of – bradycardia, hypotension, peripheral vasodilatation

Brewer Luckhardt reflex

- Stimulation of anal canal/cervix leads to vagal stimulation
- Causes Bradycardia, Laryngospasm and Bronchospasm

Oculocardiac reflex/Aschner Dagnini reflex/Aschner phenomenon

- Reflex is activated during traction applied to extraocular muscles and/or eye ball compression
- Afferents for this reflex travels through long and ciliary nerves to trigeminal nucleus
- Efferents travel through Vagus nerve to heart
- ***Characterized by Profound bradycardia***

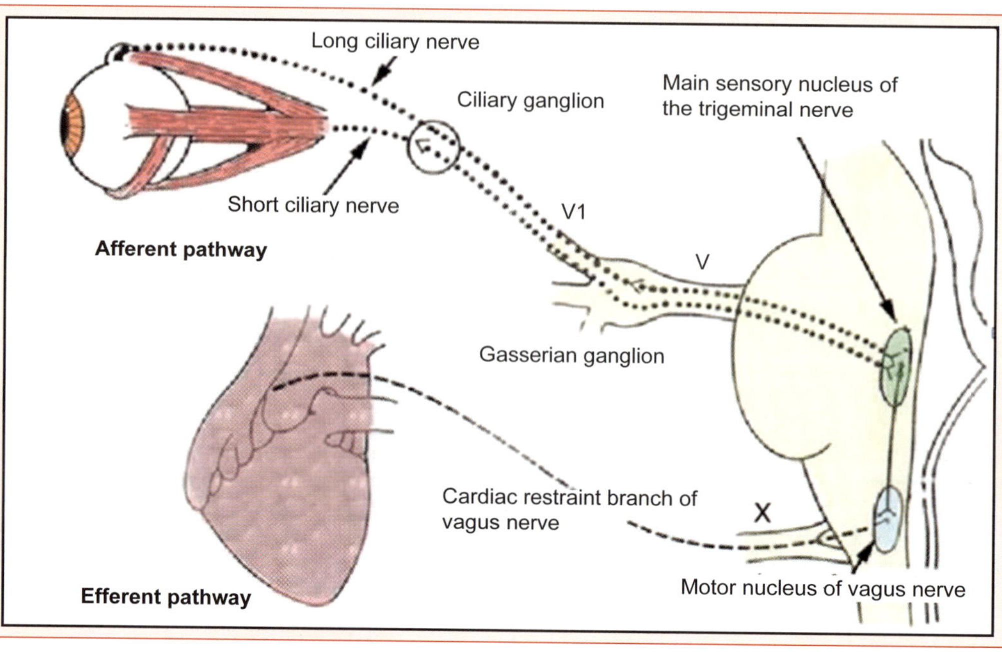

***Marey's Law:** This law states that Heart rate and BP are inversely related. This law explains reflex bradycardia associated with increase in BP.*

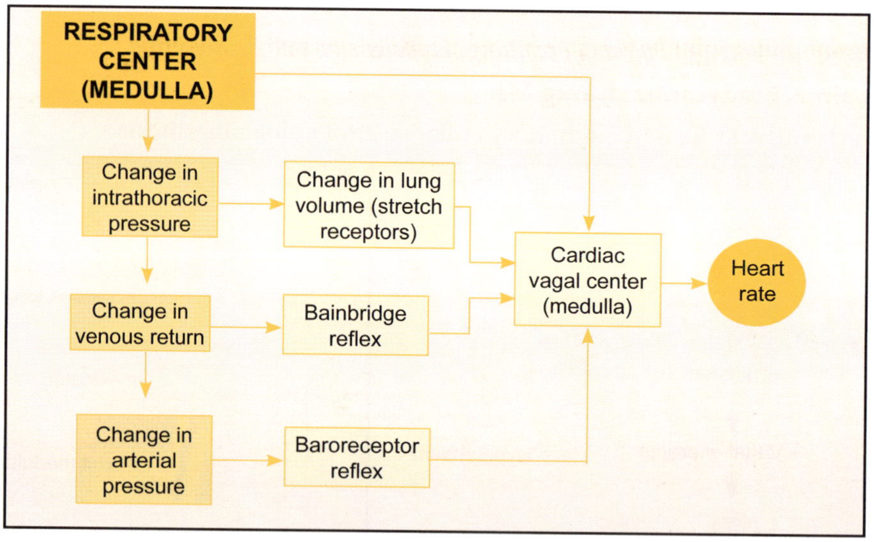

***Ref:** Guyton and Hall Textbook of Medical Physiology 13th Edition Page 539, Textbook of Human Physiology Indu Khurana Page 185, Boron Medical Physiology 2nd Edition Page 568, Comprehensive Textbook of Physiology by GK Pal Page 771*

Ans: (B) Right atrial engorgement

Chapter 3

BIOCHEMISTRY

1. Menkes disease occurs due to Defect in which of the following Enzyme?

A. Lysyl hydrolyase
B. Procollagen N peptidase
C. Lysyl oxidase
D. Prolyl oxidase

Key:

Menkes disease occurs due to Deficiency of ATP-dependent ATP7A transporter which is result of Mutations in gene for copper-binding P-type ATPase resulting in defect of Lysyl oxidase

Lysyl oxidase is an enzyme that functions in Cross linking of collagen and elastin (Deficiency leads to defect in connective tissue like bones)

Menkes Disease

- Also known as *"kinky" or "steely" hair disease.*

Genetics

- Deficiency of ATP-dependent ATP7A transporter.
- Mutations in gene for copper-binding P-type ATPase.

Pathogenesis

- X-linked recessive–Affects only male infants.
- Reflects dietary deficiency of copper required by ***lysyl oxidase*** (catalyzes key step in formation of covalent cross-links that strengthen collagen fibers).
- Disease results in copper malabsorption because copper cannot be transferred from enterocytes to the blood.

Clinical Features

- Involves CNS, Connective tissue and Vasculature.
- Characterized by kinky hair and growth retardation.
- Light skin and hair pigmentation are caused by deficient activity of tyrosinase in melanocytes, connective tissue abnormalities by impaired lysyl oxidase activity and neurological degeneration may be caused by impaired activity of Cytochrome C oxidase.

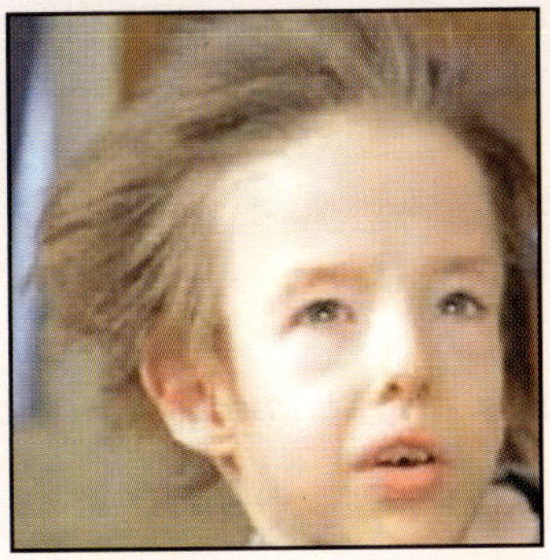

Contd.

- Clinical abnormalities are attributed to deficient activity of copper-containing enzymes.
- **Classical cases:** Disease presents about 2 months after birth with growth retardation, axial hypotonia, seizures, atrophy of gray matter in cerebral cortex and cerebellum, developmental delay or regression and coarse, lightly pigmented hair that is brittle and rubs off easily.
- **Other abnormalities:** Lax skin and joints, Bone demineralization and Characteristic jowly appearance of face.
- ***Usually fatal in infancy.***
- Untreated, this multisystem disease progresses to death at age of 3 years.

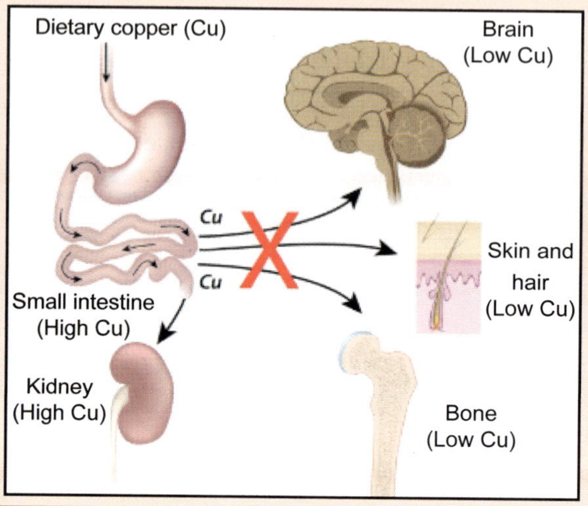

Copper levels are low in plasma, liver and brain

Treatment

- ***Menkes disease is treated by parenteral administration of copper.***
- Copper treatment provides substantial benefits only for those who have residual activity of ATP7A transporter.
- Patients with Complete deficiency will still die.

Diseases Associated with Collagen		
Disease	**Type of collagen**	**Gene or enzyme**
Menke's disease	Lysyl oxidase	Lysyl oxidase
Osteogenesis Imperfecta Osteoporosis Ehlers-Danlos Syndrome (Type VII EDS)	Type I	COL 1A1 and COL 1A 2
Chondrodysplasias Osteoarthritis	Type II	COL 2A1
Ehlers-Danlos syndrome (Type IV EDS)	Type III	COL 3A1
Alport syndrome (including both autosomal and X-linked forms)	Type IV	COL 4A3 to COL 4A6
Classical EDS	Type V	COL 5A1, COL 5A2
Hypermobile EDS (Type III EDS)	Type III	COL 3A1 Tenascin XB (TNXB)
Epidermolysis bullosa, dystrophic	Type VII	COL 7A1
Schmid metaphysial chondrodysplasia	Type X	COL 10A 1
Ehlers-Danlos syndrome (Type VI EDS) (Kyphoscoliotic EDS) Scurvy	Lysyl hydroxylase	Lysyl hydroxylase

Ref: Harper 30th Edition Page 281, Simmon's Principles of Medical Biochemistry 4th Edition Page 530

Ans: (C) Lysyl oxidase

2. A 20-year-old alcoholic malnourished patient came to hospital with respiratory distress. Pulse rate 112/min. Patient had edema, hypertension, Systolic murmur along left sternal border. High output cardiac failure was diagnosed. Which of the following vitamin deficiency could lead to this?

A. Vitamin B_1 B. Vitamin C
C. Vitamin B_2 D. Vitamin B_6

Key:

Given clinical picture shows cardiac dysfunction with dyspnea and High output cardiac failure which is typical for Beriberi (Vitamin B_1 deficiency)

THIAMINE (VITAMIN B_1)

- ***Also called as ANEURINE/ANTI BERIBERI FACTOR***
- ***Relieves neuritis***–So called Aneurine
- Contains pyrimidine and thiazole ring
- ***Source:*** Whole wheat flour and unpolished rice (High)
- Good sources include yeast, meat and legume seeds.
- ***Active form:*** Thiamine pyrophosphate/Thiamine diphosphate
- Absorbed in small intestine
- Excreted in urine
- ***Co enzyme for*** pyruvate dehydrogenase in ***carbohydrate metabolism***; α-ketoglutarate dehydrogenase in ***citric acid cycle*** and branched-chain keto-acid dehydrogenase involved in ***metabolism of leucine, isoleucine and valine.***
- ***Thiamine antagonists–Coffee, Tea, Fermented fish (Thiaminase) → Pyrithiamine and Oxythiamine***
- *RDA of thiamine is 1.2 mg/d for adult males and 1.1 mg/d for adult females.*
- Plasma levels of thiamine is about 1.0 μg/dL.

RDA	
0-6 months	0.2 mg/day
7-12 months	0.3 mg/day
1-3 years	0.5 mg/day
4-8 years	0.6 mg/day
Adult	1.2-1.5 mg/dL
Pregnancy and Lactation	1.5-2 mg/dL

Deficiency

- Plasma levels of lactate and pyruvate increase and accumulate in persons with thiamine deficiency because pyruvate dehydrogenase requires TPP for its activity.
- ***Thiamine deficiency leads to diffuse decrease in glucose utilization***
- ***Bracken disease, Chastek paralysis, Catatarulin effect and saturation effect–Animals***

  Glutamate accumulates (Impaired alpha ketoglutarate dehydrogenase activity) and along with energy deficiency leads to Excitotoxic cell damage
- ***Deficiency causes beriberi***
- Characterized by neurological disorders
- Particularly seen in persons who consume polished rice ***OR*** Highly refined wheat flour
- Occurs within 2 and 3 months of deficient intake

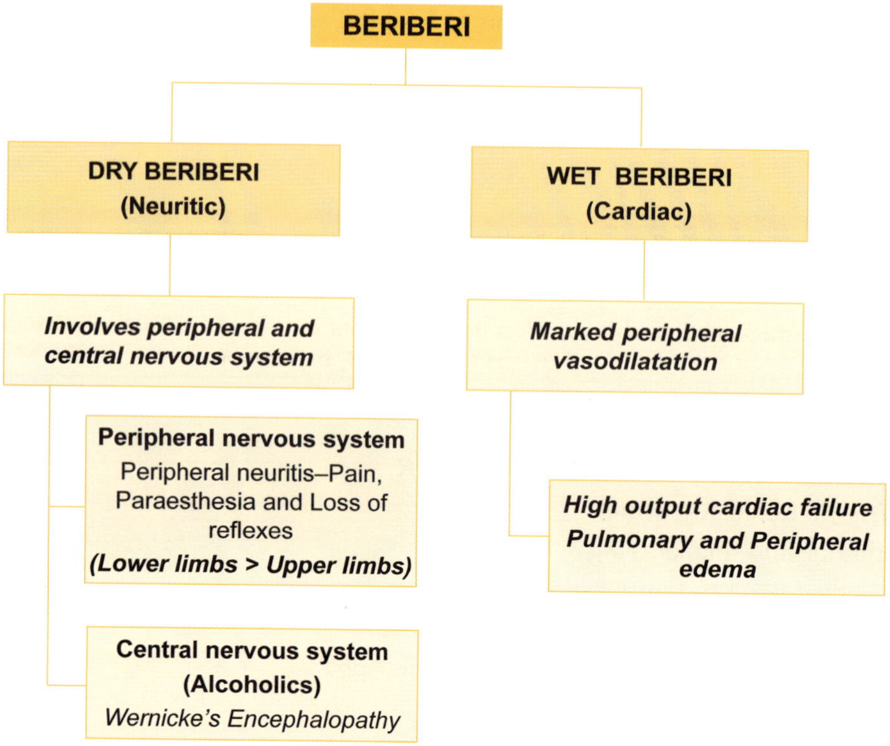

Characteristic Sign of Vitamin B_1 Deficiency
Hoarseness of voice/Aphonia that is caused by Paralysis of Recurrent laryngeal nerve

DRY BERIBERI

- Predominantly neuritic
- Involves both peripheral and central nervous system

Wernicke's Encephalopathy
• *Classical triad of Global confusion, Ophthalmoplegia (Horizontal nystagmus) and Ataxia*
Wernicke Korsakoff Syndrome
• Wernicke's Encephalopathy with additional loss of memory and confabulatory psychosis • ***Wernicke encephalopathy requires immediate treatment with thiamine injections*** to prevent development of chronic stage known as ***Korsakoff psychosis.*** This condition is dominated by severely debilitating ***anterograde amnesia.*** Patients can remember events from distant past, also immediate recall is intact, but they can't transcribe information from short-term to long-term memory. • ***Korsakoff psychosis–Most common form of amnesia→*** Attributed to focal lesions in periventricular areas of thalamus and hypothalamus, periaqueductal gray of midbrain and mammillary bodies.

WET BERIBERI

- Characterized by edema of extremities, heart enlargement, cardiac insufficiency and congestive heart failure.
- Other symptoms are dyspnoea, tachycardia and palpitation.

Diagnosis

- ***Erythrocyte Transketolase activity is a best measure of functional activity of Thiamine on addition of thiamine pyrophosphate.***
- Urinary thiamine levels.

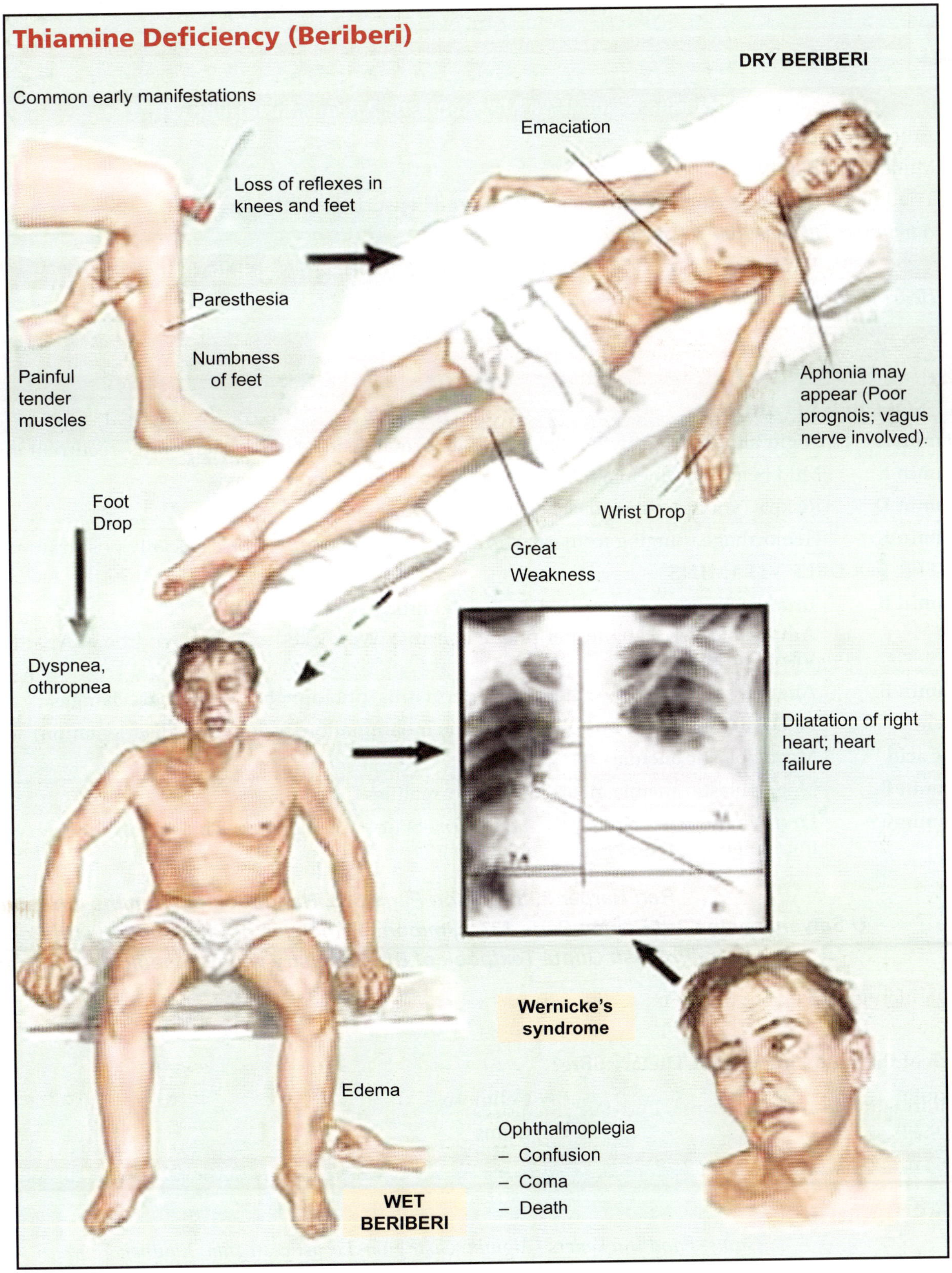

Treatment

- In chronic alcoholics intravenous glucose administration may precipitate Wernicke encephalopathy (Medical emergency–Administer thiamine before glucose administration).
- Children with cardiac failure, convulsions/coma → 10 mg IM/IV daily for 1st week followed by 3-5 mg of thiamine per day for 6 weeks.
- No known toxicity exists for Thiamine.

Thiamine Responsive Megaloblastic Anemia Syndrome (TRMA)

- Autosomal recessive disorder
- Mutation in SLC19A2
- Triad of Megalobastic Anemia, Diabetes milletus and Sensorineural hearing loss
- *Administer Thiamine 100-200 mg/day*

Acute Pernicious Beriberi (Fulminating/Shoshin Beriberi)

- ***Heart failure with metabolic abnormalities predominate***

Vitamin Deficiency

Vitamin	Clinical Picture
FAT-SOLUBLE VITAMINS	
Vitamin A_1	Night blindness, growth retardation, abnormal taste response, dermatitis, recurrent infections
Vitamin E	Mild hemolytic anemia (newborn), red blood cell fragility, ataxia
Vitamin D	Rickets (young), osteomalacia (adult)
Vitamin K	Hemorrhage (ranging from easy bruising to massive bruising), especially post-traumatic Bleeding
WATER-SOLUBLE VITAMINS	
Vitamin B_1	**Infants:** Dyspnea, cyanosis, diarrhea, vomiting **Adults:** Beriberi (fatigue, peripheral neuritis), Wernicke-Korsakoff syndrome (Apathy, Ataxia, Visual problems)
Vitamin B_2	Angular stomatitis (mouth lesions), dermatitis, photophobia, neurologic changes
Niacin	Pellagra (dermatitis, mucous membrane inflammation, weight loss, disorientation)
Folic acid	Megaloblastic anemia
Vitamin B_{12}	Megaloblastic anemia, neurologic abnormalities
Vitamin C	*First*–Vague aches and pains; ***Long term***–Scurvy (hemorrhages into skin, alimentary and urinary tract, anemia, wound healing delayed)

Ref: Harper 30th Edition Page 555, Handbook of Vitamins 4th Edition Page 253, U Satyanarayana 3rd Edition Page 137, Simmons Principles of Biochemistry 4th Edition Page 515, Prem Prakash Gupta Textbook of Biochemistry with Biomedical Significance Page 513

Ans: (A) Vitamin B_1

3. **Which of the following is not a Dietary fibre?**

A. Inulin
B. Cellulose
C. Pectin
D. Gums

Key:

Gums–Food thickeners *(Alginin, Guar gum, Locust bean gum, Xanthan gum)*
Not normally taken by diet

- All the above given options are fibers
- *Fibers are chemically complex carbohydrates which include cellulose, hemicellulose, pectins, lignin and gums*
- Question is asking about Dietary fibers
- Pectin and Cellulose→ Fruits and Vegetables
- Inulin→ Fruits, Vegetables and Herbs (Wheat, Onion, Banana, Leeks, Artichokes and Aspargus)

FIBERS

- **Soluble**
  - *Pectin*
  - *Gums*
  - *Mucilage*
- **Insoluble**
  - *Cellulose*
  - *Lignin*

DIETARY FIBER

SOLUBLE DIETARY FIBERS — **Fermentable**

- **Viscous**
  - Pectins
  - Beta-glucans
  - Gum
  - Psyllium
  - Glucomannan
- **Non-Viscous**
  - Inulin
  - Fructo-oligosaccharides
  - Resistant dextrins
  - Polydextrose
  - Resistant starch

INSOLUBLE DIETARY FIBERS — **Poorly or Non Fermentable**

- **Non-Viscous**
  - Cellulose, hemicellulose
  - Lignin
  - Resistant starch
  - Resistant protein

- Fibers digestable by Intestinal enzymes include Pectins and Gums
- Recommended daily allowance on an average is 30 gm daily
- Dietary fiber neither digested nor fermented–Lignin
- *High dietary fiber is associated with reduced risk of Diverticulosis, Cancer Colon, CAD and type 2 Diabetes mellitus*
- Digestion of dietary fibers by colonic bacteria gives rise to Small chain fatty acids (Acetate, Propionate and Butyrate).

Biochemical Effects of Fiber

- Prevents constipation
- Eliminates bacterial toxins
- Decreases GI cancers
- Improves glucose tolerance
- Reduces plasma cholesterol
- Satiety value–***Adds significantly to weight of foodstuff ingestion→ Fullness***

- Insoluble and soluble dietary fiber has Beta-1,4 glycosidic linkages that can't be hydrolyzed by amylase
- So they supply no energy, but serve several important functions in the body
- Soluble fiber (Oat bran, Psyllium seeds) has greater cholesterol-lowering effect than insoluble fiber (Wheat bran)
- Beta Glucan from oat bran fosters growth of beneficial bacteria→ ***Prebiotic effect***

Ref: Harper 30th Edition Page 153, U Satyanarayana 3rd Edition Page 509, Rapid Review of Biochemistry 3rd Edition Page 37

Ans: (D) Gums

4. In Wilson disease which of the following is decreased in urine?

A. 3-methylhistidine
B. Serine
C. Phosphotyrosine
D. Phosphorous

Key:

3-Methylhistidine present in normal human urine at a concentration of about 50 mg/dL, is unusually low in the urine of patients with Wilson's disease
Urinary levels of 3-methylhistidine are unusually low in patients with Wilson's disease–HARPER

- 3-Methylhistidine is post-translationally modified amino acid excreted in human urine.
- Urinary concentrations of 3-methylhistidine serve as a reliable index of skeletal muscle protein breakdown in humans who have been subject to muscle injury.
- ***Urinary 3-methylhistidine concentrations are also elevated from consumption of soy-based products and meat, particularly chicken.***

Wilson's Disease

- Autosomal recessive defect (Chromosome 13)
- Defect in Copper metabolism
- Usually occurs in persons <40 years age
- Accumulation of toxic levels of copper in tissues like liver, brain and eye → *Mitochondrial damage*

ATP 7B Mutation (Chr 13) → **Hepatocytes get overloaded with copper** → **Free copper splits out of liver** → **Deposited in other organs Reduced ceruloplasmin Increased free copper and urinary copper**

- Most common CNS feature–Asymmetrical tremor

CLASSIC TRIAD

- **Hepatic disease**
  - ***Acute hepatitis Fulminant hepatitis Chronic active hepatitis Cirrhosis***
- **Neurologic disease**
  - ***Deposits occur in Basal ganglia***
  - ***Asymmetrical tremor–Resting/Intention, Rigidity/Spasticity, Chorea Drooling/Dysphagia/Dysarthria***
- **Ocular disease**
  - **KF Ring**–Copper deposited in descement membrane, Doesn't interfere with vision
  - ***Sunflower cataract***

Other Systems

- *Renal:* Microscopic hematuria, Renal tubular acidosis, Nephrocalcinosis, ***Renal calculi***
- *Genital:* Free copper in intrauterine secretions, Amenorrhea, Recurrent abortions
- *Psychiatric:* Loss of emotional control, Depression, Loss of sexual activity and Hyperactivity.
- ***Coombs –ve hemolytic anemia is seen***
- ***Deiss staging is used for Wilson's disease***

Investigations

- Excessive deposition of copper in liver and brain
- Serum ceruloplasmin is low <20 mg/dL→ (90%)
- Serum copper is low
- Increased Urinary excretion of copper >100 mg/d
- Hepatic copper concentration is high→ ***Standard for diagnosis***
- 24 hours Urine copper level–Screening test
- Haplotype analysis–2 matches++ (Siblings only)
- Penicillamine challenge test–Helps to differentiate with other causes of elevated urinary copper excretion
- ***Best test/Investigation of choice***–Liver Biopsy to estimate copper content (>250 microgram/gm of dry weight)
- **Imaging:** Bilateral basal ganglia thalamic and midbrain hyperintensities

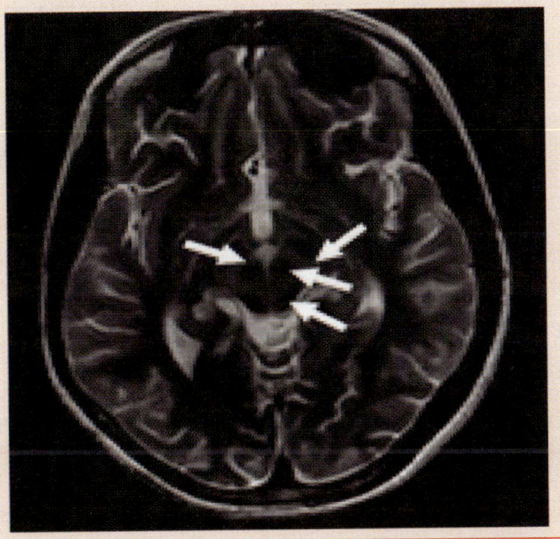
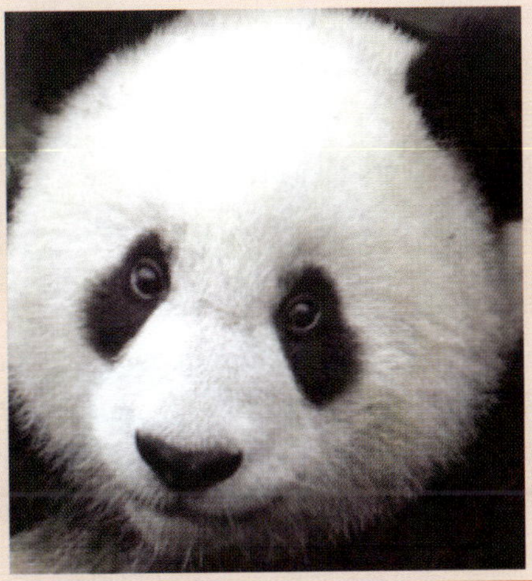

(Face of Panda Appearance)

- **Nazer Prognostic Score**–Used to guide treatment→ *Includes Serum bilirubin/SGOT/PT*

Treatment

- ***Restrict dietary copper***
- **Drug of choice–Zinc acetate** (Presymptomatic/Pediatric/Pregnant/Hepatitis without decompensation and Maintenance)
- **Drug of choice in Wilson's disease with Hepatic decompensation–Trientene**
- **Drug of choice for neurological features in Wilson disease**–Tetrathiomolybdate
- **Hepatic Transplantation**–Fulminant hepatic failure in young patients, Severe hepatic decompensation not responding to chelator therapy, Progressive and Irreversible neurologic dysfunction, Exacerbation of hepatic insufficiency acutely after stopping penicillamine.

Ref: Harper 30th Edition Page 355, Nelson 20th Edition Page 1940, Harrison 20th Edition Page 2318

Ans: (A) 3-methylhistidine

5. **Zellweger disease is due to defect in:**

A. Mitochondria
B. Golgi bodies
C. Endoplasmic reticulum
D. Peroxisomes

Key:

Zellweger's syndrome is a disorder of peroxisomes

PEROXISOMES

- Also known as microbodies.
- Single membrane cellular organelles.
- Spherical or oval in shape and contains enzyme catalase.
- Catalase protects cell from toxic effects of H_2O_2, by converting it to H_2O and O_2
- Peroxisomes are also involved in oxidation of long chain fatty acids (More than C18) and synthesis of plasmalogens and glycolipids.
- Plants contain glyoxysomes (specialized type of peroxisomes involved in glyoxylate pathway).

Peroxisome Biogenesis Disorders	
Zellweger syndrome	Pseudo-neonatal adrenoleukodystrophy
Neonatal adrenoleukodystrophy	Pseudo-Zellweger syndrome
Infantile Refsum disease	Hyperoxaluria type 1
Rhizomelic chondrodysplasia punctata	Acatalasemia, Hyperpipecolic acidemia
Adrenoleukodystrophy	Glutaryl-CoA oxidase deficiency

Zellweger's Syndrome (Hepato-Renal Syndrome)

- ***Most severe type of inherited peroxisomal disease is Zellweger syndrome.***
- ***Absence of peroxisomes*** and its enzymes ***in all tissues is the main pathology***
- Caused by mutations that are usually necessary for proper assembly or functioning of peroxisomes.
- All these events lead to Failure to oxidise long-chain Fatty acids in peroxisomes.
- Abnormal accumulation of Long chain fatty acids and abnormalities in synthesis of bile acids and marked reduction of plasmalogens.
- In its classical form, affected infants present shortly after birth with ***hypotonia, feeding difficulties, seizures and liver dysfunction.***
- ***Typical facial appearance*** (High forehead, Unslanting palpebral fissures, Hypoplastic supraorbital ridges and Epicanthal folds).
- ***Eye abnormalities:*** Cataracts, Glaucoma, Corneal clouding, Brushfield spots, pigmented retinopathy and nerve dysplasia.
- Condition is apparent at birth.
- Characterized by profound neurologic impairment.
- Victims often dying within a year.

Most severe form of peroxisomal disorder–Zellweger syndrome
Least severe form of peroxisomal disorder–Refsum disease
Most common peroxisomal disorder–X linked adrenoleukodystrophy

PEX gene mutation→*Zellweger Syndrome, Neonatal Adrenoleukodystrophy, Infantile Refsum disease*
PEX 7 gene mutationà *Rhizomelic chondrodysplasia*

Ref: Harper 30th Edition Page 241, Lehninger Fundamentals of Biochemistry 4th Edition Page 646, Textbook of Medical Biochemistry 8th Edition Page 414, Simmon's Principles of Medical Biochemistry 4th Edition Page 421, U Satyanarayana 3rd Edition Page 8

Ans: (D) Peroxisomes

6. **Which of the following is not a Ribozyme?**

A. RNase H
B. Ribonuclease
C. Peptidyl transferase
D. Poly A polymerase

Key:

Poly A polymerase is not a Ribozyme–It doesn't possess catalytic activity

Poly A polymerase–Enzyme active in post-transcriptional modification of RNA.

- Approximately 250 adenine nucleotides (AMP) are added to newly created 3′ end by a nuclear enzyme polyadenylate polymerase.

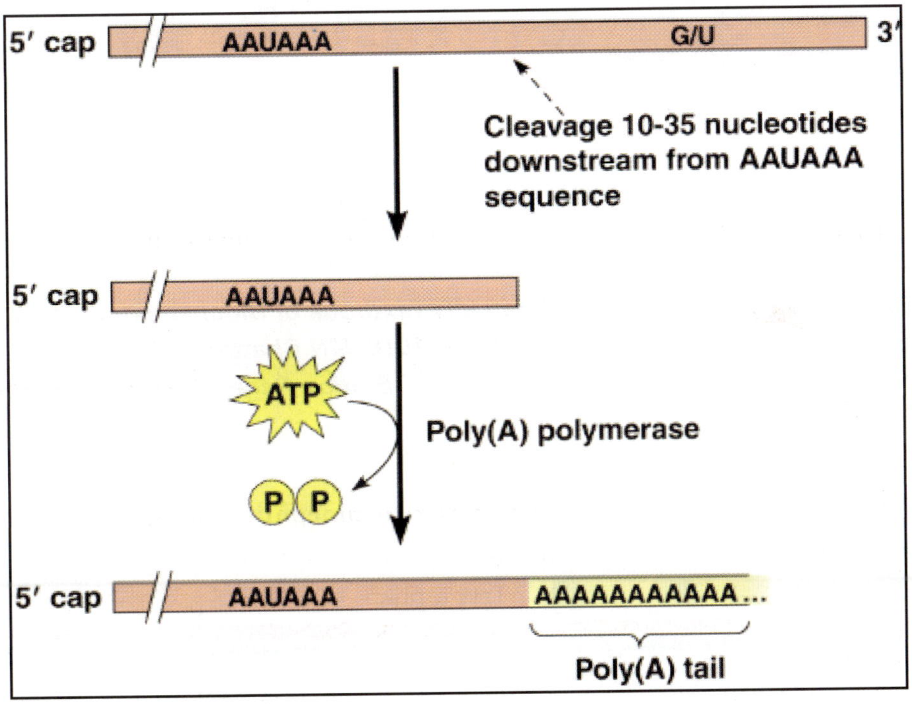

RIBOZYMES

- RNA with Special Enzymatic function ***(RNA with catalytic activity).***
- Ribozymes are involved in cleavage of nucleic acid.
- **Examples:** *SnRNA in Spliceosome, Ribonuclease P, RNase H, Peptidyl transferase*
- Best-characterized ribozymes are the self-splicing group I introns, RNase P, and the hammerhead ribozyme

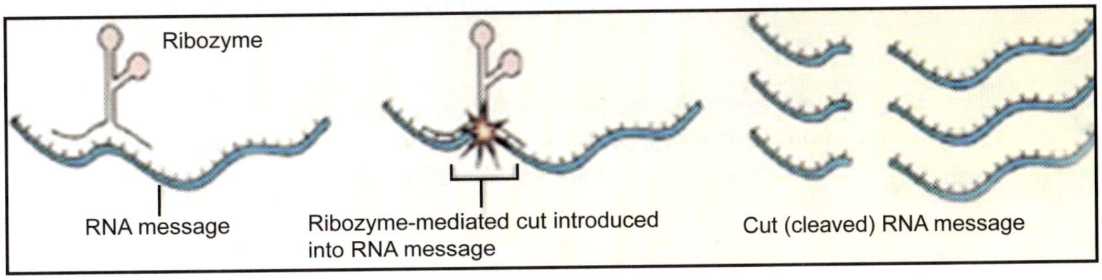

- SnRNA in Spliceosome–***Splicing of exons and Removal of Introns***

- Ribonuclease P–*Cleaves tRNA to generate mature tRNA*
- Enzyme Peptidyltransferase–*Ribozyme and component of 28Sr RNA of 60S Subunit–Forms Peptide bond.*

Role of Ribozyme in Gene Therapy

Ribozyme gene therapy aims to turn off mutated gene in cell by targeting mRNA transcripts copied from gene. This approach prevents production of mutated protein.

- Most often, they act as molecular scissors that cut RNA.
- Ribozyme gene therapy involves the following steps:
    - Delivery of RNA strands engineered to function as ribozymes.
    - Specific binding of the ribozyme RNA to mRNA encoded by the mutated gene.
    - Cleavage of the target mRNA, preventing it from being translated into a protein.

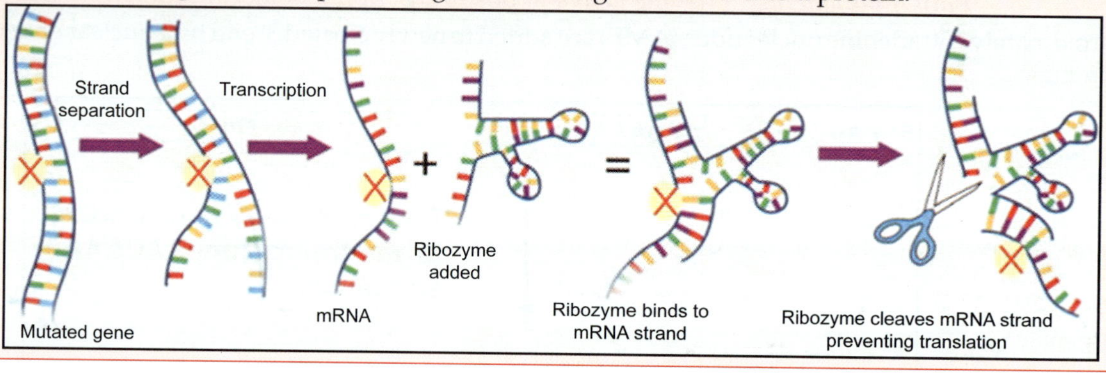

Ref: Harper 30th Edition Page 367, Rafi MD Textbook of Biochemistry 3rd Edition Page 272, Lehninger Fundamentals of Biochemistry 4th Edition Page 1018, MN Chatterjee Textbook of Medical Biochemistry 8th Edition Page 309, U Satyanarayana 3rd Edition Page 82

Ans: (D) Poly A polymerase

7. **Aminoacid required for conversion of Norepinephrine to Epinephrine is:**

A. Methionine
B. Glycine
C. Phenylalanine
D. Tryptophan

Key:

Methionine is a sulfur containing essential aminoacid. It is Glucogenic aminoacid. Participates in Transmethylation, DNA methylation and Polyamine synthesis
Transmethylation of Norepinephrine leads to formation of Epinephrine (By methylation of SAM)

- Methionine is converted to its active form S-adenosylmethionine (SAM).
- It serves as a methyl donor→*Methyl group is donated by SAM.*
- *Adrenal medulla converts Norepinephrine (noradrenaline) to Epinephrine (adrenaline) by methylation.*

Norepinephrine → *S adenosylmethionine is converted to S adenosylhomocysteine by phenylethanolamine N methyl transferase* **Donates methyl group** → **Epinephrine**

Steps of Conversion of Tyrosine to Epinephrine
1. Ring hydroxylation–***Mediated by tyrosine hydroxylase***
2. Decarboxylation–***Mediated by DOPA Decarboxylase***
3. Side chain hydroxylation–***Dopamine beta-hydroxylase***
4. N Methylation–*Phenyl ethanolamine N methyltransferase (Methylation)*

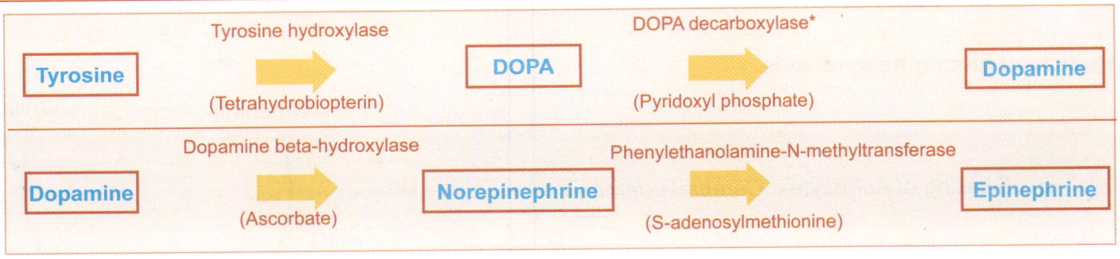

Transmethylation Function of SAM	
Acceptor of methyl group	**Methylated compound**
Norepinephrine	*Epinephrine*
Epinephrine	*Metanephrine*
Guanidioacetate	*Creatine*
Ethanolamine	*Choline*
Carnosine	*Anserine*
Acetyl Serotonin	*Melatonin*

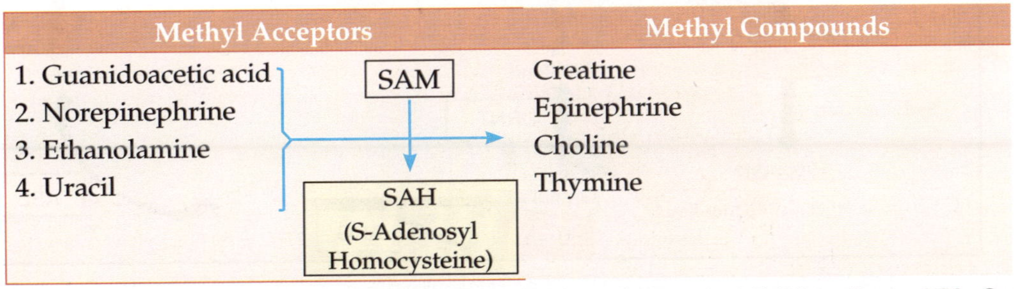

Ref: Harper 30th Edition Page 293, Rafi MD Textbook of Biochemistry 3rd Edition Page 276, Oraby's Illustrated Review of Biochemistry 12th Edition Page 106, Lehninger Principles of Biochemistry 4th Edition Page 674, Simmons Principles of Medical Biochemistry 4th Edition Page 62

Ans: (A) Methionine

8. **Accumulation of glutamine in blood, urine and CSF occurs due to which enzyme deficiency?**

A. OTC
B. ORNT 1 defect
C. Arginosuccinate synthetase
D. Arginase

Key:

In Hyperammonemia type 2, there is deficiency of Ornithine transcarbomylase
Deficiency of OTC leads defect in conversion of Ornithine to Citrulline→Leads to Increased Ammonia and Citrulline in Blood→ Hyperammonemia activates Glutamine synthetase resulting in Glutamine accumulation

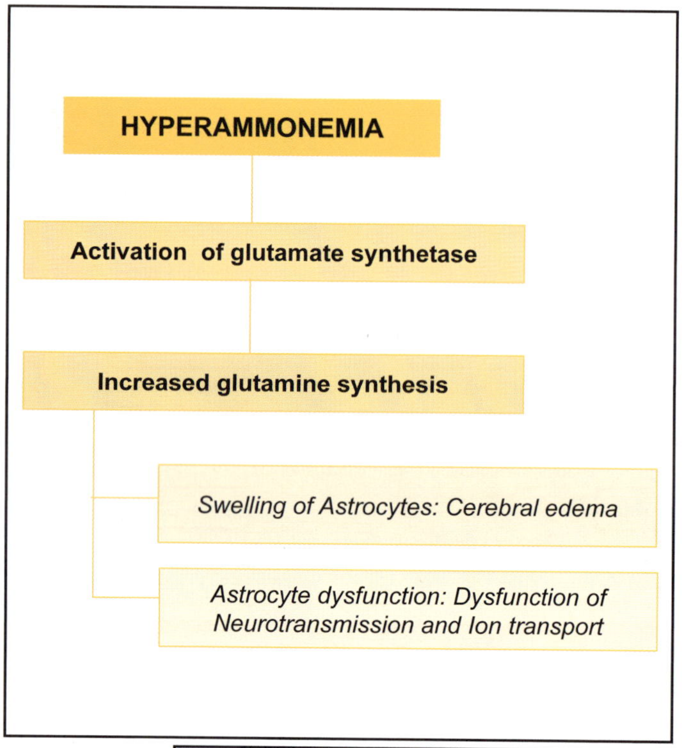

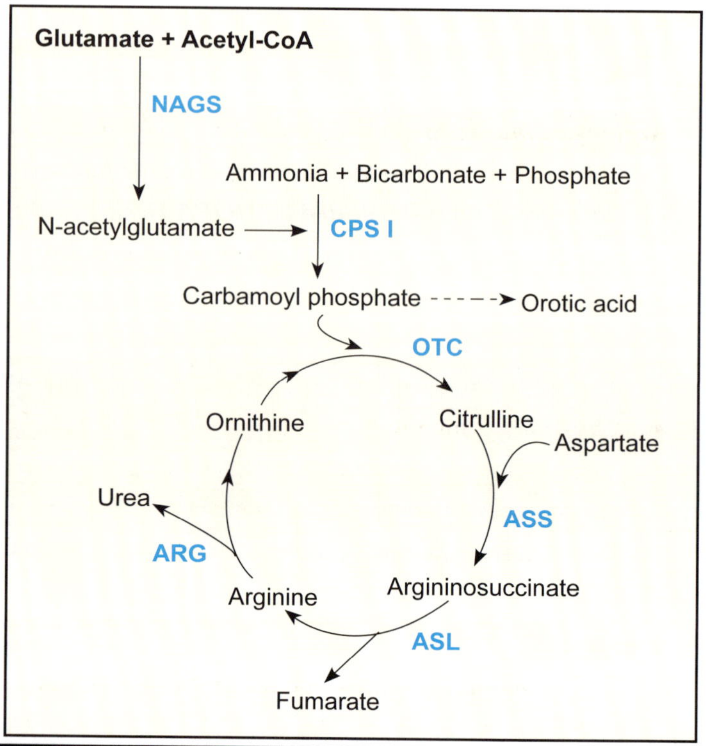

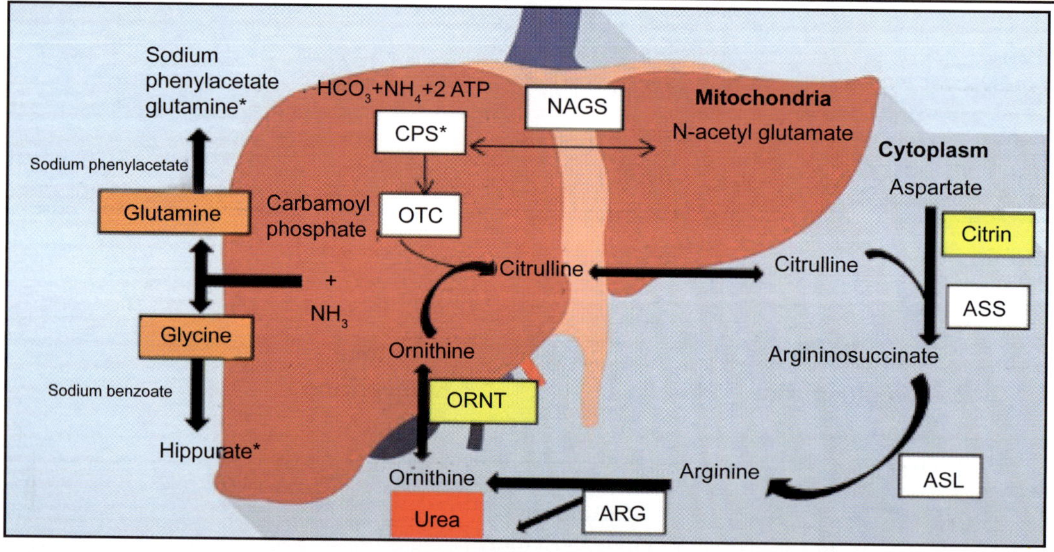

Urea Cycle Disorders				
Disorder	**Inheritance**	**Enzyme Defect**	**Clinical Features**	**Elevated in Urine**
Hyperammonemia Type 1	*Autosomal recessive*	Carbamoyl phosphate synthetase 1	Hyperammonemia–*Lethargy, Convulsions and Early death* **(Neonatal Encephalopathy)**	***Ornithine***
Hyperammonemia Type 2	*X linked recessive*	Ornithine transcarbomylase (OTC)	Blood, Urine and CSF shows increased levels of Glutamine. Increase Blood NH_3 and Ornithine levels **(Neonatal Encephalopathy)**	***Ornithine***

Contd.

Contd.

Citrullinemia Type 1/Classic Citrullinemia	*Autosomal recessive*	Arginosuccinate synthetase	**Neonatal Encephalopathy**	***Citrulline***
Arginosuccinic aciduria	*Autosomal recessive*	Arginosuccinate lyase	**Neonatal Encephalopathy,** Vomitings and Convulsions, Tufted and Friable Hair	***Argininosuccinate***
Hyperarginemia	*Autosomal recessive*	Arginase	Mental retardation	***Lysine, cystine, ornithine and arginine***

Hyperornithinemia (Hyperammonemia Hyperammonemia Hypercitrullinuria/HHH)

- Autosomal recessive disorder
- Ornithine transporter defect
- Encephalopathy and Liver dysfunction
- Elevated Ornithine, Ammonia and Citrulline in blood

Citrullinemia Type 2*–Occurs due to defect in Citrin (Defect in transport of Aspartate and Glutamate)*

Ref: Harper 30th Edition Page 295, Lehninger Principles of Biochemistry 4th Edition Page 669, Simmons Principles of Medical Biochemistry 4th Edition Page 465, Prem Prakash Gupta Textbook of Biochemistry with Biomedical Significance 2nd Edition Page 375

Ans: (A) OTC

9. Amino acid is used for synthesis of both Nitric oxide, Urea and Creatine:

A. Arginine
B. Citrulline
C. Aspartate
D. Glycine

Key:

Arginine is used for synthesis of Urea, Nitric oxide and Creatinine

- Arginine, semiessential/conditionally essential amino acid in humans.
- One of the most metabolically versatile amino acids.
- Serves as a precursor for synthesis of Urea, Nitric oxide, Polyamines, Proline, Glutamate, Creatine and Agmatine.

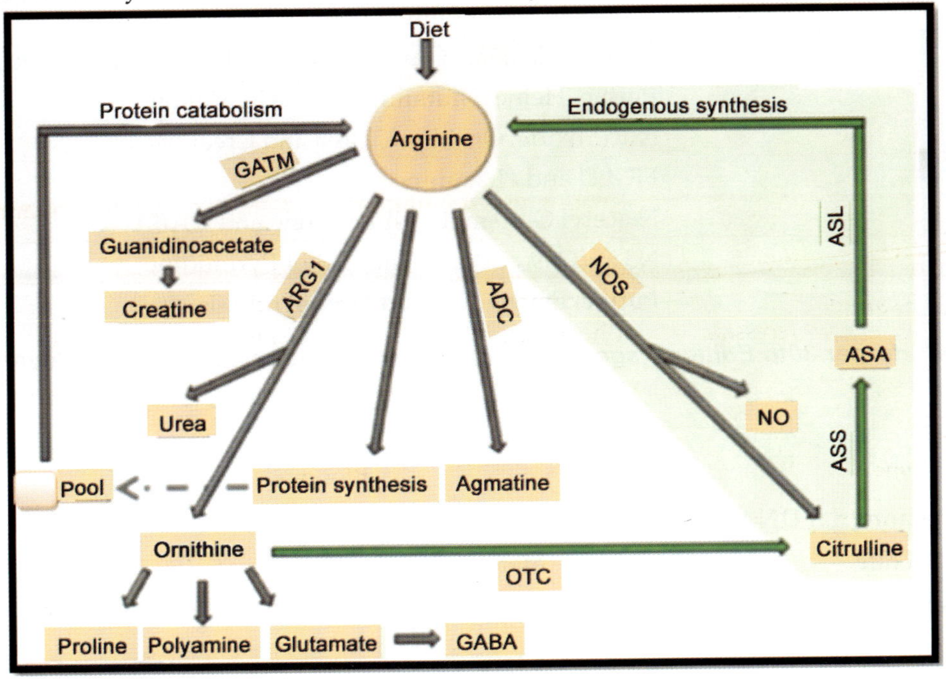

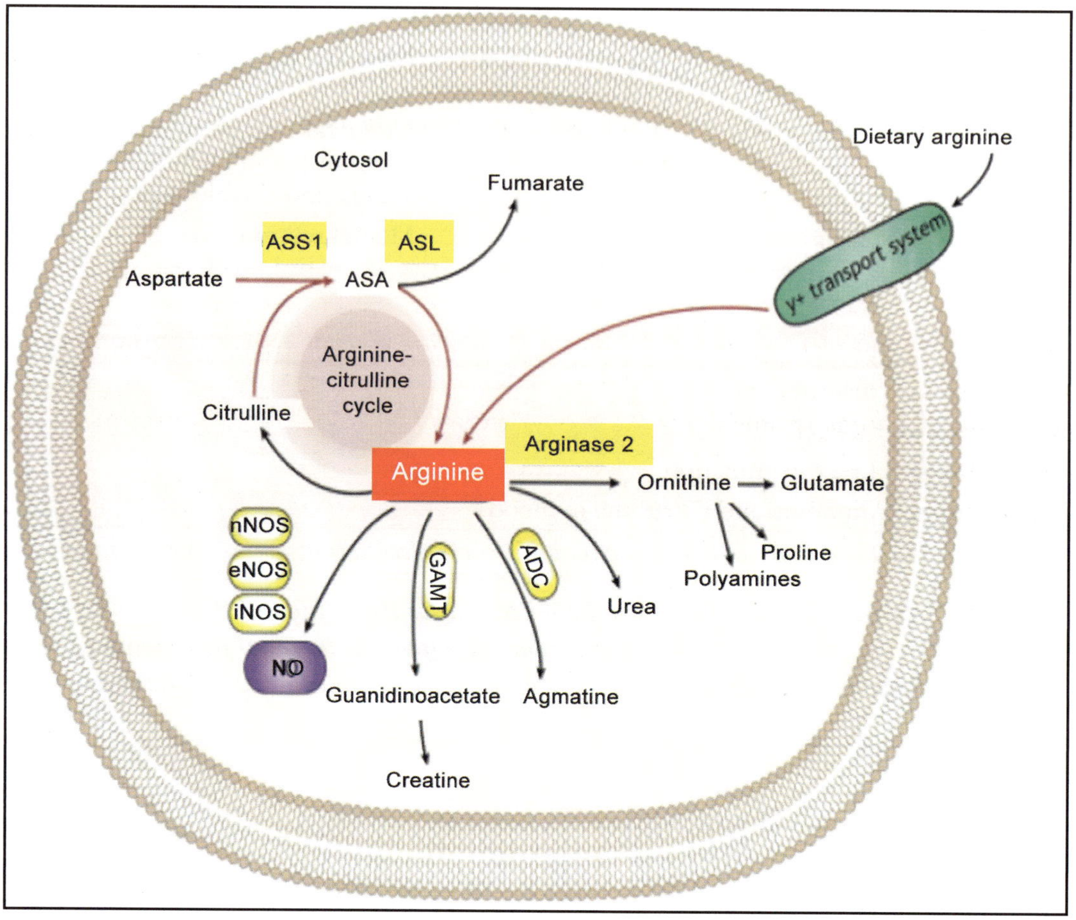

Products of Amino Acid Metabolism	
AA	**Product**
Tyrosine	Melanin, Catecholamines and Thyroxine
Tryptophan	Serotonin, Melatonin and Niacin
Cysteine	Cystine, Taurine, Glutathione and Betamercaptoethanolamine
Glycine	Purine, Heme, Glutathione and Creatinine
Arginine	Nitric oxide, Ornithine, Urea and Creatine
Histidine	FIGLU and Histamine
Glutamate	N acetyl Glutamate, Glutathione and GABA
Glutamine	N3 and N9 of Purine and N3 of Pyrimidine
Aspartate	Purine, Pyrimidine and Urea synthesis

Ref: Harper 30th Edition Page 321, Textbook of Biochemistry DM Vasudevan 7th Edition Page 537, Lehninger Principles of Biochemistry 6th Edition Page 434

Ans: (A) Arginine

10. True about mitochondrial DNA is:

A. Low mutation rate
B. Maternally inherited
C. Linear Double strand
D. All respiratory proteins are synthesized within mitochondria itself

Key:

Mitochondrial DNA transmits by maternal inheritance. It would pass disease to all her children but only her daughters would transmit trait

MITOCHONDRIAL DNA

- Human mitochondria contain 2–10 copies of small circular double standard DNA molecule.
- Mitochondrial DNA is composed of Heavy and Light chains of strands (H and L).
- Contains 16569 Base pairs.
- ***Accounts for approximately 1% of total cellular DNA.***
- Important feature of human mitochondrial DNA→***Contribution entirely by ovum during zygote formation.***
- ***Transmitted by maternal non-mendelian inheritance.***
- Thus in diseases resulting from mutations of mtDNA, an affected mother would pass disease to all her children but only her daughters would transmit trait.
- Encodes 13 polypeptides, 22 transfer RNAs (tRNAs), and the two RNAs (12S and 16S) of mitochondrial ribosomes.
- ***Mitochondrial DNA has a higher mutation rate than nuclear DNA.***
- ***Mitochondrial diseases are caused by mutations in either nuclear/mitochondrial DNA.***
- Mutations in the mitochondrial genome are present either in all copies of mitochondrial DNA (homoplasmy) or only in certain percentage (heteroplasmy).

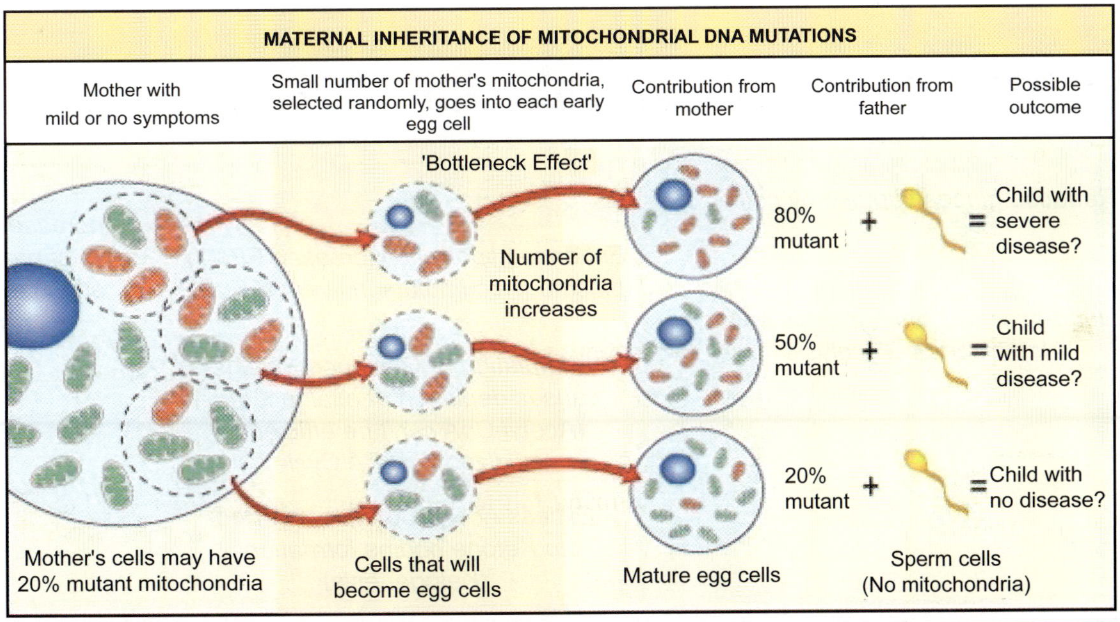

Heteroplasmy for pathogenic mutations is more common than Homoplasmy

Respiratory Proteins Encoded by Mitochondrial Genes in Humans

Complex	Number of subunits	Number of subunits encoded by mitochondrial DNA
I. NADH dehydrogenase	> 43	7
II. Succinate dehydrogenase	4	0
III. Ubiquinone: cytochrome c oxidoreductase	11	1
IV. Cytochrome oxidase	13	3
V. ATP synthase	8	2

- Proteins synthesized in cytoplasm by protein synthesizing apparatus can't pass through mitochondrial membrane.
- Hence for synthesizing proteins of mitochondrial matrix and membrane, there is a 2nd genetic system with DNA and RNA in mitochondrion itself.

Ref: Harper 30th Edition Page 378, MN Chatterjee Textbook of Medical Biochemistry 8th Edition Page 243, Lehninger Principles of Biochemistry 6th Edition Page 719, Simmons Principles of Medical Biochemistry 4th Edition Page 377, U Satyanarayana Textbook of Biochemistry Page 564

Ans: (A) Low mutation rate

11. In Type 1 Diabetes mellitus there is:

A. Decreased Hepatic glucose output
B. Increased glucose uptake
C. Decreased protein catabolism
D. Increased lipolysis

Key:

Diabetes is a state of Insulin deficiency or Insulin resistance
It results in Increased lipolysis

METABOLIC EFFECTS IN TYPE I DM

Autoimmune Etiology (Mainly)

Deranged Carbohydrate Metabolism
- *Reduced glucose uptake by cells*
- *Increased gluconeogenesis and Inhibition of Glycolysis*

Deranged Lipid Metabolism
- *Enhanced lipolysis–increased FFA in plasma (Accumulate in liver-NAFLD)*
- *Stimulation of Gluconeogenesis causes depletion of oxaloacetate (Acetyl CoA can't be efficiently oxidized by TCA Cycle)*
- *Excess Acetyl CoA is converted to Ketone bodies formation (Ketogenesis)*

Deranged Protein Metabolism
- *Increased breakdown of proteins and amino acids (Muscle wasting)*

ABSOLUTE OR RELATIVE INSULIN DEFICIENCY

⇩

Multiple metabolic effects

CHO metabolism
- ↓ Glucose uptake by certain tissues (adipose tissue and muscle)
- ↑ Glycogenolysis
- ↑ Gluconeogenesis

Lipid metabolism
- ↑ Lipolysis
- ↑ Fatty acid oxidation
- ↑ Production of Ketone bodies (in liver)

Protein metabolism
- ↓ Protein synthesis
- ↑ Protein degradation

Inulin
Well fed state-Increases TG synthesis
Starvation-Reduces TG synthesis

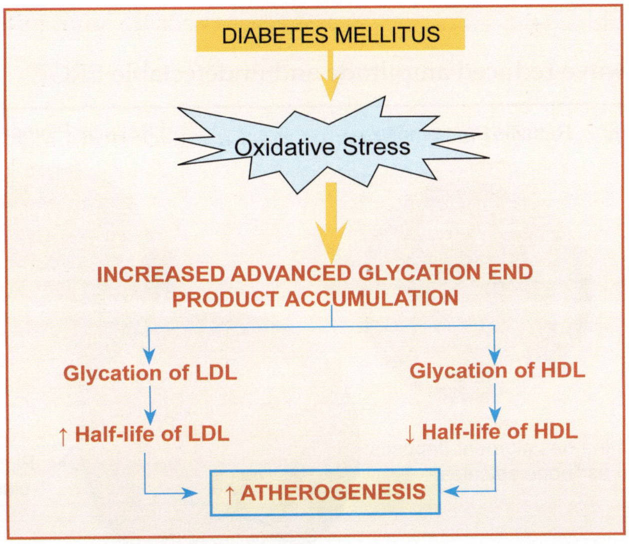

Diabetes	
Substrate	Change
FFA	⇧
Glucose	⇧
TG	⇧
ATP	⇩
Glycolysis	⇩
β-Oxidation	⇧

Ref: Harper 30th Edition Page 149, MN Chatterjee Textbook of Medical Biochemistry 8th Edition Page 583, Lehninger Principles of Biochemistry 6th Edition Page 396

Ans: (D) Increased lipolysis

12. Retinitis pigmentosa is associated with defect in:

A. Docosahexaenoic acid
B. Eicosa pentaenoic acid
C. Arachidonic acid
D. Timnodonic acid

Key:

Low blood levels of Docosahexaenoic acid is reported in patients with Retinitis Pigmentosa

DOCOSAHEXAENOIC ACID (DHA)

- Docosahexaenoic is an omega 3 fatty acid belongs to n-3 family of essential PUFA.
- Accounts for 30-40% of fatty acids in rod photoreceptor outer segments.
- Synthesized from linolenic acid (essential fatty acid) or obtained directly from maternal milk (breast milk) and fish oil.
- ***Primary structural component of human brain, cerebral cortex, skin, sperms and retina.***
- Can't be synthesized by vertebrates and therefore be obtained in diet.
- ***High level of DHA provides an optimal microenvironment for rhodopsin.***

RETINITIS PIGMENTOSA

- Familial disease characterized by degeneration of photoreceptor cells (Rods and Cons)
- Degeneration begins in Equator, Spreads posteriorly and anterior also
- *Invariably Bilateral*
- *Most common symptom–Night blindness*
- Results in progressive night blindness and constriction of peripheral vision (Functional blindness).
- Begins in childhood–Results in blindness in middle and advanced age
- Triad of Retinitis pigmentosa on Ophthalmoscopy → Attenuated blood vessels, Bone corpuscles pigmentation and Yellow waxy disc (Consecutive Optic atrophy)
- Most useful clinical tools in diagnosis–ERG and EOG

- *Gold standard investigation–ERG*
- ERG Findings–b wave prolonged time, b wave reduced amplitude and undetectable ERG

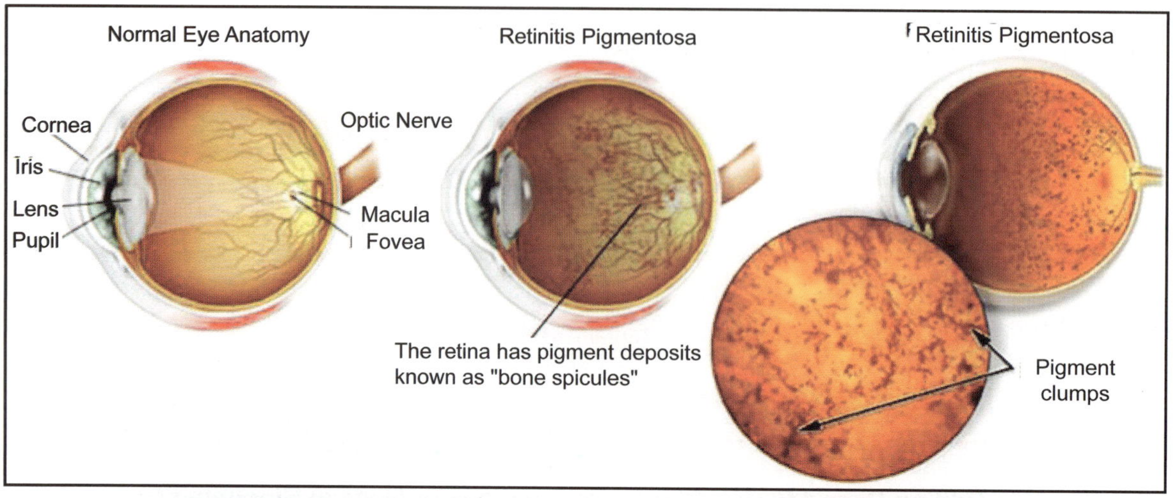

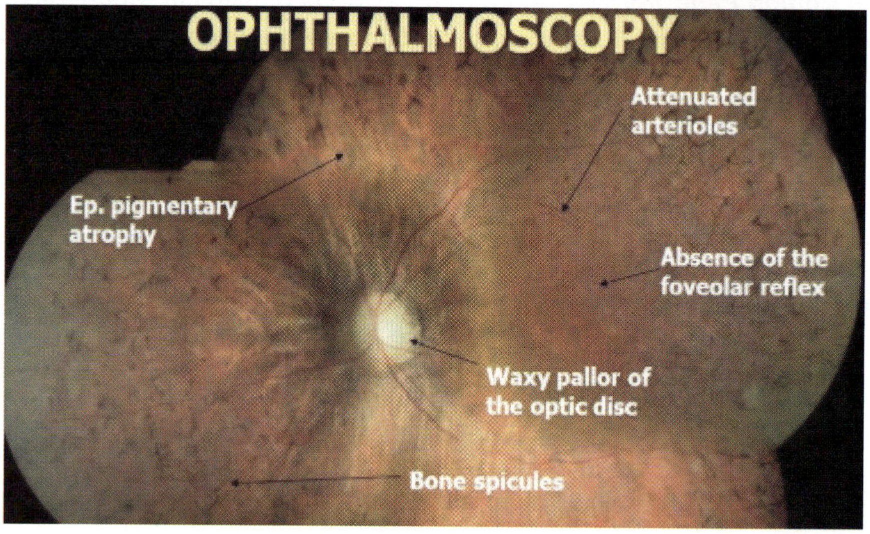

Syndromes Associated Retinitis Pigmentosa	
Laurence Moon Biedl syndrome	Autosomal recessive RP, Polydactyly, Obesity, Hypogonadism and Mental retardation
Friedrich ataxia	RP, Ataxia and Nystagmus
Refsum disease	Autosomal recessive RP, Cerebral ataxia, Deafness and Peripheral neuropathy
Cockayne syndrome	Autosomal recessive RP, Dwarfism, Ataxia, Mental retardation, Premature aging and Flexion contracture of limbs
Kearns Sayre syndrome	RP, Heart block, Chronic progressive external ophthalmoplegia
Usher syndrome	Autosomal recessive RP and Sensorineural deafness
Bassen Kornzweig syndrome	Autosomal recessive Abetalipoproteinemia–RP, Ataxia, Acanthocytosis and Fat malabsorption
Hallgren syndrome	Deafness, Mental retardation and ataxia

ATYPICAL RP

- Retinitis pigmentosa sine pigmento–Without visible pigments
- Retinitis pigmentosa albescens–Hundreds of small white dots
- Pericentric Retinitis pigmentosa–Pigmentary changes around macula
- Sectoral RP

Ref: Harper 30th edition Page 192, Chatterjea 8th Edition Page 49, AK Khurana 6th Edition Page 298, Parson 22nd Edition Page 329, Rayan's Retina 4th Edition Page 211

Ans: (A) Docosahexaenoic acid

13. Not a Source of cytosolic NADPH is:

A. Isocitrate dehydrogenase
B. ATP Citrate lyase
C. Malic enzyme
D. G6PD

Key:

Cytosolic source of NADPH include Isocitrate dehydrogenase, Malic enzyme and G6PD

SOURCES OF CYTOSOLIC NADPH

- Acetyl CoA, formed from pyruvate by pyruvate dehydrogenase.
- Pyruvate dehydrogenase is a mitochondrial enzyme and fatty acid synthesis is a cytosolic pathway.
- Acetyl CoA is made available in the cytosol from citrate synthesized in the mitochondria, transported into the cytosol, and cleaved in a reaction catalyzed by ATP-citrate lyase.
- ***NADPH is required for the energy-yielding metabolisms, but reaction of ATP-citrate lyase is not Energy-yielding reaction.***
- In hepatocytes and adipocytes, cytosolic NADPH is largely generated by the pentose phosphate pathway and by malic enzyme.
- Malate produced in cytosol generates cytosolic NADPH through malic enzyme activity.

G6PD

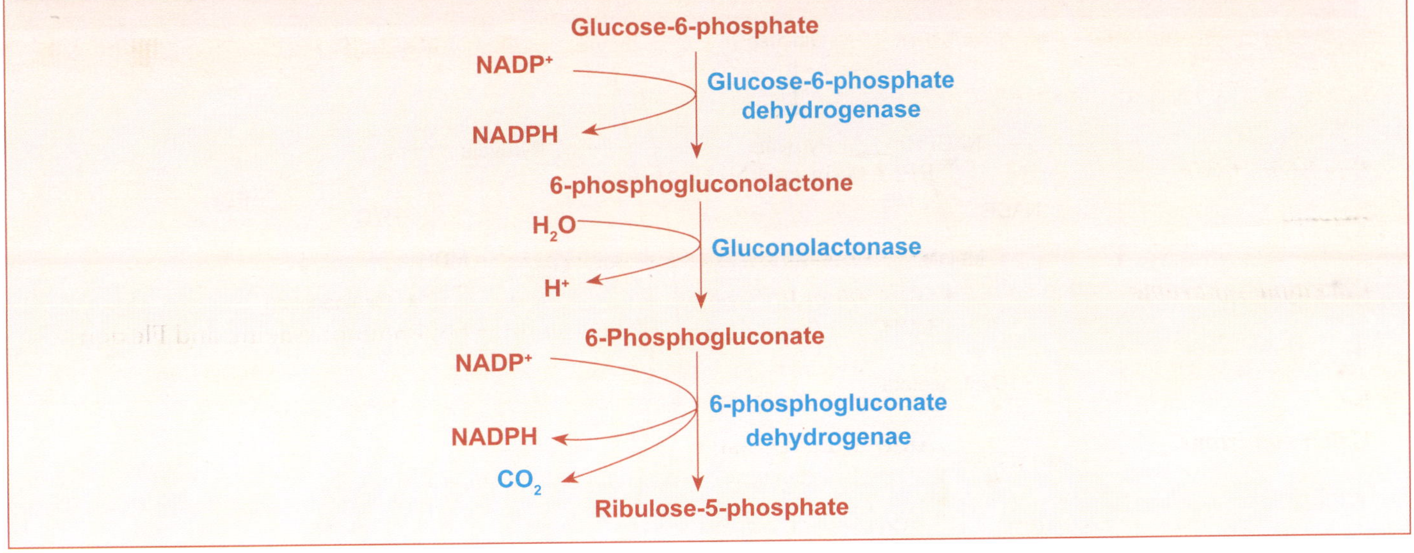

Isocitrate Dehydrogenase

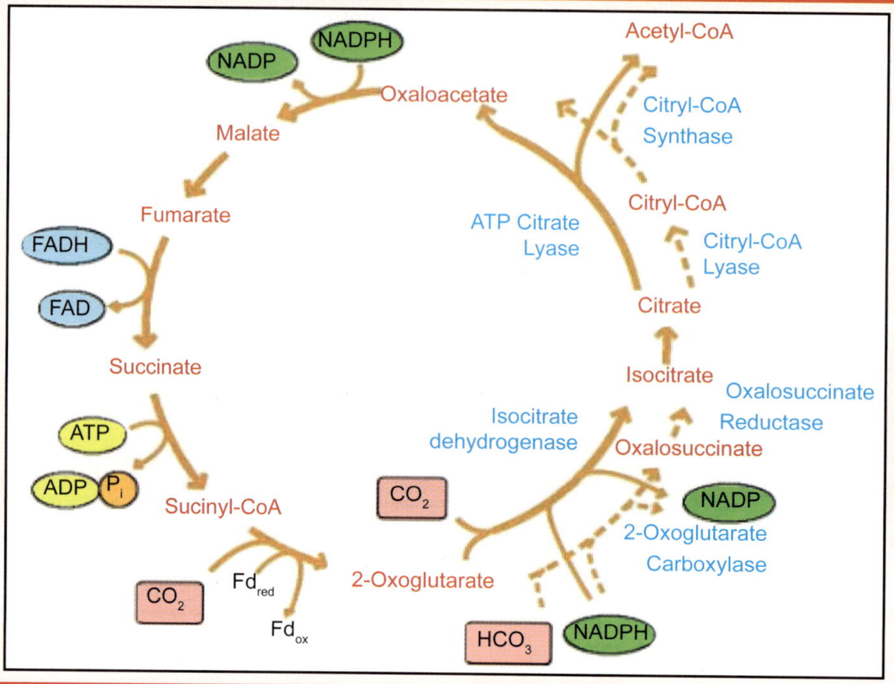

Malic Enzyme

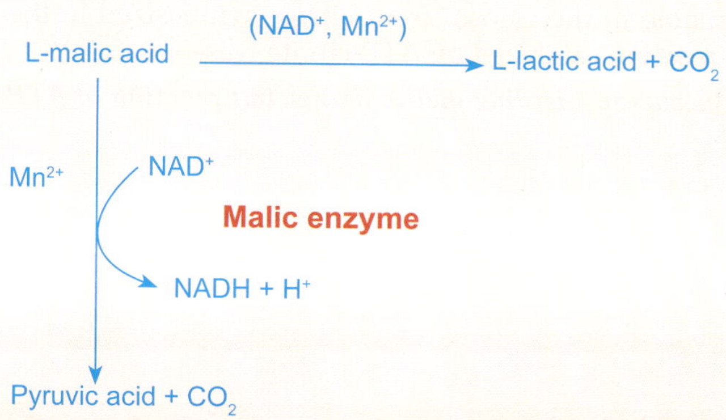

ATP Citrate Lyase

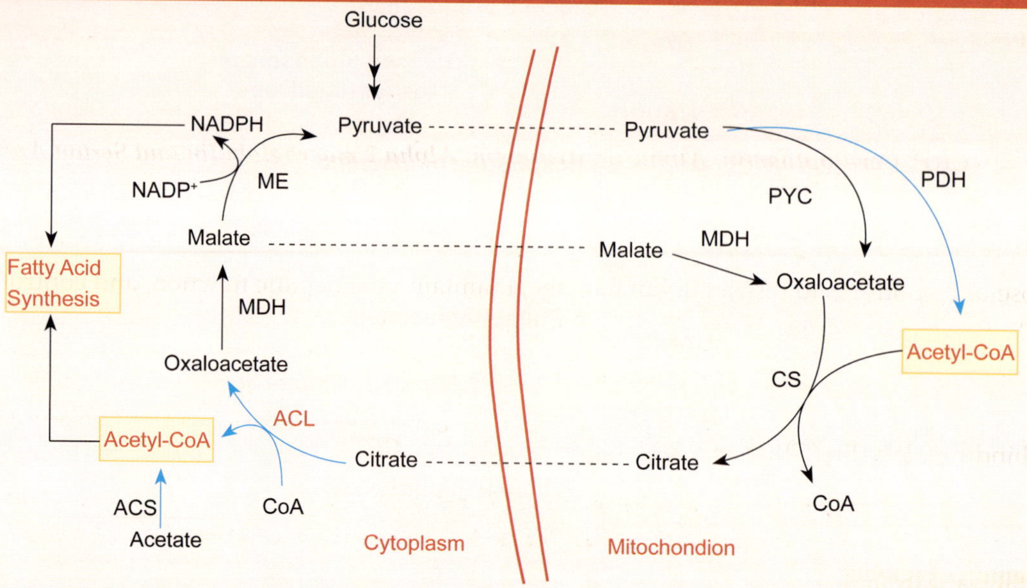

Ref: Harper 30th Edition Page 197, Lehninger Principles of Biochemistry 6th Edition Page 794, MN Chatterjee Textbook of Medical Biochemistry 8th Edition Page 340

Ans: (B) ATP Citrate lyase

14. Which of the following is not synthesized by liver?

A. Plasma protein B. Albumin
C. Acute phase reactants D. Immunoglobulin

Key:

Nearly 70-80% of all plasma proteins are synthesized by Liver Except Immunoglobulins
Immunoglobulins are secreted by plasma cells (Belong to B cells)

IMMUNOGLOBULINS

- Immunoglobulins are γ-globulins.
- Synthesized by plasma cells that belong to B-lymphocytes and participate in humoral immune response against extracellular microbes.
- Concentration of plasma γ-globulins range from 800-1500 mg/dL.

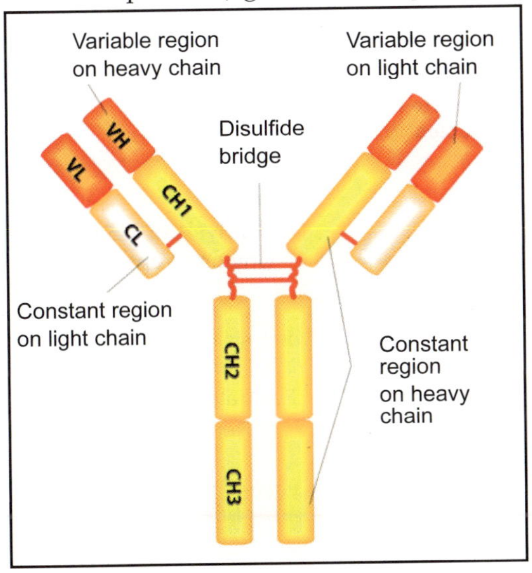

Types and characteristics of antibodies

IgG		• Highest opsonization and neutralization activities • Classified into four subclases (IgG1, IgG2, IgG3 and IgG4).
IgM		• Produced first upon antigen invasion. Increases transiently.
IgA	or / or	• Expressed in mucosal tissues. Forms dimers after secretion.
IgD		• Unknown function.
IgE		• Involved in allergy.

Acute Phase Proteins
(CRP, Ceruloplasmin, Alpha 1 antitrypsin, Alpha 2 macroglobulin and Serum Amyloid A)

- Proteins synthetic response by liver to trauma/infection.
- Proinflammatory cytokines such as IL-1, IL-6 and TNF, induce acute-phase protein gene expression in liver.
- Purpose of response is to restrict organ damage, maintain vital hepatic function, and control defense mechanisms.
- Usually occurs over in 24–48 hours, but if ongoing injury, it can be prolonged.

Examples of Carrier Proteins (Plasma Transport Proteins)
Albumin, Transthyretin, Fibrinogen, Haptoglobin, Hemoglobin A2, Transferrin, Hemopexin, TBG, Transcortin, Cortisol binding globulin (CBG) and Retinol binding protein (RBP).

Ref: Harper 30th Edition Page 670, DM Vasudevan Textbook of Biochemistry, Prem Prakash Gupta Textbook of Biochemistry, MN Chatterjee Textbook of Medical Biochemistry 8th Edition Page 110

Ans: (D) Immunoglobulin

15. **In lipoprotein lipase deficiency what will be found in body after heavy fatty meal?**

A. Lp(a)
B. Chylomicrons
C. HDL
D. LDL

Key:

Lipoprotein lipase (LPL) removes 80% to 90% of chylomicron triglycerides
So deficiency of LPL leads to reduced clearance of Chylomicrons and Increased plasma chylomicrons

- Lipoprotein lipase–Enzyme required for removing fat from chylomicrons and from VLDL.
- *LPL is activated by apoC-II on surface of chylomicron and inhibited by ApoC-III.*
- Deficiency of Lipoprotein lipase causes accumulation of Triglyceride rich chylomicrons in plasma→ *"Type 1 hyperlipoproteinemia/Type 1 hyperlipidemia".*

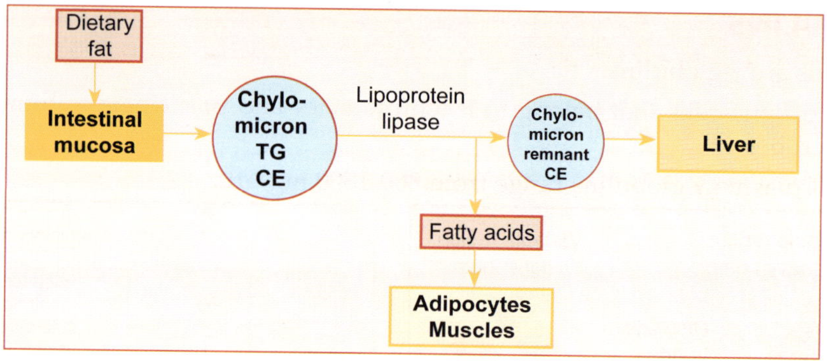

LIPOPROTEIN LIPASE ⇨	**Adipocytes, Striated muscles, Pancreatic Islets & Macrophages** ⇨	Hydrolysis of TG present in Chylomicrons and VLDL
HEPATIC LIPASE ⇨	**Hepatocytes** ⇨	Hydrolysis of TG and phospholipids in VLDL, Remnant particles and HDL Facilitates CE uptake from HDL Removal of Remnants

FAMILIAL HYPERLIPOPROTEINEMIA TYPE 1 (Familial Lipoprotein Lipase Deficiency)

- **Autosomal recessive disorder**
- Results from deficiency of LPL (Lipoprotein Lipase)
- Slow clearance of Chylomicrons and VLDL
- Patient shows eruptive xanthomas, Hepatomegaly and pancreatitis (Abdominal pain present).
- Usually manifests in young age

Lab Diagnosis	
 Creamy layer infranate clear or slightly turbid	 Heavy chylomicron band, Faint β-band pre-β-bands
Refrigeration test	***Electrophoresis test***

- Chylomicron band in fasting plasma is characteristic finding
- Low levels of LDL and HDL
- Raised plasma level of TG (hypertriglyceridemia) upto 1000 mg/dL is seen in patients with type 1 hyperlipidemia
- **Treatment:** Low fat diet

Types of Hyperlipoproteinemia

Type	Name	Cause	Inheritance	Plasma Lipids	Plasma Lipoproteins	Fraction Elevated	Clinical Features	Treatment
I	**Hyperchylomicronemia**	Inherited deficiency of LPL/Apo C2, SLE **(Familial Lipoprotein lipase deficiency)**	*AR*	Raised TG	Chylomicrons ++ Prebetalipoproteins increased, Reduced alpha and beta lipoproteins	***Chylo-microns***	*Early childhood* *Eruptive xanthomas* *Reurrent Abdominal pain*	*Low fat diet*
II	**Hyperbetalipoproteinemia/ Familial Hypercholesterolemia (Defective LDL Receptor)**	**Primary:** Familial hypercholesterolemia **Secondary:** Obesity, Poor dietary habits, Hypothyroidism, DM and Nephrotic syndrome	*AD*	Raised TG and Total Cholesterol	Raised LDL Occasionally Raised VLDL	LDL	Associated with Tendinous and Tuberous Xanthomas Premature cardiovascular disease and Atherosclerosis	Reduced Dietary cholesterol and Saturated fats
III	**Dysbetalipoproteinemia/Broad Beta disease/Remnant-Remnant disease**	Homozygosity of Apo E2 (Doesn't bind to Hepatic Apo E receptors), Combined with poor dietary habits	*AD*	Raised TG and Cholesterol	Raised VLDL, LDL and IDL Increased synthesis of Apo E and Apo B	Chylo-micron remnants, VLDL	Associated with Tuberous & Palmar Xanthomas Premature cardiovascular disease and Peripheral vascular disease	Weight reduction, Low carbohydrate diet
IV	**Hypertriglyceridemia/ Hyper prebetalipoproteinemia (FHTG)**	DM, Obesity, Alcoholism, Poor dietary habits	*AD*	Raised TG and Cholesterol	VLDL, Alpha and Beta lipoproteins subnormal	VLDL	Present in early adulthood Increased synthesis of Lipids from carbohydrates	Low cholesterol diet, Hypolipidemic drugs, Replace carbohydrate with Unstaurated fats
V	**Combined Hyperlipidaemia**	Obesity, DM, Alcoholism and OCP	*AD*	Raised TG and Chylo-microns	VLDL & Chylomicrons, Alpha and Beta lipoproteins Raised	Chylo-microns, VLDL	Xanthomas present Abnormal Glucose Tolerance	Weight reduction Diet change

Ref: Harper 30th Edition Page 275, MN Chatterjee Textbook of Medical Biochemistry 8th Edition Page 454, U Satyanarayana 3rd Edition Page 321, Prem Prakash Gupta Textbook of Biochemistry with Biomedical Significance 2nd Edition Page 162, Simmons Textbook of Medical Biochemistry 4th Edition Page 452

Ans: (B) Chylomicrons

16. Hyperammonia causes depletion of which of the following in TCA cycle?

A. Oxaloacetate
B. Alpha ketoglutarate
C. Fumarate
D. Malate

Key:

Ammonia Reacts with Alpha ketoglutarate to form Glutamate
This results in depletion of Alpha ketoglutarate levels impairing TCA cycle function in neurons

TCA CYCLE/CITRIC ACID CYCLE/KREB CYCLE

- Ammonia is produced as a result of various metabolic activities.
- It has to be detoxified immediately or else can prove toxic to brain cells and other tissues.
- ***Elevated concentration of ammonia increases amination of α-ketoglutarate by glutamate dehydrogenase (GDH) forming glutamate in brain.***
- This causes depletion of α-ketoglutarate, an intermediate of TCA cycle, in brain.
- Impairs operation of TCA cycle in neurons resulting in decreased ATP production.
- *Leads to coma since normal ATP production is required to maintain normal brain function.*

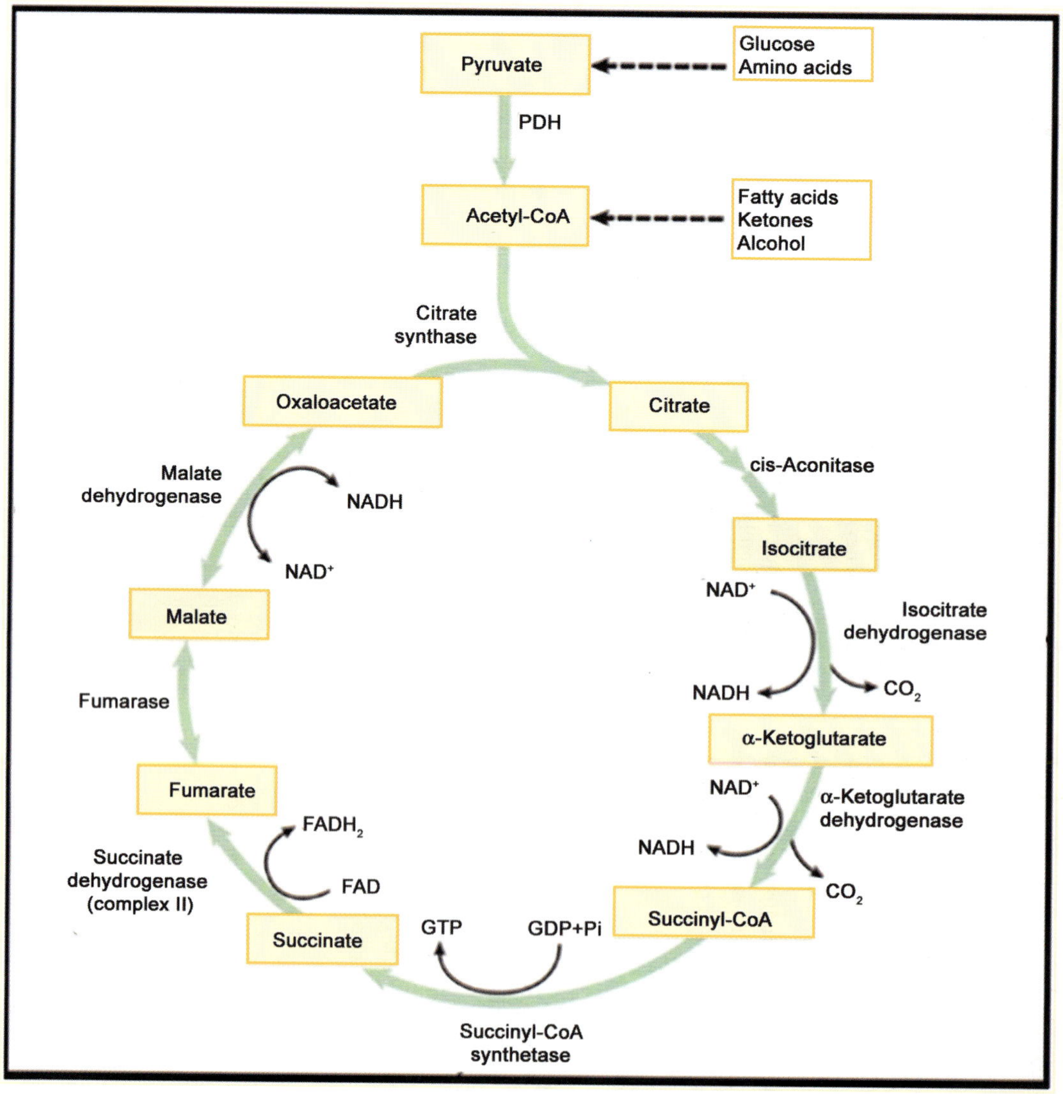

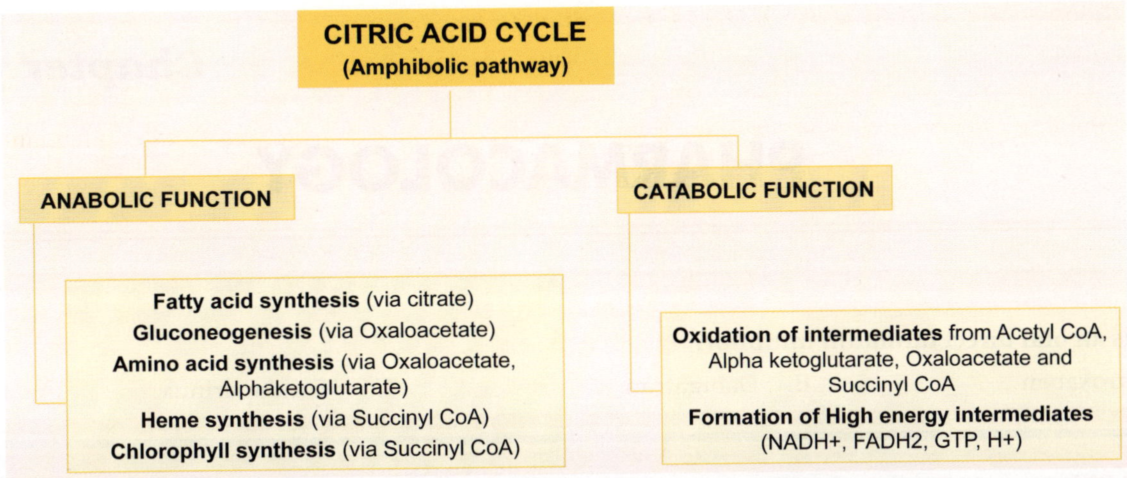

Inhibitors of Tca Cycle	
Aconitase	Inhibits Fluoroacetate
Arsenite	Inhibits Alpha ketoglutarate dehydrogenase
Malonate	Inhibits Succinate dehydrogenase
Long chain Acyl CoA and ATP	Inhibits Citrate synthase
ATP and NADH	Inhibits Isocitrate dehydrogenase
Oxaloacetate	Inhibits Succinate dehydrogenase

Ref: Harper 30th Edition Page 168, Lehninger Principles of Biochemistry 6th Edition Page 620, Prem Prakash Gupta Textbook of Biochemistry with Biomedical Significance 2nd Edition Page 211, MN Chatterjee Textbook of Medical Biochemistry 8th Edition Page 342

Ans: (B) Alpha ketoglutarate

Chapter 4

PHARMACOLOGY

1. Which is an oral direct thrombin inhibitor?

A. Rivaroxaban B. Dabigatran C. Fondaparinux D. Bivalrudin

Key:

Dabigatran is a Oral direct thrombin inhibitor that doesn't requires monitoring

Schematic Solution		
Option A	Rivaroxaban	Oral factor Xa inhibitor
Option B	Dabigatran	Oral direct thrombin inhibitor
Option C	Fondaparinux	Parenteral factor Xa inhibitor
Option D	Bivalrudin	Parenteral direct thrombin inhibitor

Mechanism of Action

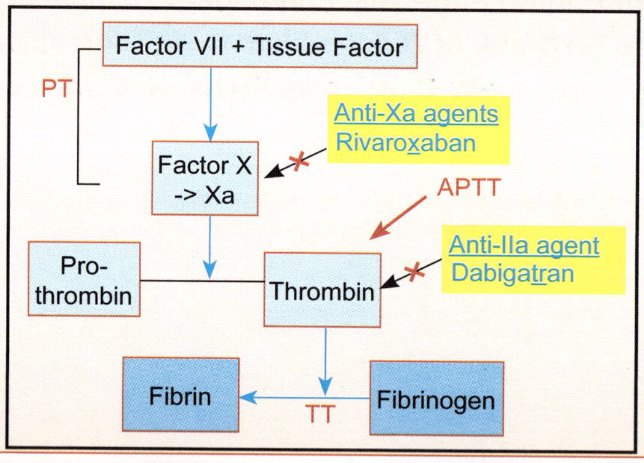

Anticoagulants

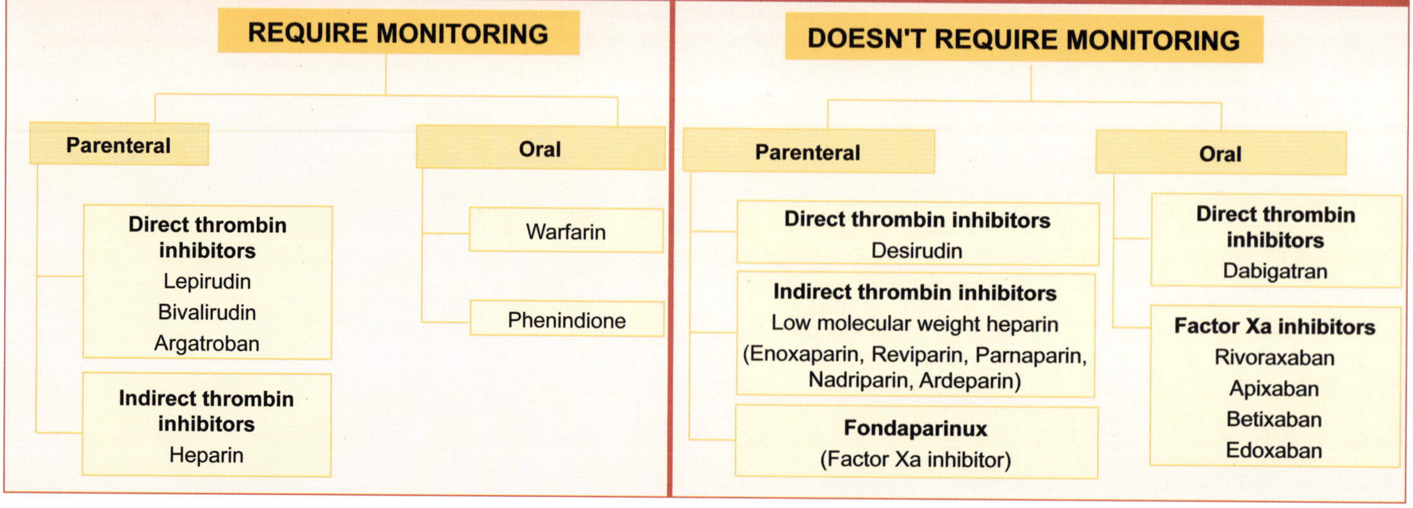

Ref: Katzung 13th Edition Page 593, Harrison 20th Edition Page 775, Goodman and Gilman 13th Edition Page 589, KDT 8th Edition Page 603

Ans: (B) Dabigatran

2. Tolvaptan is used for:

A. Central DI
B. SIADH
C. von Willebrand's disease
D. Catecholamine resistant shock

Key:

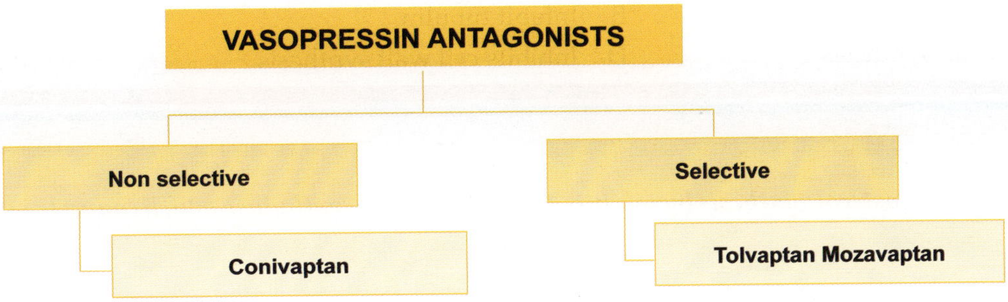

TOLVAPATAN

- Orally Active Nonpeptide Vasopressin V2 receptor antagonist.
- Half life–12 to 24 hours.
- Tolvaptan is a substrate and inhibitor of P-glycoprotein and is eliminated entirely by CYP3A4 metabolism.
- ***Drug of choice for treatment of Euvolemic hyponatremia (SIADH).***
- *Used for correction of water retention and hyponatremia in SIADH as well as advanced CHF and Liver cirrhosis.*
- Tolvaptan has afforded short-term improvement by increasing water excretion, restoring serum Na^+ and relieving dyspnoea.
- ***Tolvaptan can cause hypotension.***
- ***Tolvaptan should not be used in patients with liver disease***→ Can cause liver damage therefore tolvaptan administration generally should be limited to 30 days.
- Both tolvaptan and conivaptan can induce headaches, hypokalemia and hyperglycemia and both are contraindicated in anuria (no benefit) and in patients receiving drugs that inhibit CYP3A4 (clarithromycin, ketoconazole).

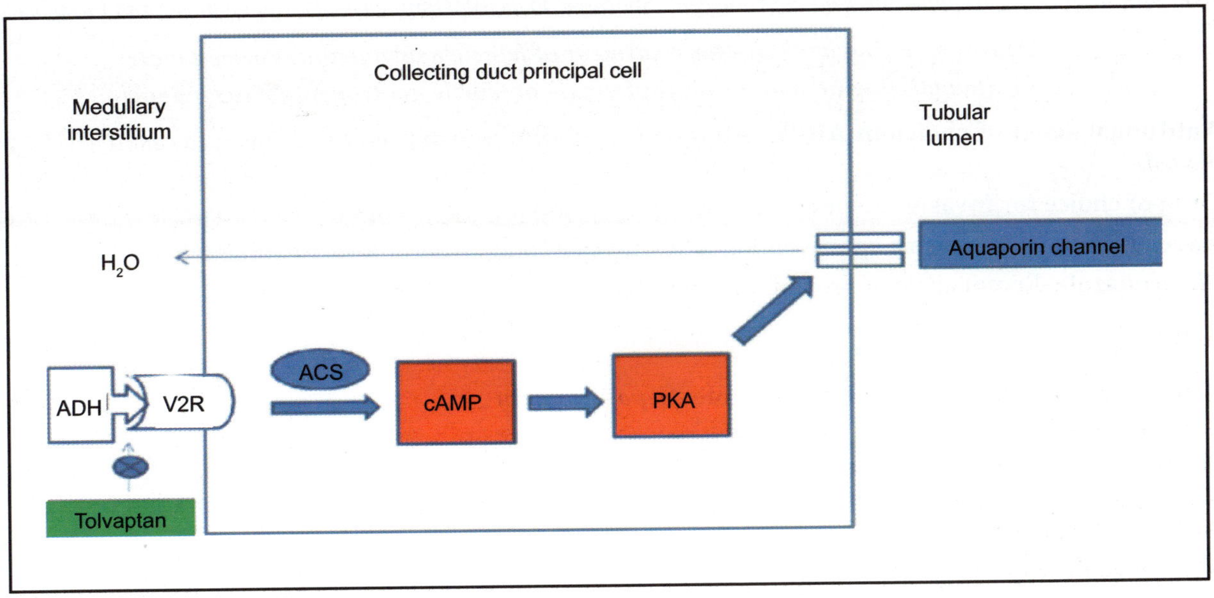

Conivaptan→ Used by intravenous route for short term management in admitted patients
Tolvaptan and Mozavaptan→ Used by oral route for long term management
Relcovaptan→ Selective V1 receptor antagonist→ Dysmenorrhea, Raynaud's disease and Tocolysis
Nelivaptan→ Selective V1b (V3) receptor antagonist→ Anxiolytic
Satavaptan and Lixivaptan→ Selective V2 antagonist approved by FDA for hyponatremia

Ref: Goodman and Gilman 13th Edition Page 468, KDT 7th Edition Page 569, Katzung 12th Edition Page 265

Ans: (B) SIADH

3. **Mechanism of action of triazoles is:**
   A. Inhibit ergosterol synthesis
   B. Inhibit tubulin
   C. Inhibits glucan synthesis
   D. Inhibits cell wall synthesis

Key:

Triazoles inhibits Ergosterol synthesis by inhibits 14 alpha sterol demethylase which converts lanosterol to ergosterol

Azoles

Mechanism of Action

- Inhibit Ergosterol synthesis by inhibiting 14 alpha sterol demethylase

Classification

- Imidazoles–Ketoconazole and Clotrimoxazole (High sterol synthesis blocking effect)
- Triazoles–Fluconazole, Itraconazole, Posaconazole, Voriconazole and Isavuconazole

Spectrum

- **Ketoconazole–***Narrow antifungal spectrum, Inhibits Cytochrome P450 and increases concentration of Warfarin, theophylline and Cyclosporine.*
- **Fluconazole–***Drug of choice for treatment of Candidiasis and Coccidiodal meningitis. Maximum oral bioavailability and CNS penetration among this group*
- **Itraconazole–***Drug of chioice for Endemic mycoses, Sporotrichosis, Blastomycosis, Histoplasmosis and Paracoccidiomycosis*

Antifungal drug of choice for treatment of febrile neutropenia–Voriconazole
Antifungal drug of choice for prophylaxis of febrile neutropenia–Fluconazole

- **Antifungal agent of choice in ABPA (Allergic bronchopulmonary aspergillosis)–***Itraconazole (Drug of choice–Steroid)*
- **Drug of choice for Invasive Aspergillosis, Scedosporium and Trichosporon–***Voriconazole (Widest spectrum)*
- **Isavuconazole**–Recent azole approved for Mucormycosis and Aspergillosis treatment
- **Efinaconazole**–Recent azole approved for fungal toe nail infection treatment

Side Effects

- **Itraconazole, Fluconazole and Voriconazole–*Hepatotoxicity***
- **Itraconazole–***CHF, Hypokalemia and Edema*
- **Fluconazole–***Alopecia*
- **Voriconazole–***QT prolongation, Visual disturbances, Peripheral neuropathy, Periostitis due to fluoride excess, Skin cancer (SCC) and Hallucinations*
- **Ketoconazole–***Antiadrogenic action→ Gynecomastia*

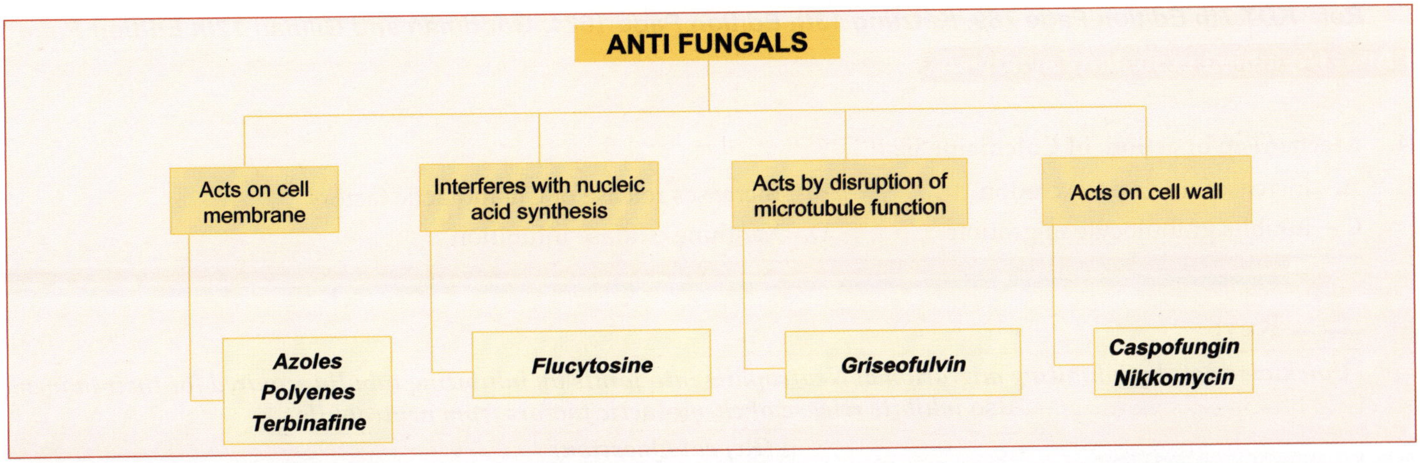

Terbinafine

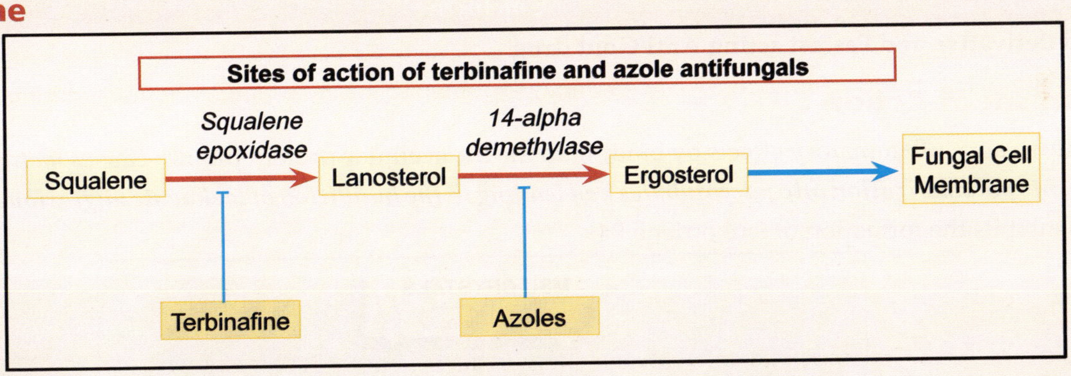

Echinocandins

Inhibits the synthesis of β-1, 3-glucan, which is a unique component of fungal cell wall.

Flucytosine

Competitive inhibitor of thymidylate synthesis

Interferes with DNA and RNA synthesis

Griseofulvin

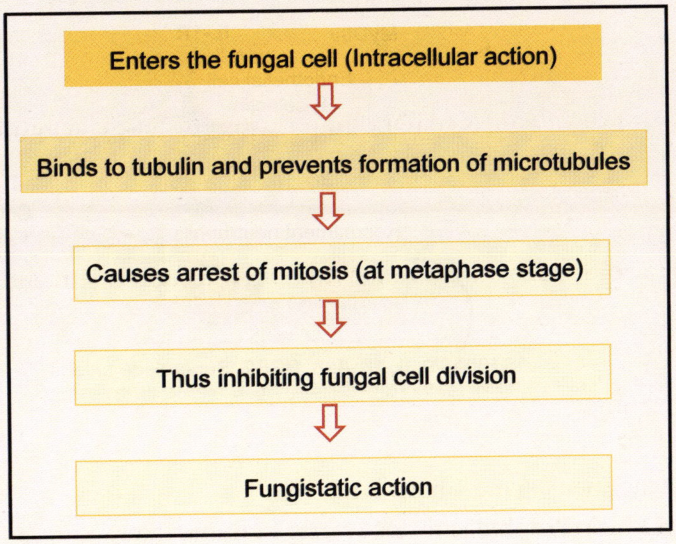

Ref: ***KDT 7th Edition Page 789, Katzung 13th Edition Page 1624, Goodman and Gilman 12th Edition Page 1573***

Ans: (A) Inhibit ergosterol synthesis

4. **Mechanism of action of Colchicine is:**

A. Increases uric acid excretion
B. Increases release of Chemotactic factors
C. Inhibits granulocyte migration
D. Xanthine oxidase inhibition

Key:

Colchicine acts by inhibiting migration of Neutrophils into joints by inhibiting tubulin required for their movement. Also inhibits release of chemotactic factors from neutrophils

(Repeat Question)

Colchicine

Alkaloid derivative and Fastest acting Anti Gout drug

Mechanism of Action

- Produces anti-inflammatory effects by binding to the intracellular protein tubulin causes *metaphase arrest.*
- ***Prevents polymerization into microtubules and leading to the inhibition of leukocyte migration and phagocytosis.***
- Also inhibits the formation of leukotriene B4.

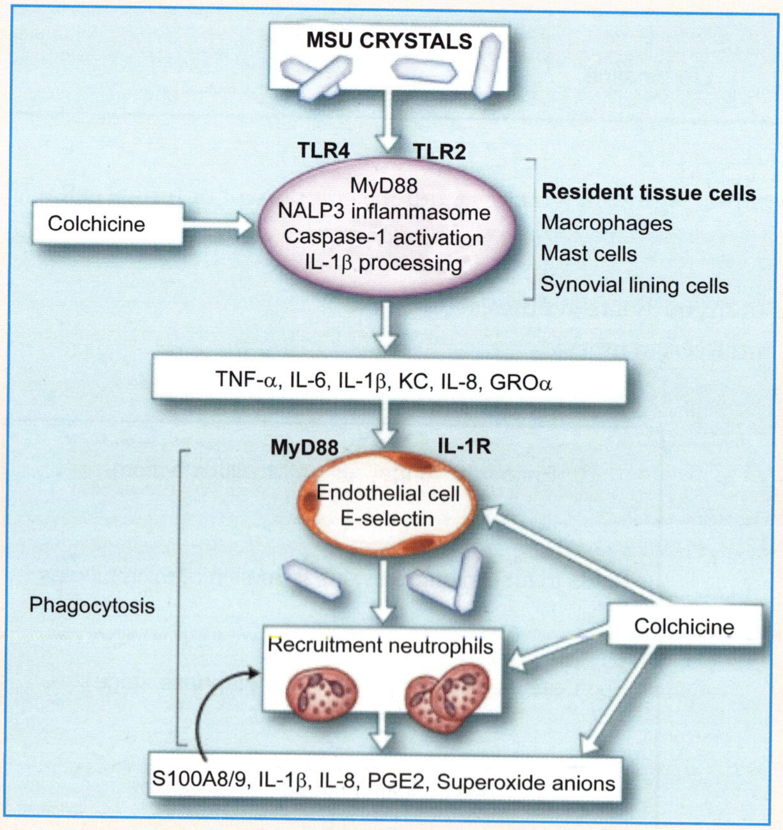

Dose

- Acute Gout attack–1.2 mg then 0.6 mg 1 hour later
- Prophylaxis–0.6 mg QD-BID (Prophylactic dose starts 12 hours later)

Contd.

Contd.

Adverse Effects: ***Most common and dose limiting toxicity is diarrhea (80% patients)***

Advantages of I.V. Administration

- Reduces the risk of GI disturbances
- Provides faster relief (6–12 hours)

Disadvantages of I.V. Administration

- Increases risk of sloughing of skin and subcutaneous tissue.
- Higher doses may (rarely) result in liver damage and blood dyscrasias.
- No direct effect as an analgesic or no effect on metabolism of urate crystals.

Daily Colchicine is Indicated

- To prevent further attacks
- Along with urate lowering therapy to suppress attacks precipitated by abrupt changes in serum uric acid

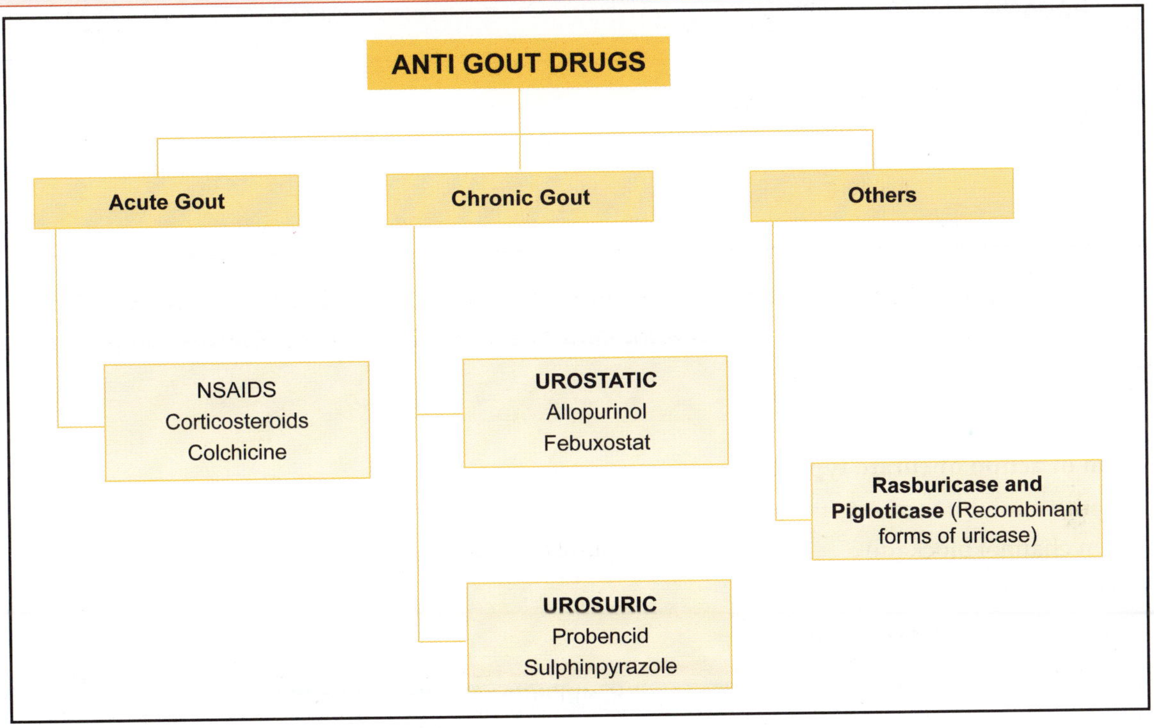

- *Drug of choice in Acute Gout–**NSAIDS (except aspirin)***
- *Drug of choice for refractory Acute Gout–**Colchicine***
- *Drug of choice for Chronic Gout–**Allopurinol***
- *Drug of choice for Chronic Gout in patients allergic to allopurinol–**Febuxostat***

(See Flowchart on the next page)

EXTRA EDGE

Colchicine is now used between attacks for prolonged prophylaxis (at low doses)–"Intercritical period"

Effective in preventing attacks of acute Mediterranean fever and may have a mild beneficial effect in sarcoid arthritis and in hepatic cirrhosis.

Colchicine treated neutrophils show a characteristic Drunken walk

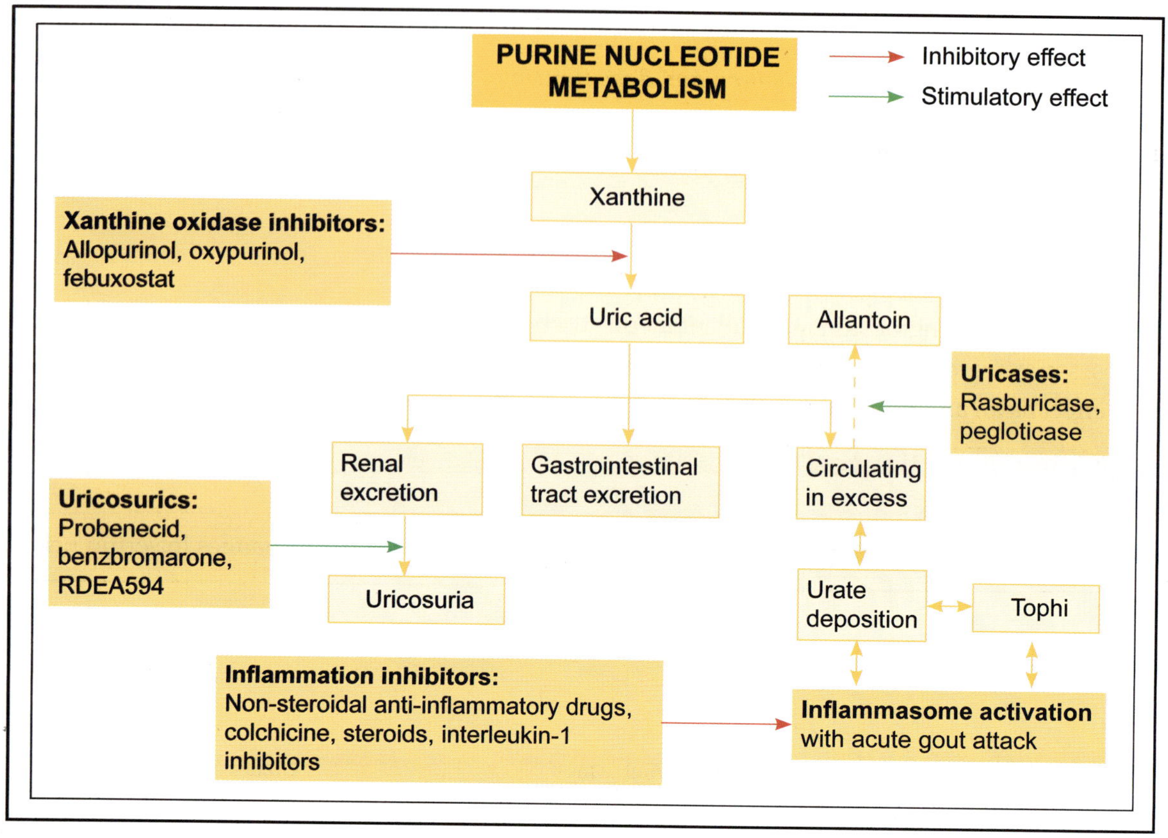

Ref: KDT 7th Edition Page 214, Katzung 14th Edition Page 660, Goodman and Gilman 13th Edition Page 702, Sharma and Sharma Principles of Pharmacology 3rd Edition Page 381

Ans: (C) Inhibits granulocyte migration

5. **Mechanism of action of curare type drugs is:**
   A. Competitive inhibitor of Acetylcholine receptors
   B. Calcium channel blockade
   C. Persistent depolarization of receptors
   D. Blocking release of Acetylcholine

Key:

Tubocurarine–Non depolarizing agent and Competitive antagonist of acetylcholine receptor

D-Tubocurarine

- Competitive antagonist of acetylcholine receptor acts as Non depolarizing agent

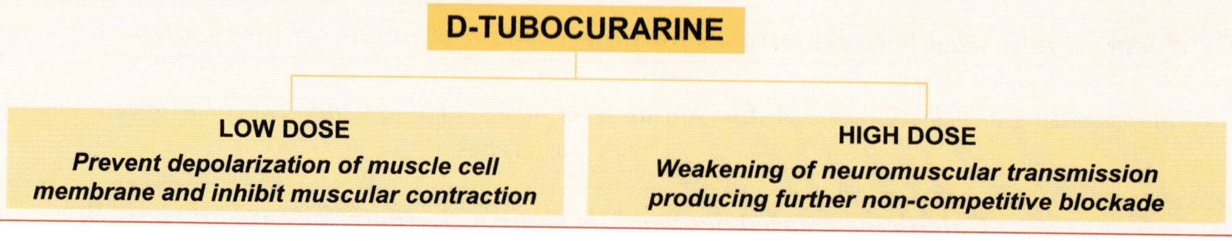

Contd.

Contd.

- Tubocurarine has prominent histamine releasing, ganglion blocking and cardiovascular actions as well as long duration of paralysis needing pharmacological reversal.
- During anesthesia, administration of tubocurarine, 0.1–0.4 mg/kg IV, initially causes motor weakness, followed by skeletal muscles becoming flaccid and inexcitable to electrical stimulation.
- Larger muscles (abdominal, trunk, paraspinous, diaphragm) are more resistant to NM blockade and recover more rapidly than smaller muscles (e.g., facial, foot, hand).
- Diaphragm is usually the last muscle to be paralyzed.
- When administration of muscle relaxants is discontinued, recovery of muscles usually occurs in reverse order, with the diaphragm regaining function first.

MECHANISM OF ACTION OF NON DEPOLARIZING AGENTS

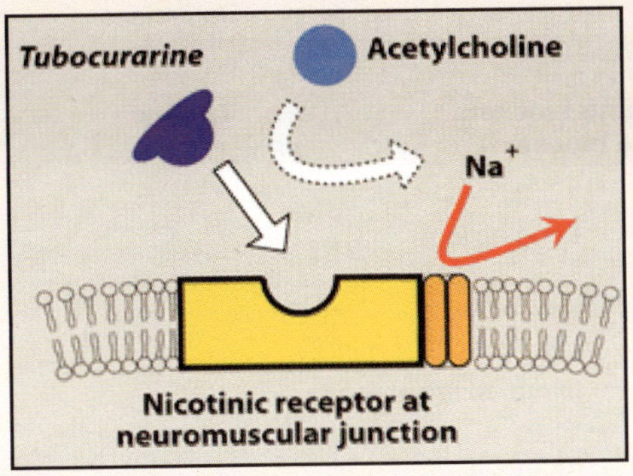

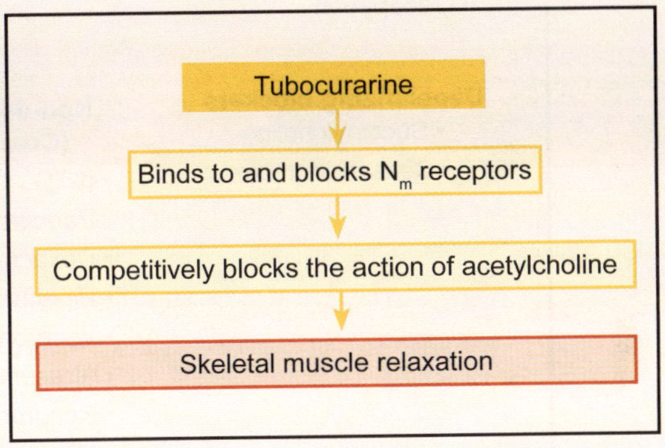

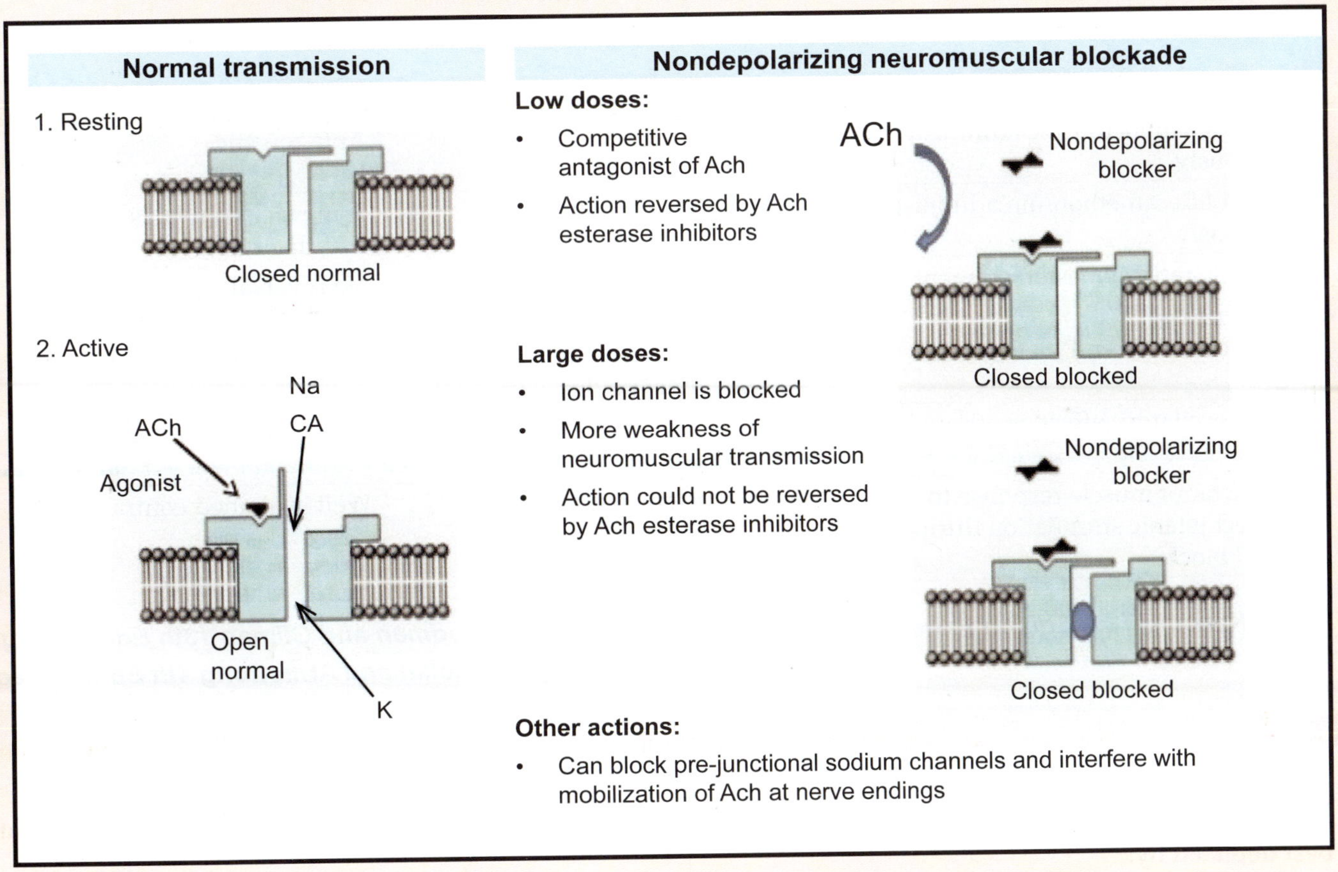

- Pharmacologic effect of tubocurarine, 0.3 mg/kg IV ***(Usually lasts 45 to 60 min).***
- Residual muscle paralysis detected using neuromuscular monitor may last for another hour, increasing likelihood of adverse outcomes like aspiration and reduced hypoxic drive.

Contd.

Contd.

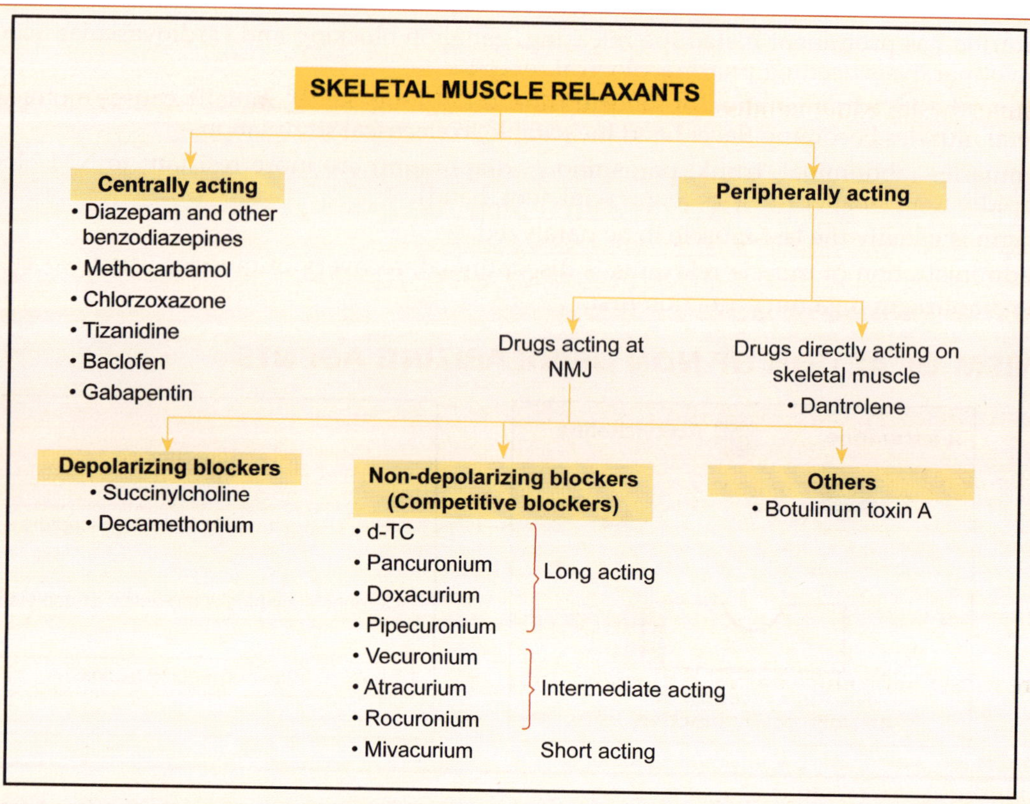

	D-Tubocurarine	Decamethonium
Effect of D-tubocurarine administered previously	Additive	Antagonistic
Effect of decamethonium administered previously	No effect or antagonistic	Some tachyphylaxis, but may be additive
Effect of anticholinesterase agents on block	Reversal of block	No reversal
Effect on motor end plate	Elevated threshold to acetylcholine; no depolarization	Partial, persisting depolarization
Initial excitatory effect on striated muscle	None	Transient fasciculations
Character of muscle response to indirect tetanic stimulation during *partial* block	Poorly sustained contraction	Well-sustained contraction

Ref: Katzung 13th Edition Page 456, KDT 8th Edition Page 374, Goodman and Gilman 13th Edition Page 181, Principles of Pharmacology by Golan and Armstrong 4th Edition Page 138

Ans: (A) Competitive inhibitor of acetylcholine receptors

6. **Increasing fraction of population that shows a specified response at progressively increasing dose concentration is best depicted by:**

A. Potency

B. Efficacy

C. Graded dose response curve

D. Quantal dose response curve

Key:

Quantal Dose-Response Curve

*Graph of increasing fraction of a population that shows a **specified response** at progressively increasing doses*

QUANTAL DOSE RESPONSE CURVE

- *Graph of increasing fraction of a population that shows a **specified response** at progressively increasing doses. **Dose response follows All or None phenomenon.***
- ***Quantal DRC are useful for determining doses to which most of population responds.***
- In a quantal dose-response relationship, percentage of the population affected increases as the dose is increased.

Graded dose–response relationship is determined in an individual and quantal dose-response relationship is determined in population

- Dose required to produce particular toxic effect in 50% → ***Median toxic dose (TD50).***
- If the toxic effect is death→ ***Median lethal dose (LD50) is determined.***
- Quantal dose-effect curve is often characterized by stating ***Median effective dose* (qED50)**, which is dose at which 50% of individuals exhibit the specified quantal effect.
- qDRC deals with Therapeutic index and Therapeutic window.

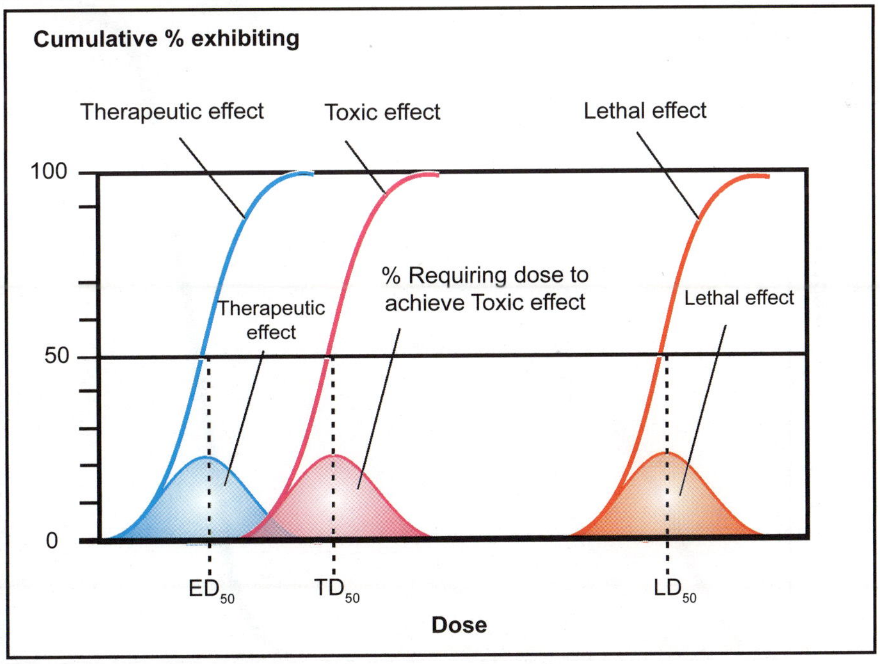

End point is set, and an individual is either a responder or a nonresponder. This response is expressed as a normal histogram or cumulative distribution profile. Normal histogram is usually bell-shaped

GRADED DOSE-RESPONSE CURVE

- Graph of increasing response to increasing drug concentration or dose in an individual.
- Graded doses of a drug given to an individual usually result in a greater magnitude of response as dose increases.
- Response in one subject or test system.

Graded responses can be transformed to quantal responses by designating a predetermined level of graded response as the point at which a response occurs or not.

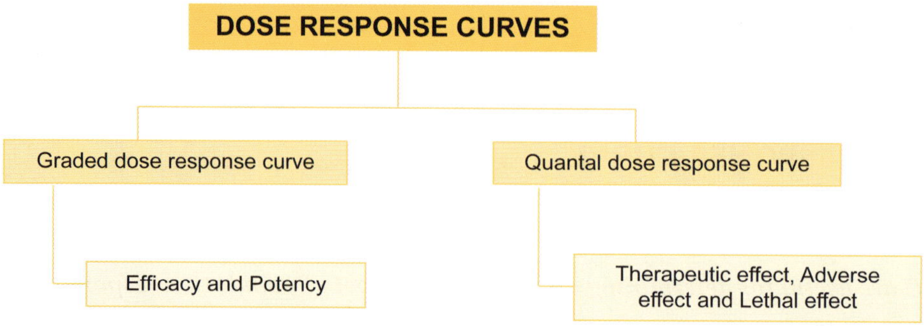

Potency

- Measure of amount of a drug needed to produce response.
- ***Drugs producing same response at lower dose are more potent whereas those requiring large dose are less potent.***
- Potency refers to concentration (EC50) or dose (ED50) of a drug required to produce 50% of that drug's maximal effect.

Efficacy

- Maximum effect produced by a drug.
- More the peak of the curve greater is the efficacy.
- It is clinically more important than potency.

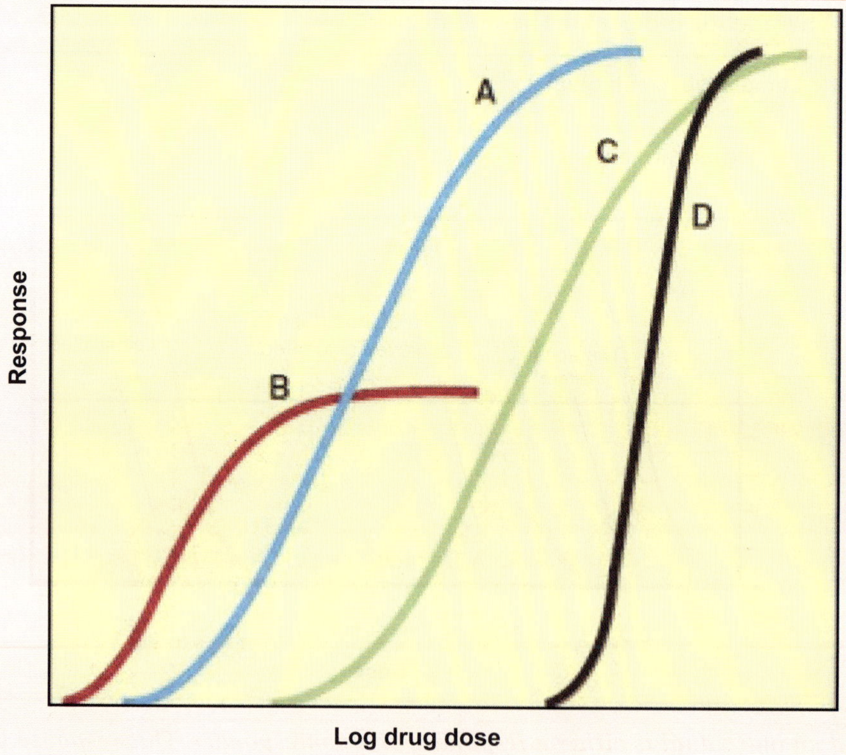

Graded dose response curve

- Drugs A and B are more potent than C and D
- Potency of drug A is less than that of drug B, partial agonist because EC_{50} of A is greater than EC_{50} of B.
- Drugs A, C and D have equal maximal efficacy and all have greater maximal efficacy than B.

Nonmonotonic Dose Response Curves

U shaped DRC *Essential vitamins and minerals*	Hockey stick shaped DRC *Toxicants and Metabolic byproducts*
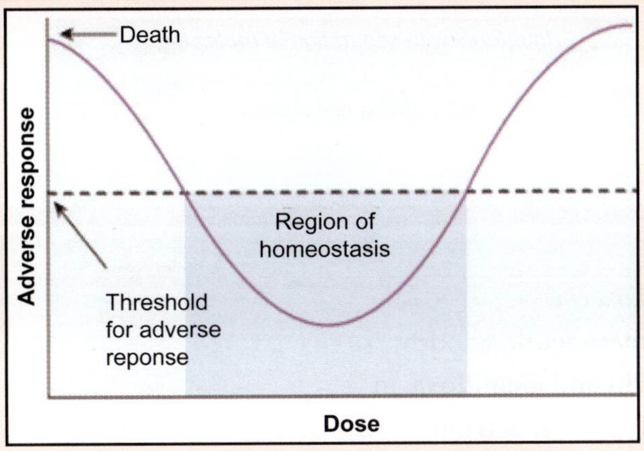	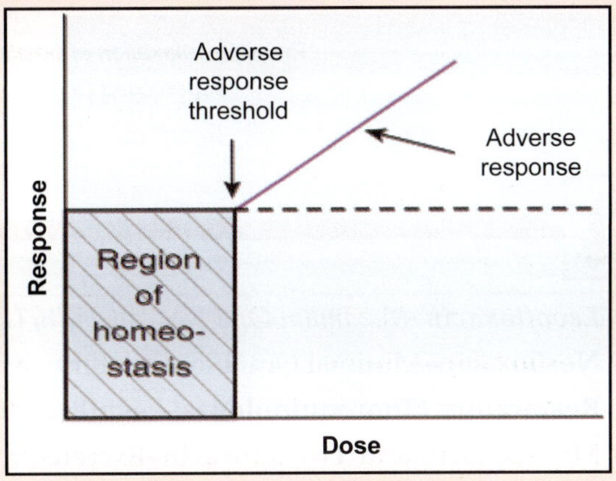

Inverted U shaped DRC

Ligands that down regulate their receptors

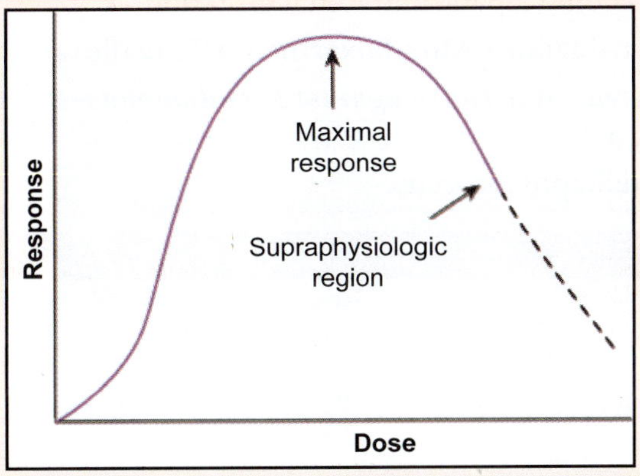

Ref: K.D.Tripathi 8th Edition Page 64, Katzung 13th Edition Page 94, Goodman and Gilman 13th Edition Page 37, Principles of Pharmacology by Golan and Armstrong 4th Edition Page 20

Ans: (D) Quantal dose response curve

7. **Fluoroquinolone with highest oral bioavailability is:**

A. Levofloxacin B. Gemifloxacin
C. Ciprofloxacin D. Norfloxacin

Key:

Gatifloxacin > Levofloxacin has highest Oral bioavailability

FLUOROQUINOLONES

Mechanism of Action

- DNA Gyrase enzyme is present in Gram –ve bacteria responsible for nicking of torsional stress area in DNA
- *Persistence of torsional stress leads to break down of DNA–Bactericidal effect*

FLUOROQUINOLONES

- **DNA Gyrase inhibitor/ Topoisomerase II inhibitor**
  - *Prevents relaxation of positively supercoiled DNA*
- **Inhibits Topoisomerase IV enzyme**
  - *Interferes with separation of replicated chromosomal DNA into respective daughter cells during cell division*

- ***Levofloxacin**–Maximum Oral bioavailability (Highest-Gatifloxacin)*
- **Norfloxacin**–Minimal Oral bioavailability and Narrow therapeutic window
- **Respiratory Fluoroquinolones**–Levofloxacin, Gatifloxacin and Gemifloxacin
- **Moxifloxacin and Trovafloxacin**–Excreted in liver and Widest spectrum
- **Longest $t_{1/2}$**→ Moxifloxacin, Trovafloxacin and Sparfloxacin
- **Overall longest $t_{1/2}$**→ Sparfloxacin
- Sparfloxacin and Pefloxacin–Both Hepatic and Renal excretion
- Fluoroquinolones Safe in Renal failure–**Moxifloxacin and Trovafloxacin**
- ***Fluoroquinolones that has greatest activity against Pseudomonas–Ciprofloxacin***
- Finafloxacin is a fluoroquinolone that has been approved recently for topical treatment of acute otitis externa caused by Pseudomonas and Staphylococcus.

Drug	Oral Bioavailabilty (%)	Oral dose (mg)
Ciprofloxacin	70%	500
Gatifloxacin	98%	400
Gemifloxacin	70%	320
Levofloxacin	95%	500
Lomefloxacin	95%	400
Ofloxacin	95%	400
Moxifloxacin	>85%	400
Norfloxacin	80%	400

Ciprofloxacin

- *Drug of choice for treatment of Anthrax, Traveller's diarrhea, Pyelonephritis.*
- *Drug of choice for Prophylaxis of contacts in meningococcal meningitis.*
- *Used in Prostatitis.*
- *Also effective against Pseudomonas.*

Norfloxacin

- Least active
- Used for Treatment of UTI and Prostatitis

Respiratory Fluoroquinolones–Levofloxacin, Gatifloxacin and Gemifloxacin

- Used as first line empirical drug for treatment of pneumonia

Moxifloxacin, Ofloxacin and Ciprofloxacin–Used as 2nd line drugs for treatment of Tuberculosis

Pefloxacin

- Most lipid soluble fluoroquinolone
- Maximum Crossing of Blood brain barrier
- Preferred for treatment of Meningitis

Side Effects

- Tendinitis–Common side effect in Elderly *(Tendon rupture)*
- Most common side effect–Nausea and Vomiting/GI distress
- Pseudomembranous colitis is maximum with Ciprofloxacin
- Cartilage defect–Arthropathy (Contraindicated in children <18 years and pregnancy)
- Pefloxacin and Moxifloxacin–Contraindicated in Liver failure
- Maximum QT prolongation–Sparfloxacin
- Maximum photosensitivity–Sparfloxacin

Gatifloxacin	Sparfloxacin and Lomefloxacin	Trovafloxacin	Grepafloxacin	Clinafloxacin	Temafloxacin
Hypoglycemia and Hyperglycemia	*QT prolongation and Photosensitivity*	*Hepatotoxicity*	*Cardiotoxicity*	*Photosensitivity*	Hemolytic anemia (Autoimmune)

Ref: KDT 8th Edition Page 760, Katzung 13th Edition Page 1139, Goodman and Gilman 13th Edition Page 1015, Principles of Pharmacology by Golan and Armstrong 4th Edition Page 628

Ans: (A) Levofloxacin

8. True statement about pegylated filgrastim is:

A. Active orally
B. GM-CSF
C. Shortens recovery time from severe neutropenia
D. Has short duration of action

Key:

Pegfilgrastim –Covalent conjugation product of filgrastim and form of polyethylene glycol
Has much longer serum half-life than recombinant G-CSF
Injected once per myelosuppressive chemotherapy cycle instead of daily for several days

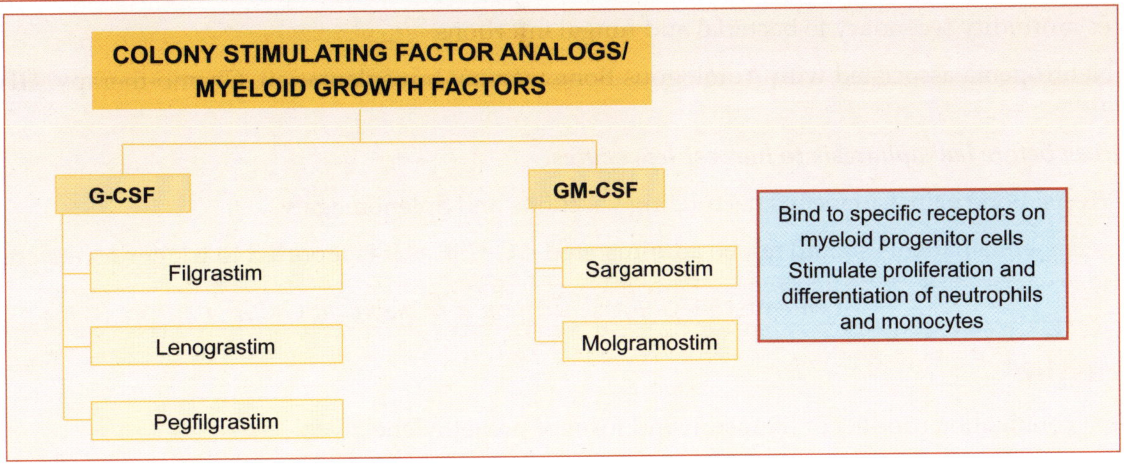

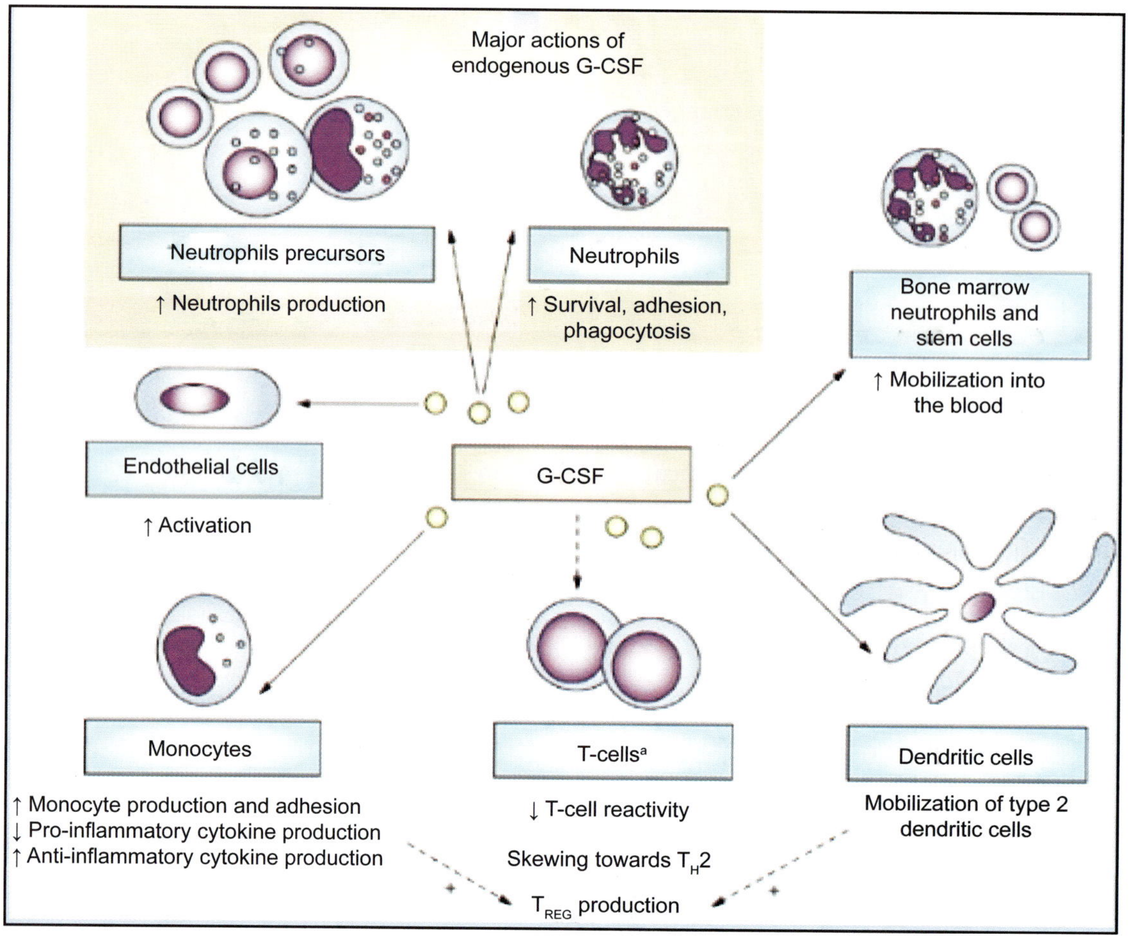

Filgrastim

- Recombinant human granulocyte-colony stimulating factor (G-CSF) produced in bacterial expression system
- Produced in E.coli by Genetic Engineering
- Contains Nonglycosylated peptide of 175 amino acids
- ***Principal action of filgrastim is stimulation of CFU-G to increase neutrophil production***
- Started one day after myelosuppressive chemotherapy and injected subcutaneous or intravenous daily → ***till neutrophil count normalizes***
- ***Filgrastim–Routinely used in patients undergoing PBSC collection for stem cell transplantation and promotes release of CD34+ progenitor cells from marrow, reducing number of collections necessary for transplant.***
- Used to shorten recovery time from neutropenia.
- Reduces morbidity secondary to bacterial and fungal infections
- **Uses:** Neutropenia associated with Autologous Bone marrow transplantation, Chemo-therapy, HIV and Aplastic anemia.
- ***Also given before leukapharesis to harvest leucocytes***
- **Side Effects:** Bone pain, Cutaneous necrotizing vasculitis and Splenomegaly
- Sickle cell anemia patients should not be administered→G-CSF as it is reported to trigger severe crises.

Lenograstim–Glycosylated form of recombinant G-CSF

Pegfilgrastim

- Covalent conjugation product of filgrastim and form of polyethylene glycol

- *Has a much longer serum half-life than recombinant G-CSF*
- Can be injected once per myelosuppressive chemotherapy cycle instead of daily for several days.

Sargramostim

- Recombinant human GM-CSF produced in a yeast expression system
- Partially glycosylated peptide of 127 amino acids
- Low dose–Increases Neutrophil only
- High dose–Increases Eosinophils and Monocytes also
- **Side Effects**–Capillary leak syndrome, Bone pain, Malaise, Flu like symptoms and Ventricular tachycardia

Hematopoietic Growth Factor	Clinical Condition Being Treated or Prevented	Recipients
Erythropoietin, darbepoetin alfa	Anemia	Patients with chronic renal failure HIV–infected patients treated with zidovudine Cancer patients treated with myelosuppressive cancer chemotherapy Patient scheduled to undergo elective, noncardiac, nonvascular surgery
Granulocyte colony-stimulating factor (G-CSF; filgrastim) and granulocyte-macrophage colony-stimulating factor (GM-CSF; sargramostim)	Neutropenia	Cancer patients treated with myclosuppressive cancer chemotherapy Patients with severe chronic neutropenia Patients recovering from bone marrow transplantation
	Stem cell or bone marrow transplantation	Patients with nonmyeloid malignancies or other conditions being treated with stem cell or bone marrow transplantation
	Mobilization of peripheral blood progenitor cells (PBPCs)	Donors of stem cells for allogeneic or autologous transplantation
Interleukin–11 (IL-11, oprelvekin)	Thrombocytopenia	Patients with nonmyeloid malignancies who receive myelosuppressive cancer chemotherapy
Romiplostim	Thrombocytopenia	Patient with idiopathic thombocytopenic purpura

Ref: KDT 8th Edition Page 936, Katzung 13th Edition Page 1139, Goodman and Gilman 13th Edition Page 756, Principles of Pharmacology by Golan and Armstrong 4th Edition Page 838

Ans: (C) Shortens recovery time from severe neutropenia

9. Which of the following is a K^+ channel opener?

A. Verapamil B. Ranolazine
C. Nicorandil D. Ivabridine

Key:

Nicorandil is an ATP sensitive K^+ channel opener that acts on myocardium thus leading to hyperpolarization and decrease in intracellular calcium→ Reduced contraction and oxygen demand of myocardium in Angina

Also has Nitric oxide releasing property (No tolerance develops for this mechanism)

DRUGS THAT ACT ON POTASSIUM CHANNEL

- **K^+ Channel openers**
  - Nicorandil, Diazoxide, Minoxidil, Hydralazine, Ezogabine, Tilisolol
- **K^+ Channel blockers**
  - Class IA and III Antiarrythmics, Sulfonylureas, Meglitinides

ANTI ANGINAL DRUGS

- **Nitrates**: GTN, Isosorbide
- **Calcium channel blockers**: Verapamil, Diltiazem
- **Beta blockers**: Propranolol, Atenolol, Metoprolol
- **K^+ channel openers**: Nicorandil
- **pFOX inhibitors**: Trimetazidine, Ranolazine
- **Na^+ channel blockers**: Ranolazine, Ivabradine

Ranolazine

- Inhibits late sodium current in Myocardial cell→Stimulates sodium calcium exchanger pumps→Depletion of intracellular calcium→Decreases contraction of myocardium and oxygen demand.
- *No effect on heart rate and blood pressure*
- Contraindicated in patients with Long QT interval, Liver and Kidney failure
- Indicated for prevention of angina when all other drugs are ineffective
- *Not used for treatment of acute angina episodes*
- Also used to decrease incidence of atrial fibrillation and decreases HbA1c.
- Safe to use with erectile dysfunction drugs like sildenafil

Ivabridine

- Inhibits I_f (funny) channels of sodium required for depolarization of cells in SA node
- *Decreases heart rate and oxygen demand (Bradycardiac agent)*
- Decreases episodes of Angina
- *Most important side effect–Visual disturbances*

Calcium Channel Blockers

- Block L type voltage gated calcium channels present in blood vessels and heart

CALCIUM CHANNEL BLOCKERS

- **Phenylalkylamines**
  - Verapamil, Nor verapamil
- **Benzothiazepines**
  - Diltiazem
- **Dihydropyridines**
  - Nifedipine, Nicardipine, Nimodipine, Nitrendipine, Isradipine, Lacidipine, Amlodipine, Felodipine

- Result in vasodilatation and decreases activity of heart (Decrease HR, AV Conduction and Contractility)
- **Long acting Dihydropyridines, Verapamil and Diltiazem**–Used in Angina
- **Short acting Dihydropyridines** (Nifedipine)–Should be avoided→Can accentuate Angina symptoms of angina by causing tachycardia.
- **So CCB are effective in treatment of both classical and variant angina**

Verapamil
• Treatment of Angina, PVST, Hypertension and HOCM
• Can cause Constipation and Ankle edema
• ***Have strong cardiodepressant activity***

- Nifedipine can cause hyperglycemia and voiding difficulty in elderly.
- **Drugs should be avoided in Sick sinus syndrome (Avoided with beta blockers)**
- CCB increase plasma digoxin by decreasing its excretion
- Nimodipine→ Subarachnoid hemorrhage

Nicardipine→Longest acting parenteral CCB
Drug of choice for Hypertensive emergencies

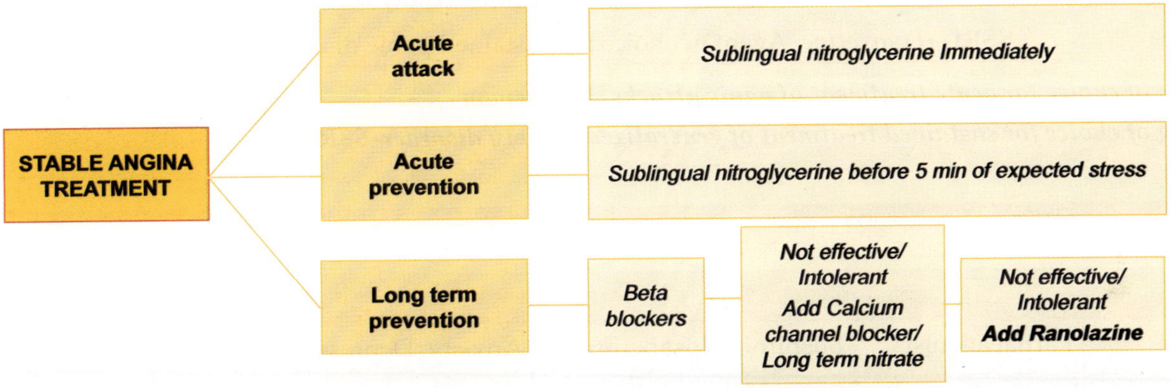

Ref: K.D.Tripathi 8th Edition Page 598, Katzung 13th Edition Page 94, Goodman and Gilman 13th Edition Page 500, Principles of Pharmacology by Golan and Armstrong 4th Edition Page 392

Ans: (C) Nicorandil

10. Buspirone acts on:

A. Negative allosteric inhibition of NMDA
B. Inhibition of GABA
C. 5 HT1A agonist
D. Excitation of GABA

Key:

Partial agonists–5HT1A agonists (Contains ONE in its name)
Buspirone, Gepirone and Ipsapirone–*Act as partial agonist of presynaptic 5HT1A receptors and decrease release of serotonin (Anxiolytic→Decreases anxiety)*

Anti Anxiety Drugs	
Benzodiazepines	Most commonly used ***Chlordiazepoxide***–Chronic anxiety state ***Oxazepam, Lorazepam, Alprazolam and Diazepam***–Short lasting anxiety state ***Oxazepam and Lorazepam***–Safe in Elderly and Liver disease patients ***Benzodiazepine***–Drug of choice for Acute panic attacks and Generalized anxiety disorder
Azapirones	***Buspirone, Gepirone and Ipsapirone***–Act as partial agonist of presynaptic 5HT1A receptors and decrease release of serotonin *Doesn't cause sedation or cognitive impairment* *Devoid of Abuse potential, Muscle relaxant and Anticonvulsant activity* *Ineffective in acute anxiety states (Panic attacks)* Indicated for mild to moderate generalized anxiety states
Beta blockers	***Propranolol–Indicated for performance anxiety*** Decreases sympathetic manifestations of anxiety
Others	***Hydroxyzine***–H1 Antihistaminic that has anti anxiety activity (Profound sedation) **SSRI→*Fluoxetine***–Agent of choice for sustained panic disorder

- *Drug of choice for acute treatment of panic attacks–Lorazepam*
- *Drug of choice for sustained treatment of generalized anxiety disorder–SSRI*

Receptor	Action	Drugs	Disorder	Comments
5HT 1A	Partial agonist	Buspirone, Ipsaperone	Anxiety, Depression	–
5HT 1D	Agonist	Sumatriptan	Migraine and Cluster headache	Short acting
5HT 2A/2C	Antagonist	Methysergide, Risperidone, Ketanserin	Migraine, Depression, Schizophrenia	–
5HT 3	Antagonist	Ondansetron	Chemotherapy induced emesis	–
5HT 4	Agonist	Cisapride	GI Disorders	–
SERT	Inhibitor (5HT transporter)	Fluoxetine, Sertraline	Depression, OCD, Panic disorder, Social phobia, PTSD	–
5HT	Dexfenfluramine		Appetite suppressant	Monitor for pulmonary HTN

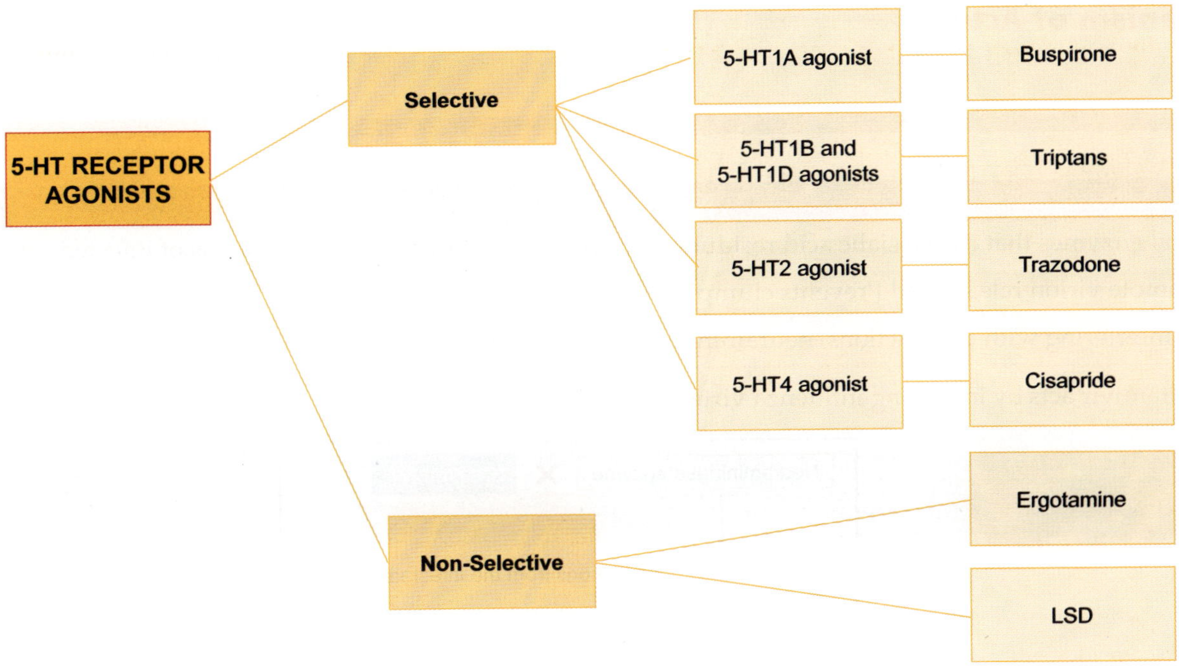

Ref: KDT 8th Edition Page 187, Goodman and Gilman 13th Edition Page 232, Katzung 13th Edition Page 576, Principles of Pharmacology by Golan and Armstrong 4th Edition Page 238

Ans: (C) 5 HT1A agonist

11. Mechanism of action of oseltamivir is:

A. Neuraminidase inhibition
B. DNA polymerase inhibition
C. Inhibiting viral mRNA
D. Uncoating of virus

Key:

Oseltamivir is a neuroaminidase inhibitor that prevents release of virus by causing clumping of mature virions by binding to neuraminidase receptors

OSELTAMIVIR

- Sialic acid analogue and an ester prodrug

Spectrum

- Broad spectrum activity against Influenza A, H5N1 and Influenza B. *(Currently active against both H3N2 and H1N1 strains)*

Pharmacokinetics

- Rapidly and nearly completely hydrolysed during absorption in intestine and by liver esterases to the active form ***oseltamivir carboxylate.***
- Oral bioavailability of ~80%.
- Excreted by kidney–***Dose reduction is needed in renal insufficiency.***
- t½ of 6-10 hours.
- Started within few hours (maximum 48 hours) of symptom onset, it reduces severity, duration and complications of the illness.
- Early initiation of therapy is critical because viral replication is maximal during the first 2 days of symptom onset.

Mechanism of Action

Neuraminidase Enzyme
• Viral enzymes that cleave sialic acid residues from viral proteins and surface proteins of infected cells.
• Promote virion release and Prevents clumping of newly released virions.
• By interfering with these actions, neuraminidase inhibitors impede viral spread.

- Oseltamivir acts by inhibiting influenza virus neuraminidase enzyme.

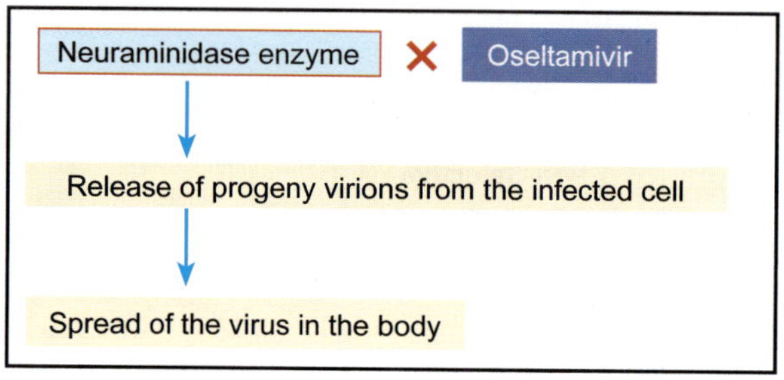

Dose

- Therapeutic 75 mg oral BD for 5 days; Prophylactic 75 mg OD for 7 days.
- Prophylactic use within 2 days of exposure prevents illness in contacts of influenza patients.

Resistance

- Develop by mutation of viral neuraminidase enzyme.

Side Effects

- Nausea and Abdominal pain due to gastric irritation (reduced by taking drug with food), headache, weakness, sadness, diarrhoea, cough and insomnia.
- Neuropsychiatric side effects are common.

ZANAMIVIR

- Inhalational route→Low oral bioavailability
- Drug of choice for Oseltamivir resistant influenza
- Therapeutic 10 mg oral BD for 5 days; Prophylactic 10 mg OD for 7 days
- *Approved for treatment in children >7 years and prophylaxis in children >5 years*
- Main side effect is Bronchospasm (Avoid in asthma and COPD)
- Neuropsychiatric side effects are common.

PERAMIVIR

- Intravenous route
- Not active against oseltamavir resistant Influenza
- Single dose 600 mg for treatment
- Only in adults (>18 years)

LANINAMIVIR

- *Longest acting*
- Inhalational route
- Given as 40 mg single dose
- Effective against Oseltamivir resistant influenza

M Protein Inhibitors

- Anti influenza drugs that prevent uncoating of virus
- **Drugs**–Amantidine and Rimantidine

Amantidine	Rimantidine
Good oral absorption	Metabolized by liver
Treatment and Prophylaxis of influenza A only	Excreted by kidney
Also effective for treatment of parkinsonism	Longer acting than amantidine
Side effects–Nausea, Vomiting, Ankle edema, ***Livedo reticularis*** and Insomnia	Most commonly GI side effects

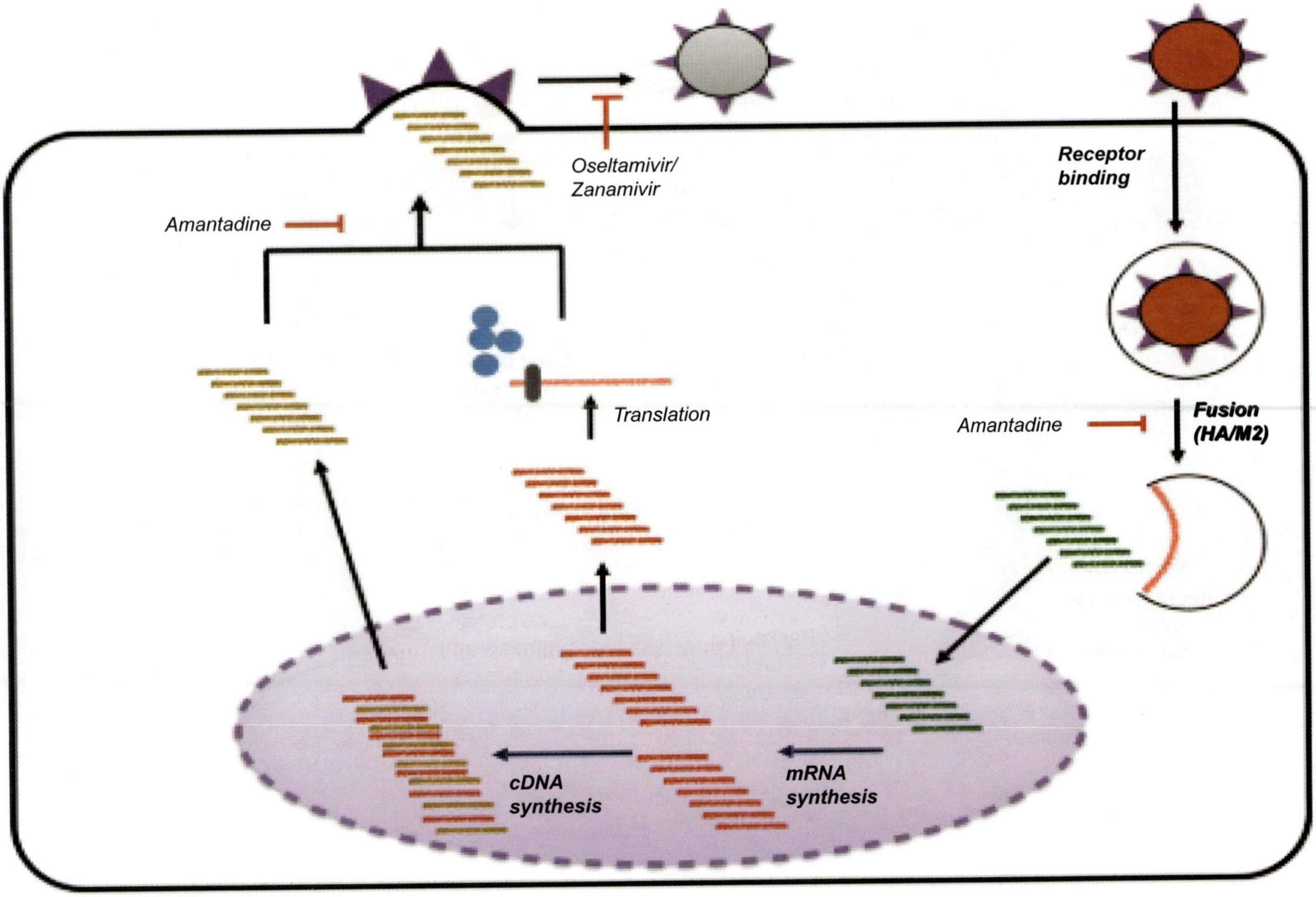

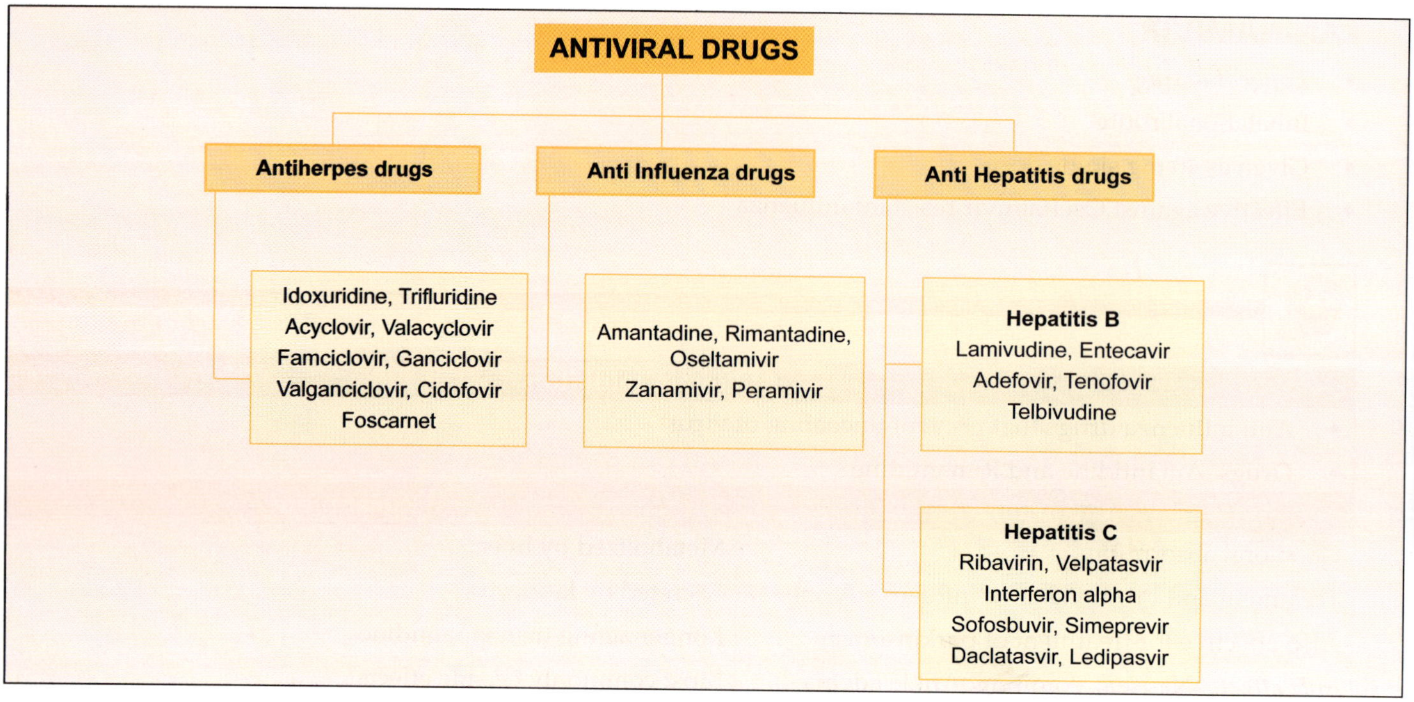

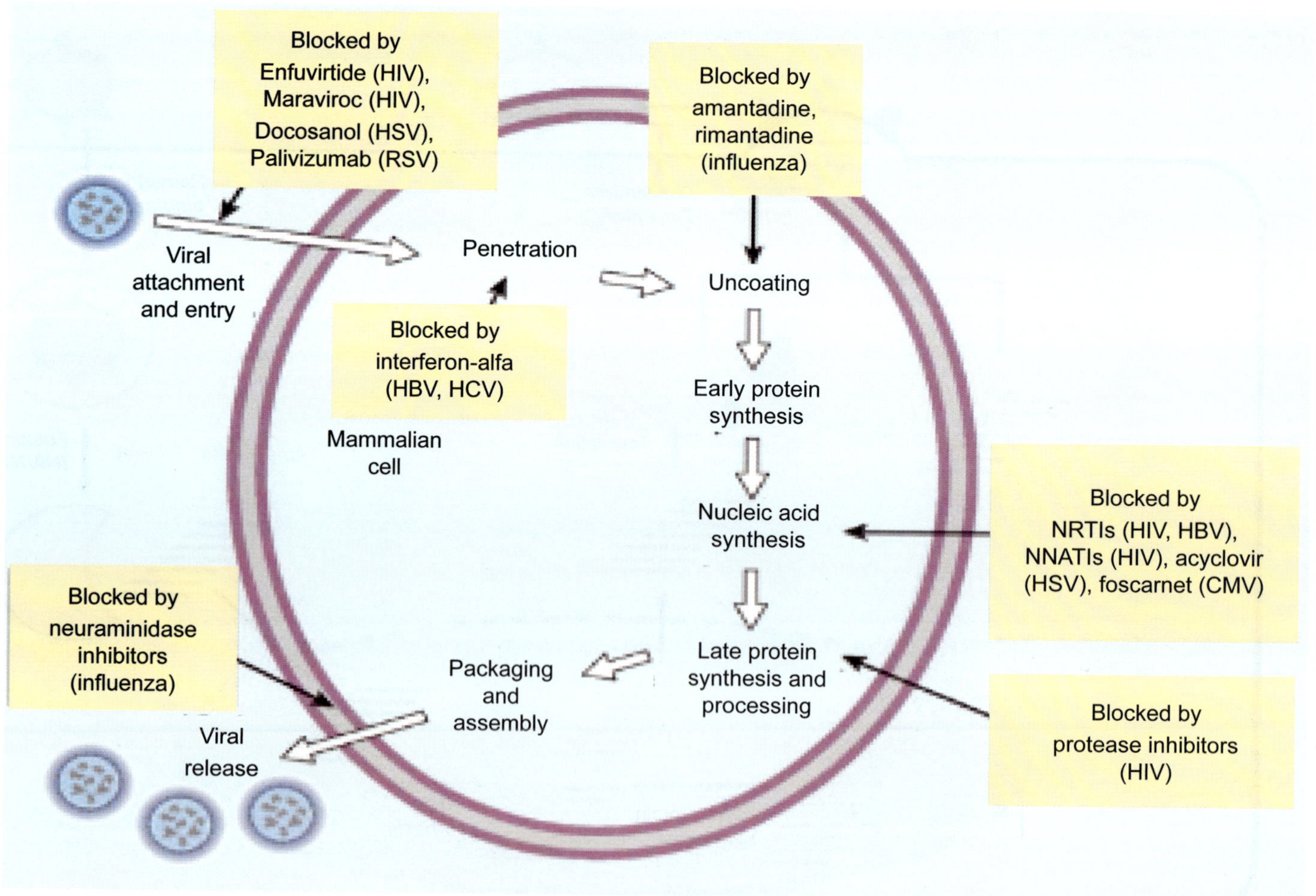

Ref: KDT 8th Edition Page 853, Katzung 13th Edition Page 1689, Goodman and Gilman 13th Edition Page 1113, Principles of Pharmacology by Golan and Armstrong 4th Edition Page 714

Ans: (A) Neuraminidase inhibition

12. High plasma protein binding of a drug result in:

A. Increase in Volume of distribution
B. Decrease in glomerular filtration
C. Increase in tubular secretion
D. Decreased drug interactions

Key:

Drugs with high plasma protein binding is less filtered via glomerular membrane

PLASMA PROTEIN BINDING

- **Directly proportional**
  - *Age, Lipid solubility of drug and Drug interactions*
- **Inversely Proportional**
  - *Volume of distribution*
- **Independent**
  - *Independent on tubular secretion of drug or tubular reabsorption*

Sequence of protein drug binding
Albumin > Glycoprotein > Lipoprotein > Globulin

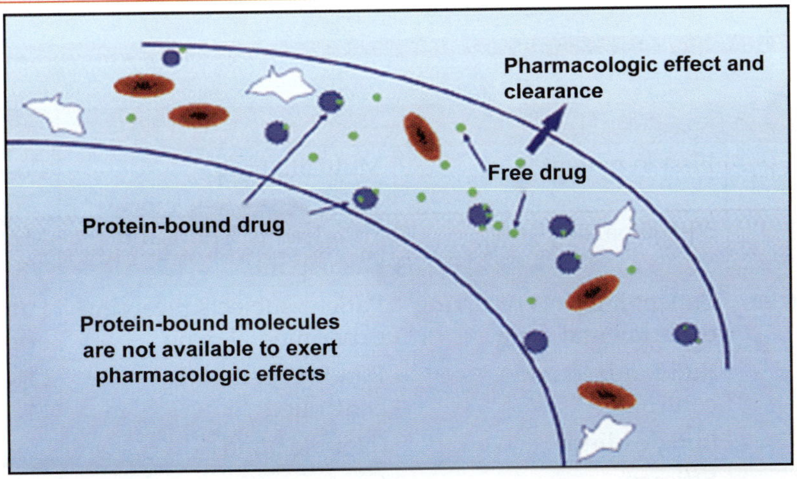

Protein Bound Drug Fraction Can't Cross Blood Brain Barrier

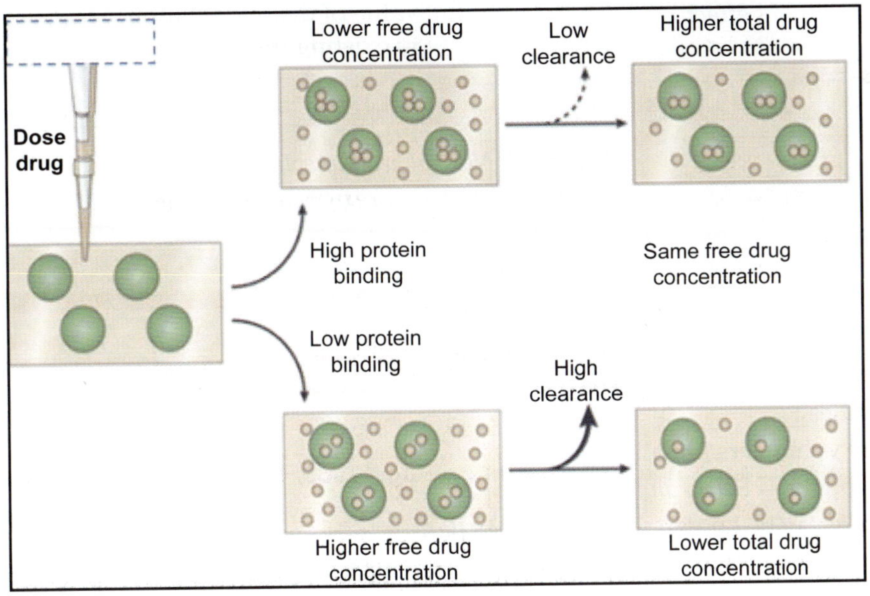

High albumin bound drugs	High alpha 1 acid Glycoprotein bound drugs
Benzodiazepines, Barbiturates, Phenytoin, Valproate, Penicillins, Tetracyclines, Sulfonamides, Warfarin and NSAIDS	Verapamil, Lidocaine, Dis opyramide, Beta blockers ***(Propranolol),*** Quinidine, Opoids, TCA, Prazosin, Bupivacaine

Ref: KDT 8th Edition Page 853, Katzung 13th Edition Page 1689, Goodman and Gilman 13th Edition Page 1113, Principles of Pharmacology by Golan and Armstrong 4th Edition Page 714

Ans: (B) Decrease in glomerular filtration

13. Which of the following statements about clinical trials is true?

A. Phase 1 is done to determine efficacy and safety in patients

B. Phase 2 is done for Toxicity

C. Randomized controlled trial in patients is done in phase 3

D. Phase 4 is a Pharmacokinetics study in animals

Key:

Phase 3 trials are Randomized and Controlled double blind trials

PHASE I	PHASE II	PHASE III	PHASE IV
First in human	First in patient	Multisite trial	Postmarketing surveillance
10-100 participants	50-500 participants	Hundred to Thousand participants	Many thousand participants
Usually healthy volunteers	Patient-subjects receiving experimental drug	Patient-subjects receiving experimental drug	Patients in treatment with approved drug
Open label	Randomized and controlled (Single blind)	Randomized and controlled (Double blind)	Open label
Safety and Tolerability Maximum tolerable dose Pharmacokinetics, Pharmacodynamics	Efficacy Dose ranging and Ceiling effect	Confirm efficacy in larger population, Establish value of drug in relation to existing therapy	Adverse events, Compliance, Drug-Drug interactions Special groups like children, pregnancy can be tested
1-2 years	2-3 years	3-5 years	No fixed duration

PHASE I: *Normal healthy volunteers*

PHASE II, III and IV: *Patients*

Phase Zero (0)

- Microdosing studies
- Done on Healthy volunteers (Small number)
- Dose is subtherapeutic→ *Safety and Efficacy can't be known*
- Movement of drug can be known when radiolabelled
- Could avoid costly phase I studies for candidate drugs with unsuitable pharmacokinetics

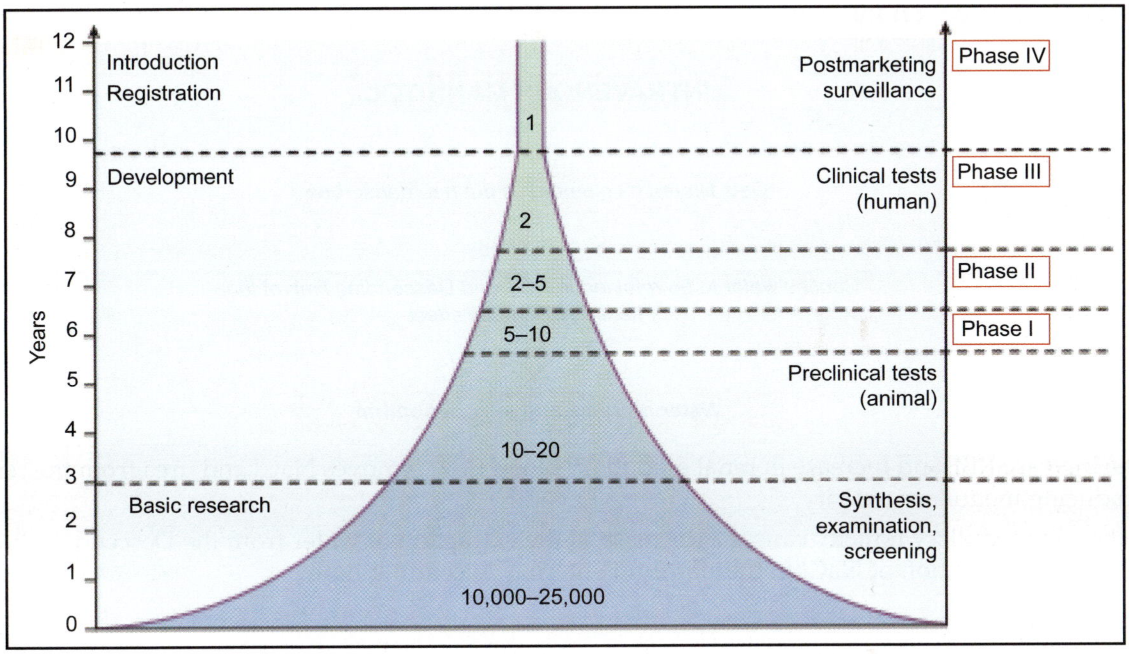

Phase V (Pharmacoepidemiology)

- Main aim of this phase is to supplement findings of phase IV trial or Pharmacovigilance
- If inconclusive Adverse drug reaction reports are found in phase IV then this phase can be helpful in confirming those signals.
- Study designs used are Case reports, Case control studies, Cohort studies and Active surviellance

Ref: Goodman and Gilman 13th Edition Page 6, Katzung 13th Edition Page 75, KDT 8th Edition Page 90

Ans: (C) Randomized controlled trial in patients is done in phase 3

14. Mannitol is used for treatment of:

A. Acute congestive glaucoma
B. Pulmonary edema
C. Acute renal failure
D. CHF

Key:

Osmotic diuretics are used to control intraocular pressure during acute attacks of glaucoma and for short-term reductions in intraocular pressure both preoperatively and postoperatively in patients who require ocular surgery

OSMOTIC DIURETICS

- **Oral agents**
  Glycerine and Isosorbide
- **Intravenous agents**
  Mannitol and Urea

MANNITOL

- Pharmacologically inert substance.

MECHANISM OF ACTION

INTRAVENOUS MANNITOL

⇩

Gets filtered by glomerulus but not reabsorbed

⇩

Causes water to be retained in PCT and Descending limb of loop of henle by Osmotis effect

⇩

Water diuresis and loss of sodium

- ***Effects:*** Increase RBF and Increase in renal medullary blood flow removes NaCl and urea from the renal medulla, thus reducing medullary tonicity.
- Reduction in medullary tonicity causes a decrease in the extraction of water from the Descending limb, which in turn limits concentration of NaCl in tubular fluid entering Ascending limb.

ADVERSE EFFECTS

MANNITOL

- **ECF volume expansion**
  - *Can complicate heart failure*
  - *May produce pulmonary edema*
- **Dehydration, Hyperkalemia and Hypernatremia**
- **Hyponatremia**
  - *Causes osmotic extraction of water from cells leading to hyponatremia*

Most common side effect is headache.

USES

- **Used in treatment of dialysis disequilibrium syndrome**
- To maintain urine volume and prevent oliguria in conditions like massive hemolysis and shock and severe trauma ***(Intravascular glycerol can cause hemolysis)***
- To reduce ***intracranial and intraocular pressure*** following head injury and glaucoma respectively.

Diuretic of choice in Cerebral edema–Mannitol

CONTRAINDICATIONS

- *Contraindicated in Renal insufficiency, Acute tubular necrosis, Anuria, Pulmonary edema; Acute left ventricular failure, CHF and Cerebral haemorrhage.*

Ref: Goodman and Gilman 13th Edition Page 452, Katzung 13th Edition Page 263, KDT 8th Edition Page 638

Ans: (A) Acute congestive glaucoma

15. Drug of choice for prophylaxis of diphtheria is:

A. Tetracycline
B. Erythromycin
C. Amikacin
D. Ciprofloxacin

Key:

Antimicrobial of Choice For Prophylaxis	
Diphtheria	*Penicillin/Erythromycin*
Meningococcal meningitis	*Rifampicin/Ciprofloxacin/Ceftriaxone*
Group B Streptococcal infection	*Ampicillin*
Tuberculosis	*Isoniazid alone or with rifampicin*
Anthrax	*Ciprofloxacin/Doxycycline*
Cholera	*Tetracycline*
Hemophilus influenza type B	*Rifampicin*
Mycobacterium avium complex (MAC)	*Azithromycin/Clarithromycin/Rifabutin*
Pertussis	*Azithromycin*
Plague	*Tetracycline*
Pneumocystis jiroveci	*Cotrimoxazole/Dapsone/Atovaquone*
Toxoplasmosis	*Cotrimoxazole*
Malaria	*Chloroquine/Mefloquine/Doxycycline*
Influenza A and B	*Oseltamivir*
Herpes simplex	*Acyclovir*
Otitis media	*Amoxicillin*
Endocarditis	*Amoxicillin/Clindamycin*
Rheumatic fever	*Benzathine penicillin*
UTI	*Cotrimoxazole*
Surgical prophylaxis	*Cefazolin*

Ref: KDT 8th Edition Page 802, Katzung 13th Edition Page 813, Goodman and Gilman 13th Edition Page 1054

Ans: (B) Erythromycin

16. Which of the following has maximum risk of seizures?

A. Imipenem
B. Meropenem
C. Ertapenem
D. Doripenem

Key:

Imipenem has maximum risk of seizures as it rapidly inactivates Renal dehydropeptidase I

CARBAPENEMS

- Contain beta lactam ring fused with five-membered penem ring
- **Drugs**–Imipenem, Doripenem, Meropenem and Ertapenem
- ***Beta lactamase resistant***–Resistant to hydrolysis by most beta lactamases
- Carbapenems penetrate body tissues and fluids well, including CSF.

SPECTRUM

- Wide spectrum against Gram +ve cocci, Gram –ve bacilli and Anaerobes
- Meropenem is most active against Pseudomonas treatment
- *Drug of choice for Enterobacter, Klebsiella Serratia and Acinetobacter*

- Only Beta lactams with reliable efficacy against ESBL (Extended spectrum betalactamase) producing organisms.
- Imipenem, meropenem or doripenem, with or without an aminoglycoside, may be effective treatment for febrile neutropenic patients.

MECHANISM OF ACTION

Carbapenems inhibit bacterial cell wall synthesis similar to penicillins.

Imipenem

- Not absorbed orally (Administered intravenously)
- Good tissue permeability
- **Imipenem is rapidly inactivated by Renal dehydropeptidase I→ *Short duration of action*** (Brush border of proximal convoluted tubule).
- Highest Seizure activity→ Imipenem.
- ***Always combined with cilastatin in order to prolong plasma half life.***
- Both imipenem and cilastatin have a *t* 1/2 of about 1 hour.
- When administered concurrently with cilastatin, about 70% of administered imipenem is recovered in urine as the active drug.
- ***Adverse effects***–Nausea and Vomiting (Most common), Diarrhea and Allergic reactions.
- ***High dose can cause Seizures.***

Meropenem

- Not destroyed by renal dipeptidase and therefore no need to combine with cilastin
- ***Risk of seizures is less than Imipenem***
- ***More potent on Gram –ve aerobes***
- Less active against Enterococcus compared to Imipenem
- Preferred treatment of meningitis when carbepenem therapy is required
- Reserve drug for treatment of serious nosocomial infections like septicemia, Febrile neutropenia, Intraabdominal and Pelvic infections.

Ertapenem

- ***Longest acting (4 hours)***
- Inactive against Pseudomonas
- Intramuscular ertapenem is irritating and for that reason drug is formulated with 1% lidocaine for administration by this route.
- Major mechanism of resistance–Upregulation of antibiotic efflux mechanism and selection of mutants with deficient porin channels.

Faropenem

- Orally effective
- Good efficacy against both gram +ve and gram –ve organisms along with anaerobes

Doripenem

- Better activity against Gram –ve aerobes than gram +ve
- Greater activity against Pseudomonas

Carbapenems are highly resistant to hydrolysis by penicillinases and cephalosporinases, but they are hydrolyzed by metallo-beta lactamase and carbapenemases

Ref: Goodman and Gilman 13th Edition Page 1035, Katzung 13th Edition Page 802, KDT 8th Edition Page 782

Ans: (A) Imipenem

17. Cilastin is given in combination with Imipenem because:

A. Synergism
B. Decreases side effect
C. Increases duration of action
D. Increased potency

Key:

Why Imipenem is Combined With Cilastatin
• **Imipenem is rapidly inactivated by Renal dehydropeptidase I→** ***Short duration of action*** (Brush border of proximal convoluted tubule). • Highest Seizure activity→ Imipenem • *Always combined with cilastatin in order to prolong plasma half life.* • Both imipenem and cilastatin have a *t* 1/2 of about 1 hour. • When administered concurrently with cilastatin, about 70% of administered imipenem is recovered in urine as the active drug.

Refer to Question Number 16 for Explanation

Ref: Goodman and Gilman 13th Edition Page 1035, Katzung 13th Edition Page 802, KDT 8th Edition Page 782

Ans: (C) Increases duration of action

18. Which drug is used for differentiating myasthenia gravis from cholinergic crisis?

A. Edrophonium
B. Neostigmine
C. Atropine
D. Pirenzepine

Key:

Edrophonium is a reversible anticholinesterase used in diagnosis of Myasthenia gravis

It differentiates between Myasthenia gravis and cholinergic crisis. Weakness due to myasthenia gets improved by Edrophonium but gets worsened if it is due to Cholinergic crisis

EDROPHONIUM

- Shortest acting synthetic reversible anticholinesterease inhibitor→ *Cholinergic drug*
- Inhibits only anionic site
- Used for diagnosis of myasthenia gravis
- Used in Tensilon test because of its short duration of action (10-30 min) and fast action.

Differentiates between Myasthenia gravis and cholinergic crisis

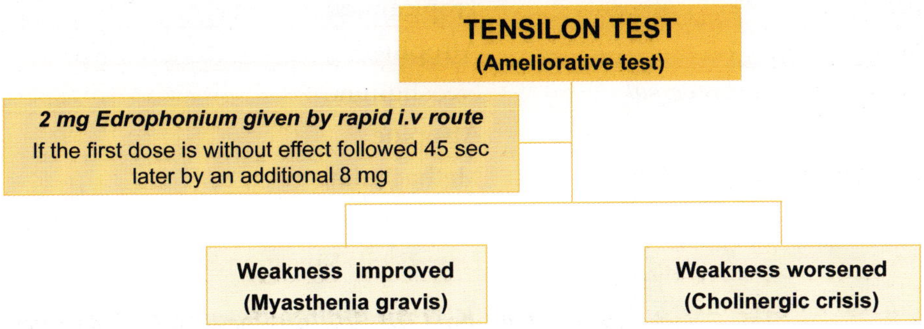

Cholinergic crisis: Results from Persistent depolarization of post synaptic membrane due to Ach excess.

Edrophonium can be used for treatment of acute attack of PVST

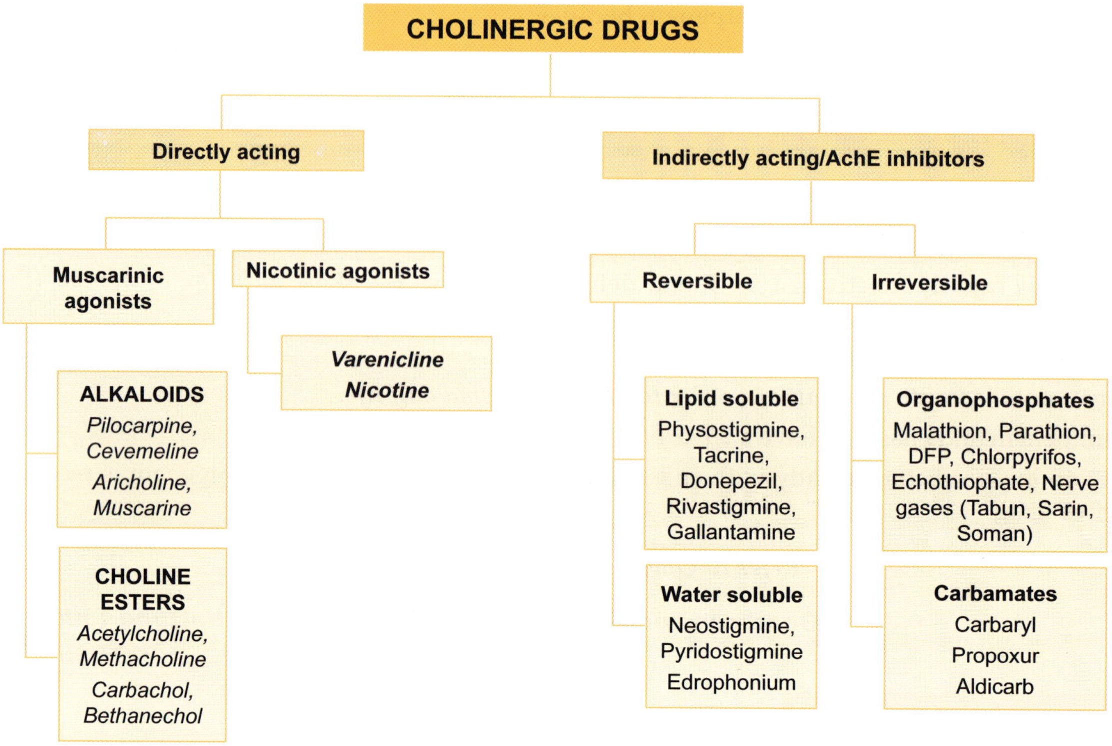

Drug of Choice	
Mushroom Poisoning	Atropine
Myasthenia gravis	Neostigmine
Belladona Poisoning	Physostigmine
Atropine poisoning	Physostigmine
Datura poisoning	Physostigmine
Bradycardia	Atropine
AV Block	Atropine
Motion sickness	Scopalamine
Myasthenic crisis	IV immunoglobulin
Drug induced Parkinsonism	Benzhexol
Colicky pain	Dicyclomine
Cycloplegia in adult	Tropicamide
Cycloplegia in children	Atropine
Non depolarizing muscle relaxant reversal	Neostigmine
Organophosphorous poisoning	Atropine
Bronchial challenge test	Methacholine
COPD	Tiotropium
Alzheimer's disease	Donepezil/Rivastigmine

Ref: KDT 8th Edition Page 119, Katzung 13th Edition Page 243, Goodman and Gilman 13th Edition Page 172

Ans: (A) Edrophonium

19. Which of the following statement is advantage of fixed dose combination of drugs?

A. Increased flexibility of dose adjustment
B. Reduction in adverse effects
C. Easy to assess side effects
D. Increases development of resistance

Key:

Fixed drug combination of drugs offer an advantage of reduction in adverse effects
Dose adjustment flexibility is reduced

FIXED DOSE COMBINATIONS

- When two or more drugs are combined to be given as a single preparation, it is called fixed dose combination (FDC).

Advantages

- Convenience and thereby better patient compliance
  Example: 2 to 3 antitubercular drugs/antiretroviral drugs are combined in single tablet.
- *Synergistic effect*
  Example: Cotrimoxazole, levodopa and carbidopa.
- *Reduced adverse effect*
  Example: Thiazides with K+ sparing diuretics.
- *Prevent development of resistance*
  Example: Antitubercular drugs.

Disadvantages

- *Reduced flexibility in dose adjustment.*
- *Difficulty to assess side effects.*
- ***Increased risk of toxic effects***—due to both drugs especially if there are overlapping side effects. For example, hepatotoxicity due to INH, rifampicin and pyrazinamide.

Ref: KDT 8th Edition Page 72, Pharmacology for Dental Students and Allied Health Sciences 4th Edition Page 26

Ans: (B) Reduction in adverse effects

20. Most specific antiemetic for chemotherapy induced vomiting is:

A. Granisetron
B. Tegaserod
C. Domperidone
D. Doxylamine

Key:

5HT3 receptor antagonist→ Drug of choice for Chemotherapy induced vomiting

MECHANISM OF EMESIS

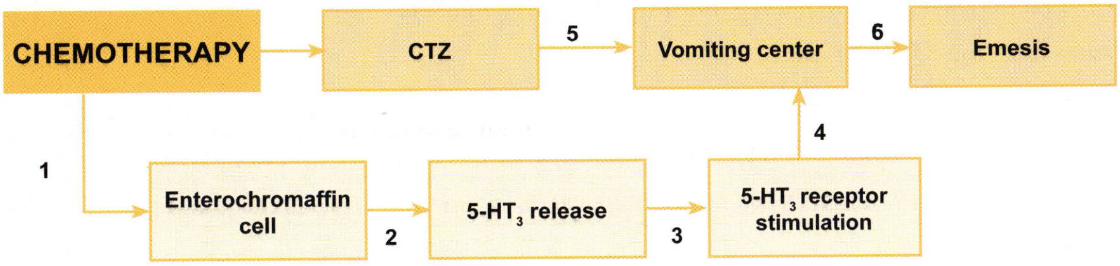

ANTIEMETICS

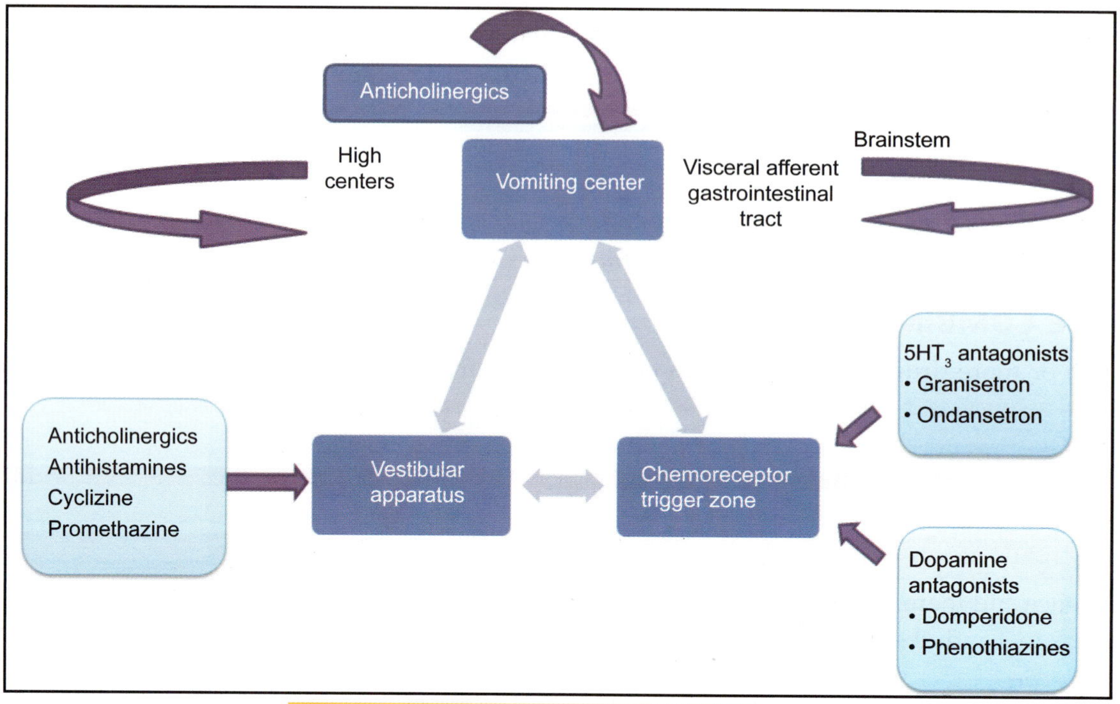

CINV TREATMENT AND PROPHYLAXIS

- **5HT3 Antagonists**: *Dolasectron, Granisetron, Ondansetron, Palonosetron*
- **NK1 Blocker**: *Aprepitant*
- **Corticosteroids**: *Methylprednisolane, Dexamethasone*
- **Dopamine antagonists**: *Prochlorperazine, Olanzapine, Metoclopramide*
- **Cannabinoids**: *Nabilane, Dronabinol*

5HT3 RECEPTOR ANTAGONISTS

- 5HT3 receptors are present in Chemoreceptor trigger zone.
- Causes nausea and Vomiting when stimulated by Serotonin released by Enterochromaffin cells in response to Chemotherapy.
- **Drugs:** Ondansetron, Granisetron, Palonosteron and Dolasetron.
- **Ondansetron–Drug of choice for Early onset chemotherapy induced Nausea and Vomiting** (Shortest acting).
- **Palonosetron–** Most potent and Longest acting (Preferred for Late onset Nausea and Vomiting).
- ***Not used for Apomorphine induced emesis (Risk of hypotension).***
- ***Effective for Hyperemesis of pregnancy and Postoperative nausea.***
- ***Dolasetron–*** Prolongs QT interval.

Drug of choice for Early onset chemotherapy induced Nausea and Vomiting–Ondansetron
Drug of choice for Late onset chemotherapy induced nausea and vomiting–Aprepitant
Preferred drugs for Postoperative vomiting–5HT3 Antagonists

Contd.

Contd.

Drug of choice for Motion sickness–Scopalamine
Drug of choice for Hiccups–Chlorpromazine

Ref: KDT 8th Edition Page 716, Katzung 13th Edition Page 583, Goodman and Gilman 13th Edition Page 935

Ans: (A) Granisetron

21. A patient is brought to casualty with acute attack of asthma after starting treatment of Glaucoma. Causative drug is:

A. Timolol B. Betaxolol

C. Clonidine D. Acetazolamide

Key:

Timolol is a Non selective beta blocker that acts against beta 2 receptors present in ciliary process and reduces secretion of Aqueous
Life–threatening bronchospasm is seen in asthmatic and COPD patients with beta blockers

Beta 2 stimulation→ Vasodilatation→ Increased secretion of Aqueous
Beta blockers inhibit this and causes vasoconstriction

ANTI GLAUCOMA DRUGS

- ***Reduced aqueous secretion***
  - **Beta blockers**
    - *Cardioselective–Betaxolol, Levo betaxolol*
    - *Non selective–Timolol, Levobunolol, Carteolol*
  - **Alpha 2 agonists**
    - *Brimonidine*
    - *Apraclonidine*
  - **Carbonic anhydrase inhibitors**
    - *Acetazolamide, Dorzolamide, Brinzolamide*
- ***Increase aqueous outflow***
  - **Increased trabecular outflow**
    - ***Miotics**–Pilocarpine, Physostigmine*
    - ***Alpha 2 agonists**–Dipivefrine*
  - **Increased Uveoscleral outflow**
    - *Latanoprost, Bimatoprost*

Drug of choice for Open angle Glaucoma–Latanoprost
Drug of choice for Closed angle Glaucoma–Acetazolamide
Drug of choice for Normal tension Glaucoma–Latanoprost

Drugs and Their Side Effects	
Pilocarpine, Physostigmine, Carbachol and Echothiophate	Ciliary body spasm (Accommodation difficulty), Induced myopia, Brow ache, Corneal edema and Retinal detachment
Echothiophate	***Iris cysts and Nasolacrimal duct stenosis***
Physostigmine and Echothiophate	***Cataract***
Latanoprost and Bimatoprost	Heterochromia iridis, Trichomegaly, Dry sandy eyes and Periorbital fat depletion
Beta blockers	Timolol–Nasolacrimal duct stenosis Can cause bronchoconstriction–*Aggravates Asthma* ***Betoxolol–Best retinal neuroprotective effect→safe in asthmatics*** ***Bradycardia, accentuation of heart block and CHF occur especially in elderly***
Apraclonidine	***Lid retraction***
Brimonidine	***CNS depression, Drowsiness***
Dipivefrine, Adrenaline	Black pigmentation of conjunctiva (Adenochrome)

Ref: KDT 8th Edition Page 169, Katzung 13th Edition Page 168, Goodman and Gilman 13th Edition Page 171

Ans: (A) Timolol

22. Teduglutide drug used for malabsorption in short bowel syndrome. True about this is:

A. It is effective orally
B. GLP2 agonist
C. It is a pancreatic enzyme
D. Bile sequestrant

Key:

Teduglutide is 33 amino acid GLP-2 analogue recently approved for treatment of short-bowel syndrome

Teduglutide

- **GLP2 Analogue**
- Gut hormone GLP-2 is secreted by L cells of ileum and colon
- *Only intestinotrophic gut peptide.*

Pharmacokinetics

- Resistant to degradation by proteolytic enzyme Dipeptidyl peptidase 4
- Longer half life than GLP2
- Well tolerated

Mechanism of Action

- Enhances growth of the intestinal mucosa through release of mediators, including IGF 1.
- Leads to restoration of intestinal functional and structural integrity through significant intetinotropic and proabsorptive effects.

Contd.

Contd.

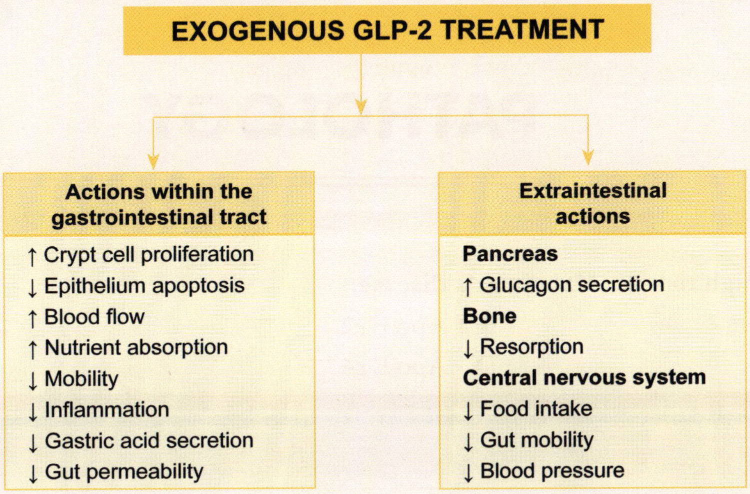

Therapeutic Uses

- Teduglutide is ***administered subcutaneously*** once daily (0.05 mg/kg).
- Helps to improve intestinal absorption of nutrients and thereby reduces need for parenteral support.

First targeted therapeutic agent to gain approval for use in adult short bowel syndrome with intestinal failure

Side Effects

- Abdominal pain, Nausea, Headache and Flu-like symptoms.
- It also has the potential to cause cancer of the bowel (Not recommended for patients with active malignancies).

Ref: Goodman and Gilman 13th Edition Page 939, Sabiston 20th Edition Page 1292

Ans: (B) GLP2 agonist

Chapter 5

PATHOLOGY

1. **Gene associated with high risk of Alzheimer's disease:**

   A. Apo E ε1 B. Apo E ε2

   C. Apo E ε3 D. Apo E ε4

Key:

Gene associated with high risk of Alzheimer's disease is Apo E ε4
Each Apo E ε4 allele present increases the risk of AD by approximately 4 fold and also appears to lower age of onset

ALZHEIMER DISEASE

- Most common cause of cortical dementia
- Most common cause of Dementia in elderly
- Predominantly affects Temporoparietal cortex *(Frontal lobe is also frequently involved)*
- Most important risk factor for Alzheimer's disease–Old age and Family history
- Earliest sites involved–Hippocampus, Entorhinal cortex and Amygdala

Risk Factors
• Increasing age, Female sex, Family history of dementia, Aluminium, Virions and Prions, APP, Adult with trisomy 21, Lower educational attainment, Past history of head trauma, Elevated homocysteine, cholesterol, HTN and Insufficient exercise
Reduced Risk
• Post menopausal estrogen use and NSAID use

GENETICS

- Most cases are sporadic, 5-10% are familial
- Individuals carrying the E4 allele are at increased risk of Alzheimer's disease compared with those carrying more common E3 allele
- Apo E2 allele is associated with decreased risk.

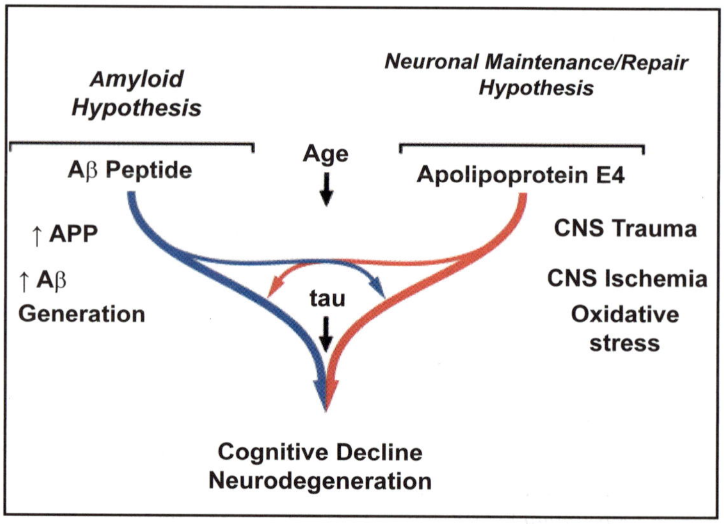

Genes causing Autosomal dominant	**APP (Chr 21), PSEN 1 (Chr 14) and PSEN 2 (Chr 1)** *All can cause early onset disease but PSEN 2 is associated with broad range of onset ages*
Susceptibility genes	**Apo E (Apolipoprotein E)→ Chromosome 19** • **Reduced risk–** *ε2 allele* • **Neutral–** *ε3 allele* • **High risk–** *ε4 allele* ***(Especially Homozygous state)*** **SORL 1**

In sporadic early onset type of Alzheimer's disease, apolipoprotein gene E4 codes for a product that cannot eliminate A beta from brain leading to early onset of neurotoxicity.

- Presence of the *APO E*4 allele is also associated with increased risk of cerebral amyloid angiopathy and age-related cognitive decline during normal ageing.
- Adults with Trisomy 21 consistently develop Neuropathologic hallmarks of Alzheimer's disease if they survive more than 40 years.

Clinical Features

- Subtle onset memory loss followed by slowly progressive dementia over several years
- Brain gets diffusely atrophied (20% or more weight reduction)
- Gradual development of forgetfulness–Major symptom.

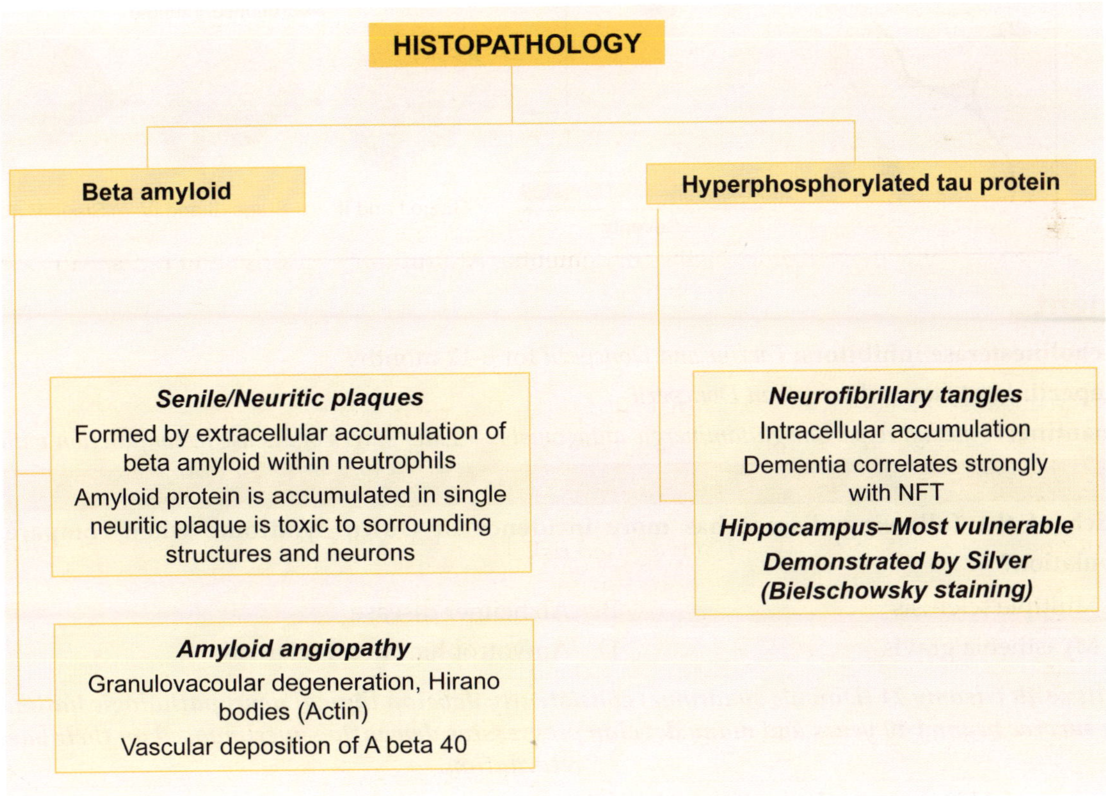

Biochemical Features

- **Decreased levels of Acetylcholine–Primary biochemical abnormality** *(Related to loss of memory).*
- **Reduced levels of Noradrenaline, Serotonin and Somatostatin** *(Related to sensory disturbance and aggressive behavior).*

BRAAK AND BRAAK STAGING

Stage (Amyloid Plaque)	Stage (Neurofibrillary Tangles)	Region Involved	Clinical Feature	Temporal Order
A	I	Along Entorhinal cortex	Memory disturbances	*Preclinical*
	II	CA1 region of Hippocampus	Memory disturbances	
B	III	Limbic structure like subiculum	Cognitive impairment	*Limbic*
	IV	Amygdala, Thalamus and Claustrum	Cognitive impairment	
C	V	Affects Association areas	Alzheimer's disease	*Isocortical*
	VI	Primary sensory motor and visual areas involved	Alzheimer's disease	

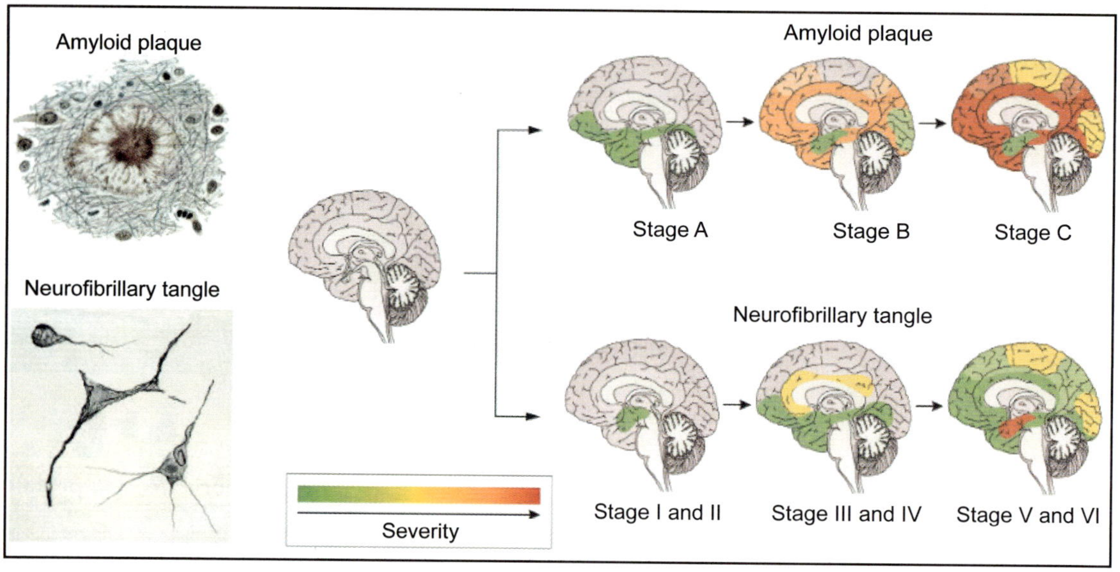

Treatment

- **Anticholinesterase inhibitors:** *Tacrine and Donepezil* for 6-12 months
- **Donepezil:** *Most favoured drug than Donepezil*
- **Memantine:** *N methyl Aspartate glutaminergic antagonists → Later stages of disease in conjunction with cholinergic drugs*

Version 2

Which of the following disease has more incidence in Down syndrome when compared with normal population?

A. Multiple sclerosis
B. Alzheimer disease
C. Myasthenia gravis
D. Amyotrophic lateral sclerosis

Adults with trisomy 21 (Down's syndrome) consistently develop typical neuropathologic hallmarks of AD if they survive beyond 40 years and many develop progressive dementia superimposed on their baseline mental retardation.

Extra dose of APP gene on chromosome 21 is initiating cause of AD in adult Down's syndrome and results in excess cerebral amyloid production.

APP gene is on chromosome 21.

Ans: (B) Alzheimer disease

Ref: Robbin's 9th Edition Page 835, Harrison 20th Edition Page 3048, Harsh Mohan 7th Edition Page 876, Harper 30th Edition Page 275

Ans: (D) Apo E ε 4

2. **Cytokines that cause Vasodilatation and Inhibits Platelet Aggregation is:**

A. PgF2 alpha
B. PgD2
C. TxA2
D. PgI2

Key:

PgI_2→ Prostacyclin–Formed by endothelial cells Causes vasodilatation and Inhibits platelet aggregation

- PgD2 and PgE2 are formed from Mast cells–Vasodilatation
- **PgD2–** *Chemoattractant for Neutrophils*
- PgF2 alpha– Contracts uterine and bronchial smooth muscle
- TxA2 formed from platelets–-Vasoconstrictor and Platelet aggregation
- LTB4– Most potent Chemotactic agent→ Activator of Neutrophils
- LTC4,D4 and E4– Increase vascular permeability and Bronchoconstriction

Action	Eicosanoid
Vasodilation	Prostaglandins PGI_2 (protacyclin), PGE_1, PGE_2, PGD_2
Vasoconstriction	Thromboxane A_2, leukotrienes C_4, D_4, E_4
Increased vascular permeability	Leukotrienes C_4, D_4, E_4
Chemotaxis, leukocyte adhesion	Leukotriene B_4, HETE

	Organ	Prostaglandin E_2 (PGE_2)	Prostaglandin F_{2a} (PGF_{2a})	Prostacyclin (PGI_2)	Thromboxane A_2 (TXA_2)
1.	Blood vessels	Vasodilation, ↓ BP	Vasodilatation (mostly), larger veins constrict, little effect on BP	Vasodilatation (marked and widespread), ↓ ↓ BP	Vasoconstriction
2.	Heart	Weak inotropic, reflex cardiac stimulation	Weak inotropic	–	–
3.	Platelets	Variable effect	–	Anti-aggregatory	Aggregation and release reaction
4.	Uterus	Contraction (*in vivo*), relaxes nongravid human uterus *in vitro*, softening of cervix	Constriction *(in vivo* and *in vitro)* softening of cervix	–	–
5.	Bronchi	Dilatation, Inhibit histamine release	Constriction	Dilatation (mild), inhibit histamine release	Constriction
6.	Stomach	↓ acid secretion ↑ mucus production	–	↓ acid secretion (week), mucosal vasodilatation	–

Contd.

Contd.

7.	Intestine	Contracts longitudinal and relaxes circular muscles, ↑ peristalsis, ↑ Cl^- and water secretion	Spasmogenic, ↑ fluid and electrolyte secretion (weak)	Weak spasmogenic, inhibit toxin-induced fluid secretion	Weak spasmogenic
8.	Kidney	Natriuresis, ↓Cl^- reabsorption, inhibit ADH action, vasodilatation, renin release	–	Natriuresis, vasodilatation, renin release	Vasoconstriction
9.	CNS	Pyrogenic, variety of effects on I.C.V. inj.	–	–	–
10.	Release of NA	↑ or ↓	↑ or ↓	–	–
11.	Afferent nerves	Sensitize to noxious stimuli → tenderness	–	Same as PGE_2	–
12.	Endocrine system	Release of ant. pituitary hormones, steroids, insulin; TSH-like action	Release of gonadotropins and prolacting, luteolysis (in animal)	–	–
13.	Metabolism	Antilipolytic, insulin like action, mobilization of bone Ca^{2+}	–	–	–

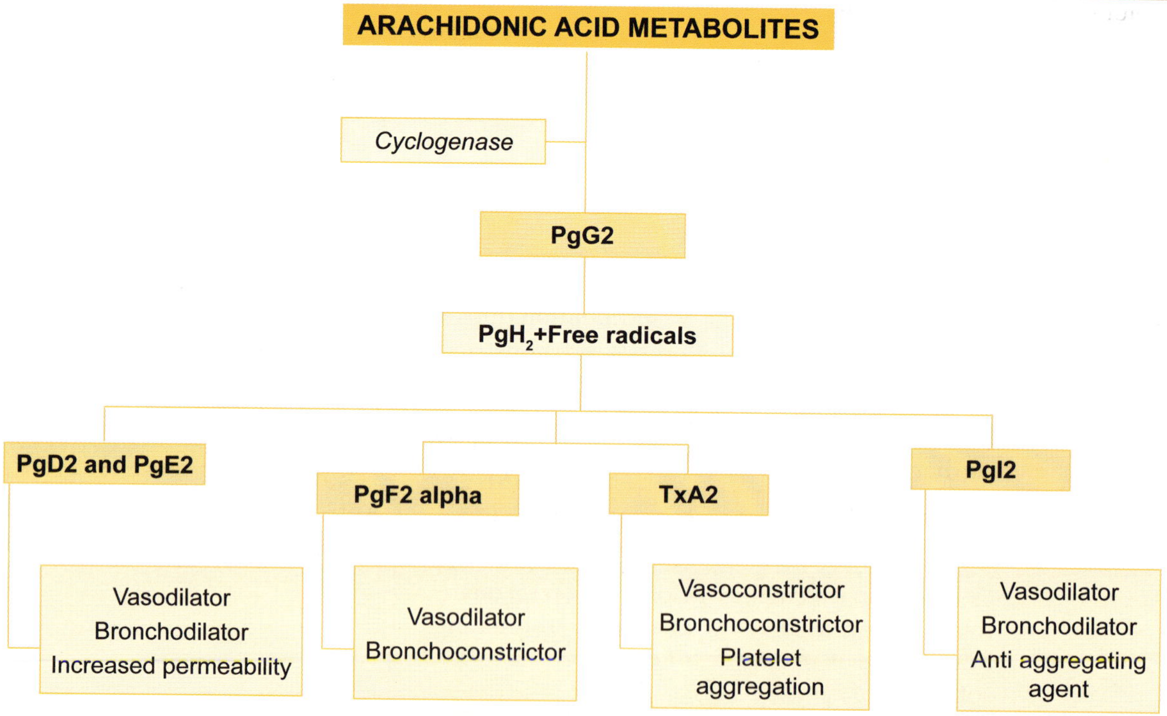

Ref: Robbin's 9th Edition Page 46, Harsh Mohan 7th Edition Page 124

Ans: (D) PgI2

3. **Glanzman thrombesthenia is due to:**

A. Gp Ib-IX deficiency
B. Gp Ib/IIa deficiency
C. Gp IIb/IIIa deficiency
D. Deficiency of ADAMTS 13

Key:

Glanzmann's thrombasthenia is an abnormality of the platelets and an extremely rare coagulopathy in which platelets contain defective/low levels of glycoprotein IIb/IIIa. Glycoprotein IIb/IIIa is an integrin that helps in platelet to platelet aggregation by binding fibrinogen

PLATELET FUNCTION DEFECTS

- *Defects in platelet adhesion*
  - *Von Willebrand disease*
  - *Bernard-Soulier syndrome*
- *Defect in platelet aggregation*
  - *Glanzmann's thrombasthenia*
- *Defect of platelet secretion*
  - *Decreased cyclo oxygenase activity*
  - *Drug induced NSAID*
  - *Granule storage pool defects*
- *Scott syndrome*

GLANZMANN THROMBASTHENIA

- Autosomal recessive inheritance
- Platelet aggregation defect disorder
- Occurs due to deficiency of glycoprotein IIb/IIIa
- Presents with increased bleeding from umbilical cord stump at birth

Lab Features

- Bleeding time prolonged.
- PT and aPTT is normal.
- ***Ristocetin adhesion test +ve.***
- Platelet aggregation with ADP, collagen or epinephrine is defective.

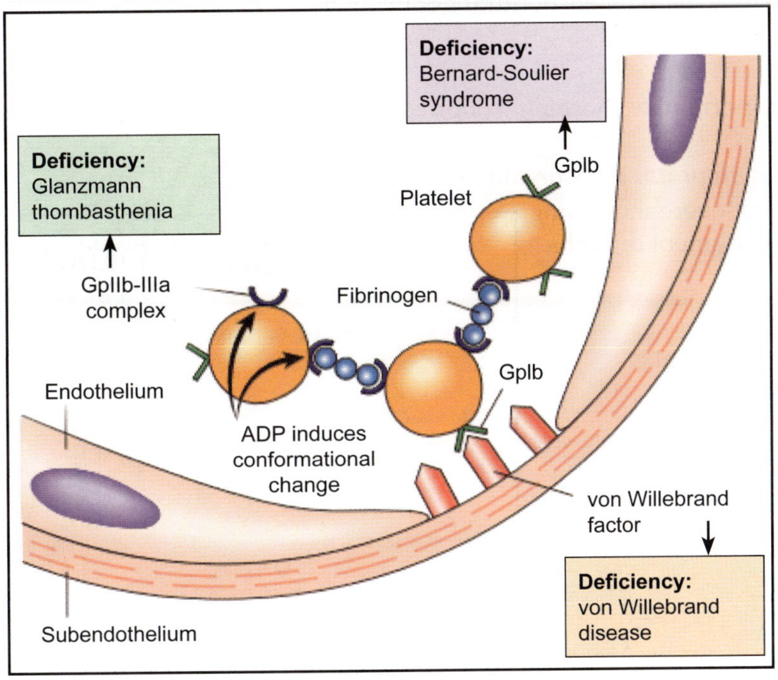

BERNARD-SOULIER SYNDROME

- **Autosomal recessive inheritance**
- Platelet adhesion defect disorder
- Occurs due to Glycoprotein Ib-IX deficiency (Gp Ib-IX→ platelet receptor for von Willebrand factor that is necessary for platelet collagen adhesion
- **Presents with mild thrombocytopenia and Giant platelets**

Lab Features

- **Bleeding time is prolonged**
- PT and aPTT is normal
- Risticetin adhesion test is –ve/Abnormal
- Platelet aggregation with ADP, collagen or epinephrine is normal

Deficiency of ADAMTS13 occurs in Thrombotic thrombocytopenic purpura→ Acquired
Upshaw Schulman syndrome–Inherited deficiency of ADAMTS13.

Ref: Robbin's 9th Edition Page 81, Harsh Mohan 7th Edition Page 334, Hoffman 4th Edition Page 847, Harrison 20th Edition Page 828

Ans: (C) Gp IIb/IIIa deficiency

4. Achondroplasia is:

A. Autosomal dominant disorder
B. Autosomal recessive disorder
C. X-linked dominant disorder
D. X-linked recessive disorder

Key:

Achondroplasia is an Autosomal dominant disorder

ACHONDROPLASIA

- **Autosomal dominant disorder**
- **Most common form of dwarfism**
- Caused by activating point mutations in FGFR3
- Affects all bones that develop by enchondral ossification

Clinical Features

- Short stature, disproportionate shortening of proximal extremities, bowing of legs and frontal bossing with midface hypoplasia.
- *Cartilage of the growth plates is disorganized and hypoplastic.*
- Disproportionate and severe shortening marked in proximal segment of limbs.
- *Trident hands.*
- Spinal stenosis.
- Mental development normal.
- **Autosomal dominant.**
- **X-Ray**; Hour glass appearance–ace tabular roof is almost horizontal.
- No treatment exists for this condition.

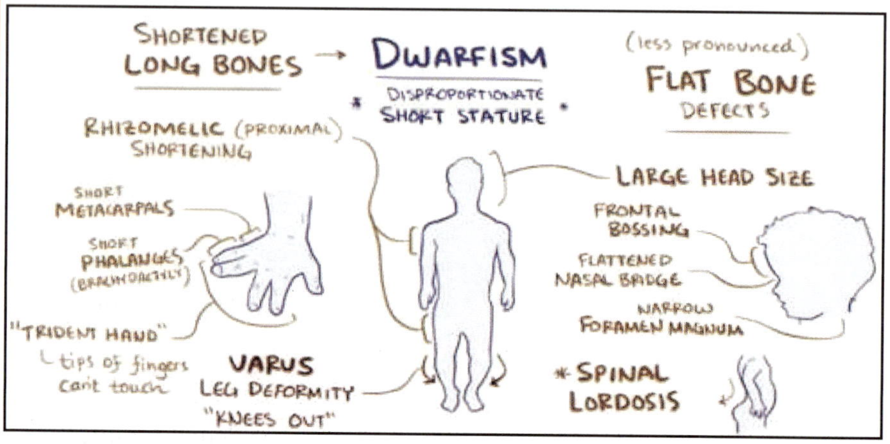

Autosomal Dominant	Autosomal Recessive
Achondroplasia	***Thalassemia***
Acute intermittent porphyria	***Sickle cell anemia***
Huntington's disease	Cystic fibrosis
Familial hypercholesterolemia	Hemochromatosis
Tuberous sclerosis	Albinism
NF	Wilson's disease
Marfan's syndrome	Xeroderma pigmentosum
Osteogenesis Imperfecta	Alkaptonuria
Osteopetrosis	Phenylketonuria
Von Willebrand disease	Fanconi's anemia
Retinoblastoma	Friedrich ataxia
Von Hippel Lindau disease	Dubin Johnson syndrome, Rotor syndrome
Myotonic dystrophy	Congenital adrenal hyperplasia
Adult polycystic kidney disease	Chediak Hegashi syndrome
FAP	Ataxia telangiectasia
Peutz Jeghers syndrome	Bloom syndrome
Ehlers Danlos syndrome	***Lysosomal storage disorders (Except Hunter and Fabrys disease)***
Hypokalemic periodic paralysis	Hurler syndrome
Hereditary spherocytosis	Sphingolipidoses–Niemann Pick, Tay sachs, Gauchers, Sandhoff, Metachromatic leukodystrophy
Osler Weber Rendu disease	Glycogen storage disorders (Type 1-7)

Autosomal Codominant
ABO Blood groups
Alpha 1 antrypsin deficiency
HLA Antigens

X Linked Dominant	X Linked Recessive
Fragile X syndrome	***Colour Blindness***
Alport syndrome	Hemophilia A
Incontinentia Pigmenti	G6PD deficiency
Rett syndrome	Diabetes insipidus
Charcot Marie tooth disease X linked	Chronic granulomatous disease
Hypophosphatemic rickets	Burton agammaglobulinemia
Goltz syndrome	Muscular dystrophy–DMD, BMD
	Hunter's disease
	Lesch Nyhan syndrome
	Wiskott Aldrich syndrome
	Ocular albinism
	Menkes disease
	Fabry's disease
	Testicular feminization syndrome

Ref: Robbin's Textbook of Pathology 9th Edition Page 767, Harsh Mohan 7th Edition Page 255, Harper Textbook of Biochemistry, Textbook of Biochemistry by DM Vasudevan 7th Edition Page 499

Ans: (A) Autosomal dominant disorder

5. **Vitamin A is stored in which cells?**

A. Ito cells
B. Kupffer cells
C. Sinusoidal cells
D. Endothelial cells

Key:

Ito cells store Vitamin A rich inclusions and secrete several extracellular matrix proteins and proteoglycans

ITO CELLS

- Also called as Stellate cells/Fat storing cells/Lipocytes/Interstitial cells
- Present in extrasinusoidal space called space of disse
- Exist in space between parenchymal cells and liver sinusoidal endothelial cells of the hepatic lobule
- ***Identified histologically by their large lipid vacuoles.***
- Helps in Vitamin A metabolism and collagen producing myofibroblast during inflammation
- ***Hepatic fibrosis/Cirrhosis occurs due to collagen Type 1 and 3 produced by Ito cells.***

Normal Liver
Collagen Type 1 and 3 is present at portal tract and around Central vein. Collagen Type 4 present in space of disse.
Cirrhotic Liver
Collagen Type 1 and 3 both are present at space of disse.

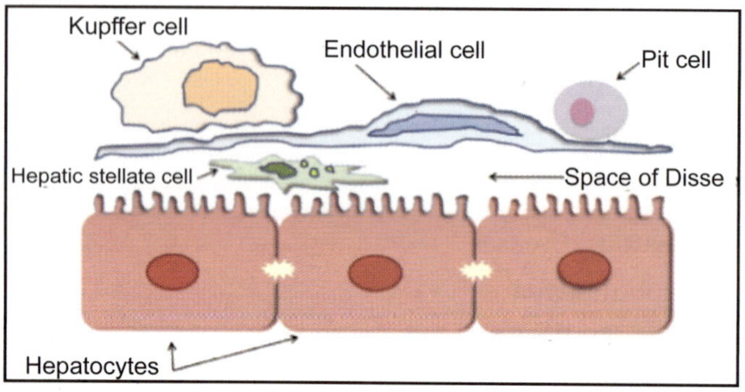

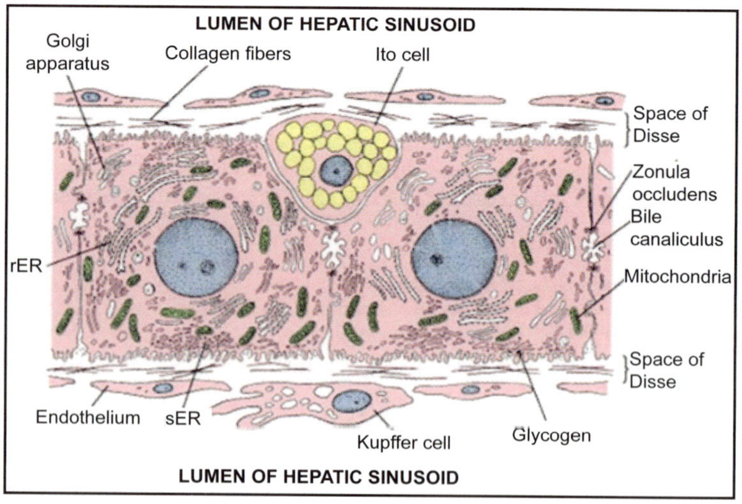

KUPFFER CELLS

- Mononuclear macrophage cells attached to luminal surface of Endothelial cells

SINUSOIDS

- Blood vessels with fenestration in endothelial lining and gaps in Basement membrane

Ref: Robbin's 9th Edition Page 436, Harsh Mohan 7th Edition Page 578

Ans: (B) Kupffer cells

6. **Which of the following is an Autosomal recessive disorder?**

A. G6PD
B. Marfan's syndrome
C. Familial hypophatemic rickets
D. Albinism

Key:

Albinism is an Autosomal recessive disorder

Autosomal Recessive Disorders	
Metabolic	**Cystic fibrois**
	Phenylketonuria
	Galactosemia
	Homocystinuria
	Lysosomal storage disorder
	Alpha 1 antitrypsin deficiency
	Wilson's disease
	Hemochromatosis
	Glycogen storage disorder
	Albinism
Hematopoietic	Sickel cell anemia Thalassemia
Endocrine	Congenital adrenal hyperplasia
Skeletal	Ehlers-Danlos syndrome Alkaptonuria
Nervous	Neurogenic muscular atrophies Friedreich ataxia Spinal muscular atrophy

Refer to above Question 4

Ref: Robbin's 9th Edition Page 141, Harsh Mohan 7th Edition Page 255, Harper Textbook of Biochemistry, Textbook of Biochemistry by DM Vasudevan 7th Edition Page 499

Ans: (D) Albinism

7. **Which of the following is an anti apoptic gene?**

A. Bcl 2
B. BAX
C. BAK
D. BAD

Key:

Anti apoptotic genes–BCL 2, BCL XL, MCL 1
Pro apoptotic genes–BAX, BAK
Sensors–BAD, BIM, BID, Puma, Noxa

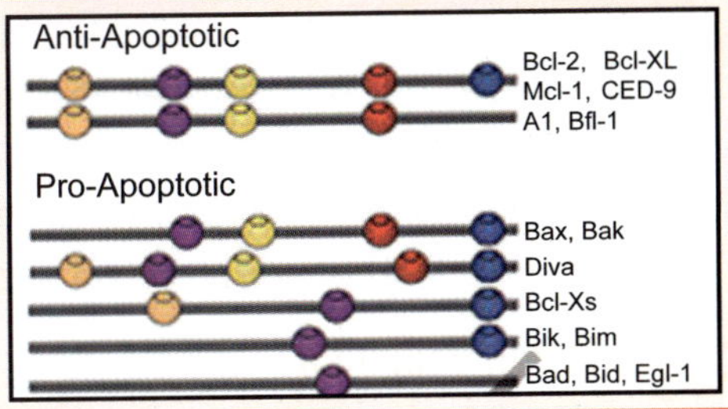

APOPTOSIS

- *Programmed cell death*
- Active process (Energy dependent process–since it involves Mitochondria)

Etiology	
Physiologic Causes	**Pathologic Causes**
• Embryogenesis, Organogenesis and Neovascularization • Hormone dependent involution of endometrium and prostate • Cell depletion in intestinal epithelium • Cell death after function of neutrophils • Deletion of harmful self reactive lymphocytes	• Cytotoxic chemotherapy • Radiotherapy • Accumulation of misfolded protein-like *Alzheimer disease*

MECHANISM OF APOPTOSIS

- **Results from activation of enzymes called caspases**
- **Marker of apoptosis**–*Presence of cleaved active caspases*

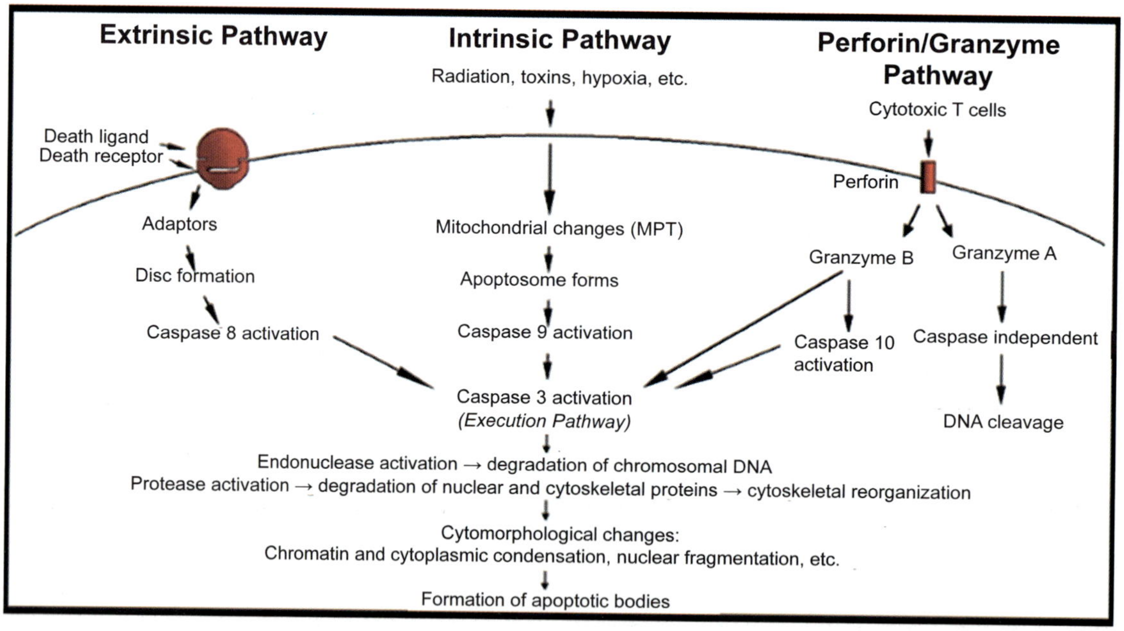

- Caspase involved in Intrinsic pathway– Caspase 9
- Caspase involved in Extrinsic pathway– Caspase 8

Morphologic Changes of Apoptosis
• ***Earliest change–Cell shrinkage***
• ***Most characteristic change–Chromatin condensation***
• Formation of cytoplasmic blebs and apoptotic bodies
• Phagocytosis of apoptotic cells/bodies by macrophages

Biochemical Changes in Apoptosis
• ***Hallmark–Caspase activation***   • ***Annexin V–Marker of Apoptosis***   • Hallmark of Neuronal Apoptosis–AIF Activation   • **Agarose gel electrophoresis–*Step ladder pattern*** *(Endonuclease induced internucleosomal damage).*

Anti apoptotic proteins	Proapoptotic proteins	Sensors (BH3 only proteins)
BCL 2, BCL XL, MCL 1 and FLIP	BAX, BAK and Smac/Diablo	BAD, BIM, BID, Puma and Noxa ***Sensors of cellular stress and damage*** ***Act as arbiters of apoptosis***

Most common anti apoptotic gene associated with drug resistance to chemotherapy–MCL 1

BCL 2
• *BCL 2 is human proto-oncogene located on chromosome 18 involved in intrinsic (mitochondrial) phase of the initiation pathway of apoptosis*   • *Normal location of BCL 2 is on the mitochondrial membrane*   • *BCL 2, BCL-XL, and MCL1 are the principal members of anti-apoptotic group*

Feature	Necrosis	Apoptosis
Cell size	Enlarged (swelling)	Reduced (shrinkage)
Nucleus	Pyknosis → karyorrhexis → karyolysis	Fragmentation into nucleosome size fragments
Plasma membrane	Disrupted	Intact; altered structure, especially orientation of lipids
Cellular contents	Enzymatic digestion; may leak out of cell	Intact; may be released in apoptotic bodies
Adjacent inflammation	Frequent	No
Physiologic or pathlogic role	Invariably pathologic (culmination of irreversible cell injury)	Often physiologic; means of eliminating unwanted cells; may be pathologic after some forms of cell injury, especially DNA and protein damage

Ref: Robbin's 9th Edition Page 55, Harsh Mohan 7th Edition Page 31

Ans: (A) Bcl 2

8. IL1 is activated by which of the following?

A. Caspase 9 B. Caspase 8

C. Caspase 1 D. Caspase 5

Key:

IL1 is activated by Caspase 1

NOD-LIKE RECEPTORS

- NOD-like receptors→ Cytosolic receptors that recognize products of necrotic cells (Uric acid and released ATP), Ion disturbances (Loss of K^+) and microbial products.
- NLRs are cytoplasmic leucine rich repeat containing proteins that serve as scaffolding and sensing elements of inflammasome.

- ***NLRs signal via cytosolic multiprotein complex called inflammasome to produce biologically active form of IL-1.***

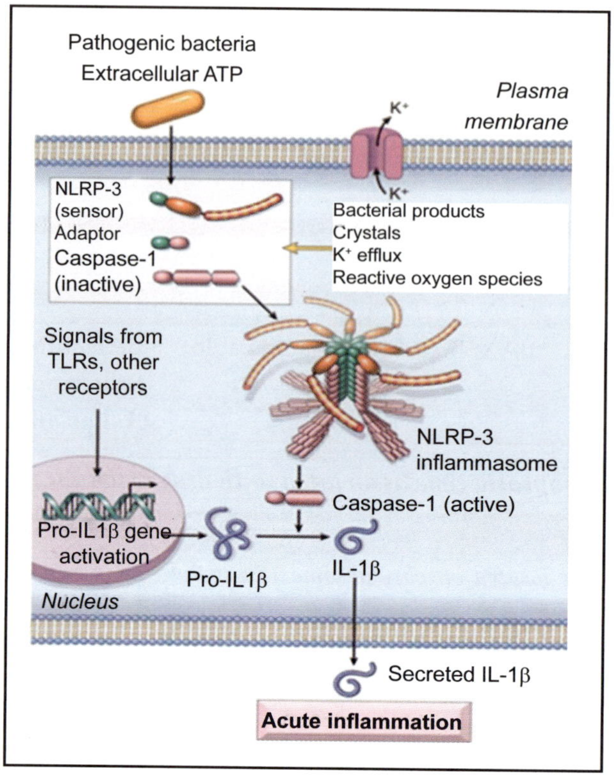

INFLAMMASOME

- Inflammasomes are large cytoplasmic complexes that contain NOD-like receptors that recognizes products of dead cells and microbes.
- Recognition of an intracellular danger signal by the inflammasome activates caspases, intracellular proteases produced as inactive zymogens which trigger inflammatory cascades expressing IL-1β and IL-18.
- Activated caspase 1 converts inactive IL 1 beta to Active form.
- ***It induces secretion of biologically active interleukin-1.***

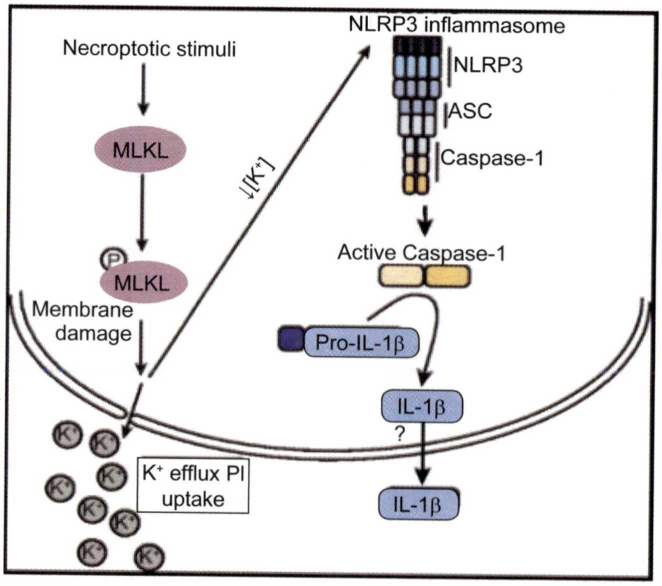

Formation of the inflammasome complex proceeds by prion-like mechanism of propagation→ ***One protein altered by activation induces conformational changes in other proteins of the same type.***

NLR-inflammasome pathway plays a role in conditions like gout, atherosclerosis and type 2 DM

Role of Inflammasome in Gout

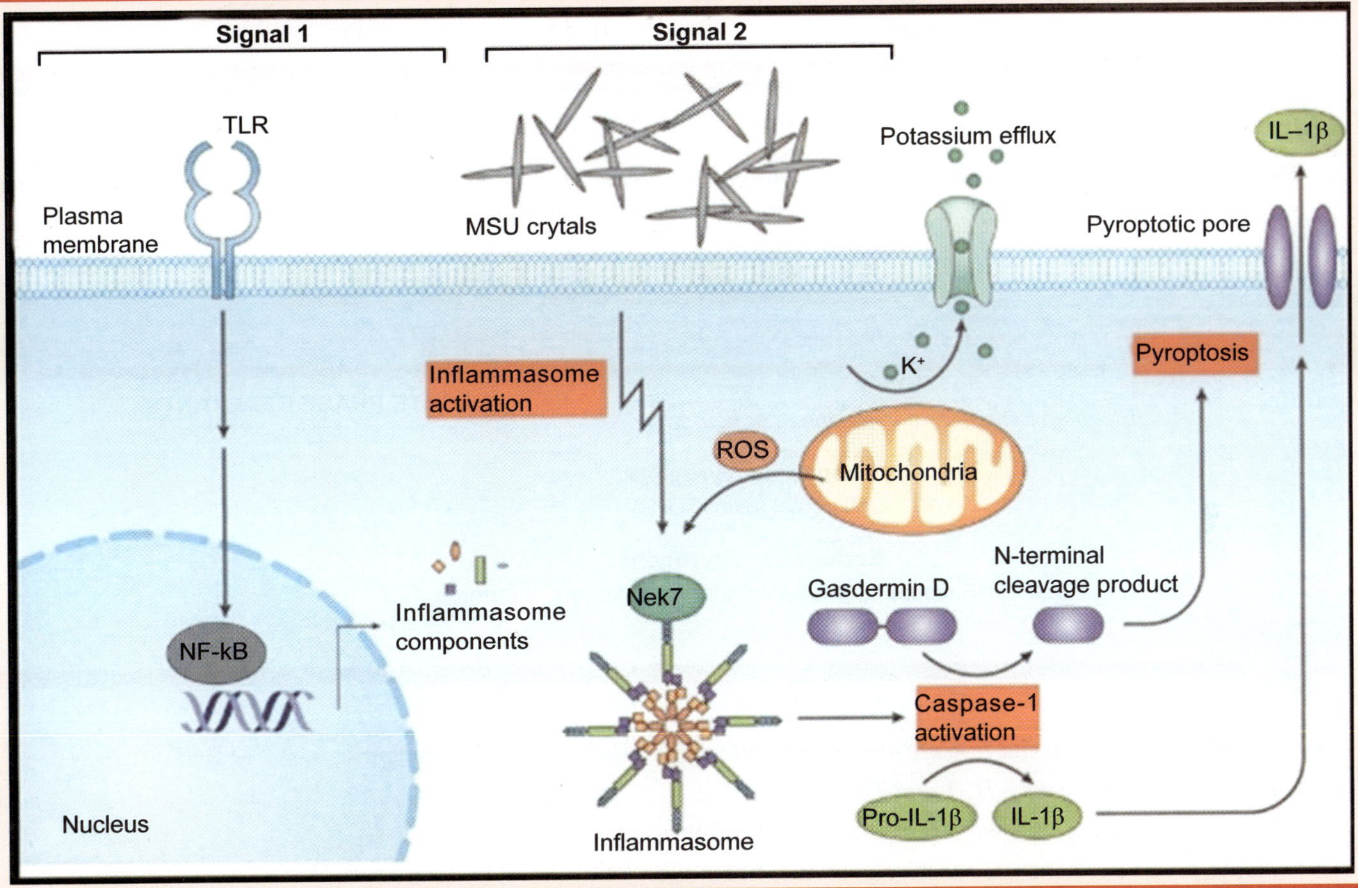

Role of Inflammasome in Rheumatic Disease

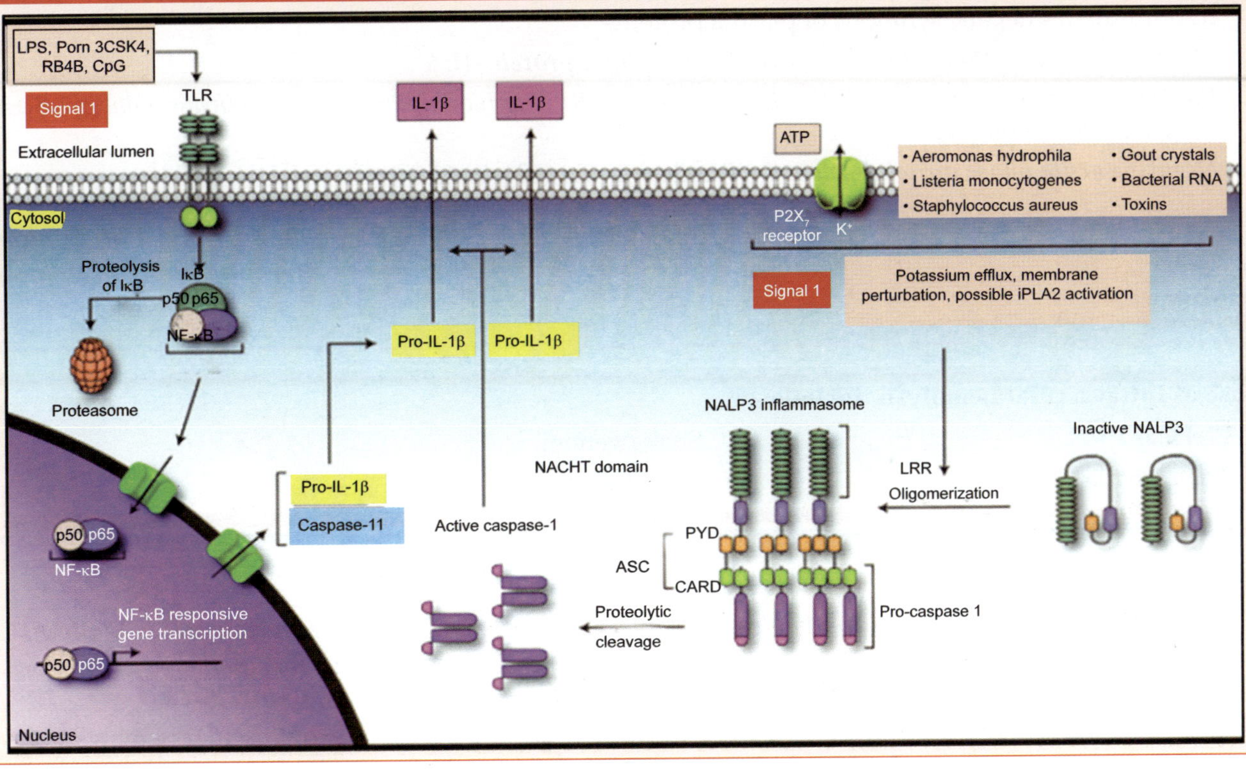

Ref: Robbin's 9th Edition Page 188, Sabiston 20th Edition Page 27

Ans: (C) Caspase 1

9. Which of the following is an Endogenous Pyrogen?

A. IL-1 B. IL-10 C. IL-12 D. IL-4

Key:

Pyrogens (LPS from bacteria) cause macrophages to release IL-1 and TNF→ increase cyclooxygenase activity in perivascular cells of hypothalamus

SYSTEMIC EFFECTS OF INFLAMMATION

- **FEVER** *(Elevated temperature in response to pyrogen)*
  - **Exogenous pyrogens** Microbial toxins (LPS)
  - **Endogenous pyrogens** IL-1, TNF alpha, IL-6, Ciliary neurotropic factors, Interferon
- **ACUTE PHASE REACTANTS**

- *Cytokines TNF, IL-1, and IL-6 are most important mediators of acute-phase reaction*
- ***Endogenous pyrogens – IL-1 and TNF***
- Exogenous pyrogens – Bacterial product→ ***Lipopolysaccharides***
- Acute phase proteins – C reactive proteins, fibrinogen–stimulated by IL-6
- Serum amyloid A protein (SAA)–stimulated by IL-1 or TNF
- IL-6 stimulates hepatic synthesis of plasma proteins
- ***Most important cytokine for synthesis of acute phase protein–IL 6***
- ***Positive acute phase proteins***–*CRP, Highly sensitive CRP, Fibrinogen, Plasminogen activator inhibitor, Serum amyloid A, Ferritin and Ceruloplasmin*
- ***Negative acute phase proteins***–*Albumin, Prealbumin, Transferrin, IGF-1*

Ref: Robbin's 9th Edition Page 99, Harrison 20th Edition Page 862
Harsh Mohan 7th Edition Page 176

Ans: (A) IL-1

10. Cause of Intravascular hemolysis include:

A. PNH B. Snake venom
C. Thalassemia D. Transfusion

Key:

PNH is acquired mutation in phosphatidyl inositol glycan complementation group A (PIGA)
Red cells deficient in GPI linked factor are abnormally susceptible to lysis by complement–Manifests as Intravascular hemolysis caused by Membrane attack complex (C5b-C9)
This is the cause of hemolysis in PNH (Rest of the options cause extravascular hemolysis)

PARAOXYSMAL NOCTURNAL HEMOGLOBINURIA

- **Acquired Intracorpuscular disorder (at stem cell level)→ Clonal stem cell disorder**
- Characterized by undue sensitivity of RBC membrane to complement

Pathogenesis

- Nomally RBC are protected from complement mediated lysis by regulatory proteins (DAF and MIRL) that attach to cell by GPI (Glycosylphosphatidylinositol)
- PGPA protein is essential for synthesis of GPI→ This process is encoded by PIGA
- PIGA gene is on X chromosome
- *Most important of all complement regulatory protein mutation–MIRL (CD59)*

MUTATION IN PIGA GENE

⇩

Reduced/Absent synthesis of PGPA protein

⇩

GPI is not formed (Glycophosphatidyl inositol)

⇩

Reduced anchorage of complementary regulatory proteins *DAF (CD55), C8 binding protein and MIRL (CD59)*

⇩

Cells become susceptible to lysis by complement

⇩

Intravascular hemolysis

***DAF–Decay accelerating factor** (Activates decay of complement), **MIRL–Membrane inhibitor of reactive lysis** (Inhibits Membrane attack complex)*

CLINICAL MANIFESTATIONS (Triad)

Hemolytic anemia
- Increased activation of complement mediated destruction
- Hemoglobinuria, Hemosiderinuria Hemoglobinemia and Elevated LDH

Thrombosis
- Stimulation of platelet aggregation and Hypercoagulability
- Involves portal, hepatic and cerebral veins (Occurs due to absence of CD59 that results in externalization of phosphatidyl serine)

Pancytopenia
- Lysis of Granulocytes and Platelets (Defect is at stem cell level)
- Granulocytopenia and Thrombocytopenia

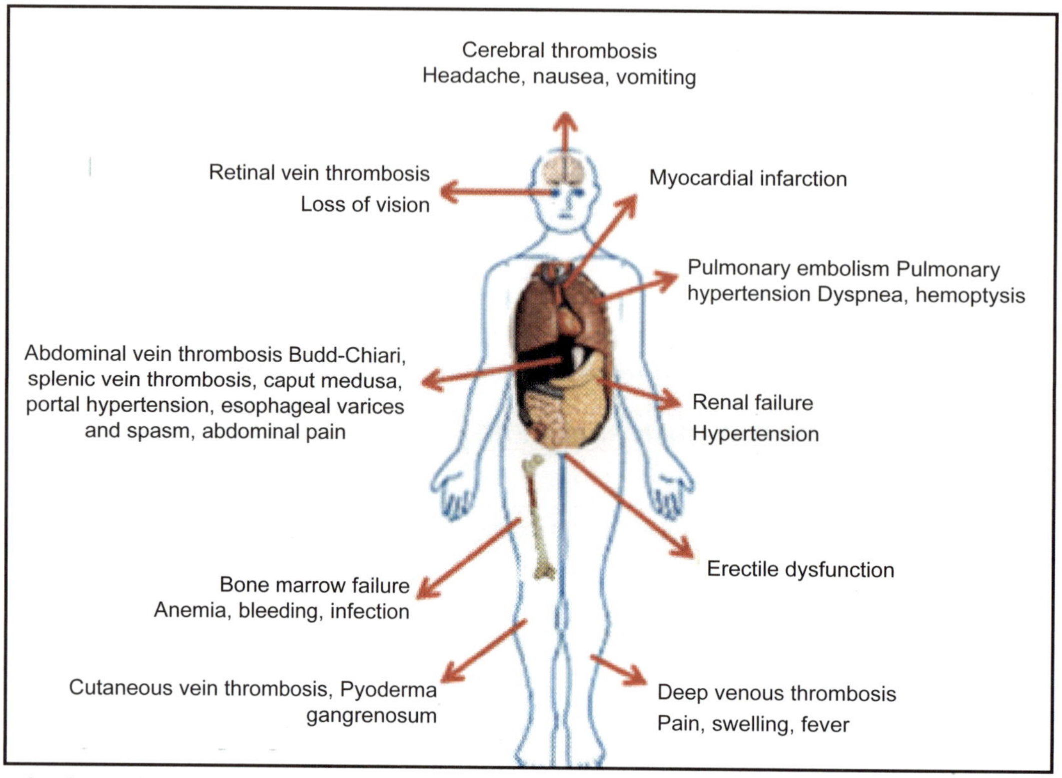

- **Intravascular hemolysis is seen but is paroxysmal and nocturnal in only 25% of cases**
- **Sleep and Exercise precipitates PNH**

Night time→Relative hypoxia→Acidosis→Enhanced complement activity→Complement mediated destruction of RBC→Paroxysm of hemoglobinuria→Identified by brown urine in morning.

- **Most common cause of death in PNH–Thrombosis**
- **Most common site of thrombosis in PNH–Abdominal veins**
- **Frank cerebral thrombosis is a grave complication of PNH**
- Level of Neutrophil/Leukocyte alkaline phosphatase (LAP) is reduced in PNH
  (LAP is GPI linked protein→ Since GPI linked protein is reduced in PNH→LAP reduced)

PNH→ Pancytopenia with cellular bone marrow, Thrombocytopenia with thrombosis

Screening Tests

- **HAM'S Test:** Best screening method→Acidic pH will activate complement pathway for RBC Lysis
- **Sucrose Lysis Test:** Sucrose will reduce pH and this will activate complement pathway

Flow cytometry–Investigation of choice Gold standard / Confirmatory test (Bimodal distribution of red cells)
Simplest method: Analysis of expression of CD59 on RBC

Treatment

- PNH can transform to AML/Myelodysplastic syndrome (20%)
- Bone marrow transplantation can be curative
- Eculizumab–Many patients have improvement

Targeted therapy with an antibody that inhibits C5b–C9 membrane attack complex is effective at diminishing both the hemolysis and the thrombotic complications but has high risk for meningococcal sepsis.

- Transfusion of filtered RBC can also be done

Hemolysis		
	Extravascular	Intravascular
Causes	Thalassemia, Hemoglobinopathies, Enzyme defects, Membrane disorders, Autoimmune hemolytic anemia, Drug induced hemolysis, DIC, HUS/TTP, Eclampsia/Pre eclampsia, Mali-gnancy ***Malaria, Infectious mononucleosis, Mycoplasma pneumonia***	PNH, PCH, Trauma, Microangiopathic hemolytic anemia, ABO mismatched transfusion, Thermal burns, Snake bites, Mechanical heart valves ***Plasmodium falciparum, Clostridium welchii, Babesiosis, Bartonellosis, Mycoplasma pneumonia***
Serum haptoglobin	Normal	*Reduced*
Serum methalbumin	-ve	+ve
LDH	Slightly increased	*Markedly increased*
Hemosiderinuria	Absent	Present
Hemoglobinuria	Absent	Present
Plasma hemoglobin	-ve	+ve
Serum bilirubin (Unconjugated)	Marked increase	Mild increase
Splenomegaly	Usual	Uncommon
Tissue iron in spleen and Liver	Increased	Reduced

Location	Mechanism	Examples	Mode
Intrinsic	Enzyme deficiency	G6PD deficiency	Hereditary
	Hemoglobinopathies	Sickle cell anemia, thalassemia	
	Membrane abnormalities	Hereditary spherocytosis	
		PNH	
	Immune-mediated	Autoimmune; drug-induced, tx rxn	
	Traumatic	MAHA; protheses (valves, TIPS)	
Extrinsic	Direct infections, toxins	Malaria, babesiosis; snake and spider venoms; Wilson's; hypotonic infusions	Acquired
	Entrapment	Hypersplenism	

Ref: Robbin's 9th Edition Page 417, Harrison 20th Edition Page 721, Harsh Mohan 7th Edition Page 314

Ans: (A) PNH

11. True about Fragile X syndrome is:

A. Trinucleotide CAG Sequence mutation
B. Males have IQ 20-40
C. 10% of females are mentally retarded
D. Gain of function mutation

Key:

> ***Fragile X syndrome is a Trinucleotide CGG mutation (Loss of function) with male IQ 20-60 and 30-50% carrier females are mentally retarded***

FRAGILE X SYNDROME

- Second most common genetic cause of mental retardation
  (Most common–Down syndrome)

GENETICS

- Caused by Trinucleotide repeats CGG mutation in familial mental retardation 1 → Loss of *FMR1* gene function (FRAXA)→ ***Cytoplasmic protein abundant in brain and testis***

GENETIC BASIS

- **Normal population** *(29-55 CGG repeats)*
- **Carrier males and females Carry pre mutations** *(55-200 CGG repeats)*
- **Full mutation** *(200-4000 repeats)*

- *Other gene protein involved:* FMR-2 protein (FRAXE)
- This Disorder occurs during Oogenesis (Other disorders like Huntington disease occur during spermatogenesis).
- ***During Oogenesis permutation is converted to Full mutation***
- 30-50% carrier females→ Mentally retarded
- 20% are male carriers

FRAGILE X-ASSOCIATED TREMOR-ATAXIA

- Phenotypically different from Fragile X syndrome (Gain of function)
- Characterized by intention tremors and cerebellar ataxia
- It may progress to ***parkinsonism.***

Clinical Features

- Long face with large mandible
- Large ears
- Large testicles (Macroorchidism)
- Hyperextensible joints
- High arched palate
- Mitral valve prolapsed
- ***Male IQ→ 20-60***

> ***Macroorchidism→ 90% of post pubertal males (Only distinctive physical abnormality)***

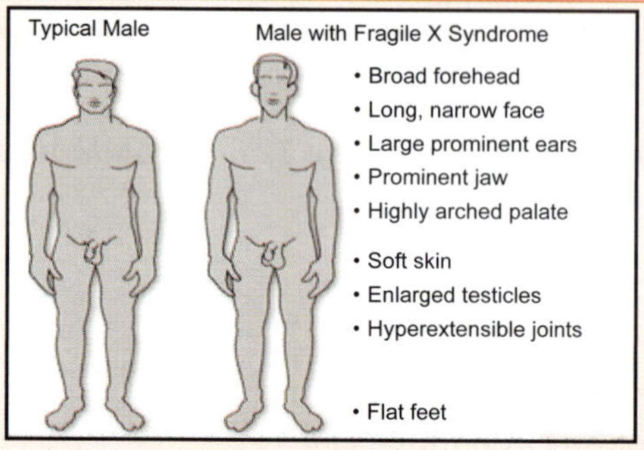

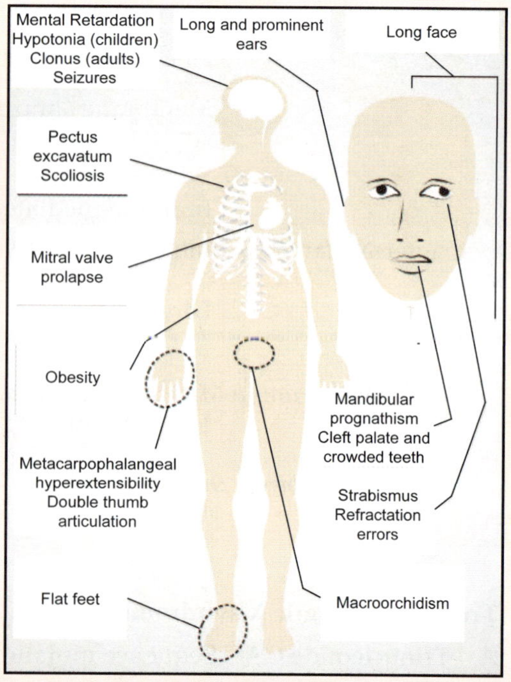

- Approximately 30% of ***females carrying premutation*** have premature ovarian failure (before 40 years).
- About one third of ***premutation-carrying males*** exhibit progressive neurodegenerative syndrome starting in their sixth decade.

Anticipation: Clinical features worsen with each successive generation as number of repeats increase with each generation ***(Symptoms at an early age)***	
Sherman's Paradox: Risk of expressing mental retardation in Fragile X syndrome increases in later generations (Risk of MR in grandson is more than in brother of transmitting male)	

- Diagnosis–*PCR*
- ***DNA analysis to identify Trinucleotide repeats–BEST TEST***
- Southern blotting is used for Genetic counselling

Disease	Gene Protein	Repeat	Inheritance
Fragile X syndrome (FRAXA)	FMR-1 protein (FMRP)	CGG	X linked recessive
Fragile X syndrome (FRAXE)	FMR-2 protein	GCC	X linked recessive
Spinobulbar muscular atrophy (Kennedy disease)	Androgen receptor	CAG	X linked recessive
Myotonic dystrophy	Myotonic dystrophy protein kinase	CTG	Autosomal dominant
Huntington's disease	Huntingtin	CAG	Autosomal dominant
Spinocerebellar ataxia type 1	Ataxin 1	CAG	Autosomal dominant
Spinocerebellar ataxia type 2	Ataxin 2	CAG	Autosomal dominant
Spinocerebellar ataxia type 3	Ataxin 3 ***(Machado Joseph disease)***	CAG	Autosomal dominant
Haw river syndrome	Atrophin 1 ***(Dentatorubro pallidoluysian atrophy)***	CAG	Autosomal dominant
Friedrich ataxia	Frataxin	GAA	Autosomal recessive

Ref: Robbin's 9th Edition Page 169, Harrison 20th Edition Page 3362, Harsh Mohan 7th Edition Page 241

Ans: (B) Males have IQ 20-40

12. MRP2 gene defect is seen with:

A. Gilbert syndrome
B. Dubin Johnson syndrome
C. Crigler-Najjar syndrome I
D. Crigler-Najjar syndrome II

Key:

Mutation in MRP2 protein (Canalicular protein) is asscociated with Dubin Johnson syndrome

DUBIN JOHNSON SYNDROME

- Autosomal recessive hereditary disorder

Genetics

- Absence of canalicular protein ***(Multidrug resistance protein 2→MRP2)***
- Defect in hepatic excretory function across canalicular membrane of hepatocyte

Clinical Features

- ***Most are Asymptomatic***
- Unexplained low grade jaundice during teenage years
- Often exacerbated by OC pills, Pregnancy and Intercurrent Illness
- **Physical examination is usually normal**

Laboratory studies	Histology
• **Conjugated hyperbilirubinemia:** Total bilirubin is typically between 2 and 5 mg/dL • Presents with conjugated hyperbilirubinemia but serum transaminases and alkaline phosphatase is normal	Darkly pigmented liver because of coarse pigmented granules within cytoplasm of hepatocytes. Pigment is located in Lysosomes and derived from Epinephrine metabolites that are not excreted normally.

Diagnosis

- Bromosulphalein test–*Investigation of choice→*

In Dubin Johnson syndrome biliary excretion of number of anionic compounds is compromised (Bromosuphalein). Disappearance of BSP from plasma is determined after IV bolus. Characteristic rise in plasma concentration at 90 min after injection occurs due to reflux of conjugated bilirubin into circulation from hepatocyte

- Corporphyrin test (Preferential urinary excretion of Coproporphyrin I)→***Urine of Dubin Johnson syndrome shows >80% of Corporphyrin Isomer I*** (Normal urine–Corporphrin III)

Crigler-Najjar Syndrome	Gilbert Syndrome
Type I: • ***Congenital total absence of UGT1A1 activity (AR)*** • Seen in neonates • Severe jaundice (>20 mg/dL) • Neurological impairment due to kernicterus • ***Death occurs in infancy/childhood (<1 year)*** **Type II:** • ***Mutation in Bilirubin UDPGT gene (AD)→Partial deficiency of UDPGT activity*** • Live into adulthood, Jaundice (6-25 mg/dL) • Susceptible to kernicterus under stress of illness/ surgery	• Mild unconjugated hyperbilirubinemia • Jaundice <6 mg/dL • Serum levels may fluctuate, jaundice is often identified only during periods of fasting • Male predominant • **Autosomal dominant** **Rotor Syndrome** • Defect in bilirubin excretion • Non-pigmented liver • No need for treatment

Disorder	Inheritance	Defects in Bilirubin Metabolism	Liver Pathology	Clinical Course
UNCONJUGATED HYPERBILIRUBINEMIA				
Crigler-Najjar syndrome type 1	Autosomal recessive	Absent UGT1A1 activity	–	***Fatal in Neonatal period***

Contd.

Contd.

Crigler-Najjar syndrome type 2	Autosomal dominant with variable penetrance	Decreased UGT1A1 activity	–	Generally mild Occasional kernicterus
Gilbert syndrome	Autosomal recessive	Decreased UGT1A1 activity	–	–
CONJUGATED HYPERBILIRUBINEMIA				
Dubin Johnson syndrome	Autosomal recessive	Impaired biliary excretion of bilirubin canalicular multidrug resistance protein 2	Pigmented cytoplasmic globules	–
Rotor syndrome	Autosomal recessive	Decreased hepatic uptake and storage Decreased biliary excretion	–	–

Ref: Robbin's 9th Edition Page 854, Harrison 20th Edition Page 2345, Harsh Mohan 7th Edition Page 600

Ans: (B) Dubin Johnson syndrome

13. Type of necrosis that occurs with Blood vessel involvement is:

A. Coagulative
B. Fibrinoid
C. Liquefactive
D. Caseous

Key:

Fibrinoid necrosis is seen in immune reactions that involve blood vessels

FIBRINOID NECROSIS

- Seen in immune reactions that involve blood vessels
- Occurs when antigen-antibody complexes are deposited in walls of arteries
- *Deposition of immune complexes and fibrin→ Bright pink and Amorphous appearance*
- **Examples: PAN, Malignant hypertension, Acute rheumatic fever, Libman Sach endocarditis, Lupus nephritis and Hyperacute graft rejection**

Types of Necrosis	
Coagulative	Most common type Architecture is preserved Mechanism–Protein denaturation Almost all solid organs *except brain* ***Most commonly affected organ–Heart***
Liquefactive	Tissue gets transformed to Viscous sac Mechanism–Enzymatic digestion Increased lysosomal permeability and release of enzymes Tissue architecture is lost Typically involves CNS (Bacterial infections)
Caseous	Consists of both coagulative and liquefactive necrosis Mechanism–Granuloma formation with collection of amorphous granular debris enclosed by inflammatory cells Mainly seen with TB, Histoplasmosis and Coccidiomycosis

Contd.

Contd.

Fat	Mechanism–Destruction of fat by lipases→Combine with calcium→ Saponification Seen with Acute pancreatitis and Breast injury
Fibrinoid	Immune reaction seen in blood vessels Seen in Malignant hypertension, Acute rheumatic fever, PAN, Libman sacks endocarditis
Gangrenous	Dry Gangrene–Coagulative Wet Gangrene–Liquefactive

Ref: Robbin's 9th Edition Page 44, Harsh Mohan 7th Edition Page 27

Ans: (B) Fibrinoid

14. Genotype for Follicular lymphoma is:

A. Bcl 1
B. Bcl XL
C. Bcl 2
D. Bcl 6

Key:

Genotype for Follicular lymphoma is Bcl 2

Follicular Lymphoma

- Most common form of indolent NHL.
- ***Arises from germinal centres.***
- Characteristically presents as painless generalized lymphadenopathy
- Frequently affects Middle age
- *Male = female*

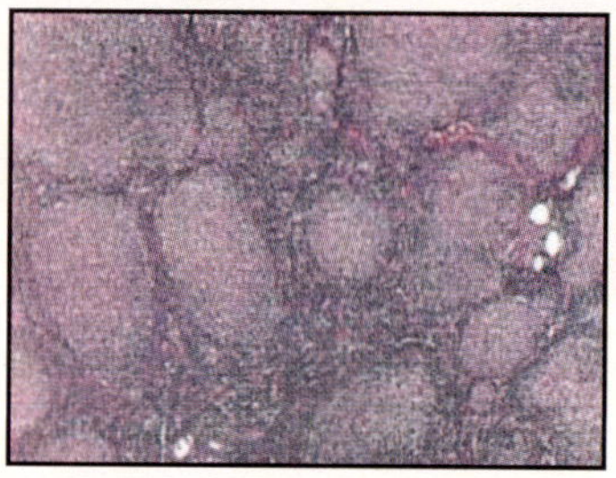

- **Immunophenotyping:**
    - >90% express Bcl 2 Protein
    - Mutations of Bcl 2 and MLL 2 genes are implicated
- **Cytogenetics:** Involves t(14;18) IGH translocation→More than 85%
    - ***Nearly 30-50% of cases will transform into DLBCL (diffuse large B cell)***
- **Treatment:** Very responsive to chemoradiation

Lymph node Biopsy:

Centrocytes *(Small cell with cleaved nuclear contours) and scant cytoplasm–Predominant*

Centroblasts *(Large cell with open nuclear chromatin, several nucleoli and modest cytoplasm*

Bone marrow Biopsy– Characteristic paratrabecular lymphoid aggregates

B CELL LYMPHOMA	
Follicular lymphoma	Bcl 2, t(14,18), CD 5-, CD 10+
Mantle cell lymphoma	Cyclin D1, Bcl 1+, t(11,14), CD 5+, CD 10-, CD 23-
Marginal zone lymphoma	CD5-, CD10-, t(11,18)
DLBCL	CD10+, Bcl 6+
SLL/CLL	CD 5+, CD 23+

Diagnosis	Cell of Origin	Genotype	Salient Features
NEOPLASMS OF IMMATURE B AND T CELLS			
B-cell acute lymphoblastic leukemia/lymphoma	Bone marrow precursor B cell	Diverse chromosomal translocations; ***t(12;21)*** involving *CBF* α and *ETV6* present in 25%	Predominantly children; symptoms relating to marrow replacement and pancytopenia; Aggressive
T-cell acute lymphoblastic leukemia/lymphoma	Precursor T cell *(often thymic origin)*	Diverse chromosomal translocations, *NOTCH1* mutations (50% to 70%)	Predominantly adolescent males; **thymic** masses and variable bone marrow involvement; ***Aggressive***
NEOPLASMS OF MATURE B CELLS			
Burkitt lymphoma	Germinal-center B cell	Translocations involving c-*MYC* and lg loci, usually ***t(8;14); EBV associated***	Adolescents or young adults with extranodal masses; uncommonly presents as "leukemia"; aggressive
Diffuse large B-cell lymphoma	Germinal center/Post Germinal center B cell	Diverse chromosomal rearrangements, most often of **Bcl 6 (30%),** Bcl 2 (10%), or c-*MYC* (5%)	All ages–Most common in adults; often appears as rapidly growing mass; *30% extranodal; aggressive*
Extranodal marginal zone lymphoma	Memory B cell	***t(11;18), t(1;14) and t(14;18)*** creating MALT1-IAP2, Bcl L10-IgH and MALT1-IgH fusion genes respectively	Arises at ***extranodal sites*** in adults with chronic inflammatory diseases; localized and indolent
Follicular lymphoma	***Germinal center B cell***	***t(14;18) creating Bcl 2-IgH fusion gene (indolent)***	***Older adults with generalized lymphadenopathy and marrow involvement***
Hairy cell leukemia	Memory B cell	No specific chromosomal abnormality	Older males with pancytopenia
Mantle cell lymphoma	Naive B cell	***t(11;14)*** creating ***CyclinD1-IgH*** fusion gene	Older males with disseminated disease; moderately aggressive
Multiple myeloma/solitary plasmacytoma	Post-germinal-center bone marrow homing plasma cell	Diverse rearrangements involving IgH; ***13q deletions***	***Myeloma:*** Older adults with lytic bone lesions, pathologic fractures, hypercalcemia and renal failure; moderately aggressive ***Plasmacytoma:*** Isolated plasma cell masses in bone or soft tissue
Small lymphocytic lymphoma/chronic lymphocytic leukemia	Naive B cell or memory B cell	***Trisomy 12, deletions of 11q, 13q and 17p***	Older adults with bone marrow, lymph node, spleen and liver disease; autoimmune hemolysis and thrombocytopenia in minority

Contd.

Contd.

NEOPLASMS OF MATURE T CELLS OR NK CELL			
Adult T-cell leukemia/ lymphoma	Helper T cell	HTLV-1 provirus present in tumor cells	Adults with cutaneous lesions, marrow involvement and hypercalcemia; Aggressive
Peripheral T-cell lymphoma, unspecified	Helper/Cytotoxic T cell	No specific chromosomal abnormality	Mainly older adults; usually presents with lymphadenopathy; aggressive
Anaplastic large-cell lymphoma	Cytotoxic T cell	Rearrangements of ALK	Children and young adults, usually with lymph node and soft-tissue disease; Aggressive
Extranodal NK/T-cell lymphoma	NK cell (common) or cytotoxic T cell (rare)	***EBV-associated;*** No specific abnormality	Adults with destructive extranodal masses, ***most commonly sinonasal;*** aggressive
Mycosis fungoides/ Sézary syndrome	Helper T cell	No specific chromosomal abnormality (indolent)	***Adult patients with cutaneous patches,*** plaques, nodules, or generalized erythema
Large granular lymphocytic leukemia	Two types: Cytotoxic T cell and NK cell	No specific chromosomal abnormality	***Adult patients with splenomegaly, neutropenia and anemia,*** accompanied by autoimmune disease

Important Cytogenetics and Immunochemistry Tables	
CD1a, S-100, CD-207 (Langherin)	• Langerhan cell histiocytois
CD 2, 3, 4, 5, 7 & 8	• T-cell markers • CD3 is pan T cell marker
CD 10 (aka CALLA antigen)	• Early pre B marker • Immature B cell marker
CD 13, 33, 117, MPO	• Myeloid series marker–AML
CD 14, 64	• Monocyte marker (AML–M4 M5)
CD 15	• RS Cell • Neutrophils
CD 13, 14, 203c	• Basophil
CD 15, 30	• RS Cell
CD 16, 56	• NK Cell
CD 19, 20, 21, 22	• B Cell markers • CD 19 is pan B cell marker
CD 23+, CD 5+	• CLL/SLL
CD 23–, CD 5+	• Mantle cell lymphoma
CD 31	• Endothelial cell marker (positive in angiosarcomas)
CD 34	• Stem cell (aslo positive in angiosarcomas)
CD 41, 61	• Megakaryocyte • Platelet marker • Positive in AML-M7

Contd.

Contd.

CD 45 RO	• Memory cell
CD 95/FAS ligand	• Apoptosis marker (extrinsic pathway)
CD 99/MIC-2	• Ewings sarcoma (FLI 1 is most senitive and specific than CD 99)
CD 117	• GIST • Mastocytosis • AML (DOG 1 is more useful than CD 117 in GIST)

Genetic Feature	Genes	Lymphoma
t(8; 14) **t(2; 8)** **t(8;22)**	*MYC/IgH* *MYC/Igκ* *MYC/Igλ*	Bukitt's lymphoma
t(11; 14)	*BCL 1 (CCND1)/IgH*	Mantle cell lymphoma; multiple myeloma
t(14; 18) **t(3; 14)**	*BCL 2/IgH* *BCL 6/IgH*	Follicular lymphoma, diffuse large B-cell lymphoma (DLBCL)
t(11; 18) **t(1; 14)** **t(14; 18)** **t(3; 14)**	*API2/MALT1* *BCL10/IgH* *MALT1/IgH* *FOXP1/IgH*	MALT lymphoma
Trisomy 3 **7q21 deletion**	*Unknown* *CDK6*	Splenic marginal zone lymphoma
t (9; 14) **6q21 deletion**	*PAX5/IgH* *Unknown*	Lymphoplasmacytic lymphoma
Inv (14) **t (14;14)**	*TCRα/TCL1*	Peripheral T-cell lymphoma, NOS; T-PLL
t (2; 5) **t (1; 2)** **t (2; 3)** **t(2; 17)** **Inv(2)**	*NPM1/ALK* *TPM3/ALK* *TFG/ALK* *CTLC/ALK* *ATIC/ALK*	Anaplastic large cell lymphoma (ALCL)
Trisomy 3 **Trisomy 5**	*Unknown* *Unknown*	Angioimmunoblastic T-cell lymphoma
Isochromosome 7q	*Unknown*	Hepatoplenic T-cell lymphoma

Ref: Robbin's 9th Edition Page 435, Harrison 20th Edition Page 776, Harsh Mohan 7th Edition Page 356

Ans: (C) Bcl 2

15. **Fish mouth appearance occurs due to:**

A. Mitral valve prolapse
B. Ashoff bodies
C. Calcification and Fibrosis of valve
D. Hypertrophy of ventricular wall

Key:

In chronic/healed phase of Rheumatic heart disease thickening of valve leaflets as a result of calcification and fibrosis of valve

Fibrous bridging across valvular commissures and calcification create "fishmouth" "buttonhole" stenoses

CARDINAL ANATOMIC CHANGES IN CHRONIC RHD

- **Leaflet thickening**
- **Commissural fusion and shortening**
- **Thickening and fusion of tendinous cords**

MORPHOLOGY

Acute

Aschoff bodies–pathognomonic/diagnostic of RHD

Aschoff bodies–Foci of T lymphocytes, plasma cells and plump activated macrophages with caterpillar like nuclear chromatin (Antischkow cells).

Antischkow cells–Modified macrophages with abundant cytoplasm and central round to ovoid nuclei in which chromatin is deposited in central slender waxy ribbon like pattern–Caterpillar cells.

- These bodies are present in all layers–Myocardium, Pericardium and Endocardium
- *Most commonly seen in Myocardium (Perivascular areas)*
- Inflammatory vasculitis is characterized by *beady fibrous vegetations (verrucae)* along lines of valve closure

Chronic

- Diffuse/Fibrous thickening of valve leaflets with fibrous commissural fusion forms ***Fish mouth/Button hole stenosis***

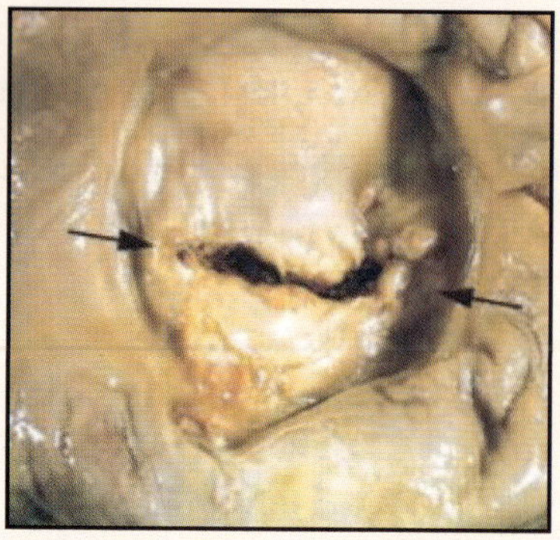

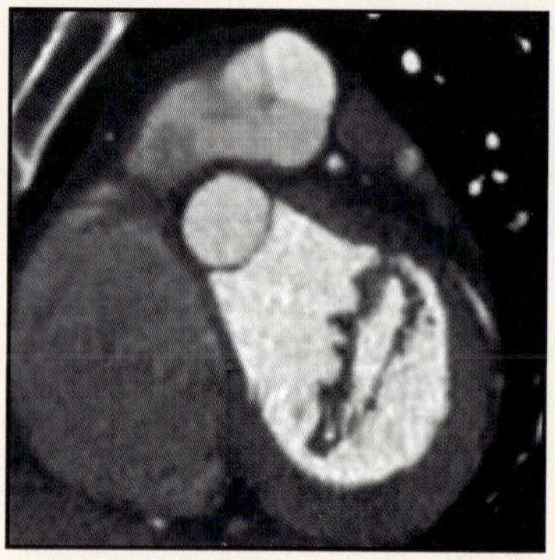

- Thickened, fused and shortened *Chordae tendinae*
- ***Mac Callum plaques*** are seen in posterior wall of left atrium consisting of subendocardial collections of Aschoff bodies
- **Aschoff bodies are rarely seen in chronic RHD**

WHO Health Criteria for Diagnosis of Rheumatic Fever and Rheumatic Heart Disease	
Major manifestations	Carditis, Polyarthritis, Chorea, Erythema marginatum, Subcutaneous nodules
Minor manifestations	*Clinical*–Fever, Polyarthralgia *Laboratory*–Elevated ESR/Leucocyte count *Electrocardiogram*–Prolonged PR interval
Essential criteria *(Supporting evidence of preceding streptococcal infections within last 45 days)*	Elevated/Rising ASO or Other streptococcal antibody or +ve throat culture or Rapid antigen test for Group A streptococcus or Recent scarlet fever

Diagnostic Categories	Criteria
Primary episode of rheumatic fever	Two major or 1 major and two minor manifestations plus evidence of preceding Group A streptococcal infection
Recurrent attack of rheumatic fever in patient without established rheumatic heart disease	Two major or 1 minor manifestations plus evidence of preceding Group A streptococcal infection
Recurrent attack of rheumatic fever in patient without established rheumatic heart disease	Two minor manifestations plus evidence of preceeding Group A streptococcal infection

- ***Most common cause of death in Acute Rheumatic Fever–CHF*** *(Caused by Endocarditis)*
- ***Overall most common cause of death–Myocarditis****
- ***Most common manifestation–Migratory polyarthritis***
- *Fibrinous/Serofibrinous pericarditis→ Bread and Butter Pericarditis*
- *Most common valvular defect in Acute rheumatic heart disease–Mitral regurgitation*
- *Most common valvular defect in chronic rheumatic heart disease–Mitral stenosis*

Fish Related Signs
• **Fish Hook Coeliac**: Median Arcuate Ligament Syndrome.
• **Fish Hook Ureter:** Benign prostatic hypertrophy, retrocaval ureter.
• **Fish Vertebrae:** Osteoporosis.
• **Fishtail deformity of the elbow:** Lateral trochlear ossification centers fails to develop or resorbs.

Ref: Robbin's 9th Edition Page 558, Chandrasoma Taylor 3rd Edition Page 347, Textbook of Cardiology 2nd Edition Page 877, Harsh Mohan 7th Edition Page 422

Ans: (C) Calcification and Fibrosis of valve

16. Not seen in cystic fibrosis:

A. Most common type is Type II

B. Abnormality in CFTR leads to defective calcium transport

C. Autosomal recessive inheritance

D. Type 5 has best prognosis

Key:

Abnormality in CFTR leads to defective Chloride transport in Cytsic fibrosis

CYSTIC FIBROSIS

- ***Autosomal recessive***
- Chromosome 7q31.2 (Apparent clinically in homozygous only)
- Cystic fibrosis gene encodes **CFTR protein** *(Cystic fibrosis transmembrane conductance regulator)*

Pathology

DEFECTS
- ENaC
- *Outwardly rectified chloride channels*
- *Inwardly rectified potassium channels (Kir 6.1)*

- ***Most common mutation***–CFTR F508 gene.
- More than 1500 CFTR polymorphisms are associated with CF

Site	Normal function	Cystic fibrosis	Effect seen in CF
Apical exocrine glands of airway and GIT	Na^+ uptake from luminal fluid	Increased Na^+ and H_2O uptake from lumen	Thick, Viscid secretions
Sweat ducts	Absorb luminal Na^+	Decreased reabsorption of Na^+ and Cl^-	Salty sweat ***(Hallmark of CF)***→ High Na^+ and Cl^-

Classification of CFTR Mutations		
Class	**Mechanism**	**Genotype**
I	Defective protein production	W1282X, Del394TT, 1717-1G to A
II	Defective protein processing	F508del (Always associated with Pancreatic Insufficiency)
III	Defective channel regulation	G551D
IV	Defective channel conductance	R117H (Substantial or full sparing of lung and preservation of exocrine function)
V	Decreased active CFTR	3849+10 kb C to T, A455E (Sweat chloride concentrations are normal and some exocrine function preserved)

Type II–Most common
Type I–Worse prognosis
Type V–Best prognosis

SYSTEMIC INVOLVEMENT

Respiratory tract

- **Upper Respiratory tract–Most common site of involvement**
- ***Hemophilus influenza and staphylococcus aureus***–First organisms recovered from lung secretions
- ***Burkholderia cepacia***–Pathognomonic organism
- ***Most common organism to cause pulmonary infection in CF***–Pseudomonas
- ***Most common organism to cause pulmonary infection in CF children–Staphylococcus***
- ***Most common organism to cause pulmonary infection in CF Adults***–Pseudomonas
- ***Most common organism to cause chronic lung disease in CF patients***–Pseudomonas
- Chronic cough and sputum production, Bronchiectasis, Atelectasis, Nasal polyps (30% of children), Infiltrates and Hyperinflation
- Most common cause of severe chronic lung disease in children–CF
- Earliest pathologic lesion in Lung–Bronhiolitis
- ***Most common symptom–Cough***

Genitourinary Tract

- ***Infertility in females***→Thick cervical secretions→Formation of cervical mucus plug (Pregnancy is well tolerated in females with good pulmonary function and can breast feed normally)
- Congenital bilateral absence or obliteration of vas deferens→***Azoospermia in males***

Gastrointestinal and Nutritional Abnormalities

- ***Intestinal***–Meconium Ileus, Distal intestinal obstruction syndrome, Rectal prolapse
- ***Pancreatic–Exocrine insufficiency (>85%)***, Recurrent Acute/Chronic pancreatitis→Osmotic diarrhea
- ***Prone for Type 1 Diabetes***
- ***Most common cause of Exocrine insufficiency in children–CF***
- ***Hepatic***–Focal biliary cirrhosis/Multilobular cirrhosis, Prolonged neonatal jaundice and Gall stones
- ***Nutritional***–Protein calorie malnutrition, Hypoproteinemia, Edema, Fat soluble vitamin deficiency
- ***Salt loss syndrome***–Acute salt depletion, Chronic metabolic alkalosis (Hypochloremic alkalosis)

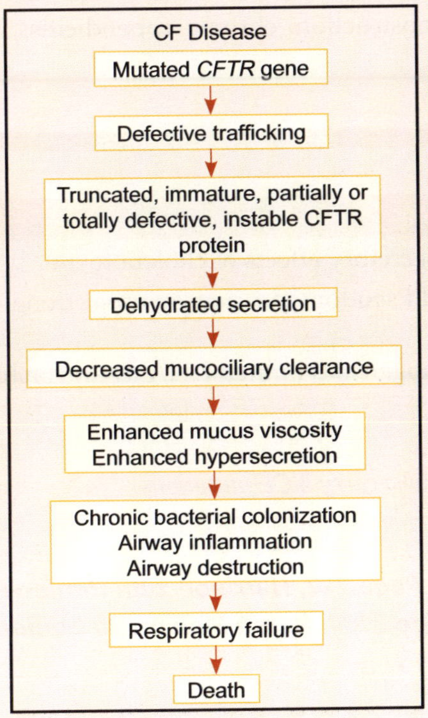

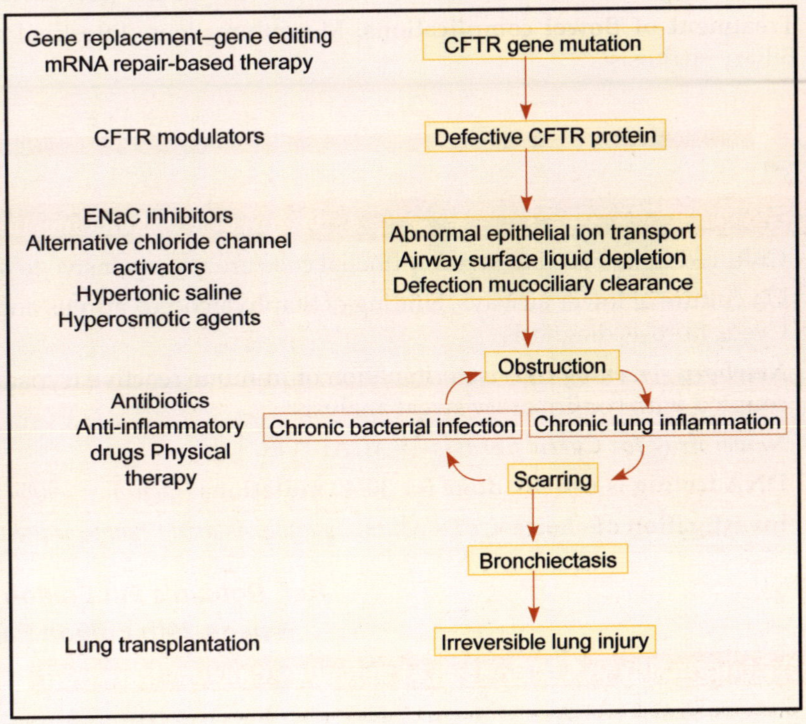

Criteria for Diagnosis of Cystic Fibrosis
One or more characteristic phenotypic features, OR a history of cystic fibrois in a sibling, OR a positive newborn screening test result AND An increased sweat chloride concentration on two or more occasions, OR identification of two cystic fibrosis mutation, OR demonstration of abnormal epithelial nasal ion transport

Sweat Chloride Test	False +ve Sweat Chloride Test
>60 mEq–Diagnostic 40-60 mEq–Borderline <40 mEq–Rules out CF	Eczema, Ectodermal dysplasia, Malnutrition, Adrenal insufficiency, Congenital adrenal hyperplasia, Celiac disease, Bylers disease, G6PD deficiency, Glycogen storage disease type 1, Nephrogenic diabetes insipidus

Abnormal Nasal potential difference measurement–*Confirms diagnosis with equivocal or frankly normal sweat chloride values by*

- Increased potential difference across nasal epithelium
- Loss of potential difference with topical amiloride application
- Absence of voltage response to beta agonist

Treatment

- **Pulmonary:** Bronchodilators, Steroids, Hypertonic saline, Aerosolized antibiotics, Ventilator assistance may be required in respiratory failure
- **Nutritional:** High caloric diet, Pancreatic enzyme replacement, Fat soluble vitamin supplementation, Mineral supplements, Correct hypoglycemia
- Lung transplantation is also recommended in end stages (few cases)
- **Treatment of Bowel complications:** Meconium ileus, Intestinal obstruction, chronic appendicitis, Pancreatitis, Biliary cirrhosis

Frequently Asked Questions

- Cultured delta F508 intestinal epithelial cells are unresponsive to secretory effects of cholera toxin
- On culture of lower airways, Finding of Staphylococcus aureus and Pseudomonas aeuroginosa strongly suggests Cystic fibrosis diagnosis
- ***Newborn screening test***–Determination of Immune reactive trypsinogen and limited DNA testing on blood spots coupled with confirmatory sweat analysis
- ***Newer drug for Cystic fibrosis***–IVACAFTOR
- **DNA testing is usually done for 30-40 mutations** *(Identifies >90% who carry 2 CF mutations)*
- **Investigation of choice**–*CFTR Mutation analysis using exonic sequencing*

Ref: Robbin's 9th Edition Page 227, Harrison 20th Edition Page 1986, Nelson 20th Edition Page 2104, Harsh Mohan 7th Edition Page 631

Ans: (B) Abnormality in CFTR leads to defective calcium transport

17. True about Class 2 MHC include:

A. Major role in Graft rejection

B. Present on APC

C. Detects intracellular organisms

D. Peptide binding site is present between Alpha 1 and 2

Key:

Class II MHC is located on APC, B cells, dendritic cells, Endothelial cells and Fibroblasts

- **Gene encoding HLA molecules are clustered on chromosome 6**
- **MHC gene is located in short arm of chromosome 6**
- ***MHC Restriction*–T cells recognise only immunogens that are bound to MHC**

MHC PROTEINS

- **Class I**
  - *Expressed virtually by all somatic cells*
- **Class II**
  - *Mixed lymphocyte reaction is used for detection of MHC Class II*

Properties	Class I MHC	Class II MHC
Location	All nucleated cells	APC, B cells, dendritic cells, Endothelial cells and Fibroblasts
Encoded by	HLA-A, B, C	HLA- DP, DQ and DR
Peptide binding cleft	Alpha 1 and 2	Alpha 1 and Beta 1
Antigens	Viral and tumor antigens intracellularly	Extracellular microbes
Major role	Graft rejection	GVHD
Recognised by	CD8+T cells	CD4+T cells

Class III MHC

Coded for C2, C4, Properdin, Factor B, TNF, HSP 70, Tyrosine hydroxylase

No role in immune system

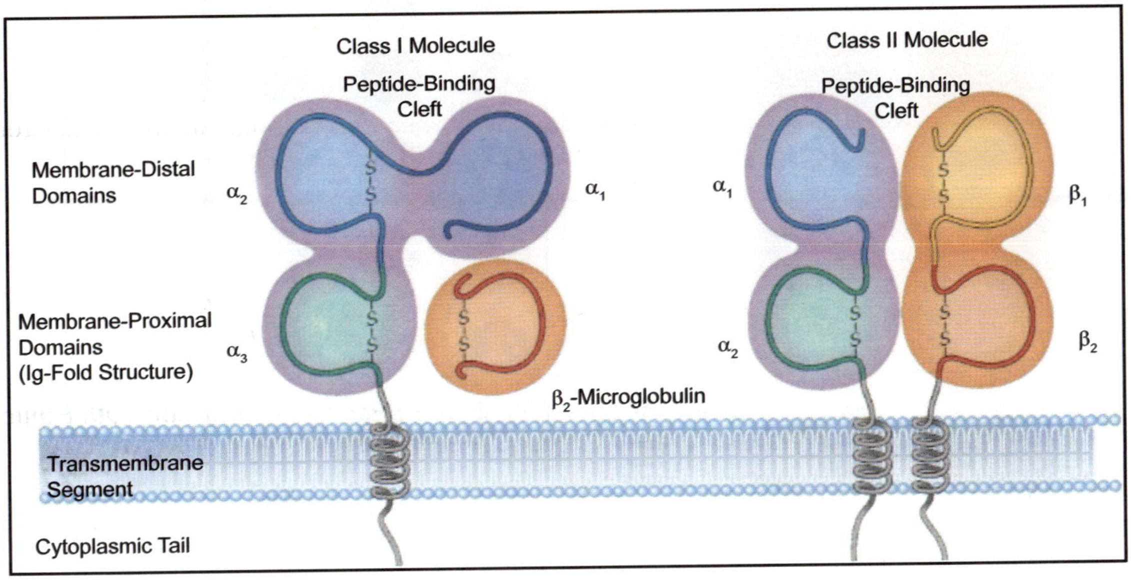

- **HLA-D is most important HLA for organ transplantation and tissue typing** *(because they are having more number of polymorphic gene).*
- Order of importance before organ transplantation or tissue typing–**HLA DR > B >A**

Uses of HLA Typing

- To resolve paternity disputes
- Compatibility between donor and host before organ/tissue transplantation
- For Anthropological studies

Ref: Robbin's 9th Edition Page 194, Harsh Mohan 7th Edition Page 49

Ans: (B) Present on APC

18. Identify Blood group based on picture shown below:

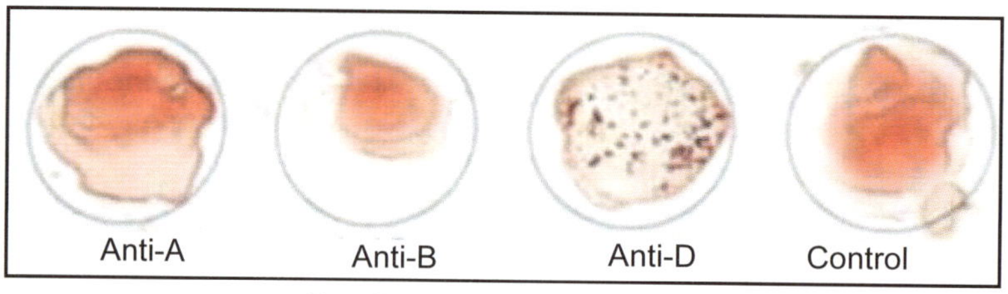

A. A +ve
B. B +ve
C. AB +ve
D. O +ve

Key:

Picture shows No agglutination in both Anti A and Anti B→ So it is Blood Group O positive

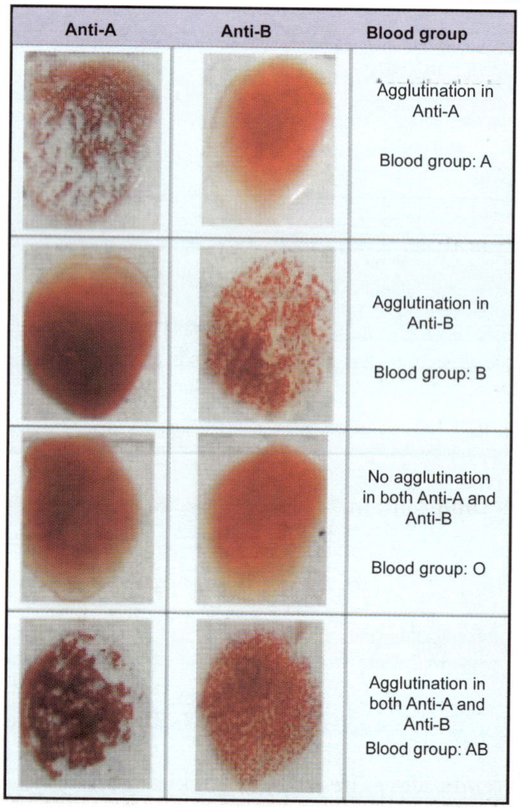

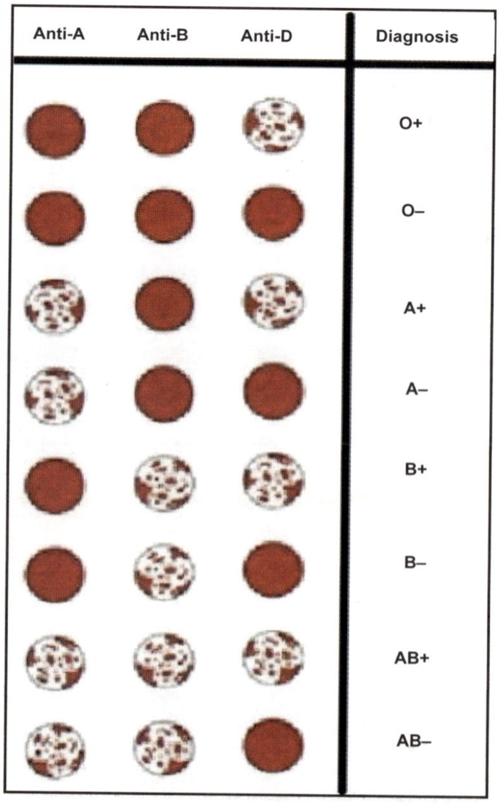

ABO Blood Grouping		
Blood grouping	**Antigen**	**Antibody**
A	*A*	*Anti-B*
B	*B*	*Anti-A*
O	-	*Anti-A and B*
AB	*A and B*	-

ABO BLOOD GROUPING

Forward grouping:
Identifies antigens on red cells.
Tests recipient or donor red cells with anti-A and anti-B sera

- Cells agglutinated only with anti-A serum are group A
- Cells agglutinated only with anti-B serum are group B
- Cells that do not agglutinate with anti-A or anti-B are group O

Reverse grouping:
Identifies presence of antibodies in serum/plasma
Tests the serum/plasma from the recipient or donor with group A and B red cells

- Agglutination with group B cells indicates presence of anti-B in plasma–Group A
- Agglutination with group A cells indicates presence of anti-A in plasma–Group B
- Agglutination with group A and B cells both indicates presence of anti-A and anti-B both in plasma–Group O

Ref: Harsh Mohan Pathology Practical Book 2nd Edition Page 202, Harsh Mohan 7th Edition Page 339, GK Pal Comprehensive Medical Physiology 1st Edition Page 120

Ans: (D) O +ve

19. CPDA advantage over ACD in improving oxygen transport by which of the following?

A. Less Fall in 2,3 DPG
B. Less acidic
C. Has low p50 value
D. Less temperature

Key:

Levels of 2,3–DPG usually decline with storage
CPDA maintains these levels since it has phosphate compared to ACD

Chemical	Function
Citrate	Chelates calcium, Prevents clotting
Monobasic sodium phosphate	*Maintains pH during storage* *Necessary for maintenance of adequate 2,3-DPG levels*
Dextrose	Substrate for ATP production (Cellular energy)
Adenine	Production of ATP *(Extends Shelf life from 21 to 35 days)*

Approved anticoagulant preservative solutions	
Name	Storage time (days)
ACD-A→ Acid citrate dextrose	21
CPD→ Citrate phosphate dextrose	21
CP2D→ Citrate phosphate double dextrose	21
CPDA-1→ Citrate phosphate dextrose adenine	35

RBC STORED

⇩

Reduced 2,3-DPG

⇩

Shift of Oxygen dissociation curve to left

⇩

Less oxygen delivered to tissues

⇩

Later 2,3-DPG is reformed in stored RBC after *in vivo* circulation

- Rate of restoration of 2,3–DPG is influenced by acid-base status of recipient, phosphorus metabolism, degree of anemia, and overall severity of the disorder.
- Stored RBCs do regain the ability to synthesize 2,3–DPG after transfusion, but levels necessary for optimal hemoglobin oxygen delivery are not reached immediately.
- Approximately 24 hours are required to restore normal levels of 2,3–DPG after transfusion.
- ***CPDA has Monobasic sodium phosphate that maintains 2,3 DPG (ACD lacks it).***

Characteristic	Change Observed on Storage
Percentage viable cells	Decreased
Glucose	Decreased
ATP	Decreased
Lactic acid	***Increased***
pH	Decreased
2,3 DPG	Decreased
Oxygen dissociation curve	Shift to left (Increase in Hb and oxygen affinity, Less oxygen delivered to tissues)
Plasma K^+	Increased
Plasma hemoglobin	Increased

- Adenine is only needed for storage beyond 3 weeks and is an ingredient of all of the additive solutions.
- Anticoagulant most often used for neonate transfusions is CPDA-1.

CPD has following advantages for blood preservation compared to ACD anticoagulant
• Isotonicity for red blood cells, thus minimizing lesion of collection and resulting in improved red blood cell survival • More physiological pH • Less citrate ion 15% • Improved red cell oxygen transport (Less fall in 2,3-DPG)

Ref: Mollison Blood Transfusion in Clinical Medicine 12th Edition 304, Textbook of Blood Banking and Transfusion Medicine Page 269, Harmening Modern Blood Banking and Transfusion Practices 6th Edition Page 9

Ans: (A) Less Fall in 2,3 DPG

20. A patient presented with Solitary lytic lesion over skull without organ damage and Urine and blood tests are normal. Diagnosis is:

A. Multiple myeloma
B. Localised myeloproliferative disorder
C. Langerhan cell histiocytosis
D. Solitary Plasmacytoma

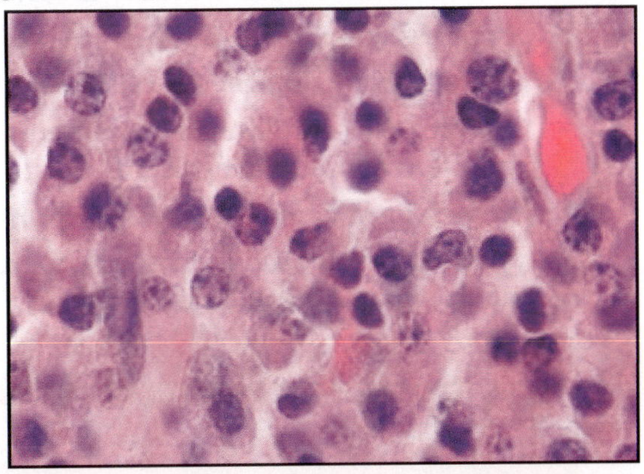

Key:

Clonal proliferation of myeloma cells with Lytic lesions of skull seen with all options except B. Picture shows large abundant cells with abundant cytoplasm and eccentric nucleus suggesting Plasma cell neoplasm of myeloma origin

Here key word is Solitary lytic skull lesion–Since there is no other organ involvement Solitary plasmacytoma is best possible answer

Osteolytic Lesions of Skull
• Metastasis • Multiple myeloma • Eosinophilic granuloma/Langerhans cell histiocytosis • Lymphoma • Tuberculosis • Osteomyelitis • Radiation • Epidermoid

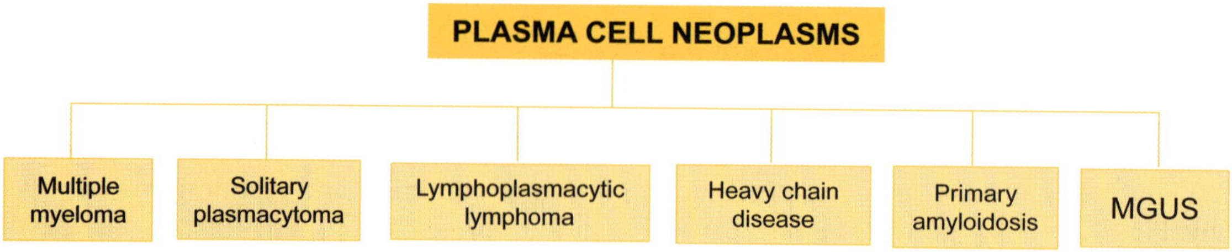

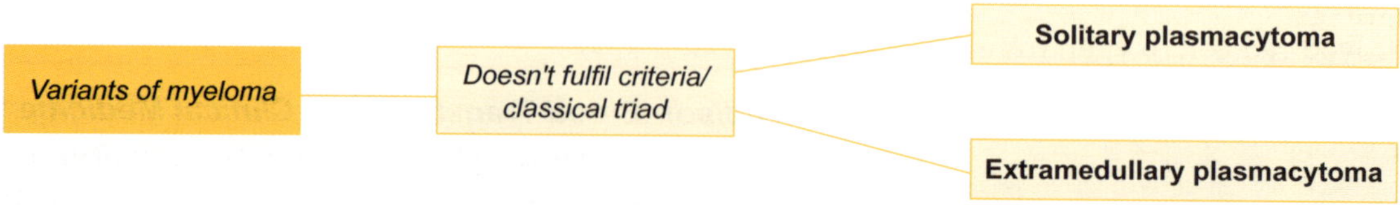

SOLITARY/LOCALISED PLASMACYTOMA OF BONE

- Account for 3-5%.
- Extraosseous lesions typically involve Lung.
- Progress to myeloma in 10-20 years.
- Plasma tumors manifest as ***solitary plasmacytomas*** involving skeleton/soft tissues.
- Solitary skeletal plasmacytomas tend to occur in same locations as does multiple myeloma and usually progress to full-blown multiple myeloma over 5 to 10 years period.
- ***Modestly elevated M proteins are present in few cases at diagnosis.***
- Adverse prognostic factors for progression to MM include persistence of paraprotein >1 year after radiotherapy, immuneparesis and lesion > 5 cm.

Diagnosis of Solitary Plasmacytoma is based on

- Histologic evidence of a tumor consisting of monoclonal plasma cells with no other lesion on skeletal survey or MRI.
- Normal bone marrow.
- Absence of M protein in blood and urine or if present therapy for solitary lesion should result in disappearance of M protein.
- Uninvolved Immunoglobulins are usually normal and there is no evidence of anemia or hypercalcemia.

Type	Features
MGUS	Most common monoclonal gammopathy Small IgG spike in elderly patients Plasma cells <3% in bone marrow No BJ proteinuria Increased risk for developing multiple myeloma, Walderstrom's macroglobulinemia
Solitary skeletal plasmacytoma	***Bone sites: Vertebrae, Ribs and Pelvis*** Slight increase in monoclonal protein ***No plasmablasts in bone marrow*** ***No BJ Proteinuria*** 75% develop Multiple myeloma

Contd.

Contd.

Extramedullary plasmacytoma	Sites–Upper respiratory tract (Nasopharynx, Sinuses and Larynx) Slight increase in monoclonal protein Absence of malignant plasma cells in bone marrow Absence of BJ Protein Small percentage may develop multiple myeloma
Lymphoplasmacytic lymphoma (Waldenstrom's macroglobulinemia)	Neoplastic lymphoplasmacytoid B cells Elderly male-dominant Major risk factor is MGUS M spike with IgM BJ Protein is present ***Generalized lymphadenopathy (Not present in Myeloma)*** ***Anemia, Bone marrow, Liver and Spleen involved (No lytic lesions like Myeloma)*** Hyperviscosity syndrome due to increased IgM, Retinal hemorrhages, Stroke, Platelet aggregation defects Plasmapheresis–Important to remove IgM
Heavy chain disease	M protein heavy chain without light chain Absence of BJ protein ***Alpha heavy chain disease***–Neoplastic infiltration of jejunum-Malabsorption/ Localized URTI ***Gamma heavy chain disease***–Presents as Lymphoma ***Mu heavy chain disease***–Often associated with CLL/Lymphoma

- *Solitary bone plasmacytoma*– Lytic bony lesion without marrow plasmacytosis.
- *Extramedullary plasmacytoma*–Involves most commonly submucosal lymphoid tissue of nasopharynx/paranasal sinuses.

Both above variants have better prognosis than classic multiple myeloma
Both are associated with M component in about a third of cases and occur in young individuals

LANGERHANS CELL HISTIOCYTOSIS

- Clonal accumulation and proliferation of immature dendritic cells called Langerhans cells
- Associated with BRAF Mutations
- ***Electron microscopy***–Tennis racket appearance
- ***Tennis racket appearance arises due to presence of Birbeck granules:*** Rod shaped cytoplasmic organelles within Langerhans cells cytoplasm
- ***Markers: CD1a, S-100 and CD207***

Letterer siewe disease	Eosinophilic granuloma	Hand Schuller Christian disease
Aggressive Age <2 years Bone destruction involving all bones of body simultaneously	***Most common–Calvarial defect (Skull defect)***	***Pulmonary Langerhan cell histiocytosis***–Adult smokers and Regress with smoking cessation

Contd.

Contd.

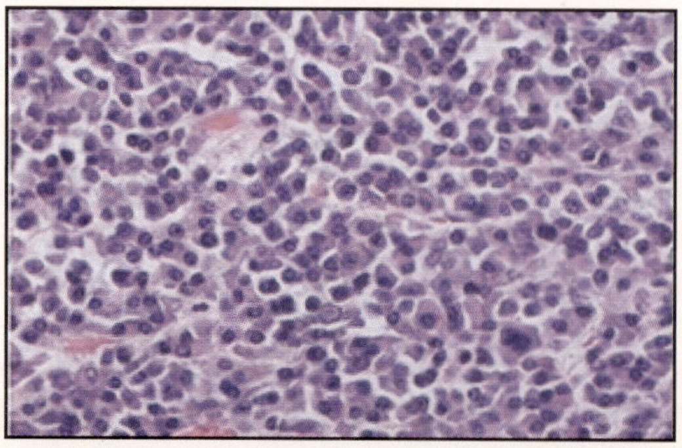 *Large cells with abundant cytoplasm and eccentric nucleus– **Suggestive of Multiple myeloma***	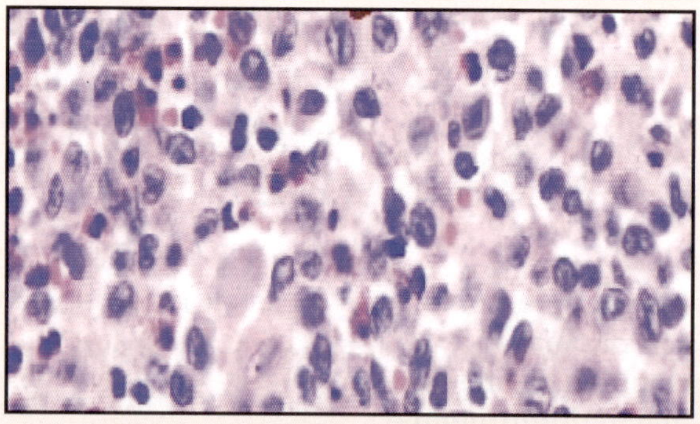 ***Picture shows Langerhans cells**–Polygonal cells with Eosinophilic cytoplasm, Oval nuclei with Longitudional grooves resembling coffee beans*

Ref: Robbin's 9th Edition Page 437, Harrison 20th Edition Page 797, Harsh Mohan 7th Edition Page 364, Atlas of Hematology 1st Edition Page 91, Oxford Handbook of Clinical Hematology 2nd Edition Page 282

Ans: (D) Solitary Plasmacytoma

21. **Alpha 1 antitrypsin works by:**
    A. Inhibition of chymotrypsin in duodenum
    B. Inhibition of trypsin activating protease
    C. Inhibition of trypsinogen activation in pancreas
    D. Inhibition of elastase in WBC of lung

Key:

*Alpha–1 antitrypsin is **produced in liver and** present in serum, tissue fluids and macrophages. Major inhibitor of proteases particularly elastase secreted by neutrophils during inflammation. **Function is to protect lungs from neutrophil elastase** (An enzyme that can disrupt connective tissue)*

- **Alpha 1 antitrypsin is synthesized by Rough endoplasmic reticulum of hepatocytes**
- α1-Antitrypsin deficiency is an ***autosomal recessive disorder*** of protein folding
- Marked by very low levels of circulating α1-Antitrypsin
- ***Caused by mutation in SERPINA 1 gene***

ALPHA 1 ANTITRYPSIN DEFICIENCY

- ***Development of pulmonary emphysema (Activity of destructive proteases is not inhibited)***
- ***Chronic liver disease (Hepatocellular accumulation of misfolded protein)***
- ***Cutaneous necrotizing panniculitis, Wegener's granulomatosis and arterial aneurysm***

- ***Gene, located on chromosome 14***
- Most common allele of protease inhibitor system-M
- PiMM–Normal and Most common form (90%)
- Z allele predisposes to clinical deficiency
- **Most common clinically significant mutation is PiZZ**
- ***Homozygous PiZZ have severe reduction (15% of normal) in enzyme levels–Most common significant manifestation→Neonatal cholestasis/Later onset cirrhosis***

- o PiMM–100% normal
- o PiMS–80% of normal serum levels of Alpha 1 antitrypsin
- o PiSS–60% of normal serum levels of Alpha 1 antitrypsin
- o PiMZ–60% of normal serum levels of Alpha 1 antitrypsin
- o PiSZ–40% of normal serum levels of Alpha 1 antitrypsin
- o PiZZ–10-15% of normal serum levels of Alpha 1 antitrypsin (Severe alpha 1 antitrypsin deficiency.

- α1AT deficiency is characterized by the presence of round-to-oval **cytoplasmic globular inclusions in hepatocytes,** which on routine hematoxylin and eosin stains are acidophilic, but are ***strongly PAS positive and diastase-resistant***
- ***Mallory Denk bodies and fibrosis of portal tract***
- Increases risk of cirrhosis and Hepatocellular carcinoma (2-3%)
- Increased risk of asthma rather than emphysema is observed in children
- **Treatment**–*Severe cases require Orthotopic Liver transplantation*
- **α1AT augmentation therapy is available for severe α1AT deficiency as a weekly IV infusion**

Diseases Caused by Misfolded Proteins

Disease	Affected protein	Pathogenesis
Caused by mutant proteins that are Degraded leading to their deficiency		
Cystic fibrosis	CFTR	Loss of CFTR leads to defect in chloride transport and death of affected cells
Familial hypercholesterolemia	LDL receptor	Loss of LDL receptor
Tay Sachs Disease	Hexosaminidase Beta	Lack of lysosomal enzyme (Storage of GM2 gangliosides in neurons)
Caused by Misfolded proteins that result in ER Stress induced cell loss		
Retinitis pigmentosa	Rhodopsin	Abnormal folding of rhodopsin causes photoreceptor loss and cell death–Blindness
Creutzfeldt Jacob disease	Prions	Abnormal folding of PrPsc causes neuronal cell death
Alzheimer's disease	A beta	Abnormal folding of A beta causes aggregation of neurons and apoptosis
Caused by Misfolded protein that result from both ER induced stress induced cell loss and functional deficiency of Protein		
Alpha 1 antitrypsin deficiency	Alpha 1 antitrypsin	Storage of non-functional protein in hepatocytes causes apoptosis, absence of enzymatic activity in lungs causes destruction of elastic tissue–*Gives rise to Panacinar Emphysema*

Ref: Robbin's 9th Edition Page 631, Harrison 20th Edition Page 1994, Harsh Mohan 7th Edition Page 613, Nelson 20th Edition Page 1933

Ans: (D) Inhibition of elastase in WBC of lung

22. Not true about Hyper IgE syndrome is:

A. Associated with defective STAT3

B. Prone for Chronic mucocutaneous candidiasis and skin infections

C. Most are of Autosomal recessive inheritance

D. Occurs due to defect in Neutrophil chemotaxis

Key:

Most cases of Job syndrome are of sporadic. In familial variety majority are of Autosomal dominant inheritance

JOB SYNDROME/HYPER IGE SYNDROME/RECURRENT INFECTION SYNDROME

- Excellent example for Complex Innate immune deficiency disorder
- Occurs due to defect in Neutrophil chemotaxis
- Most cases are sporadic

FAMILIAL
- **Autosomal dominant** — **Mutation of STAT3 gene**
- **Autosomal recessive** — **Mutations of DOCK8 gene**

Overall most common genetic cause of hyper-IgE syndrome is mutation in STAT3 gene.

Pathogenesis

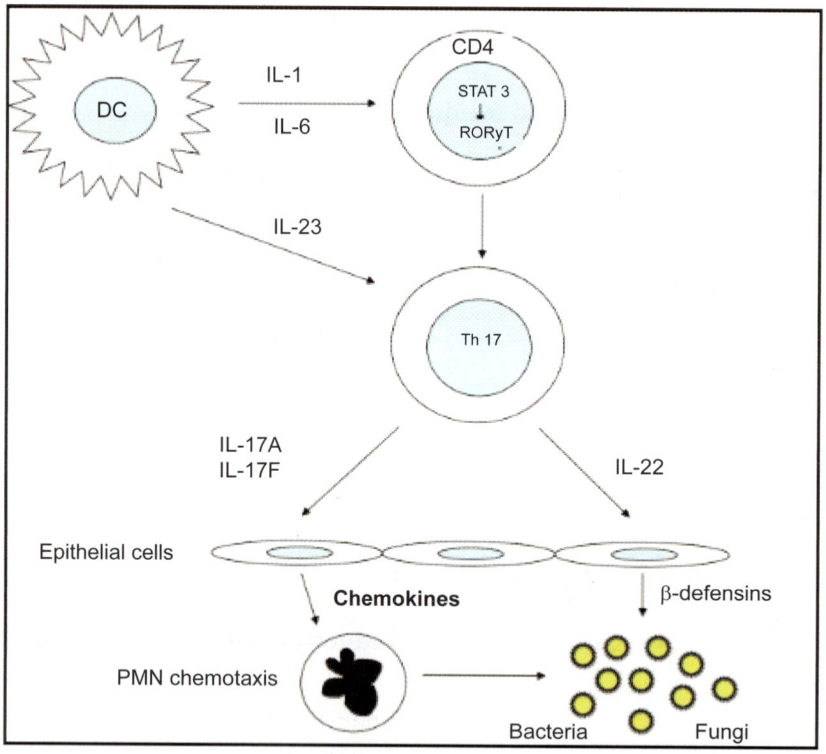

Defects in JAK-STAT signaling pathway leading to impaired Th17 function: Decreased IFN gamma production

- **STAT3 is necessary in Embryogenesis and for Cytokine production**

(IL-6, IL-10, IL-11, IL-17, IL-21, IL-22 and IL-23)

Main immunologic defect is failure to produce gamma interferon by helper T cells, which reduces ability of macrophages to kill bacteria

STAT3
- **Embryogenesis**
- **Proinflammatory (IL 6)**
- **Antiinflammatory (IL 10)**

- ***STAT3 defects result in IL-17 and other cytokine defects as well as structural changes***
- Will have defective CD14 TH_{17} responses
- ***Recurrent staphylococcal infection occur***→ *As STAT3 is defective Interleukins like IL17 and IL22 which regulate against staphyloccus also function defectively (This is also cause for Eczematous features in JOB SYNDROME)*
- Serum IgE are Elevated, Other Immunoglobulins are normal.

Clinical Features

Autosomal Dominant Inheritance	Autosomal Recessive Inheritance
Defect/Mutation of STAT3 gene	***Mutation of DOCK 8 gene***
• ***Characteristic facies (Coarse facial feature)***→ Broad nose, Osteoporosis, Facial dysmorphy, Defective loss of primary teeth, Kyphoscoliosis, Cerebral demyelinating plaques and Coronary artery aneurysms *(Abnormal calcium metabolism)* • ***Mucocutaneous candidiasis*** • Lung abscesses and Pneumatocoeles (Staphylococcal) • Atopic Dermatitis • Despite IgE patients don't present with severe allergy	• Viral infections due to CMV, HPV, HSV and allergies are particularly common. • Also an increased risk of malignancies. • Suffer from severe infections from early life.

Treatment

Mainly supportive→Antimicrobials

Defects of Humoral Immunity			
Disease	**Molecular Defect**	**Symptoms/Signs**	**Treatment**
Bruton (X-linked) agammaglobulinemia	Deficiency of the Bruton tyrosine kinase (btk) which promotes pre-B cell expansion; faulty B-cell development	Increased susceptibility to encapsulated bacteria and bloodborne viruses, low immunoglobulins of all isotypes, absent or low levels of circulating B-cells, B-cell maturation does not progress past the pre-B cells stage while maintaining cell-mediated immunity	Monthly gamma-globulin replacement, antibiotic for infection
X-linked hyper-IgM syndrome	Deficiency of **CD40L** on activated T cells	**High serum titers of IgM without other isotypes**, normal B and T-cell numbers, susceptibility to encapsulated bacteria and opportunistic pathogens	Antibiotics and gammaglobulins
Selective IgA deficiency	Multiple genetic causes	Decreased IgA levels and normal IgM and IgG with elevation of IgE. Repeated **sinopulmonary and gastrointestinal** infections, ↑ **atopy**	Antibiotics, not immunoglobulins
Common variable Immunodeficiency	Collection of syndromes; several associated genetic defects	Onsets in **late teens**, early twenties; B cells present in peripheral blood, immunoglobulin levels decrease with time; ↑ autoimmunity	Antibiotics
Transient hypogammaglo-bulinemia of infancy	Delayed onset of normal IgG synthesis	Detected in 5th to 6th month of life, resolves by 16-30 months; susceptibility to pyogenic bacteria	Antibiotics and in severe cases, gamma-globulin replacement

Defects of Phagocytic Cell		
Disease	**Molecular Defect(s)**	**Symptoms**
Chronic granulomatous disease (CGD)	Deficiency of **NADPH oxidase** (any one of 4 component proteins); failure to generate superoxide anion, other O_2 radicals	Recurrent infections with **catalase-positive** bacteria and fungi
Leukocyte adhesion deficiency	Absence of **CD18**–Common β chain of the leukocyte integrins The 3 integrins that contain CD 18: LFA-1, MAC-1 and gp 150/95	Recurrent and chronic infections, failure to form pus, and delayed separation of umbilical cord stump
Chediak-Higashi syndrome	Nonsense mutation in the lysosomal trafficking regulator, CHS1/LYST protein, leads to aberrant fusion of vesicles	Recurrent infection with bacteria: Chemotactic and degranulation defects; absent NK activity, partial **albinism**
Glucose-6-phosphate dehydrogenase (G6PD) deficiency	Deficiency of essential enzyme in hexose monophosphate shunt	Same as CGD, with associated **anemia**
Myeloperoxidase deficiency	Defect in MPO affects the ability to convert hydrogen peroxide to hypochlorite	Mild or none
Hyperimmunoglobulin E syndrome (formerly Job syndrome)	Defects in JAK-STAT signaling pathway leading to imparied Th 17 function: Decreased IFN-gamma production	Characteristic facies, severe, recurrent sinusopulmonary infections, pathologic bone fractures, retention of primary teeth, increased IgE, eczematous rash

T-Cell Deficiencies and Combined Deficiencies			
Category	**Disease**	**Defect**	**Clinical Manifestations**
Selective T-cell deficiency	**DiGeorge Syndrome**	Heterozygous deletion of chromosome 22q11. Failure of formation of **3rd and 4th pharyngeal pouches,** thymic aplasia	Characteristic facies and a clinical triad of cardiac malformations, hypocalcemia and hypoplastic thymus
	MHC class I deficiency	Failure of TAP 1 molecules to transport peptides to endoplasmic reticulum	**CD8+ T cells deficient, CD$_4$+ T cells normal,** recurring viral infections, normal DTH, normal Ab production
Combined partial B- and T-cell deficiency	**Wiskott-Aldrich Syndrome**	Defect in the WAS protein which plays a critical role in acting cytoskeleton rearrangement	Defective responses to bacterial polysaccharides and depressed IgM, gradual **loss of humoral and cellular responses, thrombocytopenia and eczema** IgA and IgE may be elevated 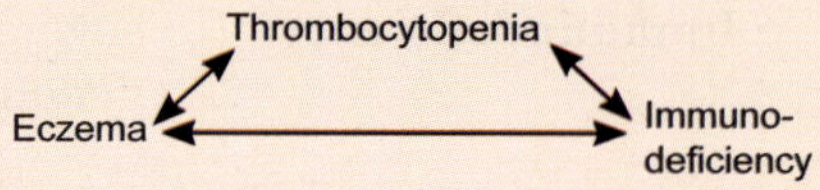

Contd.

Contd.

	Ataxia telangiectasia	Defect in the ATM kinase involved in the detection of DNA damage and progression through the cell cycle	**Ataxia** (gait abnormalities), **telangiectasia** capillary distortions in the eye), **deficiency of IgA and IgE** production
Complete functional B-and T-cell deficiency	**Severe combined immunodeficiency (SCID)**	Defects in common γ chain of IL-2 receptor (present in receptors for IL-4, –7, –9, –15), X-linked	Chronic diarrhea; skin, mouth and throat lesions; opportunistic **(fungal)** infections; low levels of circulating lymphocytes; cells unresponsive to mitogens
		Adenosine deaminase deficiency (results in toxic metabolic products in cells)	Clinical overlap with X-linked SCID plus neurologic deficiency
		Rag 1 or *rag* 2 gene nonsense mutations	Total absence B+ T-cells
	Bare lymphocyte syndrome/**MHC class II deficiency**	Failure of MHC class II expression, defects in transcription factors	T cells present and reponsive to nonspecific mitogens, no GVHD, **deficient in CD_4 + T cells,** hypogammaglobulinemia Clinically observed as a severe combined immunodeficiency

Deficiencies of Complement or Its Regulation

Deficiencies in Complement Components	Deficiency	Signs/Diagnosis
Classic pathway	C1q, C1r, C1s, C4, C2	Marked increase in immune complex diseases, increased infections with pyogenic bacteria
Both pathways	C3	Recurrent bacterial infections, immune complex disease
	C5, C6, C7, C8 or C9	Recurrent **meningococcal and gonococcal infections**
Deficiencies in complement regulatory proteins	C1-1NH **(hereditary angioedema)**	Overuse of C1, C4 or C2, edema at mucosal surfaces

Ref: David Male Immunology Textbook 8th Edition Page 272, Harrison 20th Edition Page 2494, Roitt's Essential Immunology 13th Edition Page 389, Essentials of Clinical Immunology 6th Edition Page 74

Ans: (C) Most are of Autosomal recessive inheritance

Chapter 6

MICROBIOLOGY

1. **Violent spastic paralysis in tetanus occurs due to:**

   A. Inhibition of cGMP
   B. Presynaptic inhibition of GABA release
   C. Postsynaptic inhibition of Ach release
   D. Inhibition of cAMP

Key:

Tetanospasmin–Exotoxin produced by vegetative cells at wound site. Polypeptide toxin is carried intra-axonally (retrograde). In CNS, it binds to ganglioside receptors and blocks release of inhibitory mediators (Glycine and GABA) at spinal synapses

CLOSTRIDIUM TETANI

- Gram +ve, strict anaerobe
- STATELY MOTILITY
- Tennis racket appearance
- Swarming growth on culture
- *First sign of Tetanus–Trismus*
- *Fir tree appearance on Gelatin stab culture*

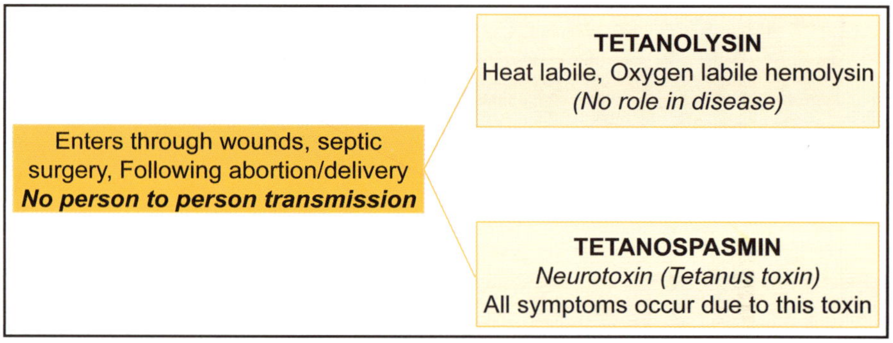

Pathogenesis

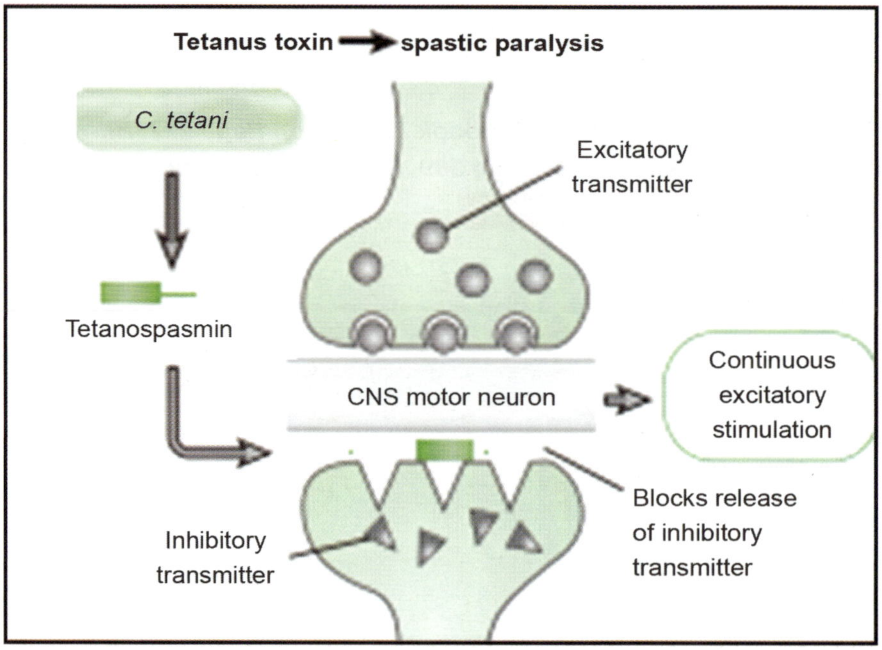

- Muscular spasms often involve first area of injury and infection. Muscle groups of shortest neuronal pathways are affected first- trismus and dysphagia are common early symptoms.
- Muscles of jaw contract so that mouth cannot be opened–Trismus, Lock jaw).
- Gradually, other voluntary muscles become involved→ Tonic spasms.
- *Any external stimulus may precipitate a tetanic generalized muscle spasm.*
- **Death**–Respiratory failure.

TETANUS

- **Generalized**
  - ***Most common form***
    Trismus, Risus sardonicus, Opisthotonous
    Severe–Autonomic nervous system involved
- **Localized**
  - Confined to musculature at primary site of infection
    Cephalic tetanus–Head
- **Neonatal tetanus**
  - ***Tetanus neonatorum (8-Day disease)***
    Initial infection at umbilical stump

Identifying Features of Clostridium Tetani

- Produces alpha hemolytic colonies initially on blood agar while on prolonged incubation becomes beta hemolytic due to tetanolysin
- Gram +ve bacilli with prominent terminal spores (Drum stick appearance)
- Motile and capsulated bacteria
- Don't ferment any sugars
- Toxigenicity testing in mouse–Reliable method for identification of Clostridium tetani toxin

- **Treatment**–Penicillin
- **Mainstay of treatment**–Antitoxin
  - *Active immunization:* Antitoxin >0.01 IU/ml
  - *Passive immunization:* Human tetanus Immunoglobulin

Tetanus→ Spastic paralysis *(strong muscle contractions)*
Botulism→ Flaccid paralysis *(weak/absent muscle contractions)*

Ref: Jawetz 27th Edition Page 185, Essentials of Medical Microbiology 2nd Edition Page 270, Murray Medical Microbiology 8th Edition Page 307, Parija Textbook of Microbiology and Immunology 2nd Edition Page 238, Sherri's Medical Microbiology 6th Edition Page 527, Levinson Review of Microbiology 13th Edition Page 313

Ans: (B) Presynaptic inhibition of GABA release

2. **Disease with which of the following shows Mononucleosis like syndrome?**

A. CMV
B. Parvo virus
C. Hepatitis B
D. HPV

Key:

Cytomegalovirus causes Mononucleosis like features

Cytomegalovirus

- Largest member of Herpes virus family
- Enlargement of the virus infected cell occurs ('cytomegalic')

Intranuclear and cytoplasmic inclusion body–owl's eye appearance

- Spread slowly and requires close contact
- Route–via secretions, sexual, blood transfusion, vertical transmission
- Exhibit strict host specificity
- CMV is present in a large percentage of medulloblastomas–most common malignant brain tumor in children.
- Most common viral cause of congenital defects.

Congenital CMV

- ***Most common intrauterine infection***
- Affects nearly 1% infants born
- Cytomegalic inclusion disease develops in 5% of infected fetus

Most common signs–Petechiae, Hepatosplenomegaly and Jaundice

- Microcephaly, Mental retardation, chorioretinitis, cerebral calcification, convulsions
- Risk is maximum if infection occurs in early pregnancy and mother is primarily infected during pregnancy
- ***Infants are highly infectious***
- Transmit the virus in urine for 3-5 years

Perinatal CMV

- Transmission to newborn occurs during
  - Delivery
  - Postnatal–through infected breast milk/secretion of mother
- Mostly asymptomatic (Shed in urine upto several years)
- Premature babies–Interstitial pneumonitis

Immunocompetent Adults *(Most common presentation)*	Immunocompromised Host *(Most common presentation)*
Mononucleosis like syndrome • Atypical lymphocytosis present • Occurs following Blood transfusion • Fever, myalgia, rash present *(No lymphadenopathy and Exudative pharyngitis)* • Heterophile Antibody test –ve	• Untreated HIV Patient–Chorioretinitis • Organ transplant recipients–Bilateral interstitial pneumonia

CMV is most common viral infection in transplant recipients

- Bilateral interstitial pneumonia in Bone marrow transplants
- Febrile leucopenia in solid organ transplants
- Obliterative bronchiolitis in Lung transplants
- Graft atherosclerosis in heart transplants
- Rejection of renal allografts

Contd.

Contd.

Group	Clinical features	Mode of infection
Congenital infections	Hepatosplenomegaly, Jaundice, Thrombocytopenic purpura, Haemolytic anaemia, Microcephaly, Permanent mental abnormalities	Transplacental
Childhood infections	Insidious hepatitis, Pneumonitis	Respiratory route
Reactivation	Hepatitis, Interstitial pneumonia	Post immunosuppression
Post perfusion syndrome	Fever, Increase in atypical mononuclear cells	Repeated transfusions

Tissue	Children/Adults	Immunosuppressed Patients
Predominant presentation	Asymptomatic	Disseminated disease, severe disease
Eyes	–	Chorioretinitis
Lungs	–	Pneumonia, pneumonitis
Gastrointestinal tract	–	Esophagitis, colitis
Nervous system	Polyneuritis, myelitis	Meningitis and encephalitis, myelitis
Lymphoid system	Mononucleosis syndrome, posttransfusion syndrome	Leukopenia, lymphocytosis
Major organs	Carditis,* hepatitis*	Hepatitis
Neonates	Deafness, intracerebral calcification, microcephaly, mental retardation	–

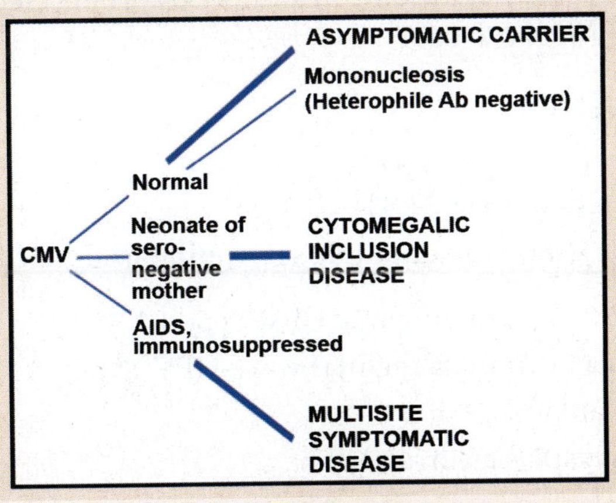

Lab Diagnosis

Test	Finding
Cytology and histology*	"Owl's-eye" basophilic nuclear inclusion body Antigen detection
	In situ DNA probe hybridization
	PCR
Cell culture	Cytologic effect in human diploid fibroblasts (slow)
	Immunofluorescence detection of early antigens (faster)
	PCR (faster)
Serology	Primary infection indicated by seroconversion, detection of IgM antibodies specific to CMV and Antigen detection

Contd.

Contd.

- **Detection of Inclusion bodies in urine**–CMV produces both perinuclear cytoplasmic and intranuclear inclusions
- **Viral isolation**–Isolated from throat washings and Urine
- **Antibody detection:**
  - IgM antibodies are indicative of active infection
  - 4-fold rise of IgG indicates recurrent infection

Antibodies are often undetectable in Immunocopromised patients

- PCR detects specific CMV DNA in blood or body fluids like CSF
- CMV Specific pp65 antigens–Highly specific and reliable method

Treatment

- **Ganciclovir**–Drug of choice form CMV inclusion disease/Retinitis/Transplant infections
- **Foscarnet**–Drug of choice in Ganciclovir resistant cases

Parvo virus	• **5th disease or Erythema infectiosum:** ○ Characterized by rash, arthralgia, lymphadenopathy ○ *Slapped cheek appearance–Rash 1st on cheek* • Causes Aplastic crisis in sickle cell anemia patients • Pregnancy–Non-immune fetal hydrops • **Polyarthropathy syndrome** in adults–50% of infected people, mainly women ***(Most common–Hand joints)***
HPV	**Carcinoma cervix** • Low risk – type 6,11–CIN • High risk – type 16,18,31,33 – Ca Cx • Risk factor – early sex, multiple sex, multiparous, OCP **Common wart /verruca vulgaris**–HPV Type 1,2,3,4 • **Condyloma acuminata /genital wart**–HPV Type 6,11 • Verruca plantaris • Epidermodysplasia verrucoplasia

Ref: Jawetz 27th Edition Page 471, Murray Medical Microbiology 8th Edition Page 442, Sherri's Medical Microbiology 6th Edition Page 259, Essentials of Medical Microbiology 4th Edition Page 413

Ans: (A) CMV

3. **Cowdry type A inclusion bodies are seen with:**

A. HIV
B. HBV
C. HSV
D. Polio

Key:

Cowdry type A bodies are seen in HSV infection

Inclusion Bodies

- Inclusion bodies are morphological changes produced by virus inside tissue

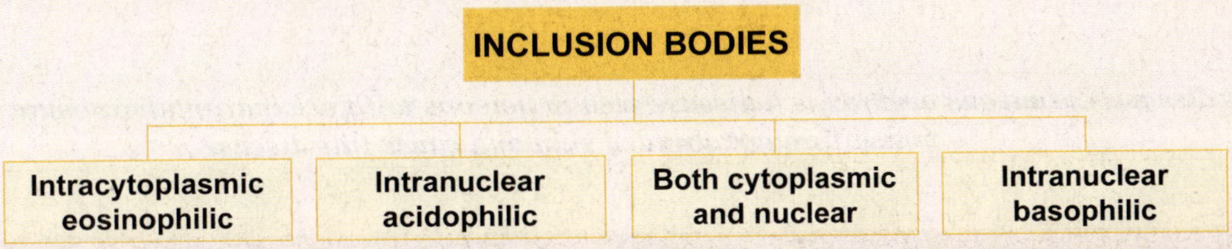

Intracytoplasmic eosinophilic	
Negri bodies	Rabies
Guarnieri bodies	Vaccinia
Paschen bodies	Variola
Bollinger bodies	Fowlpox
Henderson-Peterson bodies, Molluscum bodies	Molluscum contagiosum
Perinuclear cytoplasmic acidophilic bodies	Reo virus

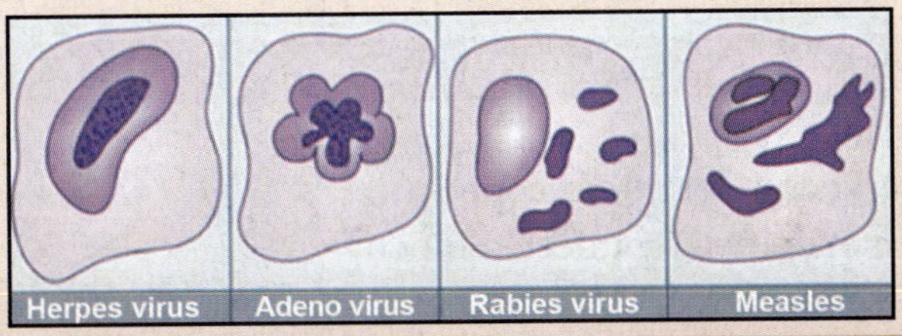

Intranuclear acidophilic	
Cowdry Type A	Herpes, Chickenpox, CMV, Yellow fever
Torres bodies	Yellow fever
Lipschultz bodies	HSV
Cowdry Type B	Polio

Intranuclear basophilic	
Cowdry type B	Adenovirus

Both nuclear and cytoplasmic	
Wartin Finkeldey cells	Measles
Owl's eye inclusion bodies	CMV

EXTRA EDGE

Both intracytoplasmic and intranuclear inclusion bodies are seen in Measles and CMV

Ref: Jawetz Textbook of Microbiology 27th Edition Page 408, Ananthanarayan and Paniker 10th Edition Page 518, Essentials of Medical Microbiology 4th Edition Page 318, Essentials of Microbiology 2nd Edition Page 437, Textbook of Microbiology and Immunology by Parija 2nd Edition Page 444

Ans: (C) HSV

4. A 38-year-old veterinarian has painless swelling in finger which was ulcerated and develops blackish eschar in weeks. What could be the causative organism?

A. Brucella abortus
B. Leptospira
C. Bacillus anthracis
D. Bacillus cereus

Key:

Hideporter's disease/Cutaneous anthrax is a disease seen in persons with occupational exposure to animals–Spores travel through abraded skin and cause this disease

Malignant Pustule
Painless coal black necrotic eschar surrounded by non pitting indurated edema
Anthrax means coal (This comes from black color of eschar) *Occupations involved include Dock worker, Butcher, Abattoir and Farmer*

Bacillus Anthracis

- 1st bacterial attenuated vaccine
- 1st pathogenic bacteria observed under microscope
- 1st Communicable disease transmitted by infected blood
- 1st bacteria to get isolated in culture
- **Selective Media**–PLET medium
- **Ascoli thermoprecipitation test**–detects antigen
- **Mc Faydeans reaction**–staining with polychrome methylene blue demonstrates capsule
- **Sterne, Mazucchi strains**–Live attenuate spore vaccine
- **Duckering**–Spore destruction by formaldehyde

Identifying features of Bacillus anthracis

1. Macroscopic appearance of serpentine chains of bacterial colony (medusa head colony).
2. Nonhemolytic colonies on blood agar.
3. Sticky consistency of colonies on blood agar.
4. No growth on chloral hydrate agar.
5. Large, Gram-positive, spore-forming bacilli in the Gram-stained smear of the colony.
6. Nonmotile and capsulated bacteria.
7. Lysis by gamma-phage positive.
8. String-of-pearls test positive.

Must Know Points

- *Medusa head appearance of colonies*
- *Bamboo stick or box car appearance on culture*
- *Frosted glass appearance in agar plate*
- *Inverted fir tree appearance on Gelatin stab culture*
- *String of pearls on solid media*
- *Cut glass appearance on transmitted light*

Contd.

Contd.

Virulence factors of *Bacillus anthracis*	
Virulence factors	**Biological functions**
Bacterial capsule	Protects anthrax bacilli against leukocytic phagocytosis and lysis; if engulfed, resist killing and digestion
Anthrax toxin complex	Anthrax toxin complex is plasmid-encoded and comprises the following three proteins
Protective antigen (PA)	Entry of the bacilli into the host cell. Binds the complex to receptors on macrophage surface
Edema factor (EF)	Causes cellular edema within the target tissue and also inhibits neutrophil function. Blocks adenyl cyclase pathway within cells
Lethal factor (LF)	Release of tumor necrosis factor-α and interleukin-1 by macrophages

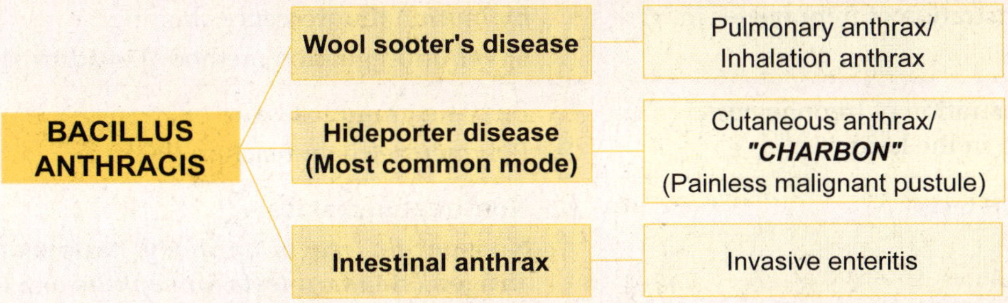

Treatment

- Drug of choice is Penicillin.
- ***In Penicillin allergy*** – Ciprofloxacin, erythromycin, tetracycline or chloramphenicol.

Anthracoid bacilli–PSEUDOANTHRAX–*B. subtilis, B. licheniformis and B. mycoides.*

- *Geobacillus stearothermophilus spores*–**Used to test efficiency of sterilization by autoclaves.**
- *Bacillus species*–**Used for production of antibiotics like bacitracin and polymyxin.**
- *Bacillus subtilis*–**Opportunistic pathogen, causing eye infections and septicemia.**
- *Bacillus licheniformis*–**Food poisoning.**

Bacillus cereus	*Food poisoning*
Leptospira	*Weil's disease*
Brucella abortus	*Brucellosis/Typhoid like illness*

Ref: Jawetz Textbook of Microbiology 27th Edition Page 180, Rapid Review of Microbiology and Immunology 3rd Edition Page 76, Essentials of Medical Microbiology 4th Edition Page 184, Textbook of Microbiology and Immunology by Parija 2nd Edition Page 223

Ans: (C) Bacillus anthracis

5. **Investigation of choice for diagnosis of neurosyphilis is:**

A. FTA-ABS B. RPR
C. VDRL D. TPI

Key:

Test of choice for diagnosis of neurosyphilis–VDRL of CSF
Most commonly used test for syphilis–VDRL

Diagnostic Tests

A. Demonstration of treponemes	
a. Demonstration of treponemes in the exudate	1. Dark ground microscopy 2. Direct fluorescent-antibody staining for *Treponema pallidum* (DFA-Tp)
b. Demonstration of treponemes in tissues	1. By immunofluorescence staining 2. Silver impregnation method (Levaditis stain)
c. Demonstration of treponemes antigen in the lesion	1. Enzyme immunoassay 2. Polymerase chain reaction (PCR)
B. Serological tests	**A. Non-treponemal tests** **Nonspecific *(reagin antibody)* tests using the cardiolipin antigen *(standard tests for syphilis or STS)*** a. Wassermann CF reaction b. Kahn flocculation test c. Venereal Disease Research Laboratory (VDRL) test d. Rapid Plasma Reagin (RPR) test e. Toluidine Red Unheated Serum Test (TRUST) **B. Treponemal tests** a. **Group specific test using cultivable treponemal (Reiter strain) antigen** Reiter Protein CF (RPCF) test b. **Specific tests using pathogenic treponemes *(T. pallidum)*** I. **Test using live *T. pallidum*** *Treponema pallidum Immobilization* (TPI) test II. **Tests using killed *T. pallidum*** a. *Treponema pallidum agglutination* (TPA) test b. *Treponema pallidum* immune adherence (TPIA) test c. Fluorescent Treponemal antibody absorption (FTA-ABS) test III. **Test using *T. pallidum* extract** a. *Treponema pallidum* Hemagglutination Assay (TPHA) Microhemagglutination test for *Treponema pallidum* (MHA-TP) b. *Treponema pallidum* Enzyme Immunoassays (TP-EIA)

Contd.

Contd.

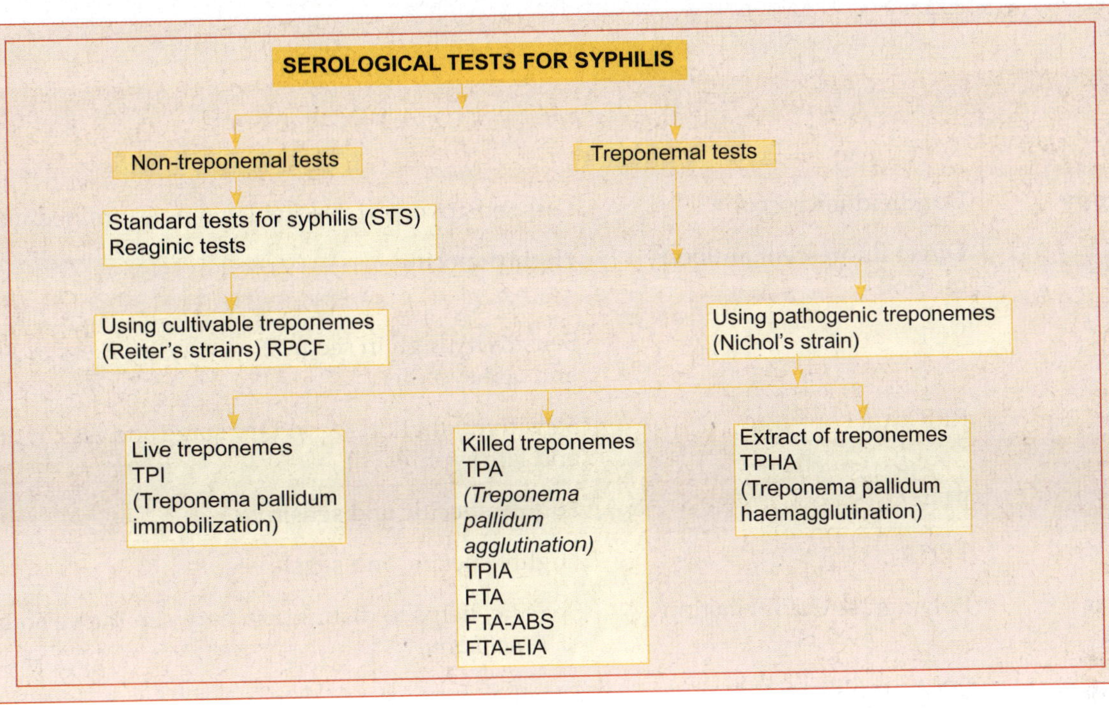

Sensitivity of serological tests for syphilis

Syphilis	VDRL	RPR	FTA-Abs	TPHA
Stage of syphilis				
Primary	+/–	–	+	–
Late primary	+	+	+	+/–
Secondary	+	+	+	+
Tertiary	+	+	+	+
Late	+	+	+	+
Latent	+/–	+/–	+	+
Treated syphilis	–	–	+	+
Cogenital syphilis	+	+	+	+

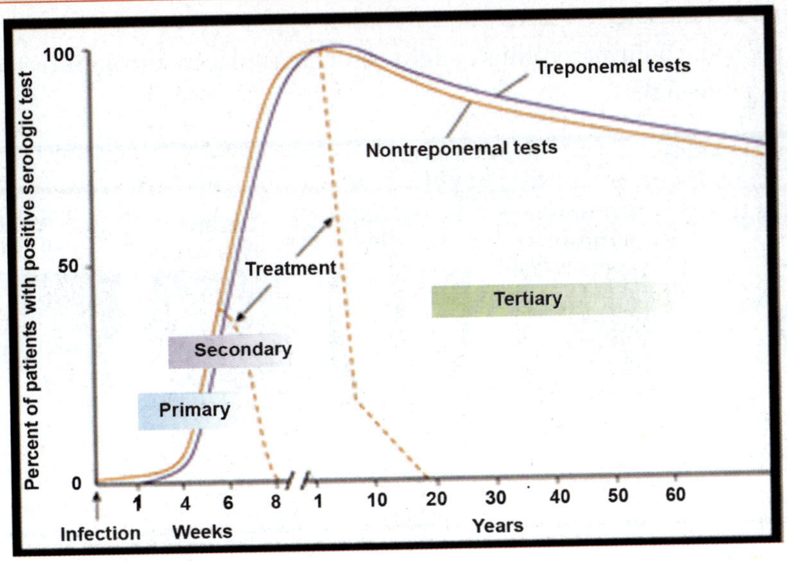

Diagnostic tests for syphilis		
Diagnostic test	**Method**	**Test accuracy**
Microscopy	Darkfield microscopy	Less sensitive; test is reliable when examined immediately
	Direct fluorescent antibody method	Highly specific
Serology	VDRL	Sensitivity high in secondary stage and less in primary stage and late syphilis
	RPR	Sensitivity high in secondary stage and less in primary stage and late syphilis
	FTA-Abs	Highly specific and sensitive
	TPHA	Highly specific and sensitive
Molecular methods	Polymerase chain reaction	Specific; helps to distinguish between the various subspecies of *T. pallidum*
	DNA amplification	Specific

Serological Tests in Syphilis

- Most sensitive for Primary syphilis–Western blot and Enzyme immunoassay
- Secondary syphilis–All tests are equally sensitive (100%)
- Most Sensitive for Latent syphilis–All treponemal tests
- Most Sensitive for Late syphilis–FTA ABS
- ***Overall most specific test–TPHA***
- First test to be positive–FTA ABS
- Rapid and mass screening–VDRL/RPR
- Test of choice for diagnosis of neurosyphilis–VDRL of CSF
- Most commonly used test for syphilis–VDRL/RPR
- Ideal test for Monitoring treatment–VDRL
- Presence of IgM in neonate confirms syphilis as IgM can't cross placenta from infected mother to newborn
- Reagin antibody in syphilis–IgG

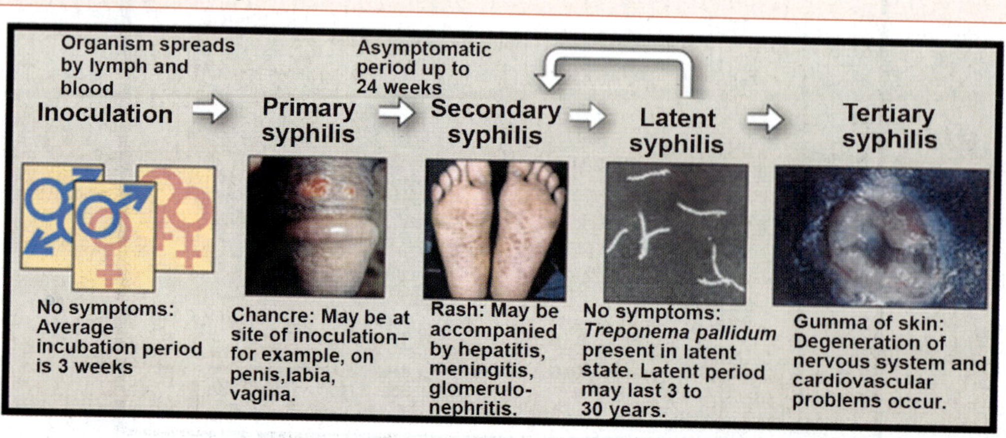

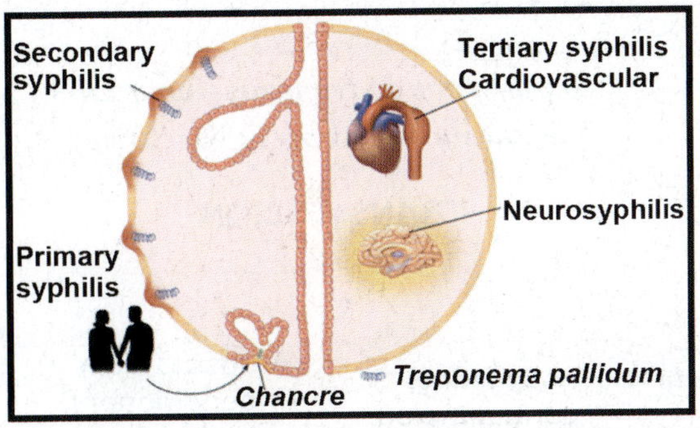

Human infections caused by most common spirochetes	
Bacteria	**Diseases**
Treponema pallidum subspp. *pallidum*	Syphilis
Treponema pallidum subspp. *endemicum*	Bejel and endemic syphilis
Treponema pallidum subspp. *pertenue*	Yaws
Treponema carateum	Pinta
Borrelia recurrentis	Epidemic relapsing fever
Many *Borrelia* species	Endemic relapsing fever
Borrelia burgdorferi	Lyme disease
Leptospira interrogans	Leptospirosis

Ref: Jawetz Textbook of Microbiology 27th Edition Page 324, Murray Medical Microbiology 8th Edition Page 325, Textbook of Microbiology and Immunology by Parija 2nd Edition Page 378, Sherri's Medical Microbiology 6th Edition Page 645

Ans: (C) VDRL

6. Culture medium of choice for Legionella pneumophila is:

A. Thayer Martin media
B. BCYE Agar
C. Bordet Gengou media
D. Cary Blair medium

Key:

Culture media of choice for Legionella is BCYE agar

Legionella

- Fastidious gram –ve short bacilli
- Associated with Respiratory syndromes–Pontaic fever and Legionnaire's disease
- ***Most cases are associated with Serogroup 1 followed by 4 and 6***
- **Reservoir**–Inhabits on Aquatic bodies–Rivers, Even inside amoebae and Air conditioners

Contd.

Contd.

No man to man transmission occurs
No animal reservoir & No carrier

TRANSMISSION

- Aspiration (Most common)
- Drinking contaminated water
- Aerosols from Air conditioners, Nebulizers and Humidifiers
- Direct instillation into lungs during respiratory tract manipulations

Pathogenesis

- Respiratory tract disease caused by Legionella species develops in susceptible people who inhale infectious aerosols.

AFTER ENTERING LUNGS
↓
Bacteria Attaches and Invasion to respiratory mucosa occurs
↓
Coiling phagocytosis
↓
Evades intracellular killing by inhibiting phagosome-lysosome fusion

Clinical Features

LEGIONELLA

- **Pontaic fever**
  - *Acute flu like illness*
- **Legionnaire's disease**
  - *Interstitial atypical pneumonia*
  - *4th most common cause of Community acquired pneumonia*
  - *Serotype 6 is more commonly involved in hospital outbreaks*
- **Extra pulmonary legionellosis**
  - *Most common lesion– Myocarditis > Pericarditis > Prosthetic valve endocarditis*

Characteristic Epaidemiology	Legionnaires Disease	Pontiac Fever
Presentation	**Epidemic, sporadic**	**Epidemic**
Infection rate	<5%	>90%
Person-to-person spread	No	No
Time of onset	Epidemic disease in late summer and fall; endemic disease throughout the year	Throughout the year
Clinical Manifestations		
Incubation period	2-10 days	1-2 days
Pneumonia	Yes	No
Resolution	Requires antibiotic therapy	Self-limited
Mortality rate	15%-20% (untreated); higher with late diagnosis	<1%

Contd.

Contd.

Lab Diagnosis

- **Gram stain**–Reveals numerous neutrophils but no organisms
- **Culture**–BCYE agar is recommended media
- **Antibody detection**–Used for epidemiological purpose
- **PCR**–Isolation from Environmental water
- **Urinary antigen**–Rapid, cheaper, easy to perform, Remains +ve even after antibiotic usage

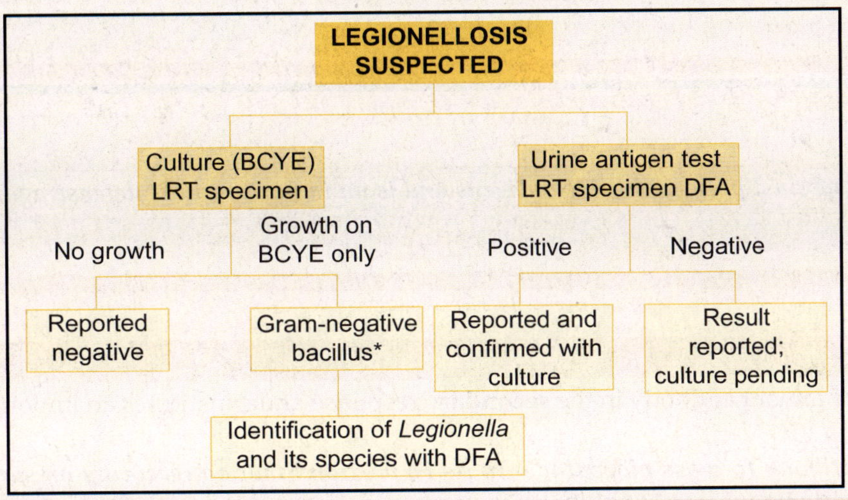

Treatment

- Macrolides and Quinolones–Antibiotic of choice

Common Phenotypic Characteristics of Legionella Species

- Slow growth (3–5 days)
- Characteristic "ground glass" colony morphology
- Lightly staining, gram-negative bacillus
- ***Best seen with Dieterle silver stain or fluorescent stain***
- Requires L-cysteine for primary isolation
- No growth on unsupplemented sheep blood agar
- Asaccharolytic
- Catalase or oxidase: Weakly positive

EXTRA EDGE

Classification Based on Autofluorescence

Yellow-Green	*L. micdadei*	**Blue-White**	**Blue-White or Yellow-Green**	*L. feeleii*
Legionella birminghamensis	*L. oakridgensis*	*L. bozemanii*		*L. lansingensis*
L. cincinnatiensis	*L. pneumophila*	*L. dumoffii*	*L. anisa*	*L. londiniensis*
L. hackeliae	*L. sainthelensi*	*L. gormanii*	**Red**	*L. nagasakiensis*
L. jordanis	*L. wadworthii*	*L. lytica*	*L. rubrilucens*	
L. longbeachae	**Yellow/Blue-White**	*L. parisiensis*	**No Color**	
L. maceachernii	*L. steelei*	*L. tusconensis*	*L. cardiac*	

Legionella micdadei–*Pittsburgh pneumonia agent and Acid fast*

Ref: Jawetz Textbook of Microbiology 27th Edition Page 303, Murray Medical Microbiology 8th Edition Page 299, Textbook of Microbiology and Immunology by Parija 2nd Edition Page 403, Sherri's Medical Microbiology 6th Edition Page 645

Ans: (B) BCYE Agar

7. **What is the Immunoglobulin deficiency that causes Capsulated microorganisms infection among the following?**

A. IgG1 B. IgG2

C. IgG4 D. IgG3

Key:

IgG2 is directed against polysaccharide antigens and is an important host defense against encapsulated bacteria

Immunoglobin G

- IgG is the predominant antibody in the **secondary response** and constitutes an important defense against bacteria and viruses.
- ***IgG is only antibody to cross placenta; only its Fc portion binds to receptors on surface of placental cells. It is therefore most abundant immunoglobulin in newborns.***
- IgG1 represents 65% of the total IgG.

IgG2 is directed against polysaccharide antigens and an important host defense against encapsulated bacteria.

- IgG3 is an effective activator of complement due to its rigid hinge region.
- IgG4 does not activate complement due to its compact structure.
- IgG1, IgG3 and IgG4 are special because these are only immunoglobulins with ability to cross placental barrier (Play an important role in protecting fetus against infections).

IgG3, IgG1 and IgG2 in order of their efficiency are effective in activation of complement.

- IgG1 and IgG3 bind with high affinity to Fc receptors on phagocytic cells and thus mediate opsonization.
- IgG4 has an intermediate affinity for Fc receptors and IgG2 has an extremely low affinity.
- IgG1 and IgG3 are more effective opsonizers than are IgG2 and IgG4.

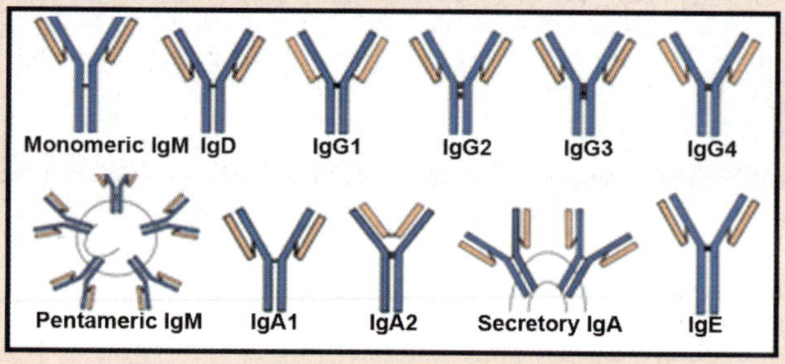

IgG – protects the body fluids

IgA – protects the mucosal surfaces

IgM – protects the blood stream

IgE – mediates reaginic hypersensitivity

IgD – recognition molecule on the surface of B lymphocytes

Characteristics	IgG	IgA	IgM	IgD	IgE
Structure	Monomer	Dimer	Pentamer	Monomer	Monomer
Percentage of total serum	80%	10-13%	5-8%	0.2%	0.002%

Contd.

Contd.

Location	Blood, lymph and intestiner	Blood, lymph and B cell surface	Secretions	B cell surface, blood and lymph	Bound to mast and basophil cell
Sedimentation coefficient	7	7	19	7	8
Molecular weight (kDa)	150	160	900	180	190
Cabohydrate (%)	3	8	12	13	12
Serum concentration (mg/mL)	12	2	1.2	0.03	0.00004
Half-life (days)	23	6-8	5	2-8	1-5
Heavy chain	$\gamma_1, \gamma_2, \gamma_3, \gamma_4$	α_1, α_2	μ	Δ	ε
Light chain	κ or δ	κ or δ	κ or δ	κ or δ	κ or δ
Complement binding	Classical pathway	Alternate pathway	Classical pathway	None	None
Placental transport	+	–	–	–	–
Present in milk	+	+	–	–	–
Seromucous secretion	–	+	–	–	–
Heat stability (56°C)	+	+	+	+	–
Binding to tissue	Heterologous	None	None	None	Homologous

EXTRA EDGE

- *Maximum molecular weight–IgM*
- *Most effective in Opsonization–IgM*
- *Most effective in complement fixation–IgM*
- *Maximum valency–IgM*
- *Presence of J chains–IgM and IgA*
- *Maximum Half life–IgG*
- *Minimum Half life–IgE*
- *Maximum distribution in Intravascular compartment–IgG*
- *Maximum distribution in Extravascular compartment–IgM*
- *Maximum presence in external secretions–IgA*
- *Antibody on surface of B cells–IgM*
- *1st Antibody to appear in Acute stage of infection–IgM*
- *Antibody as a marker of in utero infection–IgM*
- *Antibody that can cross placenta–IgG*
- *Antibody that appears in Chronic stage of infection–IgG*
- *Antibody that activates complement by classical pathway–IgG and IgM*
- *Antibody that can be transmitted through human milk–IgA and IgG*
- *Antibody primarily on Epithelial surfaces–Secretory IgA*
- *Reagenic antibody–IgE*
- *Heat labile antibody–IgE*
- *Antibody responsible for Type 1 Hypersensitivity reaction–IgE*
- *Antibody that leads to degranulation of mast cells and basophils–IgE*
- *Antibody with maximum carbohydrate content–IgE*
- *Antibody that display homocytotropism–IgE*

Contd.

Contd.

- *Antibody of ABO Incompatibility–IgM*
- *Antibody of Rh Incompatibility–IgG*
- *Antibody of Rheumatoid arthritis–IgM*
- *Antibody of Biological false positives–IgM*

Ref: Jawetz Textbook of Microbiology 27th Edition Page 137, Murray Medical Microbiology 8th Edition Page 7 Textbook of Microbiology and Immunology by Parija 2nd Edition Page 97, Sherri's Medical Microbiolog 6th Edition Page 645, Review of Medical Microbiology and Immunology 13th Edition Page 11

Ans: (B) IgG2

8. Contact isolation should be done for:

A. Influenza
B. Mumps
C. Pertussis
D. MRSA

Key:

Control of MRSA requires strict adherence to infection control practices including barrier protection, contact isolation and handwashing compliance. Other options are spread respiratory tract by droplet infection or aerosols airbone needing respiratory isolation (Just contact isolation alone will not help in these cases)

Staphylococcus

- Anterior nares is most frequent site of colonization in humans (30%)
- Most human infections are caused by biotype A
- Disease causing ability is due to iron acquisition from host
- Novobiocin sensitivity differentitates saprophyticus from epidermidis
- ***"Nutrient Agar: Oil paint appearance of colonies"***
- ***Ludlam's media: Black colour (Selective media)***
- Production of coagulase is most common association with virulence
- Most of them grow in 10% Nacl
- **Blood Agar:** Distinct zone of hemolysis around colonies
- Ferments mannitol but no gas is produced
- Produces thermonuclease enzyme
- Sensitive to lysostaphin
- Most common enterotoxin is type A
- ***Enterotoxin acts by vagal stimulation.***

Staphylococcus aureus is most common cause of	
• Acute endocarditis • Acute osteomyelitis • Spinal epidural abscess • Nosocomial pneumonia • Septic intracranial thrombophlebitis	• Botryomycosis • Pyomyositis • Psoas abscess and epidural abscess • Folliculitis, Furuncle, Carbuncle • Breast abscess

Cont

Contd.

• Paronychia • Skin, soft tissue infections • Surgical wound infection	• Septic arthritis • Pneumatoceles • Dermatitis herpetiformis

Treatment

Condition	Drug
Penicillin sensitive	*Penicillin G*
Penicillinase production but sensitive to penicillin	*Oxacillin or Nafcillin*
MRSA	*Vancomycin > Daptomycin*
VRSA	*Quinpristine, Dalfopristin, Linezolid*
Topical treatment for MRSA	***Mupirocin Ointment (Carriers)***
Food poisoning	*Supportive treatment*
Toxic shock syndrome	*Clindamycin*

Drug Resistance

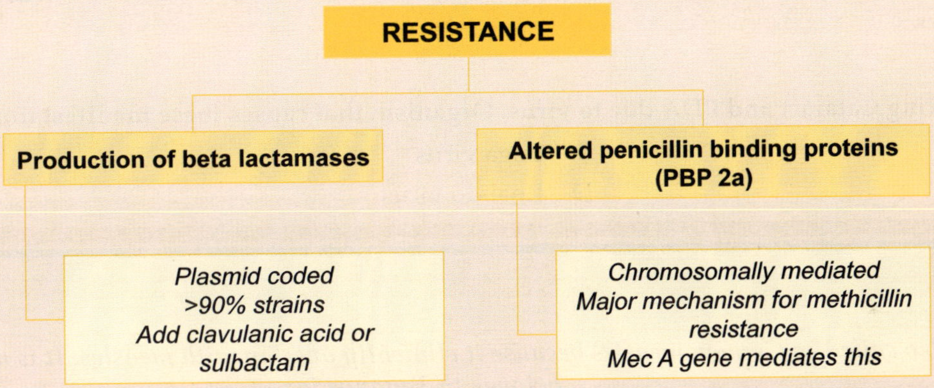

Resistance	Screening Test
Penicillin resistance	Nitrocefin test
MRSA	Disk diffusion susceptible test
VRSA	Vancomycin screen agar

- **MRSA**–*Methicillin MIC 8 μg/ml or more, Oxacillin MIC 4 μg/ml or more*

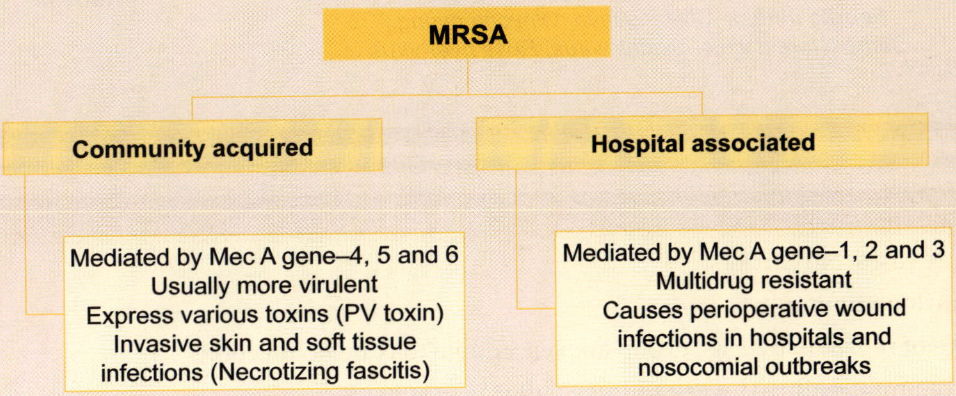

- **BORSA**–Borderline Oxacillin resistant S. aureus–MIC is Mildly elevated, occurs due to hyper production of β lactamase

Contd.

Contd.

- **VRSA**–Vancomycin Resistant *Staphylococcus aureus*–MIC 32 µg/ml or more–***Thickened cell wall***
- **VISA**–Vancomycin Intermediate *Staphylococcus aureus*–MIC 8-16 µg/ml

EXTRA EDGE

- Most common method for spread of infection in hospital–through ***hands of hospital staff***
- Most effective way to prevent the hospital infection–***hand washing***

Most common method for typing of S. aureus – Phage typing (pattern method)

- Mechanism of Penicillin resistance–production of β ***lactamase***
- Penicillin resistance in S. aureus transferred by–***Transduction (Most common)***
- MC site of colonization–Anterior nares and ***Skin*** (perineum, axilla, groins)

Ref: Jawetz Textbook of Microbiology 27th Edition Page 204, Murray Medical Microbiology 8th Edition Page 172, Textbook of Microbiology and Immunology by Parija 2nd Edition Page 181, Sherri's Medical Microbiology 6th Edition Page 443, Review of Medical Microbiology and Immunology 13th Edition Page 251

Ans: (D) MRSA

9. Newborn suffering Cataract and PDA due to virus. Organism that causes these manifestations belong to:

A. Myxo virus B. Toga virus
C. Arbo virus D. Rhabdo virus

Key:

Rubella is also called as German measles because it clinically overlap with measles. It is not a Myxovirus and belongs to Togaviridae

TOGAVIRIDAE

- **Alpha virus** *(Transmitted by mosquitos)*
  - ***Encephalitis***–*Western equine, Eastern equine and Venezuelan equine*
  - ***Febrile illness***–*Chikungunya, O'nyong nyong, Semiliki forest virus, Sindbis virus, Ross river virus*
- **Rubi virus**
  - ***Rubella***

Rubella

- **Source**–Only cases, No carriers
- Provides life long immunity
- 40% females of reproductive age group are susceptible to rubella infection
- Period of communicability–1 week to 1week after rash subsides
- **Incubation period**–2 to 3 weeks
- **Transmission**–Droplet, Contact, Sexual and In utero

Contd.

Contd.

Clinical Features

- **Rash on day 1 (Face) Lasts for 3 days**
- Subclinical infections–50%
- Lymphadenopathy–Occipital and Post auricular
- **Forschheimer spots**–Pin head sized petechiae seen on Soft palate and Uvula→Appears after onset of rash

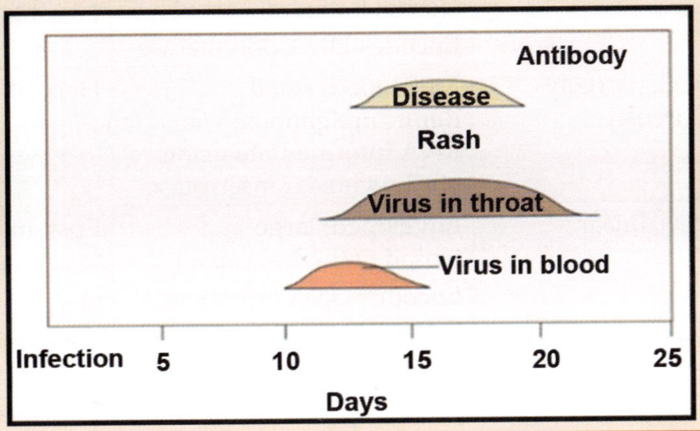

Congenital Rubella Syndrome

- Risk of transmission and severity is maximum in 1st trimester of pregnancy
- After 5th month, risk is negligible

Triad of Congenital Rubella Syndrome

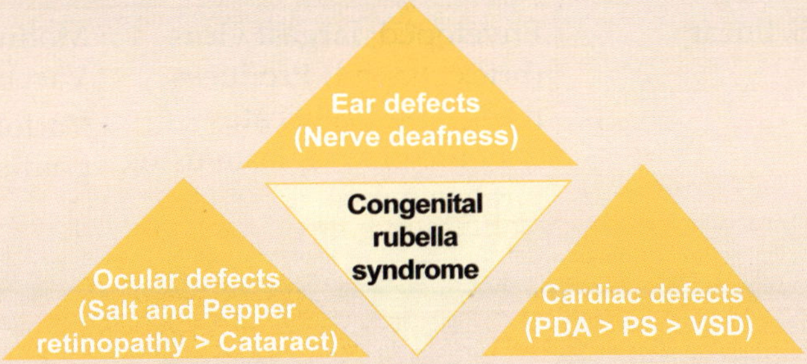

- *Most common defect of CRS–Ear defects (Nerve deafness)*
- *Most common ocular defect–Salt and Pepper retinopathy*
- *Cardiac defects: PDS (Most common) > PS > VSD*
- **Others:** *Microcephaly, Retinopathy, Microphthalmia, Cryptorchidism, Inguinal hernia and Diabetes mellitus*

- **Transient congenital changes**–*Hepatosplenomegaly, Bone lesions, IUGR and Thrombocytopenia with petechiae (Blueberry muffin syndrome).*

Diagnosis

- IgM at birth or persistent IgG that doesn't fall 2-fold dilution/month. Virus isolation within 6 months, RT-PCR for viral RNA detection.
- **Lab diagnosis–Hemagglutination inhibition test and ELISA (Most widely used)**

Ideal specimen–*Nasopharyngeal/Throat swabs*

Ideal cell line–*Monkey/Rabbit origin cell lines*

DNA Virus

Family	DNA Genome	Other Properties	Clinically Important Members
Adenoviridae	DS, linear	Nonenveloped; midsize Icosadeltahedral capsid Encodes DNA polymerase	Adenovirus Possible vector for gene therapy
Hepadnaviridae	DS, partially circular	Enveloped; small Replicates genome via RNA intermediate using viral reverse transcriptase	Hepatitis B virus
Herpesviridae	DS, linear	Enveloped; large Icosadeltahedral capsid Encodes DNA polymerase that replicates genome in nucleus	Epstein-Barr virus Herpes simplex virus 1 Herpes simplex virus 2 Human herpesvirus 6, 7 Human herpersvirus 8 Varicella-zoster virus
Papillomaviridae	DS	Nonenveloped; small, icosahedral capsid	Human papillomavirus
Polyomaviridae	DS, circular	Nonenveloped, small Icosahedral capsid	JC, BK virus
Parvoviridae	SS, linear	Nonenveloped; small Icosahedral capsid	B_{19} parvovirus
Poxviridae	DS, linear	Enveloped; largest virus (brick shaped) Produces mRNA and replicates genome in cytoplasm using viral enzymes	Molluscum contagiosum virus Vaccinia virus (used in vaccines) Variola (smallpox) virus (now eradicated)

RNA Virus

Family	RNA Genome	Other Properties	Clinically Important Members
Arenaviridae	(–) SS, circular, segmented	Enveloped; midsize Helical capsid, Carries RDRP in virion	Lymphocytic choriomeningitis virus Lassa fever virus
Bunyaviridae	(–) SS, linear, segmented	Enveloped; midsize Helical capsid, Carries RDRP in virion	California encephalitis virus Hanta virus
Caliciviridae	(+) SS, linear	Nonenveloped; small Icosahedral capsid, Genome functions as mRNA	Norwalk virus
Coronaviridae	(+) SS, linear	Enveloped; large Helical capsid Genome functions as mRNA	Coronaviruses and severe acute respiratory syndrome virus
Filoviridae	(–) SS, linear	Enveloped; mid-size Helical capsid Carries RDRP in virion	Ebola and Marburg viruses

Contd.

Contd.

Family	RNA Genome	Other Properties	Clinically Important Members
Flaviviridae	(+) SS, linear	Enveloped; small Icosahedral capsid Genome functions as mRNA	Dengue virus Hepatitis C virus St. Louis encephalitis virus Yellow fever virus
Orthomyxoviridae	(–) SS, linear, segmented	Enveloped; large Helical capsid Carries RDRP in virion	Influenza viruses (types A-C)
Paramyxoviridae	(–) SS, linear	Enveloped; large Helical capsid Carries RDRP in virion	Measles virus Mumps virus Parainfluenza virus Respiratory syncytial virus Metapneumovirus
Picornaviridae	(+) SS, linear	Nonenveloped; small Icosahedral capsid Genome functions as mRNA	Coxsackieviruses Echovirus Hepatitis A Poliovirus Rhinoviruses
Reoviridae	(+/–) DS, linear, segmented	Nonenveloped; midsize Double capsid Carries RDRP in virion	Rotavirus
Retroviridae	(+) SS, Linear (two copies)	Enveloped; midsize Helical capsid Reverse transcriptase in virion converts genome to cDNA; host enzymes form viral mRNAs and progency genomes	Human immunodeficiency virus Human T lymphotropic virus
Rhabdoviridae	(–) SS, linear	Enveloped; midsize, bullet shaped Helical capsid Carries RDRP in virion	Rabies virus
Togaviridae	(+) SS, linear	Enveloped; small Icosahedral capsid Genome functions as mRNA	Rubella virus Eastern, Western and Venezuelan equine encephalitis viruses

Ref: Jawetz Textbook of Microbiology 27th Edition Page 543, Murray Medical Microbiology 8th Edition Page 519, Textbook of Microbiology and Immunology by Parija 2nd Edition Page 538, Sherri's Medical Microbiology 6th Edition Page 281

Ans: (B) Toga virus

10. Cryptococcus stained by:

A. Giemsa stain
B. Mucicarmine stain
C. Ziehl Nelson stain
D. Gram stain

Key:

Mucicarmine stain is a special stain for Cryptococcus
Other stains include Masson Fontana stain and Alcian blue stain

Cryptococcus

- Only pathogenic yeast
- Has yeast form but no hyphal or pseudohyphal forms
- **Able to cross blood brain barrier (Trojan Horse)**
- ***Oval, budding yeast surrounded by a wide polysaccharide capsule***
- ***Urease +ve***
- Pigeon droppings contain serotype A and D, Eucalyptus tree contains serotype B

Transmission

- Human infection results from **inhalation** of organism–Most common
- No human-to-human transmission
- Grows abundantly in soil containing bird (especially pigeon) droppings

Virulence Factors

- ***Polysaccharide capsule***–Inhibits phagocytosis by WBC
- Ability to make melanin by producing phenyl oxidase enzyme
- Production of Phospholipase and Urease

Risk Factors

- *Advanced HIV infections with CD4 Counts < 200/uL*
- Hematological malignancies
- Transplant recipients
- Steroid therapy

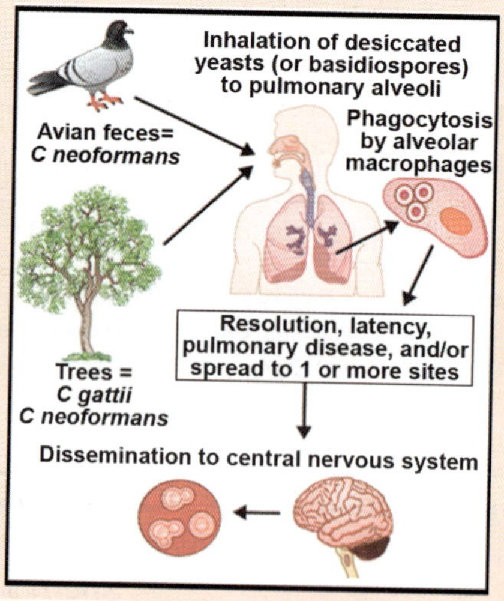

Clinical Features

Pulmonary

- **Most common site of lodgement–Lung**
- *Most common presentation–Pulmonary cryptococcosis (Mostly asymptomatic). Most common symptomatic presentation is* ***Meningitis****

Contd.

Contd.

CNS

- Affects CNS (Meninges, Cortical grey matter and Basal nuclei).
- Cryptococcosis is most common, life-threatening invasive fungal disease worldwide.
- Cryptococcus neoformans causes cryptococcosis, especially cryptococcal meningitis.
- Cryptococcal meningitis is the most serious type of infection and can resemble tuberculous or other chronic types of meningitis.

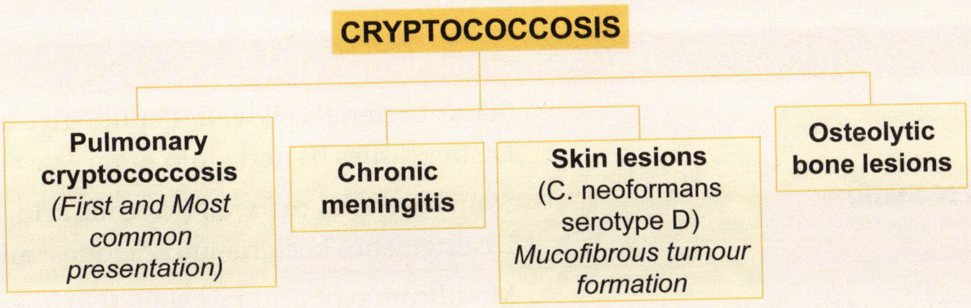

- Disseminated cryptococcosis includes the skin, prostate and medullary cavity of bones, next only to the lungs and CNS, and it occurs most commonly in patients with AIDS and other immunosuppressed conditions.

Torulosis–Cryptococcal CNS infection (Old terminology)
European blastomycosis–Cryptococcosis

Lab Diagnosis

- Specimens include spinal fluid, tissue, exudates, sputum, blood and urine.
- *Thick gelatinous polysaccharide capsule–Intense red with PAS and Mucicarmine*
- Detected by Antibody coated beads in an agglutination assay
- Most useful immunological test–Latex agglutination test
- CSF analysis–Single most useful diagnostic test
- **India ink or nigrosine preparation:**
  - In unstained, wet preparations of CSF mixed with a drop of India ink or nigrosine, the capsule can be seen as a clear halo around the yeast cells.
  - Yeast cells→ Round and surrounded by muco polysaccharide capsule.

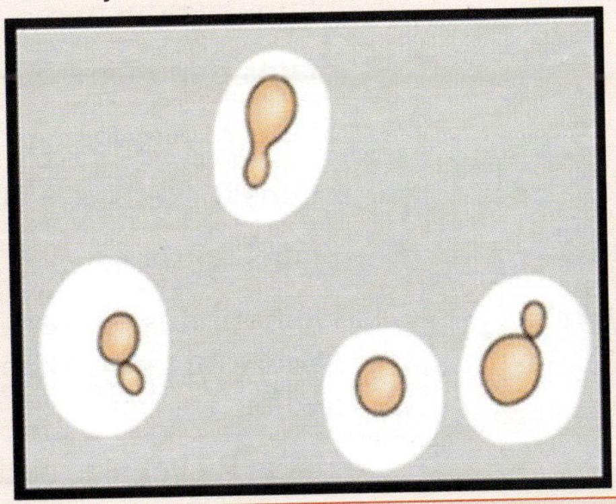

Differentiation of pathogenic (C. neoformans) from other nonpathogenic cryptococci by ability to

- Grow at 37°C.
- Hydrolyze urea.
- Produce phenol oxidase—produce black colonies on niger seed agar, bird seed agar and caffeic acid agar.
- Produce disease in mice on intracerebral and intraperitoneal inoculation (animal inoculation test positive). Capsulated budding yeast cells can be demonstrated in the brain of infected mice.

Niger seed (bird seed) agar is a differential medium for presumptive identification of C. neoformans.

Contd.

Contd.

Treatment

- Combination therapy of amphotericin B and flucytosine has been considered standard treatment for cryptococcal meningitis.
- Drug of choice for Cryptococcosis without CNS involvement–Fluconazole

Important Stains in Microbiology	
Gram stain	Stains bacterial cell wall (Peptidoglycan) Distinguishes bacteria into gram +ve and -ve
Acid fast stain (ZN Stain)	Stains bacterial cell wall (Mycolic acid Distinguishes bacteria into Acid fast and Non acid fast
Kinyoun stain	Modification of acid fast stain (No use of heat)
Auramine O stain	Fluorescent stain for Mycobacteria tuberculosis
Schaeffer Fulton stain	Stains bacterial endospores
Albert stain, Ponder stain, Lofflers methylene blue stain, Neisser stain, Pugh stain	Stains metachromatic granules of Corynebacterium diphtheria
Indian Ink stain (Nigrosin)	Stains bacterial capsules and Cryptococcus
Methylene blue with Anticapsular sera	Stains capsules of Streptococcus pneumonia ***(Quellung reaction)***
Silver impregnation method, Leifson stain, Gray method, Silver method	Stains bacterial flagella
Giemsa stain	Stains Intracellular pathogens (Chlamydiae, Rickettsiae, Mycoplasma) Also used for staining Treponema pallidum and H. pylori and Malaria
Fontana stain	Stains treponemes
Levaditi stain	Stains treponemes in tissue sections
Diene's stain	Stains Mycoplasma
Macchiavello stain	Stains Rickettsia
Warthin Starry stain, Dieterle stain	Stains Spirochetes
Bipolar staining–Safety pin appearance	Hemophilus ducreyi, Vibrio parahemolyticus, Yersinia pestis, Donovani granulomatosis, Pseudomonas pseudomallei and mallei
Castaneda stain	Stains Rickettsiae and Chlamydiae

Ref: Jawetz Textbook of Microbiology 27th Edition Page 687, Murray Medical Microbiology 8th Edition Page 655, Textbook of Microbiology and Immunology by Parija 2nd Edition Page 607, Sherri's Medical Microbiology 6th Edition Page 748, Essentials of Microbiology by Surinder Kumar Page 522

Ans: (B) Mucicarmine stain

11. Diagnostic test for Leptospirosis is:

A. Widal test
B. Paul-Bunnell test
C. Microscopic agglutination
D. Weil-Felix test

Key:

Diagnostic test of choice for Leptospirosis–Microscopic Agglutination test
Gold standard method for diagnosis of Leptospirosis–MAT
Reference Test of choice for Diagnosis of Leptospirosis–MAT

Leptospirosis/Weil's Disease

- Leptospira–Actively mobile spirochete with hooked end
- Zoonotic disease

Mode of transmission

- Indirect contact with water, Moist soil and wet surfaces contaminated with animal urine
- Direct contact with urine and products of parturition, placenta of infected animals

Direct human to human transmission doesn't occur

- **Sources of infection**–Rats, Dogs, Cattle and Pigs

Rodents, Rainfall and Ricefield–Epidemiological determinants for Leptospirosis

Clinical Features

- **Incubation period:** Around 5-14 days
- High grade fever
- Jaundice and Raised Liver enzymes
- ***Pulmonary–Most common*** (Hemorrhages)
- Kidney–Raised serum urea and creatinine

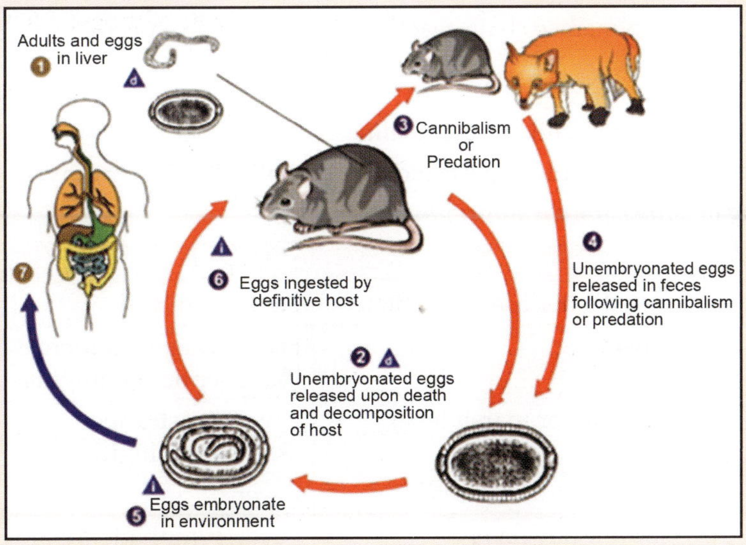

LEPTOSPIROSIS

- Anicteric febrile illness
  - *Most common (90%)*
    Mild form
    Most common finding–Fever with conjunctival suffusion
- Weil's disease
  - *Hepatorenal form (5-10%)*
    High grade fever, Jaundice and Raised Liver enzymes,
    Hemorrhagic diathesis, Hepatosplenomegaly

Contd.

Contd.

Lab Diagnosis

- ***Gold Standard serodiagnostic method–Microscopic agglutination test***
- It is specific but has inherent complexity (Alternative screening tests–ELISA, IHA and Macroscopic slide agglutination test)
- ***Definite diagnosis is based on either isolation of organism from patient or on seroconversion or rise in antibody titer in MAT***

Diagnostic test	Method	Test accuracy
Microscopy	Gram stain	Organisms too thin to be detected
	Darkfield examination	Insensitive, nonspecific
	Silver impregnation stain	Insensitive, nonspecific
	Direct fluorescent antibody	Insensitive, specific
Culture	Blood	Positive during first 10 days
	Cerebrospinal fluid	Positive during first 10 days
	Urine	Positive after first week
Serology	Indirect hemagglutination	Insensitive, nonspecific
	Slide agglutination	Insensitive, nonspecific
	ELISA	Insensitive, nonspecific
	Microscopic agglutination test	Sensitive, specific, serovar specific
Molecular methods	Direct hybridization	Insensitive, specific
	Polymerase chain reaction	Sensitive, specific

Treatment

- **Mild cases**–Doxycycline/Ampicillin/Amoxicillin
- **Moderate to severe cases**–Penicillin G/Ampicillin/Amoxicillin/Erythromycin
- ***Doxycycline–Drug of choice for chemoprophylaxis***

Serotype	Disease	Clinical picture	Animal reservoir
Icterohemorrhagiae	Weil's disease Canicola	Fever, jaundice	Rat
Canicola	fever	Hemorrhages influenza like, aseptic-meningitis	Dog
Grippotyphosa	Swamp or marsh fever	Fever, prostration, aseptic-meningitis	Field mice
Pomona	Swineherd's disease	Fever	Pig
Hebdomadis	Seven-day fever	Fever, lymphadenopathy	Field mice
Fortbragg	Pretibial fewver, Fort Bragg fever	Fever, rash over tibia	Not known
Pyrogenes	Febrile spirochetosis	Fever	Pig
Bataviae	Indonesian Weil's disease	Fever	Rat
Hardjo	Dairy farm fever	Fever	Cattle

- **Vasculitis–***Most important manifestation of Kidney and Liver disease*
- *When antibodies are formed, Leptospira gets eliminated from all sites except Eye, Proximal renal tubules and Brain.*

Ref: Jawetz Textbook of Microbiology 27th Edition Page 330, Murray Medical Microbiology 8th Edition Page 333, Textbook of Microbiology and Immunology by Parija 2nd Edition Page 385, Sherri's Medical Microbiology 6th Edition Page 651, Essentials of Microbiology by Surinder Kumar Page 346

Ans: (C) Microscopic agglutination

12. Regan Lowe medium is used for culture of which of the following organism?

A. Bartonella B. Brucella

C. Legionella D. Bordetella

Key:

Regan Lowe medium is culture medium for Bordetella

Pertussis

- Caused by Bordetella pertussis–Gram –ve, Capsulated, fimbriated, Non motile coccobacillus
- Bipolar metachromatic granules on toluidine blue stain
- Strict aerobes and Biochemically inactive (Non fermenters)
- **Culture:**
  - Bordet Gengou glycerine potato-blood agar medium–Commonly used
  - Nasopharyngeal aspirate–Gold standard specimen
  - Colonies–Mercury drops/Bisected pearls
  - Colony appearance–**Aluminium paint appearance***
- 100-day cough
- Source of Infection–Case of pertussis (No carrier/Subclinical state)
- Disease of Infants and Children
- ***Incidence and Fatality more among female children***
- Mode of transmission–Mainly by Droplet infection
- Incubation period–1 to 2 weeks
- Each stage lasts for 1-2 weeks

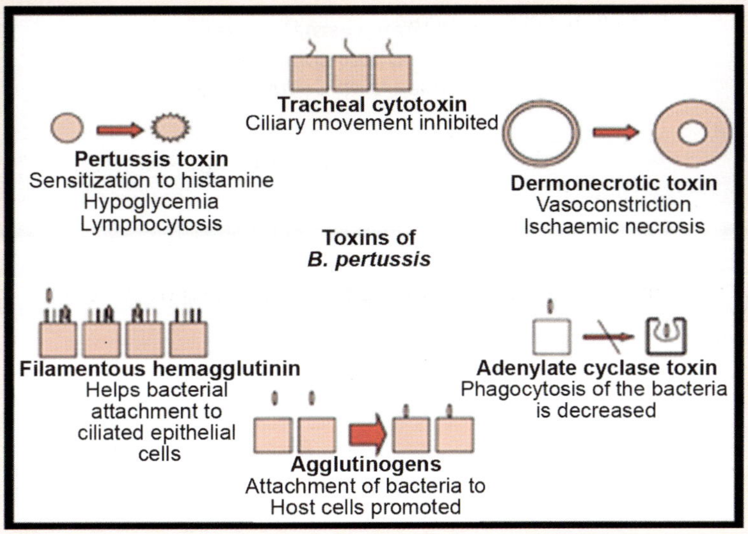

Contd.

Contd.

	Incubation	Catarrhal	Paroxysmal	Convalescent
Duration	7-10 days	1-2 weeks	2-4 weeks	3-4 weeks (or longer)
Symptoms	None	Rhinorrhea, malaise, fever, sneezing, anorexia	Repetitive cough with whoops, vomiting, leukocytosis	Diminished paroxysmal cough, development of secondary complications (pneumonia, seizures, encephalopathy)
Bacterial culture	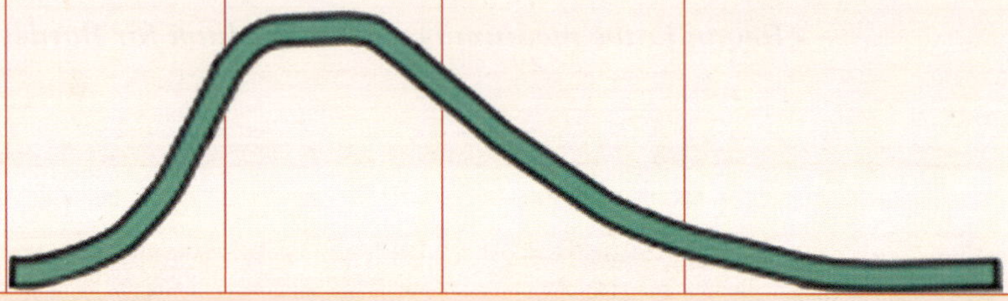			

Toxin	Biologic effects
Pertussis toxin (A-B type exotoxin)	Toxic A subunit enters cell and **ADP-ribosylates inhibitory G protein**, turning it off. The subsequent **increased cAMP level** leads to loss of fluids and electrolytes, lymphocytosis, and massive **mucus secretion** in the respiratory tract
Adenylate cyclase toxin	Enters host cell and **increases cAMP** production, which blocks immune effector function and prevents clearance of the bacteria
Tracheal cytotoxin	Inhibits and **damages ciliated tracheal cells**
Endotoxin	Causes fever and other **pyrogenic responses**

Catarrhal Stage:
Most Infectious Stage
Lasts for 1-2 weeks
Cultures are likely to be +ve

↓

Paroxysmal stage:
Maximum complications
Smear and Culture are -ve

↓

Convalescent stage:
Antibody in serum,
Severity decreases

- ***Complications***–*Atelectasis, Bronchiectasis, Pneumothorax, Encephalopathy. Non cerebellar ataxia, Subconjunctival hemorrhage, Intracranial hemorrhage and Severe malnutrition*
- Drug of choice–Erythromycin for 1 to 2 weeks
- Macrolide resistance–Co trimoxazole
- Chemoprophylaxis–Erythromycin is drug of choice

Bordetella parapertussis–*silent copy pertussis toxin gene*
Bordetella Bronchiseptica–*Kneel cough and pneumonitis*

Organism	Selective/Enrichment media
Staphylococcus aureus	Mannitol agar, Milk salt agar Ludlam's medium
Beta hemolytic streptococcus group A	Crystal violet agar
Neisseria (Gonococci/Meningococci)	Thayer Martin medium, Chocolate agar
Corynebacterium Diphtheria	Loffler's serum slope, Potassium tellurite agar
Mycobacterium Tuberculosis	**LJ Medium, Middlebrook's medium, Dorset egg medium**
Bordetella	***Regan Lowe medium,*** Bordet Gengou medium, Lacey's DFO medium
Leigonella	BCYE Medium
Bacillus anthracis	PLET (Polymyxin Lithium EDTA Thallous acetate)
Bacillus cereus	MYPA (Mannitol egg yolk phenol red polymyxin agar)
Burkholderia	Ashdown's Medium
Campylobacter	Skirrow's medium, Campy BAP Medium, Butzler's Medium
Leptospira	EMJH Medium, Fletcher Medium, Korthof Medium, Stuart's Medium
Pseudomonas	Cetrimide Agar
Plating media for Vibrio Cholera	Thiosulfate Citrate Bile Salt sucrose, Gelatin Taurocholate Tellurite Agar, Alkaline Bile salt Agar
Enrichment media for Vibrio Cholera	Alkaline peptone water, Monsur's Taurocholate peptone water
Reiter's Treponema	Smith Noguchi Medium
Anaerobes	Robertson Cooked Meat broth, Thioglycollate, Smith Noguchi Medium
Lactose Fermenting Enteric pathogens (E.coli)	Mac Conkey Agar, Eosine Methylene Blue, Deoxycholate Agar
Hemophilus	Blood agar with staphylococcal streak, Levinthal's medium, Fildes Agar, Chocolate Agar
Listeria	PALCAM Agar
Salmonella, Shigella	Deoxycholate Medium, Hektoen Enteric Agar, XLD Agar
Salmonella	Tetrathionate broth, Selenite F broth
Streptococcus Agalactiae	Told Hewitt Broth with Antibiotics
Mycoplasma pneumoniae	PPLO Medium
Clostridum difficile	Cefoxitin Cycloserine Fructose Agar, Cefoxitin Cycloserine Egg Yolk Agar
Enterococcus	Bile Esculin Agar
Yersinia	Cefsulodine Irgasan Novobiocin Medium
Actinomyces	Thioglycollate Medium, Brain Heart Infusion Agar

Organism	Transport media
Streptococcus Pyogenes	Pike Medium
Neisseria	Stuart's Medium, Amies Medium

Contd.

Contd.

Vibrio Cholera	VR Medium, Cary Blair Medium, Stuart Medium
Salmonella, Shigella	Sach's Buffered glycerol saline
Bordetella	Modified Stuart's Medium, Mischulow's Charcoal Agar

Ref: Jawetz Textbook of Microbiology 27th Edition Page 266, Murray Medical Microbiology 8th Edition Page 292, Textbook of Microbiology and Immunology by Parija 2nd Edition Page 330, Sherri's Medical Microbiology 6th Edition Page 563, Essentials of Microbiology by Surinder Kumar Page 324

Ans: (D) Bordetella

13. Hand foot mouth disease is caused by:

A. Hepatitis A
B. Human papilloma virus
C. Coxsackie B
D. Coxsackie A

Key:

Hand foot mouth disease is caused by Coxsackie A virus (Enterovirus 71)

Coxasackie Virus	
Manifestations of Group A	**Manifestations of Group B**
• Aseptic meningitis (A7,A9) • Herpangina (Vesicular pharyngitis) • ***Hand foot mouth disease (Enterovirus 71)*** • Acute hemorrhagic conjunctivitis (Coxsackie A24 and Enterovirus 70)	• Aseptic meningitis (B1-6) • Pleurodynia (Epidemic myalgia/Bronholm disease) • Myocarditis, Pericarditis • Hepatitis and Pneumonia • Pancreatitis and Juvenile diabetes ***(Coxsackie B4)*** • Generalized disease of Infants

Ref: Jawetz Textbook of Microbiology 27th Edition Page 543, Murray Medical Microbiology 8th Edition Page 519, Textbook of Microbiology and Immunology by Parija 2nd Edition Page 538, Sherri's Medical Microbiology 6th Edition Page 281

Ans: (D) Coxsackie A

14. Method that follows disc diffusion is:

A. Broth dilution method
B. Agar dilution method
C. E test
D. Kirby Bauer method

Key:

Kirby Bauer method is a disc diffusion method of Antibiotic sensitivity testing

- Antibiotic sensitivity testing is carried out to determine appropriate antibiotic to be used for a particular strain isolated from clinical specimen.

Disc Diffusion Method

- Most commonly used method to determine antibiotic susceptibility
- Disc impregnated with known concentration of antibiotics are placed on culture medium that has been inoculated with culture of bacterium to be tested
- Antibiotic sensitivity is determined by ***Zone of Inhibition*** of bacterial growth around disc
- Mueller Hinton Agar is most commonly used medium for Antibiotic sensitivity testing

Dilution Tests

- ***Used to determine Minimum Inhibitory Concentration (MIC) of antibiotics***

Disc diffusion method and E test

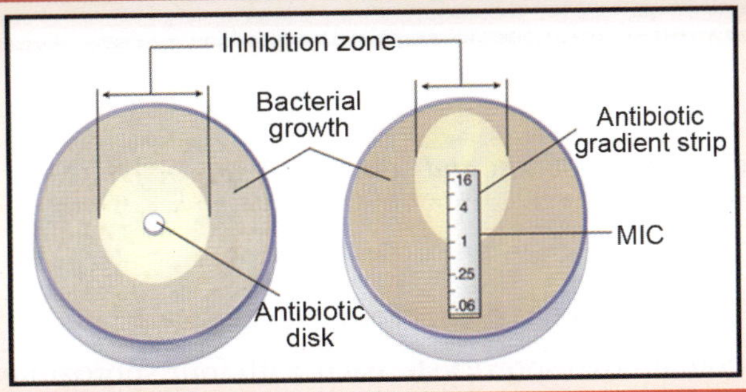

Kirby Bauer method

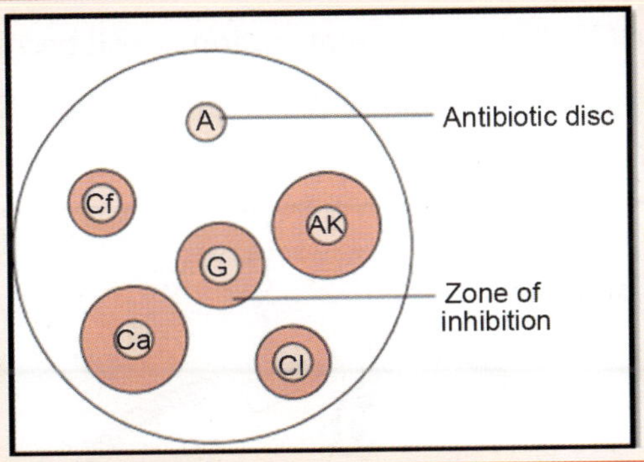

ANTIBIOTIC SENSITIVITY TESTING

- **Disc diffusion tests**
  - **Kirby Bauer disc diffusion method**
  - **Stoke disc diffusion method**
  - **Primary disc diffusion test**
- **Dilution tests**
  - **Broth dilution method**
  - **Agar dilution method**
  - **Epsilometer test**

E test–*Quantitative method detecting MIC using principles of both dilution and diffusion of Antibiotic into medium*

Automated methods–*VITEK 2, Phoenix system and Microscan walk away system*

Molecular methods–*PCR detecting drug resistant genes*

Ref: Ananthanarayan 9th Edition Page 635, Murray Medical Microbiology 8th Edition Page 160, Textbook of Microbiology and Immunology by Parija 2nd Edition Page 70, Sherri's Medical Microbiology 6th Edition Page 421

Ans: (D) Kirby Bauer method

15. **In a 45-year-old male HIV patient came with complaints of diarrhea of 10 episodes. Stool examination shows Acid fast Oocytes (25-30 microns) are shown below. What is the best treatment of this condition?**

A. Paramomycin
B. Septran
C. Albendazole
D. Metronidazole

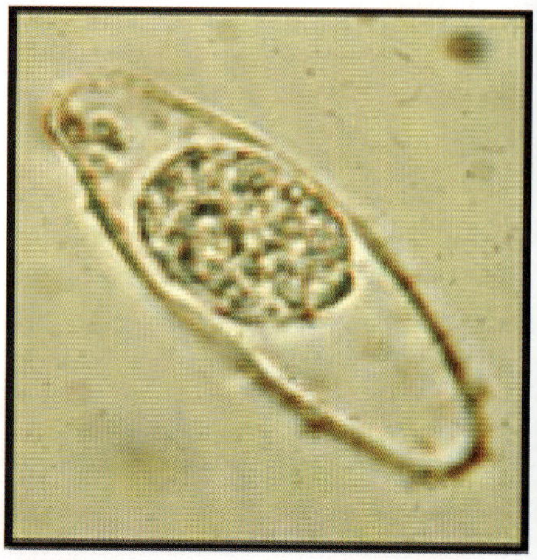

Key:

Isospora Oocyst is of 23-36 μm and contains 2 sporocyst (Each having 4 sporozoites)

Isospora

- Isospora belli, now named Cysto isospora belli, Protozoan closely related to Toxoplasma.
- Like Toxoplasma, oocysts contain two sporocysts, each with four sporozoites.
- *Infective form–Sporulated Oocyst.*
- Oocysts are much larger in size *(25-30 μm)* after maturation in soil become infective.
- ***Almost football shaped.***
- Can be stained with acid-fast procedures.

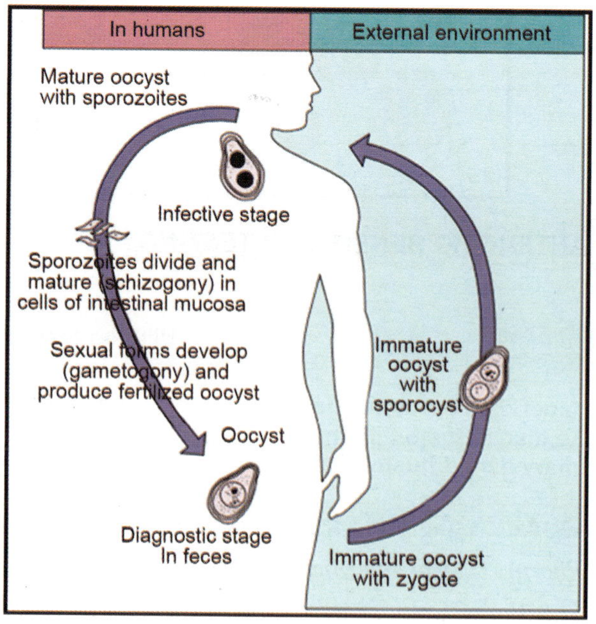

- Clinical disease resembles that of cryptosporidiosis
- Diagnosed by Acid fast Oocysts in feces
- ***Responds to treatment with trimethoprim–sulfamethoxazole.***

Property	Cryptosporidium	Cyclospora	Isospora
Infective form	Sporulated Oocyst	Sporulated Oocyst	Sporulated Oocyst
Sporulated Oocyst	*4-6 μm, Round* *Contains 4 sporozoites*	*8-12 μm, Round* *Contains 2 sporocyst (Each having 2 sporozoites)*	*23-36 μm,* Contains 2 sporocyst *(Each having 4 sporozoites)*
Acid fastness	Uniformly acid fast	Variable acid fast	Uniformly acid fast
Autofluorescence	No	++	+/-
Sporulation of Oocyst	Occurs inside host cell	Occurs in soil	Occurs in soil
Diagnostic form	Sporulated Oocyst	Unsporulated Oocyst	Unsporulated Oocyst
Autoinfection	Seen	Not seen	Not seen
Treatment	Nitazoxanide	Cotrimoxazole	Cotrimoxazole
Outbreaks	Common	Common	Less

Cryptosporidium, Microsporidia and Isospora–Most common opportunistic protozoa that can infect GIT and can cause Diarrhea in HIV patients

Version 2

A HIV patient with chronic diarrhea. Stool examination stained with special stain shows oocyst of Cryptosporidium parvum. Treatment of this condition:

A. Albendazole
B. Trimethoprim + Sulphamethazole
C. Metronidazole
D. Paramomycin

Key:

Cryptosporidia, microsporidia and Isospora belli are the most common opportunistic protozoa that infect the GI tract and cause diarrhea in HIV-infected patients
Treatment of Cryptosporidiasis is Paramomycin

Cryptosporidial Infection

- May present in a variety of ways, ranging from self-limited or **intermittent** diarrheal illness in patients in early stages of HIV infection to severe, life-threatening diarrhea in severely immunodeficient individuals.
- Cryptosporidia may also cause ***Biliary tract disease*** in HIV-infected patient, leading to **Cholecystitis** with/without accompanying **Cholangitis and Pancreatitis** secondary to papillary stenosis.
- ***Diagnosis is made by Stool examination/Biopsy of small intestine.***
- Treatment with up to 2000 mg/d of **nitazoxanide** is associated with improvement in symptoms or a decrease in shedding of organisms in about half of patients.
- **Paromomycin** may alleviate some of the diarrhoeal symptoms.

Contd.

Contd.

- Cryptosporidia are found within epithelial cells and are associated with distortion of the villus architecture. Inflammatory changes may be present.
- Progressive morphological and functional abnormalities of the small intestine occur as parasite numbers increase, although intensity of infection and inflammation does not correlate well with the severity of clinical disease.
- The immune response associated with cryptosporidiosis involves cellular and humoral components. The T-lymphocyte cellular responses are important in controlling infection, as evidenced by the increased disease severity in HIV-infected patients with CD4 counts less than 100 cells/microliter.

Ref: Harrison 20th Edition Page 1435

Ans: (D) Paramomycin

Ref: Textbook of Parasitology by Parija 6th Edition Page 104, Murray Medical Microbiology 8th Edition Page 724, Sherri's Medical Microbiology 6th Edition Page 811, Levinson Review of Microbiology and Immunology 13th Edition Page 976

Ans: (B) Septran

16. Which of the following test doesn't use labelled antibody?

A. ELISA
B. Hemagglutination
C. Radioimmunoassay
D. Immunofluorescence

Key:

Hemagglutination inhibition test is detected by inhibition of hemagglutination of anti RBC antibody present in patient's serum with respective RBC antigen
So it doesn't use Labelled antibody

LABELLED ANTIBODIES

Antibody detection
Labelled anti human gamma globulin is used to detect human gamma globulin present in patients serum

Antigen detection
Labelled specific antibodies are used to detect corresponding antigens from sample

Methods that use labeled antibodies for diagnosis
Radioimmunoassay, Enzyme immunoassay, Immunofluorescence, Chemiluminescence immunoassay, Immunochromatographic tests, Immunoferritin test and Immunoenzyme test

RADIOIMMUNOASSAY

- **Principle:** Competitive binding of radiolabeled antigen and unlabeled antigen to high affinity antibody.
- RIA involves separation of protein using specificity of antibody-antigen binding and quantitation using radioactivity.

MIXTURE IS PREPARED OF RADIOACTIVE ANTIGEN AND ANTIBODIES AGAINST THAT ANTIGEN

↓

Known amounts of unlabeled antigens are added to samples of mixture

↓

These compete for binding sites of antibodies

↓

At increasing concentrations of unlabeled antigen, increasing amount of radioactive antigen is displaced from antibody molecules

↓

Antibody bound antigen is separated from free antigen in supernatant fluid and radioactivity of each is measured

ELISA

- **Principle:** Similar to RIA but depends on enzyme rather than radioactive label
- Enzyme conjugated with an antibody reacts with a colorless substrate to generate colored reaction product→ Chromogenic Substrate
- Test sera are incubated in wells precoated with purified target antigen, bound antibodies are detected via an Enzyme conjugated anti human immunoglobulin antibody followed by color visualization with appropriate enzyme substrate

> ***Enzymes used***–*Alkaline phosphatase, Beta galactosidase and Horseradish peroxidase*
> ***Variants of ELISA***–*Direct ELISA, Indirect ELISA, Sandwich ELISA, Competitive ELISA and Elispot ELISA*

IMMUNOFLOURESCENCE

- Fluorescent compounds like fluorescein and rhodamine are used to tag antibody molecules.
- Immune complexes formed are detected by colored light emission when excited by light of appropriate wavelength.

Test that used labeled molecules	Molecules used	Effect
Radioimmunoassay (RIA)	Radioactive Isotope	Emits Beta and Gamma rays Detected by radiation counters
Chemoilluminescence linked immunoassay (CLIA)	Chemiluminescent compounds	Emits light detected by luminometer
Immunohistochemistry (IHC)	Enzyme/Fluorescent dye	Color change (Naked eye) Fluorescence microscope
Western blot (WB)	Enzyme	Color band (Naked eye)
Immunoeferritin electron microscopy (IEM)	Electron dense molecules (Ferritin)	Appears as black dot under electron microscope
Enzyme linked immunosorbent assay (ELISA)	Enzyme	Color change is detected by Spectrophotometer
Immunofluorescence assay (IFA)	Fluorescent dye	Emits light detected by Fluorescence microscope

Test	Uses
Flocculation test	Detection of reaginic antibodies in syphilis by VDRL test
Radial immunodiffusion	Detection of fungal antigen and antibodies
Counter-current immunoelectrophoresis	Detection of both antigen and antibodies in bacterial, viral, fungal and parasitic diseases
Slide agglutination test	Identification of bacterial isolates, such as *Salmonella, Shigella, Vibrio*, etc.
Tube agglutination test	Detection of antibodies in bacterial infection, e.g., Widal test for enteric fever
Latex agglutination test	Quantitation and detection of antigen and antibodies
Hemagglutination test	Detection of both antigens and antibodies in viral and parasitic infections
Coagglutination test	Detection of microbial antigens
Complement fixation test	Quantitation and detection of antibodies
Direct immunofluore-scence Test	Detection and localization of antigen in a cell or tissue
Indirect immunofluore-scence Test	Detection of specific antibodies in the serum
Sandwich ELISA	Detection of antigens and antibodies
Indirect ELISA	Quantitation and detection of antibodies
Radioimmunoassay	Quantitation of hormones, drugs, etc.
Western blot	Detection of antigen-specific antibody

Ref: Parija Textbook of Microbiology and Immunology 2nd Edition Page 103, Sherri's Medical Microbiology 6th Edition Page 71, Levinson Review of Microbiology and Immunology 13th Edition Page 1179, Rajesh Bhatia Essentials of Medical Microbiology 4th Edition Page 106

Ans: (B) Hemagglutination

17. Cysticercosis is caused by which larvae of Helminthes (Adult worm is shown in below picture)?

A. Sparganum
B. Cysticercus cellulosae
C. Precercoid larvae
D. Plerocercoid larvae

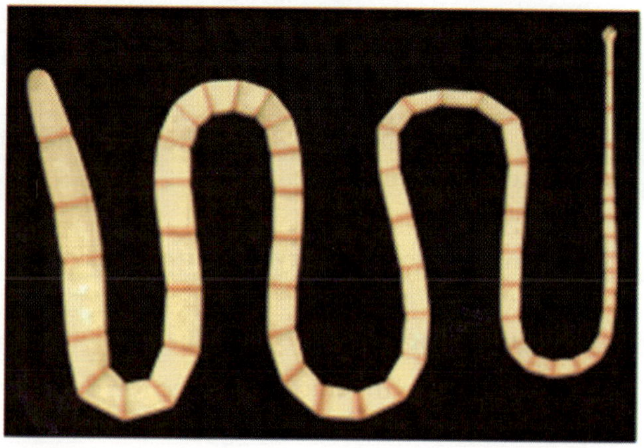

Key:

Picture depicted shows adult form of Tenia solium. Cysticercosis occurs due to Cysticercus cellulosae. Larval form of Tenia solium is Cysticercus cellulosae

- *Larval form of Tenia solium is Cysticercus cellulosae.*
- *Develops in muscles of pig.*
- *Found in man when infection is caused by ingestion of eggs to cause Cysticercosis.*
- *Most Common site of infection is Subcutaneous tissues and muscles.*

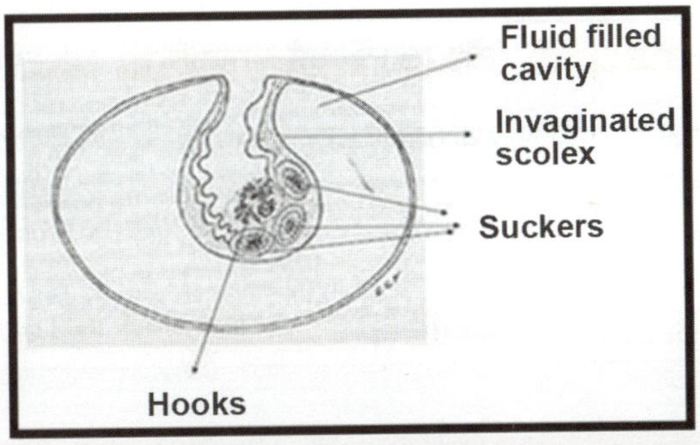

Cysticercus cellulosae is Ovoid larval form that contains fluid filled bladder with protoscolex invaginated into lumen.

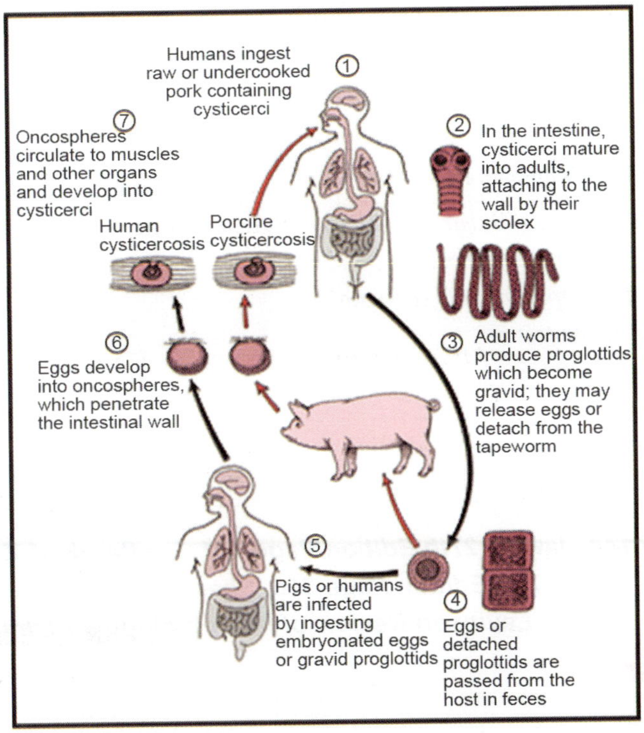

Larval Forms	
Tenia Saginata	*Cysticercus Bovis*
Tenia Solium	*Cysticercus cellulosae*
Spirometra	*Sparganum*
Echinococcus	*Hydatid cyst*
Multiceps	*Coenuerus*
Hymenolepis, Dipyllidium	*Cysticercoid*
Diphyllobothrium	*L1- Coracidium, L2- Procercoid, L3- Plerocercoid*

Infective Forms

EGGS	CYSTICERCUS	PLEROCERCOID
• Tenia solium • E.granulosus • H.Nana • Ascariasis • Enterobius • Trichuris trichiura	• T.Solium • T.Saginata	• Diphyllobothrium latum

METACERCARIA	CERCARIA	LARVA
• Fasciola • Clonorchis • Paragonimus	• Schistosomia	• Strongyloides • Ancylostoma • Trichinella • Wucheraria & Brugia malayi • Loa loa & Onchocerca • Dracunculus

EXTRA EDGE

- *Most common parasitic CNS infection–Neurocysticercosis*
- *Most common cause of Adult Onset Epilepsy in world–Neurocysticercosis*
- *Most common manifestation of Neurocysticercosis–Seizures*
- *Treatment of choice for Neurocysticercosis–Albendazole*
- ***Del Brutto criteria is used for Neurocysticercosis***
- *Most common site (Neurocysticercosis)–Subarachnoid space* ***(Arachnoiditis)***
- *Human acts as Definitive and Intermediate host*
- *Largest helminth and worm–Beef tapeworm (T. saginata)*
- *Broad tapeworm–Diphyllobothrium latum*
- *Dwarf tapeworm–Hymenolepis Nana*
- *Beef tapeworm–Tenia saginata*
- *Pork tapeworm–Tenia solium*
- *Fish tapeworm–Diphyllobothrium latum*

Ref: Paniker 6th Edition Page 148, Jawetz 27th Edition Page 731, Textbook of Microbiology and Immunology by Parija 2nd Edition Page 326, Sherri's Medical Microbiology 6th Edition Page 885, Levinson Review of Microbiology and Immunology 13th Edition Page 983

Ans: (B) Cysticercus cellulosae

18. Chronic Dysentry with abdominal pain, tenesmus and rectal prolapsed in children is caused by:

A. Ascarisis
B. Enterobius
C. Trichinella
D. Trichuris

Key:

Chronic Dysentry with abdominal pain, tenesmus and rectal prolapsed in children is caused by Massive infestation of trichuris trichiura in Intestine

TRICHURIS TRICHIURA

- **Whipworm and Intestinal Nematode** *(Buggy whip appearance)*
- **Infective stage:** Eggs

- **Route of transmission:** Oral route
- **Location:** Large intestine (Cecum and colon)
- **Clinical features:** *Dysentry, Iron deficiency anemia, Rectal prolapse, Growth retardation*

INGESTION OF CONTAMINATED FOOD/WATER

↓

Eggs hatch in small intestine

↓

Larva differentiate into immature adults

↓

Immature adults migrate to colon where they mature, mate and produce fertilized eggs

↓

Eggs deposited in warm, moist soil form embryos

↓

Adult worm burrows into intestine causes diarrhea, but doesn't cause significant anemia

↓

RECTAL PROLAPSE
(Increased peristalsis in effort to expel worms from body)

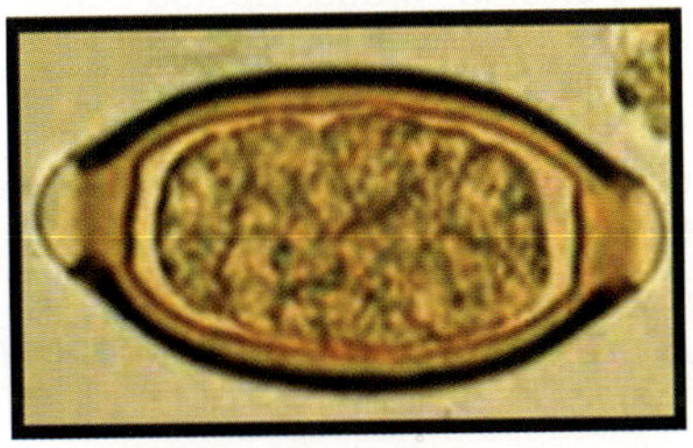

- *Heavy infection→Abdominal pain, Anorexia, Bloody/Mucoid diarrhea resembling Inflammatory bowel disease*
- *Rectal prolapse→ Massive infection with Trichuris in children (Malnourished and diarrheal)*

- **Diagnostic stage:** Unembryonated eggs in stool
- **EGGS:** Barrel shaped with Mucous plug at ends–***Bile stained***
- **Treatment of choice: Albendazole**

Ref: Jawetz 27th Edition Page 724, Paniker Textbook of Parasitology 6th Edition Page 135, Murray Medical Microbiology 8th Edition Page 754, Sherri's Medical Microbiology 6th Edition Page 851, Levinson Review of Microbiology 13th Edition Page 1022

Ans: (D) Trichuris

19. A patient recently visited a new place and developed cough with hemoptysis. Sputum is golden yellow in colour. He also gives history of Ingestion if fresh water crab. What could be most likely organism causing this disease?

A. Tuberculosis
B. Paragonimus
C. Blastomycosis
D. Histoplasmosis

Key:

Pulmonary symptoms with history of fresh water crab suggests Paragonimus westermani infestation. Hemoptysis occurs due to rupture of capsule due to Ovodeposition inside cavity

PARAGONIMUS

- **Oriental Lung fluke**
- **Route of transmission:** Eating raw or undercooked crab meat/cray fish
- **Infective stage:** Metacercariae
- **Habitat:** Cystic space of lung
- **Intermediate host: Snail**
- **2nd Intermediate host:** *Raw fresh water crab/cray fish*

Pathogenesis

INGESTION OF CONTAMINATED CRAB/CRAY FISH

↓

Encystation occurs in small intestine

↓

Immature fluke penetrates intestinal wall

↓

Migrates through diaphragm to lung parenchyma

↓

Worms exist in fibrous capsule communicating with bronchiole

↓

Eggs, released by adult worms, move up trachea to pharynx, are expectorated/swallowed and then passed in feces. Eggs in lung induce an inflammatory response forming granulomas around eggs.
Secondary bacterial infection

↓

HEMOPTYSIS AND GOLDEN YELLOW SPUTUM
(Eggs liberated disrupt capsule)

- **Extrapulmonary:** *GI type with Abdominal pain and diarrhea, Cerebral type resembling cysticercosis, Glandular type with fever and multiple abscess.*

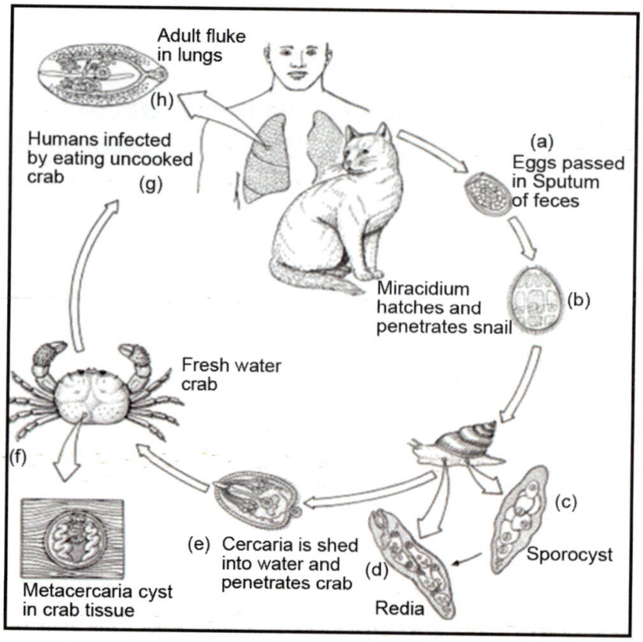

- **Diagnosis:** Made by finding the typical operculated eggs in sputum or feces
- **Treatment:** Praziquantel is drug of choice

Ref: Jawetz 27th Edition Page 735, Paniker Textbook of Parasitology 6th Edition Page 135, Murray Medical Microbiology 8th Edition Page 771, Sherri's Medical Microbiology 6th Edition Page 900, Levinson review of Microbiology 13th Edition 1010

Ans: (B) Paragonimus

Version 2

An Information technology worker presents with cough, rusty sputum, dyspnea for 2 days. He has history of travel to China and consumption of pickled crab. Two consecutive sputum samples are negative for AFB. Most likely cause:

A. Paragonimus Westermani
B. Fasciola hepatica
C. Fasciola buski
D. Histoplasmosis

Key:

Paragonimiasis is a disease caused by Lung fluke after consumption of raw, pickled, or poorly cooked crustaceans

PARAGONIMIASIS

- Parasitic lung infection caused by ***Lung flukes*** of Genus Paragonimus
- Most important endemic areas are in Far East, principally **Korea, Japan, Taiwan,** highlands of **China** and the **Philippines.**
- Paragonimus species require **2 intermediate hosts:**
  - ***First,*** Fresh water snail and
  - ***Second,*** Freshwater crustacean (Fresh water crab).
- **Life Cycle:**
  - Eggs passed in sputum or feces develop for 2 to 3 weeks in fresh water before **miracidia (first larval stage)** hatch. Miracidia invade snails; there they develop, multiply and eventually emerge as **cercariae (free-swimming larvae**).
  - Cercariae penetrate fresh water crabs/crayfish and encyst to form **metacercariae.**
  - Humans become infected by eating raw, pickled, or poorly cooked crustaceans.
  - Metacercariae excyst in human GI tract, penetrate intestinal wall, and move into peritoneal cavity, then through diaphragm into pleural cavity; they enter lung tissue, become encapsulated, and develop into hermaphroditic adult worms, which produce eggs.
  - Adult worms grow to about **7.5 to 12 mm by 4 to 6 mm.**
  - From the lungs, eggs exit body in sputum that is coughed up and spit out or swallowed and passed in stool.

Contd.

Contd.

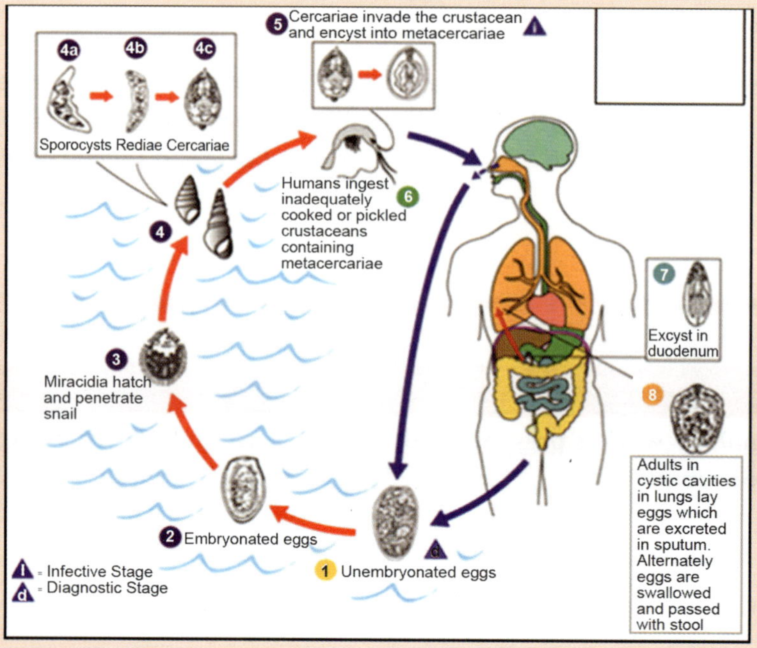

- Anamnestic information about the consumption of **raw or undercooked freshwater crabs** by immigrants, expatriates and returning travelers.
- Humans are infected by eating raw, pickled, or poorly cooked fresh water **crustaceans**.
- **Clinical features:** *Fever, Cough, Hemoptysis and Peripheral Eosinophilia,* Chronic cough, chest pain, dyspnea and hemoptysis. Allergic skin reactions and CNS abnormalities due to ectopic flukes, including seizures, aphasia, paresis, and visual disturbances, can also occur.
- Diagnosed by detection of parasite ova in sputum and/or feces.

Diagnosis is by identifying eggs in sputum, stool, or pleural or peritoneal fluid

- ***Praziquantel is Treatment of choice.***

Ref: Harrison 20th Edition Page 1641

Ans: (A) Paragonimus Westermani

20. Drug of choice for cyclospora infection is:

A. Cotrimoxazole
B. Albendazole
C. Paromomycin
D. Metronidazole

Key:

Drug of choice for cyclospora infection is Cotrimoxazole

Cyclospora (Intestinal Sporozoa)

- *Cyclospora cayetanensis* is an intestinal protozoan that causes watery diarrhea in both immunocompetent and immunocompromised individuals.
- **Cyclospora Cayetanensis–**Classified as a member of the Coccidia.
- Life cycle is similar to Cryptosporidium and involves only single host.

Contd.

Contd.

- It differs from Cryptosporidium in that Cyclospora oocysts are not immediately infectious when passed in stools.
- ***Cryptosporidium oocysts are infectious in the feces, Cyclospora oocysts take days or weeks to become infectious.***
- Direct person-to-person transmission through fecal exposure is unlikely to occur.

Pathogenesis

ALTERED MUCOSAL ARCHITECTURE WITH SHORTENED INTESTINAL VILLI

↓

Diffuse edema and infiltration of inflammatory cells

↓

Diarrhea, Anorexia, Fatigue and Weight loss

- Incubation period for *Cyclospora* infection–1 week.
- Organism is found within vacuoles in the cytoplasm of jejunal epithelial cells, and its presence is associated with inflammatory changes, villous atrophy, and crypt hyperplasia.
- ***Immunocompetent***–Diarrhea is self limited.
- ***Immunocompromised***–Severe and Prolonged diarrhea (Associated with High rate of recurrence).
- Concentrated with modified zinc sulfate centrifugal flotation technique/Sheather sugar flotation procedure.
- ***A distinguishing feature of Cyclospora is its variable appearance on acid-fast staining (ranges from unstained to mottled pink to deep red).***
- *Cyclospora* organisms appear resistant to chlorination, treatment of water supplies with chlorination and filtration remains a reasonable option.

Salient Points–Cyclospora

- **Infective form**–*Sporulated oocyst*
- **Sporulated Oocyst**–Round, contains 2 sporocyst (Each having 2 sporozoites)
- **Sporulation of oocyst**–Occurs in soil
- **Route of spread**–Contaminated food and water
- **Acid fast staining–Variable**
- **Autofluorescence ++**
- **Diagnostic form**–Unsporulated Oocyst
- **Autoinfection**–Not seen
- **Drug of choice**–Cotrimoxazole

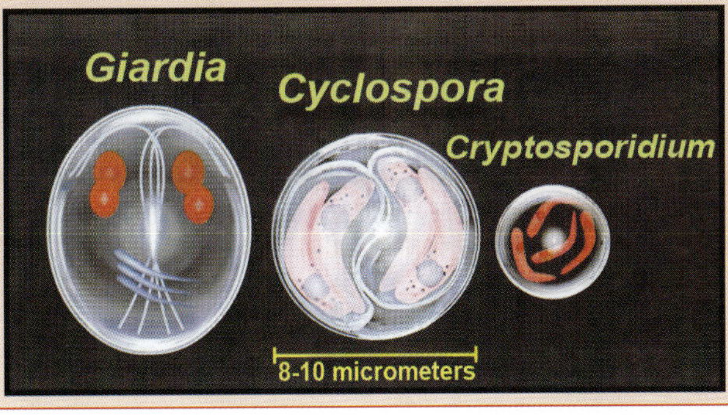

Ref: Parija Textbook of Parasitology 6th Edition Page 107, Jawetz 27th Edition Page 717, Sherri's Medical Microbiology 6th Edition Page 810, Levinson Review of Medical Microbiology and Immunology 13th Edition Page 976, Murray Medical Microbiology 8th Edition Page 786

Ans: (A) Cotrimoxazole

21. A young lady complains of fever, headache, neck stiffness for past 24 hours. These complaints are preceded by history of sore throat for 3 days. Similar history was present 1 year back. On examination patient is severely dehydrated and rash is present. Blood pressure is found to be 90/50 mm Hg on distal aspect of cuff. What could be most common etiological agent causing these symptoms?

A. Brucella abortus
B. Neisseria meningitis
C. Neisseria gonorrhea
D. Staphylococcus aureus

Key:

Given history is suggesting meningitis with sore throat, severe dehydration and rash– Typical of Meningococcemia resulting from Neisseria meningococci

MENINGOCOCCI

- Capsulated Gram –ve diplococci and Lens shaped
- Transport medium–Stuart's medium
- Selective medium–Modified Thayer Martin medium
- Ferments both glucose and maltose

VIRULENCE FACTORS

Polysaccharide Capsule of Meningococci
• Enhances virulence by anti phagocytic action • Antigen that defines serologic groups • Antigen detected in spinal fluid of meningitis patients • Antigen in vaccine

Serogroup	Comment
A	Usually responsible for massive epidemics in developing countries
B	Doesn't elicit effective immune response
B, C	Responsible for most endemic meningitis in US
A, C, Y, W 135	Effective capsular vaccine
Most common strain in India Epidemics is Group A (Meningococci)	

Most important factor that predisposes to Meningococcal infection–Complement deficiency
C5 to C9 deficiency→ Both meningococcal and gonococcal infections
C3, Properdin and Factor D deficiency→ Meningococcal infection only

ROUTE OF SPREAD

- Carrier is most important source of infection
- Humans are only reservoirs
- Disease is more common in dry and cold months of year
- Affects children between 3 months to 5 years age
- Acquired by ***droplets through respiratory route***
- Cases rapidly loose their infectiousness within 24 hours of specific treatment

Clinical Features

Waterhouse Freiderschein Syndrome

- *Fulminant meningococcemia*–Septic shock+ DIC+ MODS–*Bilateral adrenal hemorrhage*
- Most rapidly lethal form of septic shock
- Prominence of hemorrhagic skin lesions (petichae, purpura) and DIC
- Occurs due to Endotoxin (LPS) released by Autolysis

Purpura Fulminans

- Hemorrhagic skin lesions (due to Endotoxin LPS)

Postmeningococcal reactive disease–Urethritis, Conjunctivitis and Endocarditis

Lab Diagnosis

- Best specimen for case–CSF by lumbar puncture
- **Best specimen for carrier–Nasopharyngeal swab**
- **PCR amplification of DNA in buffy coat or CSF samples is the most sensitive method**
- Generalized and localized schwartzman reaction

Most commonly used method for diagnosis is Isolation on culture from specific specimen

Treatment

- 3rd generation cephalosporin such as cefataxime or ceftriaxone is *DOC* for initial therapy.
- Drug of choice for carriers and prophylaxis–Ceftriaxone.
- **Prophylaxis–**Rifampin is *DOC* for meningococcal prophylaxis.

Identifying Features of Neisseria Meningitidis

- *Gram –ve diplococci arranged in pairs*
- *Blood agar–Convex, gray and translucent colonies*
- *Catalase +ve, Oxidase +ve*
- *Ferments glucose and maltose with acid production*
- *Doesn't ferment sucrose or lactose*

Version 2

A patient presenting with features of meningitis. Lumbar puncture specimen sent for gram stain which showed Gram -ve diplococcic. What could be most likely causative organism?

A. Listeria
B. CMV
C. Meningococcus
D. Pseudomonas

Ans: (C) Meningococcus

Pyogenic Meningitis	
Neonates/ <2 months	E. coli, Group B Streptococcus, Listeria monocytogenes, Klebsiella pneumoniae
2-20 years	***Most common–Neisseria meningitidis*** Hemophilus influenza, Streptococcus pneumoniae
>20 years	***Most common–Streptococcus pneumonia*** Hemophilus influenza, Neisseria meningitidis
Overall	***Most common–Streptococcus pneumonia***

Character	Normal	Pyogenic	Tuberculous	Viral
CSF pressure (mm H_2O)	50-150 mm H_2O	>180 (High elevation)	Moderate elevation	Slight elevation
Total leukocyte count	0-5	100-10,000	10-500	25-500
Predominant cell	Lymphocyte	Neutrophil	Lymphocyte	Lymphocyte
Glucose	40-70 mg%	< 40 mg%	20-40 mg%	Normal
Total proteins	15-45 mg%	> 45 mg% *(Usually >250)*	100-500 mg% *(Moderate to markedly elevated)*	20-80 mg% *(Normal to slightly elevated)*

Ref: Ananthanarayan 9th Edition Page 230, Murray Medical Microbiology 8th Edition Page 237, Textbook of Microbiology and Immunology by Parija 2nd Edition Page 207, Sherri's Medical Microbiology 6th Edition Page 539, Rajesh Bhatia Essentials of Medical Microbiology 4th Edition Page 205

Ans: (B) Neisseria meningitis

22. Causative organism for Epidemic typhus is:

A. Rickettsia rickettsi
B. Rickettsia prowazeki
C. Rickettsia typhi
D. Rickettsia conorii

Key:

Epidemic typhus is caused by Rickettsia prowazekii

EPIDEMIC TYPHUS

- **Caused by Rickettsia prowazekii**
- Transmitted by inoculation into skin of feces of infected louse or inhalation of louse feces or dust
- **Man–Main Reservoir**
- **Disease is characterized by fever, chills, myalgia, headache and rash**
- No eschar
- Rash is seen all over the body
- Reactivation of latent infection in epidemic typhus causes Recrudescent typhus *(Brill Zinsser disease)*

ENDEMIC/MURINE TYPHUS/FLEA BORNE TYPHUS

- **Caused by Rickettsia typhi**
- *Transmitted by inoculation into skin with feces of infected flea. Inhalation of dried infective feces may also transmit this disease*
- Rodents are major reservoir
- Disease is characterized by fever, headache, myalgia and rash
- No eschar.
- ***Rash is seen on Trunk***
- ***Drug of choice–Doxycycline***

SCRUB TYPHUS

- **Caused by R. tsutsugamushi**
- Vector–Thrombiculid mite
- Transmitted by bite of infected mite
- Nymphal and Adults are free living in soil and don't feed on vertebrate hosts
- Chigger-Larval form feeds on vertebrate hosts and picks up Rickettsial organism
- Clinical features–Fever, Headache, Rash with Eschar and Lymphadenopathy

Q FEVER (QUERY FEVER)

- Caused by Coxiella burnetti
- Bandicoot–Primary reservoir
- Zoonotic disease
- No arthropod is involved in transmission to man
- Acquired by inhalation of infected dust, aerosol transmission, entry through abrasions/Ingestion of contaminated foods like meat, milk, milk products.
- ***No arthropod vector is involved for transmission to man***
- No rash

TRENCH FEVER

- 5-day fever/Quintan fever
- **Caused by Bartonella Quintana**
- Human–Only known reservoir
- Vector–Pediculus humans corporis
- Classical trench fever–Febrile illness lasts for 5 days. It is followed by remission and recurrence after 5 days.

Disease	Agent	Vector	Reservoir
Epidemic typhus	R. prowazekii	Louse	Humans
Endemic/Murine typhus	R. typhi	Flea	Rodents
Scrub typhus	R. tsutsugamushi	Mite	Rodents
Indian tick typhus	R. conorii	Tick	Rodents, Dogs

Contd.

Contd.

Rocky mountain spotted fever	R. rickettsii	Tick	Rodents, Dogs
Rickettsial pox	R. akari	Mite	Mice
Q fever	Coxiella burnetti	-	Cattle, Sheep, Goats
Trench fever	Rocholimaca	Louse	Humans

Ref: Ananthanarayan 9th Edition Page 407, Jawetz 27th Edition Page 342, Murray Medical Microbiology 8th Edition Page 340, Textbook of Microbiology and Immunology by Parija 2nd Edition Page 409, Sherri's Medical Microbiology 6th Edition Page 679, Levinson Review of Microbiology and Immunology 13th Edition Page 476

Ans: (B) Rickettsia prowazeki

Chapter 7

FORENSIC MEDICINE

1. Punishment for perjury is under IPC:

A. 190
B. 191
C. 192
D. 193

Key:

Punishment for perjury is under IPC 193

Perjury and Related Sections	
IPC 191	Definition of Perjury–Giving false evidence under oath
IPC 192	Fabricated false evidence
IPC 193	Punishment for perjury (7 Years Imprisonment)
IPC 194	Punishment of perjury leading to capital punishment (Life imprisonment or 10 years RI)
IPC 195	Punishment of perjury leading to Non-capital punishment (Life imprisonment or 7 years Imprisonment)

IPC Sections	
IPC Sec 44	*Definition of Injury*
IPC Sec 46	*Definition of Death*
IPC Sec 82	*Criminal responsibility of person < 7 years (not liable)*
IPC Sec 83	*Criminal responsibility of person 7-12 years (Liability depends on mental maturity)*
IPC Sec 84	*Criminal responsibility of insane person (not liable)*
IPC Sec 85	Criminal responsibility of involuntary drunkenness (not liable) ***Intoxicating substance is given without the knowledge of person***
IPC Sec 86	Criminal responsibility of voluntary drunkenness (liable) ***Intoxicating substance is taken with intent*** Consent for an act not intended to cause death/grievous hurt
IPC Sec 87	***Minimum age for consent of major procedures: 18 years***
IPC Sec 89	Act done in good faith for child < 12 years ***Minimum age for Consent of physical examination – 12 years*** ***Person below 12 years and an insane person can't give valid consent to suffer any harm***
IPC Sec 90	Consent given under insanity/fear of injury/intoxication – Invalid
IPC Sec 92	Act done in good faith without consent of the person In emergency situations, consent not required
IPC Sec 93	Communication made in good faith – Not an offence

Contd.

Contd.

IPC Sec 166 B	Punishment for not treating a rape victim in Govt./ Private hospitals 1 year imprisonment
IPC Sec 172	Punishment for avoiding summon Simple imprisonment for 1 month
IPC Sec 197	Punishment for Issuing false certificates (7 years)
IPC Sec 198	Punishment for using false certificates (7 years)
IPC Sec 201	Causing disappearance/ destruction of evidences (upto 10 years) Suspected articles of poison to be preserved (noncompliance – Sec 201 IPC) Embalming in poisoning case before autopsy
IPC Sec 202	Intentional omission to give information regarding offence by person bound to give (6 months)
IPC Sec 203	Giving false information regarding the offence (2 years)
IPC Sec 204	Destruction of documentary evidence (2 years)
IPC Sec 228 A	Punishment for disclosing the identity of rape victim – 2 years
IPC Sec 269	Punishment for Negligent act likely to spread infection of disease dangerous to life
IPC Sec 270	Punishment for Malignant (Willful) act likely to spread infection of disease dangerous to life
IPC Sec 272	Punishment for adulteration of food
IPC Sec 274	Punishment for adulteration of drug
IPC Sec 275	Punishment for sale of adulterated drug
IPC Sec 284	Punishment for Negligent act in handling poisonous substances
IPC Sec 290	Frotteurism
IPC Sec 294	Exhibitionism
IPC Sec 297	Necrophagia/ necrophilia (1 year)
IPC Sec 299	Definition of culpable homicide not amounting to murder
IPC Sec 300	Definition of murder (culpable homicide amounting to murder)
IPC Sec 302	Punishment for Murder – Death or Imprisonment for life
IPC Sec 304	Culpable homicide not amounting to murder
IPC Sec 304 A	Punishment for Death caused by rash and negligent act – 2 years
IPC Sec 304 B	Punishment for Dowry death (death of a female within 7 years of marriage)
IPC Sec 306	Punishment for Abetment of suicide
IPC Sec 307	Punishment for Attempt to murder
IPC Sec 308	Punishment for Attempt to commit culpable homicide
IPC Sec 309	Punishment for suicide attempt (This act has been repealed)
IPC Sec 312	Punishment for Criminal abortion with consent
IPC Sec 313	Punishment for Criminal abortion without consent
IPC Sec 314	Punishment for Criminal abortion leading to death of mother
IPC Sec 316	Punishment for Causing death of quick unborn child
IPC Sec 317	Punishment for abandoning a child < 12 years
IPC Sec 319	Definition of Hurt
IPC Sec 320	Definition of Grievous Hurt
IPC Sec 323	Punishment for voluntarily causing hurt (1 year)
IPC Sec 324	Punishment for Voluntarily causing hurt with dangerous weapon (3 years)
IPC Sec 325	Punishment for Voluntarily causing grievous hurt – 7 years

Contd.

Contd.

IPC Sec 326	Punishment for Voluntarily causing grievous hurt by dangerous weapon–10 years
IPC Sec 326 A	Punishment for acid throwing (vitriolage)–life imprisonment
IPC Sec 326 B	Punishment for Attempt to acid throwing–5 years
IPC Sec 328	Punishment for giving stupefying drug with intent to cause hurt–10 years
IPC Sec 330	Torture (Voluntarily causing hurt to extort information/confession)–7 years
IPC Sec 331	Torture (Voluntarily causing grievous hurt to extort information/ confession)–10 years
IPC Sec 334	Voluntarily causing hurt on provocation (1 month imprisonment)
IPC Sec 335	Voluntarily causing grievous hurt on provocation (4 years imprisonment)
IPC Sec 337	Causing hurt to any person by doing rash or negligent act (6 months imprisonment)
IPC Sec 338	Causing grievous hurt to any person by doing rash or negligent act (2 years imprisonment
IPC Sec 351	Assault Definition
IPC Sec 352	Punishment for assault
IPC Sec 354 A	Punishment for sexual harassment (1 – 3 years)
IPC Sec 354 B	Use of criminal force on woman to disrobe (3 – 7 years)
IPC Sec 354 C	Voyeurism
IPC Sec 354 D	Stalking (1st offence – Cognizable, bailable; 2nd offence–cognizable and non bailable)
IPC Sec 359	Kidnapping Definition
IPC Sec 362	Abduction definition
IPC Sec 363	Punishment for Kidnapping ***(364–369 punishment for kidnapping under various circumstances)***
IPC Sec 375	Rape Definition
IPC Sec 376	Punishment for rape (7 years to life)
IPC Sec 376 A	Victim suffers death or PVS due to rape (20 years to life/death)
IPC Sec 376 B	Sex with wife during separation (2-7 years)
IPC Sec 376 C	Custodial rape (upto 10 years)
IPC Sec 376 D	Gang rape (20 years to life/death)
IPC Sec 376 E	Punishment for repeated offenders (Life imprisonment or death)
IPC Sec 377	Unnatural sexual offences–10 years
IPC Sec 497	Adultery
IPC Sec 498 A	Subjecting a married woman to cruelty
IPC Sec 509	Word, gesture or act intended to insult the modesty of a woman – 3 years
IPC Sec 510	Misconduct in public by a drunken person – simple imprisonment upto 24 hours

Ref: Textbook of Forensic Medicine by P.C. Dikshit Page 8, Textbook of Forensic Medicine by Krishna Vij 5th Edition Page 11, Textbook of Forensic Medicine and Toxicology by NG Rao 2nd Edition Page 15

Ans: (D) 193

2. **In Alleged history of gun shot injury there is burning, blackening, tattooing around the wound Dirt collar, the injury is:**

A. Close shot
B. Contact
C. Distant shot entry wound
D. Distant shot exit wound

Key:

Buring, blackening, tattooing around the wound are features of close shot entry wound

Rifled Fire Arm Injuries				
Characteristics	**Contact shot**	**Close shot**	**Near shot**	**Distant shot**
Range	*Touch with skin*	*2.5 to 7.5 cm*	*30-60 cm*	*>60 cm*
Size	*Largest*	*Bullet size*	*Smaller*	*Smallest*
Shape	*Stellate*	*Circular*	*Circular*	*Circular*
Muzzle end imprint	*+ve*	*-ve*	*-ve*	*-ve*
Edge eversion	*+ve*	*-ve*	*-ve*	*-ve*
Blackening	*-ve*	*+ve*	*-ve*	*-ve*
Tattooing	*-ve*	*+ve*	*+ve*	*-ve*
Singeing	*-ve*	*+ve*	*-ve*	*-ve*
Abrasion collar	*-ve*	*+ve*	*+ve*	*+ve*
Grease collar	*-ve*	*+ve*	*+ve*	*-ve*

Short Gun Injuries					
Characteristics	**Contact shot**	**Close range**	**Near range**	**Intermediate range**	**Distant range**
Distance	Contact with skin	**<1 m**	1-2 m	2-4 m	**>4 m**
Wound	Single entrance wound Stellate or circular	Single circular entrance wound	Single entrance wound ***Irregular margins*** ***Rat hole ppearance***	Central hole due to mass surrounded by individual pelet hole	Individual pellet holes due to complete dispersion
Other features	Muzzle impression present Burns/Blackening/Tatooing along wound track	Burns/Singeing, Balckening, Tattooing present at wound site	-	-	-

FEATURES OF CLOSE SHOT INJURY

- *Victim is within range of flame in rifled fire arm injuries*
- *Close range–within a distance of <1 m in Shot gun injury*
- Burning, blackening, tattooing around the wound are features of close shot entry wound site
- *Wound is circular in shape*
- *Abrasion collar is present*

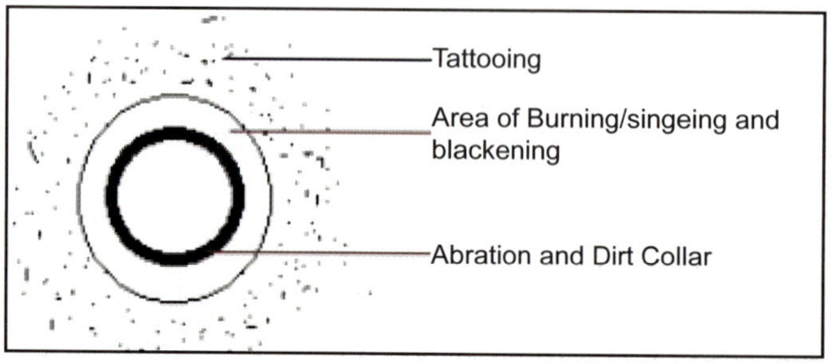

Contact shot	Close shot	Near shot	Distant shot
Contact with skin (Point blank)	**Victim in range of flame**	**Victim in range of Gun powder**	**Beyond range of gun powder**
Stellate irregular shaped Burns, Blackening, Tattooing inside track of wound	Bullet hole, ***Abrasion collar,*** Burns, Blackening and Tattooing	Bullet hole, Abrasion collar and Tattooing	Bullet hole Abrasion collar

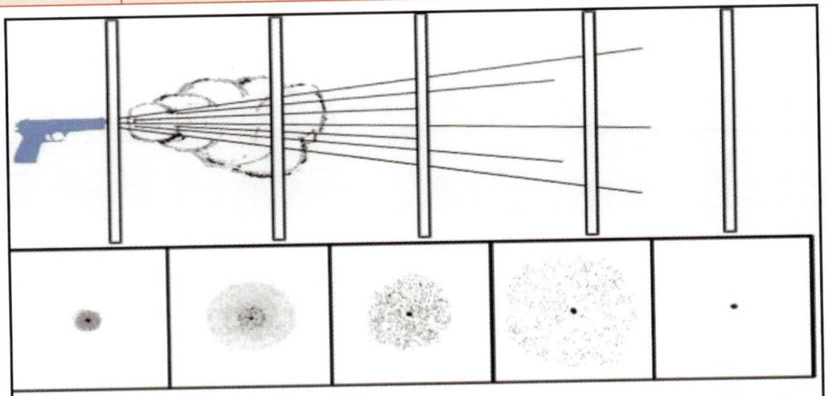

Ref: KSN Reddy 33rd Edition Page 216, Textbook of Forensic Medicine and Toxicology by NG Rao 2nd Edition Page 284, Principles of Forensic Medicine and Toxicology by Rajesh Bardale Page 211, Parikh 6th Edition Page 4.10

Ans: (A) Close shot

3. **Rigor mortis occur first in:**
   A. Myocardium
   B. Jaw
   C. Eyelids
   D. Lower limbs

Key:

Rigor Mortis

- **Synonyms:** *Cadaveric rigidity, Postmortem rigor, Postmortem rigidity, Postmortem stiffening*
- State of muscles in dead body when they become stiff or rigid with some degree of shortening.
- **Occurs due to depletion of ATP stores after death**
  - Onset: ATP level 85% of normal (Critical level)
  - **Maximum rigidity:** ATP level 15-30%

Mechanism

- Continuous and Progressive hydrolysis of ATP
- Once ATP stores are exhausted muscle goes into state of contraction
- Reduction in ATP causes stiffness and Rigidity

Muscle Involvement

- All muscles of body are involved, i.e., voluntary or involuntary
  - **Involuntary muscles earlier than Voluntary muscles**
- Occurs independent of nervous system–Even in Hemiplegic limb

Contd.

Contd.

Order of Appearance

- **Involves myocardium initially within 1 hour, then spreads externally**
- **External**–First in eyelids, Muscles of face, jaw, neck, upper limbs and lastly lower limbs

Sequence of Muscles Involvement Is As Follows
Heart > *upper eyelid* > *neck* > *jaw* > *face* > *chest* > *upper limb* > *abdomen* > *lower limb* > *finger and toes.*

Order of Disappearance

- Disappears in same order as appearance
- Begins in 1-2 hours, progress in 3-4 hours and complete in 6-12 hours

EXTRA EDGE

RULES OF RIGOR MORTIS

- **Nysten rule:** Rigor mortis usually develops sequentially
- **Shapiro rule:** Rigor mortis usually develops proximodistal (Descending pattern)
- **Rule of 12:** Takes roughly 12 hours to appear, Persists for another 12 hours and Disappears in another 12 hours

Factors Influencing Rigor Mortis–Onset and Duration	
Early Onset	**Late Onset**
Usually short duration	*Usually longer duration*
Muscle fatigue and Exhaustion before death	Muscles that are healthy and at rest before death
Death from wasting diseases	Asphyxia, Hemorrhage and Pneumonia
Hot weather	Cold weather
OP poisoning, HCN, Strychnine	CO poisoning

Rigor mortis doesn't occur in fetus <7 months old
Early onset and Longer duration rigor mortis is seen in HCN and Strychnine poisoning

Ref: KSN Reddy Essentials of Forensic Medicine 33rd Edition Page 321, Parikh 6th Edition Page 3.9, SK Shanghal 4th Edition Page 92

Ans: (A) Myocardium

4. Gastric lavage is not contraindicated in which of the poisoning?

A. Nitric acid
B. Sulphuric acid
C. Carbolic acid
D. Hydrochloric acid

Key:

Gastric lavage is contraindicated in all corrosive poisonings except phenol

Gastric Lavage

- **Tube**–Ewald/Boas tube
- **Diameter**–1 cm
- **Mark at** 50 cm
- **Openings**–Lateral

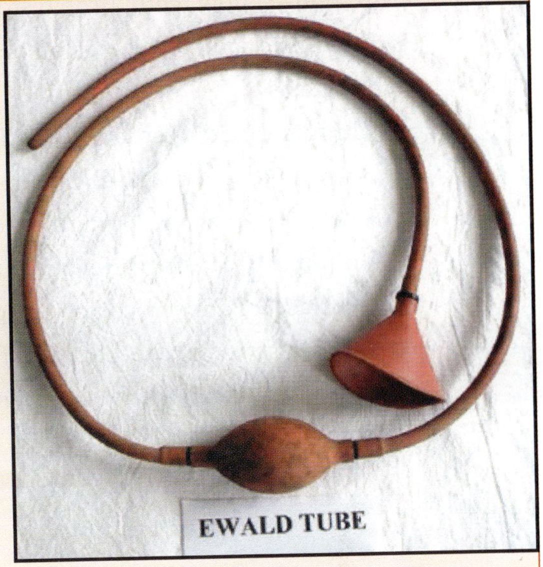

EWALD TUBE

A nasogastric tube used for gastric aspiration is inadequate and should never be used.
In a child, diameter should be at least 22 to 28 French* (Ryle's tube *may be sufficient)

- **Patient position**–Left lateral/Prone
- **Material**–Potassium permanganate, Sodium bicarbonate, Tannic acid, Sodium and potassium iodide, Calcium lactate and Saturated lime water/Starch
- ***Useful within 3 hours of poison ingestion***

Containdications for Gastric Lavage

- Corrosive (Absolute contraindication except carbolic acid)
- Convulsants/CNS stimulants use with precaution
- Comatose patient
- Volatile poison
- Upper GI Pathology (Esophageal varices)
- Hypothermic patient
- Severe heart disease and Advanced pregnancy

- ***Water/Normal saline*** is most commonly used solution for Gastric lavage
- ***$KMnO_4$****: Used for Oxidisable poisons,* ***Not useful for heavy metal poisoning****, Used in high concentrations for Opium poisoning*

Specific Substances Used For Gastric Lavage in Poisoning

Arsenic–Freshly prepared hydrated ferric oxide

Mercury–Sodium Formaldehyde

Copper–Potassium ferrocyanide (Non toxic salt of cyanosis)

Iron–Desferrioxamine

Oxalate–Calcium gluconate

Cyanides–Sodium thiosulphate

☞ EXTRA EDGE (CORROSIVES)

- Acid that causes **liquefactive necrosis–Hydroflouric acid**
- **Sulphuric acid**–Chalky white teeth, Black tongue, Black stomach (Charred), Blotting paper stomach
- **Nitric acid**–Yellow teeth, Brown stomach, Xanthoproteic reaction, yellow discolouration of tissues (Picric acid).
- **Hydrochloric acid**–No corrosion of skin, No change in teeth, No stomach perforation
- **Vitriolage:**
  - Throwing acid over face to disfigure (Sulphuric acid–Most commonly used)
  - Attempt of Vitriolage–IPC Sec 326 (5-7 years)
  - Visual impairment/Disfigurement–IPC Sec 320
  - Voluntarily causing grievous hurt–IPC Sec 326 A
- **Magenstrasse:** Pathway corrosive agents follow in food filled stomach
  - *Along lesser curvature–Location of greatest damage*
  - *In empty stomach–Lower half of stomach (Fundus spared)*

Phenol poisoning	Oxalic acid poisoning	Boric acid poisoning
Carbolism, Green urine (carboluria), Miosis, Corneal deposition, Cartilage deposition, Proximal convoluted tubule damage, CNS depression, Delayed puterefaction ***White leathery stomach***	Ink remover solution Coffee ground vomitus, Hypocalcemia (Tetany), Oxaluria, Tubular necrosis, ***Black coloured stomach***	Boiled lobster syndrome-Massive erythema, Desquamation and Exfoliation on Palms, Soles and Buttocks

Ref: KSN Reddy Essentials 33th Edition Page 516, Modern Medical Toxicology VV Pillay 4th Edition Page 20, Parikh 6th Edition Page 10.5, Katzung 11th Edition Page 396

Ans: (C) Carbolic acid

5. **Which of the following is not same in identical twins?**

A. DNA fingerprint
B. Fingerprint of hand
C. Blood group
D. Iris

Key:

Fingerprints are different even in identical twins (Not same)

Dactylography

(Fingerprint system, Galton system, Dermatoglyphycs)

- *Most reliable method of Identification of person*
- First used in India by William Herschel
- First systematized by Francis Galton
- Minutiae are principal features used to compare 2 fingerprints.

Contd.

Contd.

- 10-12 points of comparison are accepted as proof of identity
- Minimal number of points in establishing proof of identity-8
- Histological sections upto 6 mm from skin surface yields satisfactory fingerprints

Advantages

- Most reliable
- Absolutely individualistic
- Different even in identical twins (Adolphe Quetelet's rule of biological variation*)
- Not inherited
- Persistence–Don't change with time

Types

- Loops–Most common (60-70%)→ Left> Right
- Whorls
- Arch
- Composite

Chemical Reagents

- Reagents used for fingerprint collection–Ninhydrin and Cyanoacrylate
- **O-FTIR:** Optical frustrated Total internal reflection→Most commonly used to capture liver scan fingerprints

Categories of Fingerprints

- Latent fingerprints: Barely visible
- Plastic fingerprints: Prints made on soft surface (Soap, Cheese)
- Visible fingerprints: Stained with blood, greese

Modification of Fingerprints

Permanent alteration:

- Leprosy, Electrocution, Radiation and Skin graft

Ridge atrophy and Loss of pattern:

- Coelic disease

Intentional alteration (Criminals):

- Corrosives, Burns, CO_2 Snow and Rubbing against hard surface

RELATED TERMS

- Poroscopy–Study of pore structure–Unique and Permanent
- Podography–Study of foot prints (Maternity hospitals for preventing exchange of infants)
- Cheiloscopy–Study of lip prints (Suzuki classification)
- Rugoscopy/Palatoprint/Palatoscopy–Study of palatal rugae (Anterior third of palate)

- **DNA Fingerprinting is used for proving Paternity–Developed by Jeffrey**
  - Based on variable number of Tandem repeats
  - Ideal sample–Blood
  - Most common sample–Buccal smear (dead)
  - Preservative–EDTA at–20°C
- Brain fingerprinting invented by Lawrence Farrel
- Iris and Blood group can be same in between identical twins

(Indians have dark or brown iris. Europeans have blue or grey iris).

Ref: KSN Reddy Essentials 33rd Edition Page 86, Textbook of Forensic Medicine by P.C. Dikshit Page 120, Textbook of Forensic Medicine by Krishna Vij 5th Edition Page 63

Ans: (B) Finger print of hand

6. **Which of the following is not used as a preservative in Chemical analysis?**

A. Rectified spirit
B. Formalin
C. Salt solution
D. Glycerine

Key:

Formalin is not used as preservative for Chemical/Toxicological analysis as extraction of poison becomes difficult

Preservatives	
Rectified spirit	Best preservative for viscera preservation *Useful in Acid poisoning (Except phenol)* Contraindicated for Alcohol, Kerosene, Chloral hydrate, Phosphorous, Formaldehyde and Paraldehyde
Supersaturated solution of common salt	Most commonly used preservative Easily available and Cheap *Almost all poisoning except Corrosive acids*
Sodium fluoride	Blood, Urine and Vitreous *Poisonings like Alcohol, Cocaine, CO, Cyanide* Toulene is best preservative for Urine examination
Glycerine	*Virological study (Rabies)*
Formalin	**Not used as preservative for chemical analysis** Histopathological and Museum specimen
Liquid paraffin	CO, HCN poisoning (Usually no preservative if fresh)

EXTRA EDGE

Routine viscera preserved during autopsy	Viscera preservation
• Stomach and its contents • Upper part of small intestine (30 cm length) • Liver (Right lobe) >500 gm • Kidney (Half of each kidney) • Blood 10 ml and Urine 100 ml	• Suspected poisoning deaths • To rule out drug intoxication • Cause of death not found after autopsy • Advanced decomposition • Any case if requested by magistrate

Preserved Viscera	Specific poisoning
Liver	Most important tissue
Bile	Opioids, Benzodiazepines, Cocaine, Acetaminophen and Heavy metals

Contd.

Contd.

Spleen culture	Septicemia
Brain	Organophosphorous, Opiates, CO, Cyanide, Barbiturates, Rabies and Alkaloids
Spinal cord	Strychnine
CSF	Alcohol
Vitreous	Alcohol (Particularly decomposed bodies)
Fatty tissues	Pesticides–Endrin, DDT
Skin	Injected poisons, Snake bite and Firearm injuries
Heart	Strychnine, Digitalis
Lungs	Gaseous poisons, HCN, Alcohol and Chloroform
Bone	Arsenic, Antimony, Thallium and Radium
Muscle	Internal organs are badly putrified ***Skeletal muscle of buttocks is best specimen for toxicology in embalming***

Ref: Principles of Forensic Medicine and Toxicology by Rajesh Bardale Page 123, Textbook of Forensic Medicine by P.C. Dikshit Page 157, Textbook of Forensic Medicine by Krishna Vij 5th Edition Page 26

Ans: (B) Formalin

8. Test based on the principle of suspect's reaction, if he witnesses an event then he behaves in a certain way is:

A. Narcoanalysis
B. Brain fingerprinting
C. Truth serum testing
D. Polygraph

Key:

Test based on the principle of suspect's reaction, if he witnesses an event then he behaves in a certain way is Polygraph
Reaction is dealt by autonomic nervous system–So test applied in this suspect is Polygraph

Polygraph/Lie Detector Test

- Measures and Records Physiological actions of human body
- Deals with Autonomic nervous system
- Subject is asked questions relating to crime scene and he answers them
- If he tries to tell lies, then autonomic nervous system response changes are observed ***(Since it is beyond control of suspect)***
- Records blood pressure, pulse, respiration and skin conductivity while the subject is asked and answers a series of questions.
- Test has high false +ve results
- ***Usually not more than 10 questions are asked to a person at any single setting.***
- Three types of questions are asked as:
  - ***Irrelevant questions:*** Having no relation with the incident.
  - ***Relevant questions:*** Having relation with the incident
  - ***Control questions.***

Contd.

Contd.

Narcoanalysis

• Narko=Anaesthesia/Torpor/Numbness/Apathy/Dormancy
• Test carried on patient or suspect after administration of truth serum
• Patient comes in sleep like state
• His/Her repressed feelings are brought to light
• **Drugs used:**
  o Sodium amytal
  o Sodium Pentothal
  o Scopolamine hydrobromide
  o Sodium secnol
  o Benzodiazepines
• Mechanism of action of the drug is by binding GABA(A) receptors in brain and spinal cord.
• **Amobarbital is associated with Laryngospasm.** Now Diazepam is drug of choice for Narcoanalysis.

Brain Mapping/Fingerprinting
• Measures P300 Evoked potential • Suspect is made to sit in evoked potential recording machine • He/She is shown objects relating to crime scene • Sensors pick up potentials from brain • Accuracy is almost 100%

Ref: KSN Reddy Essentials 33rd Edition Page 478, Principles of Forensic Medicine and Toxicology by Rajesh Bardale Page 408, Textbook of Forensic Medicine by Krishna Vij 5th Edition Page 572, VV Pillay Modern Forensic Medicine and Toxicology 4th Edition Page 200

Ans: (D) Polygraph

Chapter 8

PREVENTIVE AND SOCIAL MEDICINE

1. Possibility that a person has actually having a disease when study is in doubt is best indicated by:

A. Sensitivity
B. Specificity
C. Positive predictive value
D. Negative predictive value

Key:

Possibility that a person has actually having a disease when study is in doubt is best indicated by POSITIVE PREDICTIVE VALUE

- If the test is abnormal, post-test probability is same as **PREDICTIVE VALUE OF POSITIVE TEST**.
- "Predictive value of a positive test" indicates the probability that a patient with a positive test result has, in fact, the disease in question.
- Positive predictive value is the proportion of individuals with a positive test result who have the disease.
- The more prevalent a disease is in a given population, the more accurate will be the predictive value of a positive screening test.
- Predictive value reflects the diagnostic power of the test.
- Sensitivity is the ability of a test to identify correctly all those who have the disease, that is **"true-positive"**.
- Specificity is the ability of a test to identify correctly those who do not have the disease, that is, **"true-negatives"**.
- Negative predictive value is the proportion of individuals with a negative test result who do not have the disease.

Sensitivity

- Ability of a test to identify correctly all those who have the disease–True Positive (TP).
- Statistical index of diagnostic accuracy.

$$\textit{Sensitivity} = \frac{\text{True positive [TP]}}{\text{True positive [TP]} + \text{False negative [FN]}} \times 100 \quad \text{or} \quad \frac{\textit{True positive [TP]}}{\textit{Total diseased}} \times 100$$

Specificity

- Ability of test to identify correctly all those who don't have the disease (healthy)–True Negative (TN)

$$\textit{Specificity} = \frac{\text{True negative [TN]}}{\text{True negative [TP]} + \text{False positive [FN]}} \times 100 \quad \text{or} \quad \frac{\text{True negative [TN]}}{\text{Total not diseased}} \times 100$$

EXTRA EDGE

- *If Sensitivity increases if TP increases and FN decreases*
- *If Specificity increases if TN increases and FP decreases.*
- ***Sensitivity and specificity are inversely related.***
- False +ve error is more serious than false –ve error
- For screening tests sensitivity is important whereas for diagnostic tests specificity is very important
- **High false +ve** → Low specificity, Low prevalence, High specificity

Contd.

Contd.

False-Positive

- It means patients who do not have the disease are told that they have.
- **A screening test with a high specificity will have few false positives**
- Causes burden to diagnostic facility; discredit to the screening programme
- A test which has very high sensitivity (though at the cost of low specificity) will have high FP.

$$\text{False Positive Rate} = \frac{b}{b+d} \times 100 = \frac{FP}{FP+TN} \times 100$$

$$\text{False positive rate } (\alpha) = 1 - \text{specificity}$$

False Negative

- It means patients who actually have the disease are told that they do not have the disease.
- A screening test which is very sensitive has few "false negatives".
- Patient ignores signs / symptoms → postponement of treatment →↑ morbidity and mortality

$$\text{False Negative Rate} = \frac{c}{a+c} \times 100 = \frac{FN}{TP+FN} \times 100$$

$$\text{False negative rate } (\beta) = 1 - \text{sensitivity}$$

$$\text{Power of a test (sensitivity)} = (1-\beta) = 1 - \text{False negative rate}$$

Positive Predictive Value (PPV)

- PPV is the probability that a person with positive test result truly have disease
- Proportion of patients with positive test results who are correctly diagnosed.

$$PPV = \frac{a}{a+b} \times 100 = \frac{TP}{TP+FP} \times 100$$

PPV α Prevalence; Specificity; Sensitivity

- If sensitivity and specificity of test are constant, predictive values are largely dependent on prevalence of disease in population in which diagnostic test is being applied.

Negative Predictive Value (NPV)

- NPV is the probability that a person with -ve test result does not have disease
- Proportion of patients with negative test who are correctly diagnosed

$$NPV = \frac{d}{c+d} \times 100 = \frac{TN}{TN+FN} \times 100$$

- **NPV is inversely related to the Prevalence of the disease in population**

$$\textit{Predictive value of positive test} = \frac{\text{True positive [TP]}}{\text{True positive [TP]} + \text{False Positive [FP]}} \times 100 \text{ or } \frac{\textit{True positive}}{\textit{Total positive declared by test}} \times 100$$

$$\textit{Predictive value of negative test} = \frac{\text{True negative [TN]}}{\text{True negative [TN]} + \text{False negative [FN]}} \times 100 \text{ or } \frac{\textit{True negative [TN]}}{\textit{Total negative declared by test}} \times 100$$

Accuracy

- Degree of closeness of a measured or calculated quantity to its true value
- Predictive accuracy reflects the diagnostic power of the test.

$$\text{Accuracy} = \frac{TP+TN}{TP+FP+FN+TN} \times 100$$

$$\text{Accuracy} = [(\text{sensitivity}) \times (\text{prevalence})] + [(\text{specificity}) \times (1 - \text{prevalence})]$$

Contd.

Contd.

Bayes Theorem

- It is statement of conditional probability of a disease for an individual with a positive screening test.

$$\text{PPV} = \frac{[\text{Sensitivity} \times \text{Prevalence}]}{[\text{Sensitivity} \times \text{Prevalence}] + (1 - \text{Specificity})(1 - \text{Prevalence})} \times 100$$

$$\text{NPV} = \frac{[\text{Specificity} \times (1 - (\text{Prevalence})]}{[\text{Specificity} \times (1 - \text{Prevalence})] + [(1 - \text{Sensitivity}) \times \text{Prevalence}]} \times 100$$

Ref: Self Assessment and Review of Statistics 1st Edition Page 116, Park's Textbook of Preventive and Social Medicine 25th Edition Page 153

Ans: (C) Positive predictive value

2. Below data representation is named as:

A. Frequency polygon
B. Histogram
C. Compound bar diagram
D. Component bar diagram

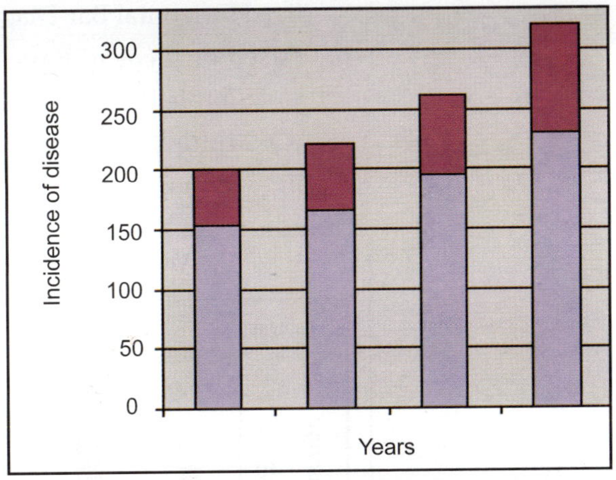

Key:

Given diagram contains Components–Component bar diagram
Each bar is divided into 2 or more parts, each part representing a certain item and proportional to the magnitude of that particular item

Multiple bar chart/Compound bar chart is a type of bar chart where two or more bars can be grouped together

PRESENTATION OF DATA

Qualitative Data

Tables Diagrams

i. Bar diagram
ii. Pie Chart
iii. Pictogram
iv. Spot Map
v. Shaded Map
vi. Cartogram

Quantitative Data

Tables Graphs

i. Histogram
ii. Frequency Polygon
iii. Frequency curve
iv. OGIVE–Cumulative Frequency curve
v. Line Chart/Line Graph
vi. Scatter diagram
vii. Box and whisker plot
viii. Stem leaf plot

Bar Chart

- **Use:** To compare the frequency distribution of Categorical Variables (Qualitative Data)
- **Horizontal X** axis (Abscissa) = ***Categories of Variables***
- **Vertical Y** Axis (Ordinate) = ***Frequency (Number or %)***
- Length of bars = Frequency of the variables
- ***Width of bars must be Equal.*** Equal Space or Gap is present between the bars

Type of Bar Diagrams

A. Based on Direction of Bars:

i. Vertical Bar Diagram

ii. Horizontal Bar Diagram

B. Based on Type of Bars:

i. Simple Bar Diagram

ii. Multiple (or) Compound Bar Diagram

iii. Component and Proportional Bar Diagram

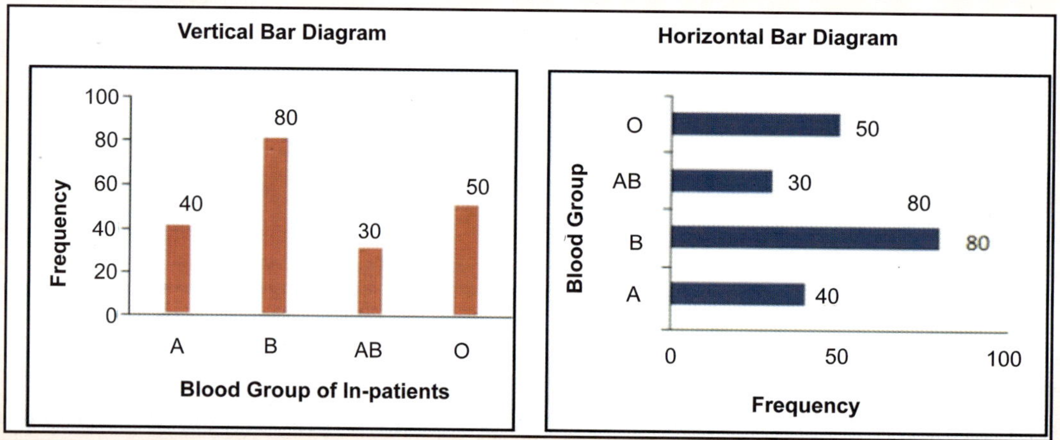

Simple Bar Diagram

- Depicts the frequency of Categories of a **Single Variable.**
- Consists of bars of a **single colour** or shade.
- **Equal Space between the bars is present**

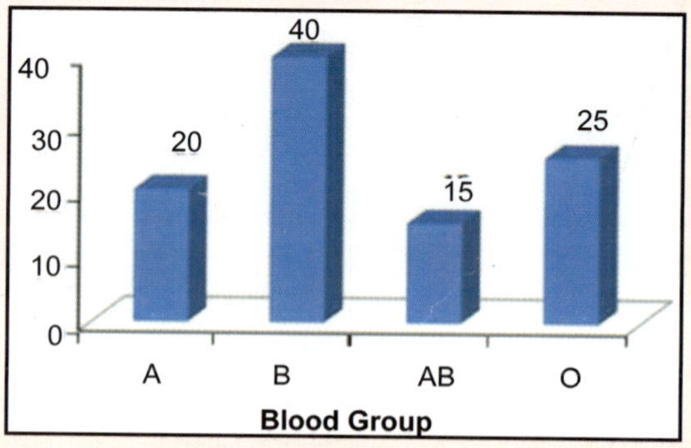

Multiple / Compound Bar Diagram

- **Use:** To compare frequency of ≥ 2 sub-groups within the Categories of a variable.
- Bars are placed adjacent to each other – **Adjacent Bar Diagram**
- Bars are of Multiple colours or shades
- Horizontal X axis = ≥ 2 groups within Categories

Contd.

Contd.

- Vertical Y axis = Frequency (Number or %)

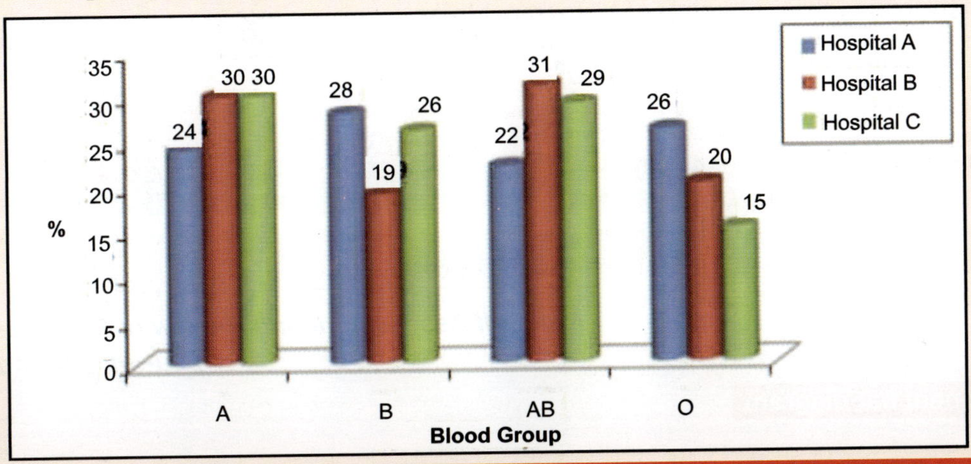

Component Bar Diagram

- Simple bar diagram externally and Multiple bar diagram internally
- X axis: Categories of variables; Y axis: Frequency (Number)
- Length of bars = Total Frequency of a category
- Height of the bars vary according to the frequency of the variables
- Each bar is divided into 2 or more parts depending on the no. of sub-groups in a category
- Each part within a bar has a different colour and so every bar is Multicoloured
- Equal Space between the bars is present

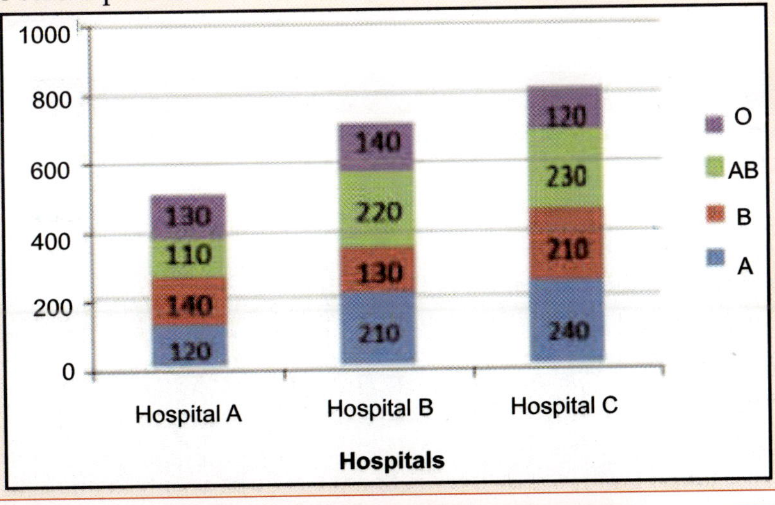

Histogram

- Consists of a series of blocks where the class intervals are given along the horizontal axis and the frequencies along the vertical axis.
- ***NO GAPS or SPACE between the Bars***
- ***Histogram is useful for graphical presentation for 'continuous quantitative data'***

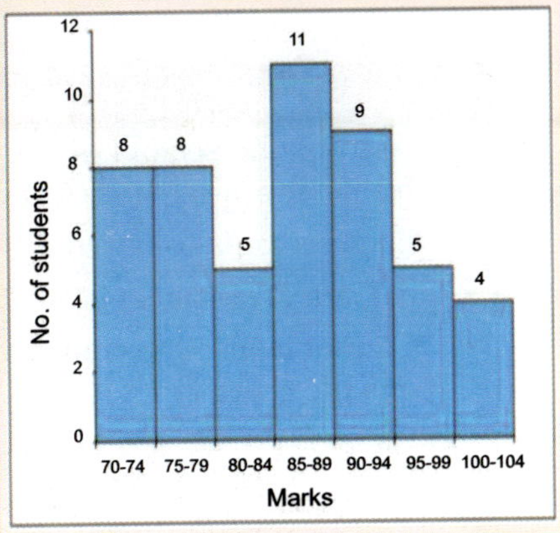

Contd.

Contd.

Frequency Polygon	
• Obtained by joining the mid-points of histogram blocks. • AREA DIAGRAM of frequency distribution. • X axis: Class-Midpoints • Y axis: Frequency/Relative frequency • Touches X-axis on both ends. • Comparison of ≥ 2 groups of continuous variable- possible	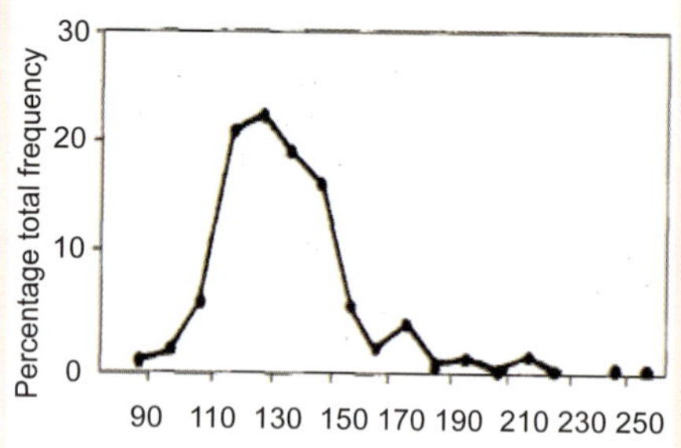

Ref: Self Assessment and Review of Statistics 1st Edition Page 16, Park's SPM 25th Edition Page 846

Ans: (D) Component bar diagram

3. Which representation is best to indicate the trend of events over a period of time?

A. Histogram B. Pie chart

C. Line diagram D. Scatter diagram

Key:

Line diagram is used to show trend of events with passage of time

Line Diagram/ Line Chart/Line Graph	
• **Type of Frequency Polygon:** Basically frequency polygon where the class intervals are in terms of time. • *Use: to show the TREND OF EVENTS over a period of time (TIME TREND)* • Presents variations of frequency by line • **X axis:** TIME (Years/Months/Weeks/Days/Hrs/Mins) • **Y axis:** Frequency (Number) • *Line DOES NOT touch the X axis*	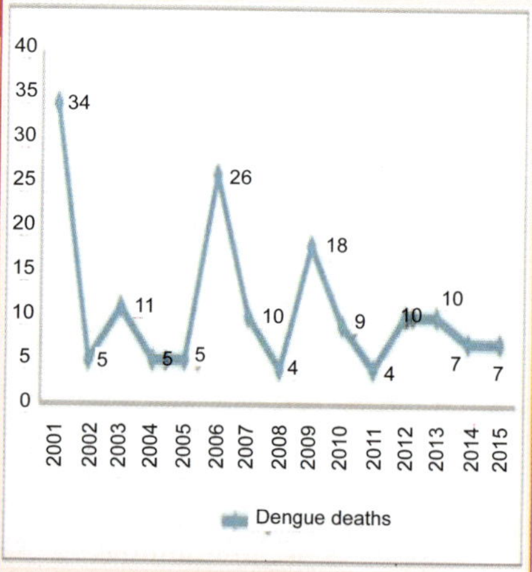

Pie Chart	
• Area of the sectors of the circle and their angulations are proportional to frequency of categories of the variable. • Each sector is coloured differently. • *All categories must be Mutually Exclusive (Total must be 100% = 360°)* • Cannot be used to compare frequency distribution of 2 different variables in one pie chart.	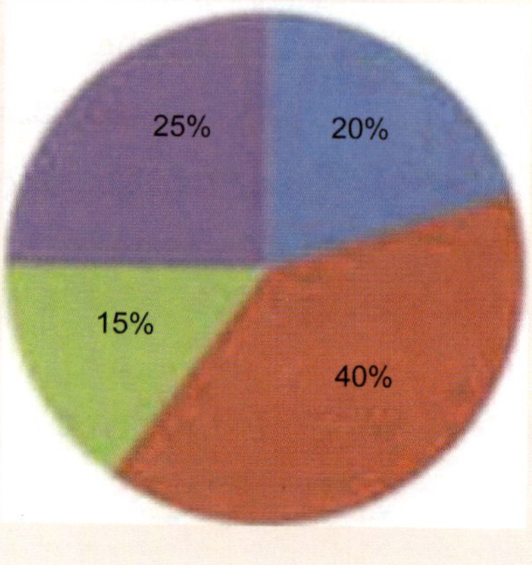

Contd.

Contd.

Histogram

- Consists of a series of blocks where the class intervals are given along the horizontal axis and the frequencies along the vertical axis.
- ***NO GAPS or SPACE between the Bars***
- ***Histogram is useful for graphical presentation for 'continuous quantitative data'***

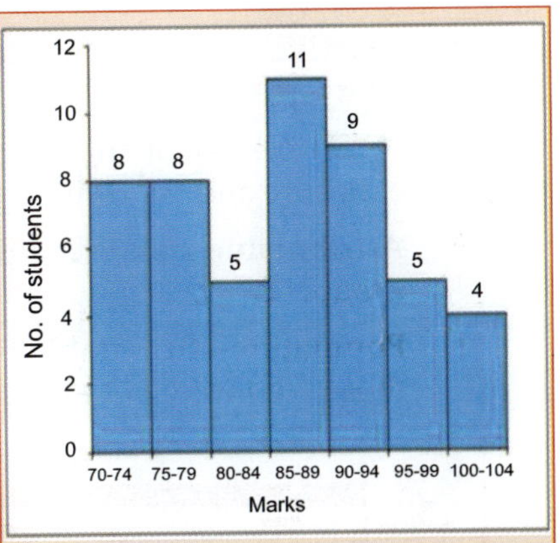

Scatter Diagram

- **Use:** To depict the **Correlation** (relationship) between **2 continuous variables (Quantitative Data)**
- **X axis:** Independent Variable or Exposure Variable
- **Y axis:** Dependent Variable or Outcome Variable
- **Trend line** drawn along the distribution of dots / scatter, shows **Direction** of relationship.
- Also called as "**Correlation Diagram**"

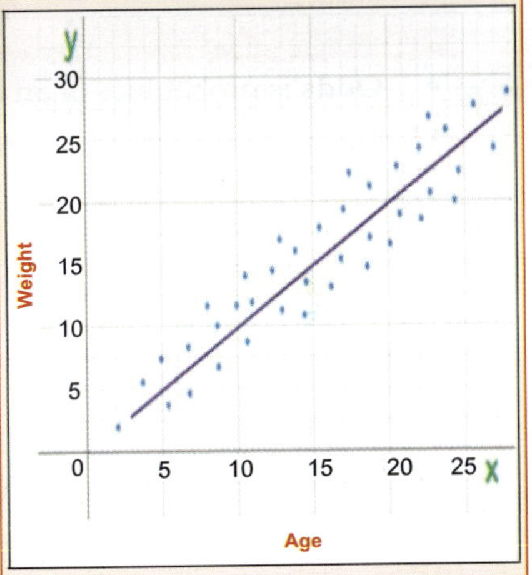

Ref: Self Assessment and Review of Statistics 1st Edition Page 18, Park 25th Edition Page 846

Ans: (C) Line diagram

4. Cross product ratio is calculated in:

A. Case control study

B. Cross sectional study

C. Cohort study

D. Ecological study

Key:

Cross product ratio/Odds ratio is calculated in Case control study

Cross Product Ratio/Odd's Ratio

- **Cross product ratio (Odds ratio)** is a measure of the strength of the association between risk factor and outcome in a case control study.
- **Derivation of odds ratio is based on three assumptions:**
  - Disease being investigated must be relatively rare
  - Cases must be representative of those with the disease
  - Controls must be representative of those without the disease

Contd.

Contd.

- **Relative risk** is direct measure of the strength of the association between suspected cause and effect in a cohort study.
- A relative risk of one indicates no association, whereas greater than one suggests "positive" association between exposure and the disease under study.
- **Attributable risk** is the difference in incidence rates of disease between an exposed group and non-exposed group.
- **Population-attributable risk** is incidence of the disease in the total population minus incidence of disease among those who were not exposed to the suspected causal factor.

Application of case control study

- **Odds** is probability of an event occurring vs probability of it not occurring, in other words
- OR is a measure of the **strength of association** between a risk factor and an outcome.

$$\text{Odds Ratio} = \frac{\text{Odds that case was exposed}}{\text{Odds that control was exposed}}$$

Odds ratio= ad/bc

Three Assumptions to Calculate OR

- Disease must be relatively rare.
- Cases must be representative of the diseased.
- Controls must be representative of the non-diseased.

- Incidence of the disease in exposed and unexposed are not available, hence relative risk cannot be calculated in a case control study.
- So Odds Ratio is calculated as **'an estimate of Relative Risk'**

Interpretation of Odds Ratio

OR value	Association	Interpretation
OR <1	Negative association	**Negative association** exists between the disease and exposure (exposure is protective)
OR = 1	No association	**No association** exists between the disease and exposure (no role of exposure on outcome)
OR > 1	Positive association	**Positive association** exists between the disease and exposure (exposure is harmful)

Application of Cohort Study

Relative Risk (Risk Ratio)

- Ratio of the incidence rates between exposed group and non-exposed group
- Can only be calculated from prospective studies (cohort studies)

Contd.

Contd.

- **Ratio that measures strength of association**

$$RR = \frac{\text{Incidence rate among exposed}}{\text{Incidence rate among non-exposed}}$$

Interpretation of RR
RR > 1 = Increased risk of outcome among "exposed" group RR < 1 = Decreased risk, or protective effects, among "exposed" group RR = 1 = No association between exposure and outcome

Attributable Risk (AR)

- Indicates to what extent the disease under study can be attributed to the risk / exposure
- It is additional incidence of disease that can be attributed to the risk factor in question.
- Amount of disease that might be eliminated if factor under study is controlled/eliminated.
- Usually expressed as a percentage

Attributable risk [Risk difference]

$$= \frac{[\text{Incidence of disease/death among exposed} - \text{Incidence of disease/death among non-exposed}]}{\text{Incidence of disease or death among exposed}}$$

Population Attributable Risk

- It indicates the risk in the total population that can be attributed to the exposure.

$$\frac{\text{Incidence of disease in total population} - \text{Incidence of disease among non-exposed}}{\text{Incidence of disease in total population}}$$

Ref: Self Assessment and Review of Statistics 1st Edition Page 149, Park Textbook of Preventive and Social Medicine 25th Edition Page 73

Ans: (A) Case control study

5. **Confounding factor in a study:**
   A. It itself is an independent risk factor for causation of disease
   B. It is present in study group and not in control group
   C. It is associated with the exposure not with the disease
   D. It is associated with the disease not with the exposure

Key:

Confounding factor is itself is an independent risk factor for causation of disease

Confounding Factor

- **Confounder is** any factor associated with both **exposure and outcome,** and has an **independent effect** in causation of outcome (thus it is a risk factor by itself).
- Confounder is found **unequally** distributed between the study and control groups
- **Measures to reduce confounding during the study:**
  - Randomization

Contd.

Contd.

- Restriction
- Matching

- **Features of confounding factor:**
  - Associated both with exposure and disease.
  - Distributed unequally in study and control groups.
  - Associated with exposure under investigation, it itself is an independent risk factor for disease.
- **Example:** Study of role of alcohol in oesophageal cancer, smoking is a confounding factor
  - Associated with consumption of alcohol
  - Independent risk factor for oesophageal cancer

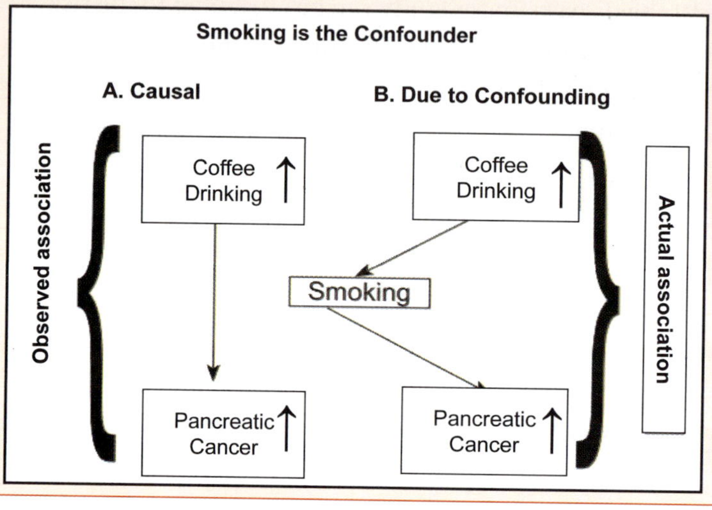

Confounding is Controlled By Following Methods

- **Randomization** – ensuring confounding variables are equally distributed among groups being compared
- **Restriction** – limiting the study to people who have particular characteristics
- **Matching** – ensuring potential confounding variables are evenly distributed in 2 groups being compared
- **Stratification** – confounding occurring during analysis phase rather than design phase – measurement of strength of association in well defined and homogenous categories (strata)
- **Statistical modeling** – multivariate analysis – done to estimate strength of associations while controlling for number of confounding variables

Method	Utility to control confounding
Randomization	*Most ideal method*
Restriction	Limiting study to people who have particular characteristics
Matching	Mostly useful in case control studies
Stratification	Useful for larger studies
Statistical modeling	When many confounding variables exist simultaneously

Ref: Self Assessment and Review of Statistics 1st Edition Page 159, Park 25th Edition Page 80

Ans: (A) It itself is an independent risk factor for causation of disease

6. **Significance of difference between proportions is better compared by:**
   A. Chi-square test
   B. Z square test
   C. Paired t test
   D. Unpaired t test

Key:

Chi-square test offers an alternate method of testing the significance of difference between two proportions

Chi-Square Test (X2) - Developed By Karl Pearson

- Type of non parametric test ***used for qualitative data* in form of proportions.**
- Alternate method of testing the significance of difference between two proportions.
- **Used as a test of goodness of fit:** It determines whether the observed frequency distribution differs from theoretical distribution [i.e., normal, binomial or Poisson] by chance or sample is drawn from different population.
- Chi-square test has the advantage that it can also be used when more than two groups are to be compared.
- **Null Hypothesis** states that there is no difference between the two proportions.
- ***Degree of freedom (d.f.)*** *depends upon the number of columns and rows in the original table, and given by the formula : d.f. = (c — 1) (r — 1)*
- Used to find whether any association between 2 events/discrete attributes is real/chance.
- *Advantage:* can also be used when more than two groups are to be compared.
- ***Yates correction:*** *Applied when expected frequency in any cell of 2 x 2 contingency table is < 5.*

Applications of Chi-Square Test

- *Test of proportions*
- *Test of association*
- *Test of goodness of fit*

- **Unpaired t-test** is used to assess the difference between two unrelated measurements.
- **Paired t-test** is used to assess the difference between two paired measurements.

Condition	Dependent Variable	Parametric Test	Non-Parametric Test
Comparisons between 2 independent groups	Continuous	Z test, (in >30) unpaired t test (n ≤ 30)	Wilcoxon rank sum test (Mann Whitney 'U' test)
	Discrete	Z test, (n >30) unpaired t test (n ≤ 30)	Chi-square X_2) test
Comparisons between 2 paired groups	Continuous	Paired t test	Wilcoxon signed rank test
	Discrete	Paired t test	Mc Nemar's (X_2) test

Contd.

Contd.

Comparisons among > 2 independent groups	Continuous	One way ANOVA	Kruskal Wallis 'H' test
	Discrete	One way ANOVA	Chi-square (X_2) test
Comparisons among > 2 paired groups	Continuous	Repeated measures ANOVA	Friedman's test
	Discrete	Repeated measures ANOVA	Mc Nemar's (X_2) test
Correlation between 2 quantitative variables	Continuous/ Discrete	Pearson's correlation coefficient (r)	Spearman's correlation coefficient (p)

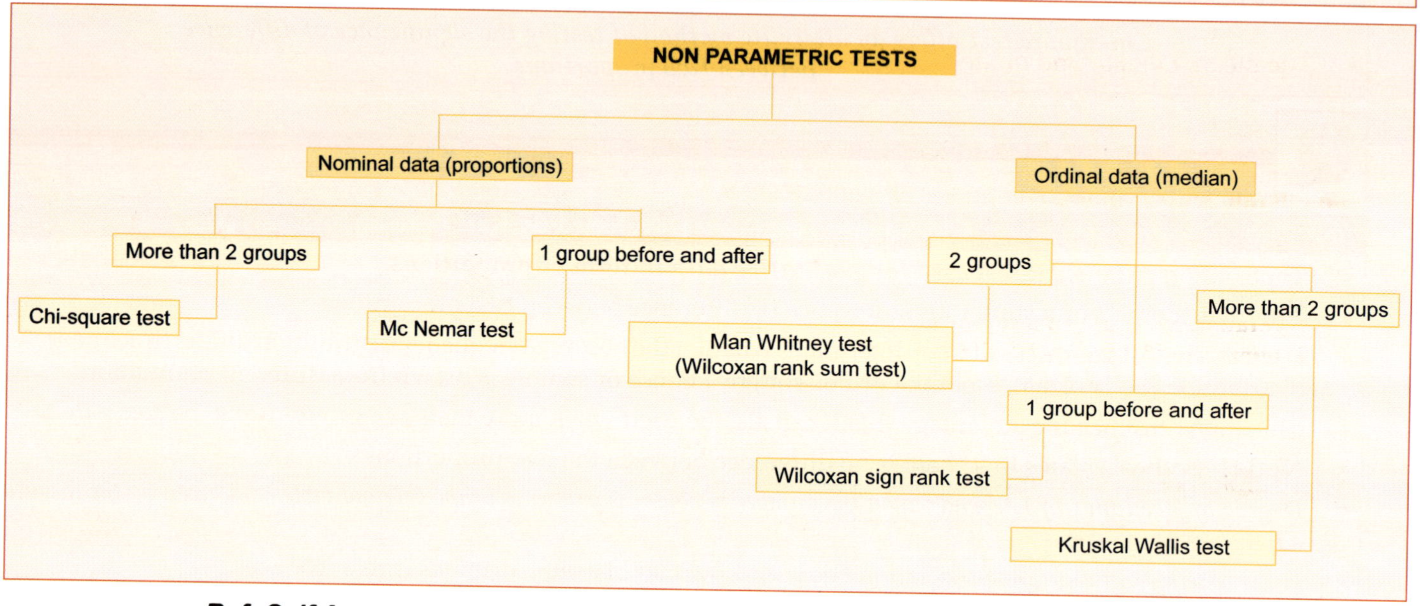

Ref: Self Assessment and Review of Statistics 1st Edition Page 82, Park 25th Edition Page 915

Ans: (A) Chi-square test

7. Area included 1 standard deviation on either side of mean value is:

A. 33% B. 68% C. 95% D. 98%

Key:

- ***Mean ± 1 SD covers 68.3% of values, hence called as 68% confidence limit***
- ***Mean ± 2 SD covers 95.4% of values, hence called as 95% confidence limit***
- ***Mean ± 3 SD covers 99.7% of values, hence called as 99% confidence limit***

- Area between one standard deviation on either side of mean will include approximately 68% of the values in the distribution.

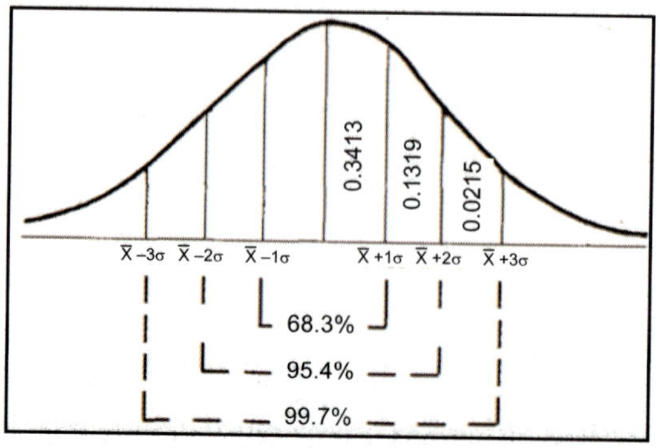

- Area between two standard deviations on either side of the mean will cover approximately 95% of the values.
- Area between three standard deviations will include 99.7% of the values.
- These limits on either side of the mean are called "confidence limits".

Characteristics of Standard Normal Distribution Curve

- **Smooth, bell-shaped, perfectly symmetrical curve**, based on an infinitely large number of observations.
- The total area of the curve is **1**
- Its **mean** is **zero**
- Its **standard deviation** is **1**
- The mean, median and mode all coincide.
- Distance of a value (x) from mean of the curve in units of standard deviation is called "relative deviate or standard normal variate" and is denoted by Z.

Skew Distribution

- **Asymmetric Distribution**
- It is a measure of asymmetry of a probability distribution of random variable.
- One tail of the curve is longer than other
- **A relative measure of skewness as given by Karl Pearson is:**
  Skewness = [3(Mean – Median)] / SD.

If the skewness so calculated:

- **"+ve" →Mean > Median→** Skewness is to the right (Tail is towards right side and there are large number of low scores, small number of high scores)
- **" –ve" →Mean < Median→**Skewness is to the left (Tail is towards left side and there are large number of high scores, small number of low scores)

Distribution	Central tendency
Normal (Gaussian) distribution	Mean = Median = Mode (coincide)
Right (Positive) skew distribution	Mean > Median > Mode
Left (Negative) skew distribution	Mean < Median < Mode

- Pearson's mode or First Skewness coefficient = (Mean – Mode)/SD
- Pearson's median or Second Skewness coefficient = 3(Mean – Median)/SD
- Quartile skewness = (Q3 – 2Q2 + Q1)/ Q3 – Q1

Negatively skewed distribution (Asymmetric Distribution)	Standard Normal Distribution	Positively skewed distribution (Asymmetric Distribution)
Left skewed (or) left tailed distribution	Symmetric distribution	Right skewed (or) Right tailed distribution

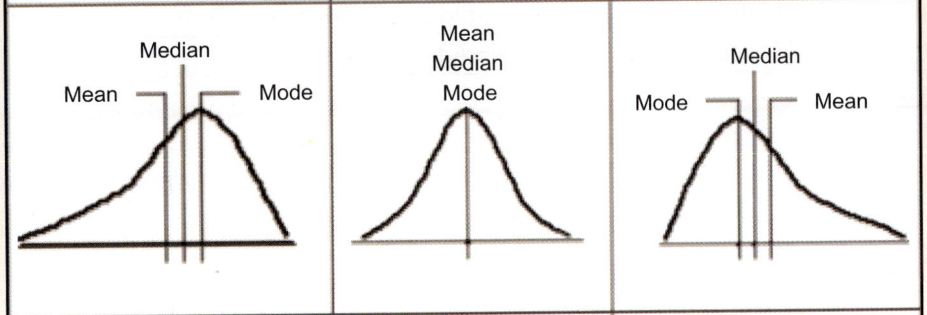

Mean < Median < Mode	Mean – Median – Mode	Mean > Median > Mode

Ref: Self Assessment and Review of Statistics 1st Edition Page 70, Park 25th Edition Page 912

Ans: (B) 68%

8. **Test applied when separate observations are made on means of individuals of two separate groups, and these need to be compared:**

A. Paired T test
B. Unpaired T test
C. Chi-square test
D. Wilcoxon signed-rank test

Key:

- **Unpaired T test** is applied to compare means of two different groups.
  Example: Length at one year of a group of infants who were breastfed, compared with a group who were not breastfed
- ***Before applying the Unpaired T test, data needs to meet few requirements and assumptions as follows:***
  - Variable is being compared between two different groups in the hypothesis
  - Variable is measured on quantitative scale
  - Variable follows normal distribution
  - *Equality of variance :* Data in both groups have the same variance
  - Sample size in either of the two groups is less than 30
- **Paired t-test** is used to assess the difference between two paired measurements.
  - e.g., weight measurements from the same subjects at a 6-month interval
- If the data are clearly not normally distributed, non-parametric tests can be used.
  - Wilcoxon signed-rank test – replaces the paired t-test
  - Mann-Whitney U-test or Wilcoxon rank-sum test – replaces the unpaired t-test
- **Chi-square test** offers an alternate method of testing the significance of difference between two proportions.

Condition	Dependent Variable	Parametric Test	Non-Parametric Test
Comparisons between 2 independent groups	Continuous	Z test (n > 30) unpaired t test (n ≤ 30)	Wilcoxon rank sum test (Mann Whitney 'U' test)
	Discrete	Z test (n > 30) unpaired t test (n ≤ 30)	Chi-square (χ^2) test
Comparisons between 2 paired groups	Continuous	Paired t test	Wilcoxon signed rank test
	Discrete	Paired t test	Mc Nemar's (χ^2) test
Comparisons among > 2 independent groups	Continuous	One way ANOVA	Kruskal Wallis 'H' test
	Discrete	One way ANOVA	Chi-square (χ^2) test
Comparisons among > 2 paired groups	Continuous	Repeated measures ANOVA	Friedman's test
	Discrete	Repeated measures ANOVA	Mc Nemar's (χ^2) test
Correlation between 2 quantitative variables	Continuous/ Discrete	Pearson's corrleation coefficient (r)	Spearman's correlation coefficient (p)

Ref: Self Assessment and Review of Statistics 1st Edition Page 82, Park 25th Edition Page 915

Ans: (B) Unpaired T test

9. **Paradoxical carrier is defined as:**

A. A person not suffering from disease acts as carrier
B. A person as carrier acquired from carrier
C. Who acquires disease from patient
D. Who spreads infection to normal people

Key:

Paradoxical carrier is a carrier who acquires infection from carrier

Carriers

- **Paradoxical carrier** refers to carrier who acquires pathogen from another carrier.
- **Incubatory carriers** are carriers who shed the infectious agent during the incubation period of disease, e.g., measles, mumps, polio.
- **Convalescent carriers** are those who continue to shed the disease agent during the period of convalescence, e.g., typhoid fever.
- **Healthy carriers** are subclinical cases who have developed carrier state without suffering from overt disease, but are nevertheless shedding the disease agent, e.g., poliomyelitis.
- **Pseudo-carriers** are those carriers who shed avirulent organisms.
- ***Carriers are less infectious than cases, but epidemiologically, they are more dangerous than cases, e.g., Typhoid Mary.***

Elements of Carrier

- Presence in the body of the disease agent
- Absence of recognizable symptoms and signs of disease
- Shedding of the disease agent in the discharges or excretion.

Ref: Park Textbook of Preventive and Social Medicine 23rd Edition Page 95, Ananthanarayan and Paniker 9th Edition Page 72

Ans: (B) A person as carrier acquired from carrier

10. Disease with bird-arthropod-Man transmission:

A. Japanese encephalitis
B. Malaria
C. Plague
D. Paragonimus

Key:

Disease with bird-arthropod-Man transmission is seen with Japanese Encephalitis

JAPANESE ENCEPHALITIS

- Mosquito-borne encephalitis caused by **a group B arbovirus (Flavivirus).**
- **Vectors of JE include C. tritaeniorhynchus (Most common), C. vishnui and C. gelidus**
- Basic cycles of transmission are:
  - **Pig–mosquito—pig;**
  - Ardeid bird-mosquito-Ardeid bird
- JE virus is mainly amplified in pigs and birds and are transmitted by Culex mosquitoes between vertebrates
- **Incubation period:** 5 to 15 days

- Case fatality rate→ 20-40%
- *Cattle and buffaloes may act as "mosquito attractants" but not natural hosts of JE virus*
- Disease is transmitted to man by the bite of infected mosquitoes.
- Man is an incidental "dead-end" host.

JE Vaccine	Strain
Mouse brain derived, purified and inactivated vaccine	*Nakayama strain, Beijing strain*
Cell culture derived, Inactivated vaccine	*Beijing P3 strain*
Cell culture derived, Live attenuated vaccine	*SA 14-14-2 strain (India)*

Vector borne disease classification based on transmission chain

- Man—Arthropod—Man **(Malaria)**
- Man—Snail—Man **(Schistosomiasis)**
- Mammal—Arthropod—Man **(Plaque)**
- Bird—Arthropod—Man **(Encephalitis)**
- Man—Cyclops—Fish—Man **(Fish tape worm)**
- Man—Snail—Fish—Man **(Clonorchis sinensis)**
- Man—Snail—Crab—Man **(Paragonimiasis)**

Ref: Park 25th Edition Page 311, Greenwood Medical Microbiology 18th Edition Page 530, Jawetz 27th Edition Page 548

Ans: (A) Japanese encephalitis

11. **"Healthy individual → risk factors→ Diseased→ clinical features → Death, disabled or Recovery" . What is this known as?**

A. Natural history of disease
B. Disease process
C. Levels of prevention
D. Phase of disease

Key:

"Healthy individual → risk factors → Diseased → Clinical features → Death, disabled or Recovery" represents Natural history of disease

- **Natural history of disease** signifies the way in which a disease evolves over time from the earliest stage of its pre-pathogenesis phase to its termination as recovery, disability or death, in the absence of treatment or prevention.
- ***Natural history of disease is best established by cohort studies.***

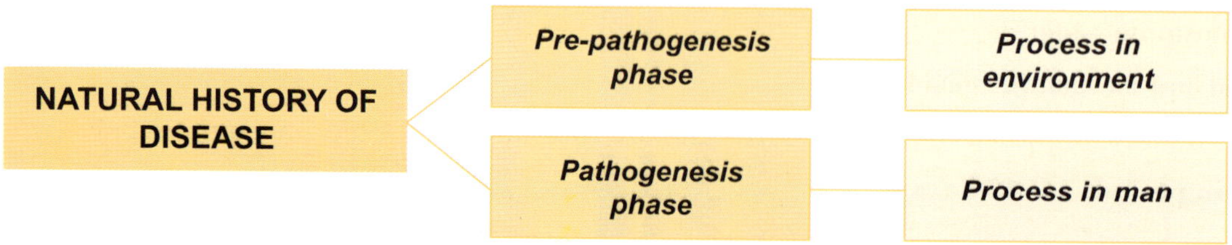

Pre-pathogenesis Phase

- **Pre-pathogenesis phase** refers to the phase where the disease agent has not yet entered man, but the factors are already existing in the environment.
- Pre-pathogenesis situation is frequently referred to as "man in the midst of disease" or "man exposed to the risk of disease".

Pathogenesis Phase

- In pathogenesis phase, disease agent multiplies, disease progresses through a period of incubation and later through early and late pathogenesis which may result in recovery, disability or death.

- **Levels of prevention** is categorized in terms of four level:
  - Primordial prevention
  - Primary prevention
  - Secondary prevention
  - Tertiary prevention
- Disease process is initiated by the interaction of 3 factors in epidemiological triad namely, agent, host and favourable environmental factors.

Ref: Park 25th Edition Page 346, Gordis Epidemiology 6th Edition Page 123

Ans: (A) Natural history of disease

12. In the disaster triage system:

A. First come first served

B. Green code indicates person needs prior treatment and transport

C. To benefit the greatest number injured

D. To mobilise the moribund patients

Key:

Triage is the only approach that can provide maximum benefit to the greatest number of injured in a major disaster situation

Triage

- **Triage** is the only approach that can provide maximum benefit to the greatest number of injured in a major disaster situation.
- In Disaster triage system, the principle of "first come, first treated", is not followed in mass emergencies.
- Triage consists of rapidly classifying injured on basis of severity of their injuries and likelihood of their survival with prompt medical intervention.
- **Most common classification uses the four color code system:**
  - **Red** indicates *high priority treatment or transfer*
  - **Yellow** signals *medium priority*
  - **Green** indicates *ambulatory patients*
  - **Black** for *dead or moribund patients*
- *Second Wednesday of October is designated as World Disaster Reduction Day*

- *Triage sieve:* Quick survey to separate dead and walking from injured
- *Triage sort:* Remaining casualities are assessed and allocated to categories
- *Tagging:* In procedure, where identification, age, place of origin, triage category, diagnosis and initial treatment are tagged onto every victim of disaster through colour coding.

Simple Triage

- Used in scene of mass casuality in order to sort patients into those who need critical attention and immediate transport to hospital and those with less serious injuries
- Step is required before transportation becomes available
- Categorization is based on severity of injuries and can be aided with printed tags/colored flags

Rapid Triage

- **S.T.A.R.T.**– Simple Triage and Rapid Treatment
- Simple triage system performed by lightly trained lay and emergency personnel in emergencies
- May serve as instructive example
- Has been field proven in mass casualty incidents like trench wrecks and bus accidents

Reverse Triage

- Less wounded are treated in preference to more severely wounded
- *Example:* War–Requires soldiers as quickly as possible.

Ref: Park 25th Edition Page 857

Ans: (C) To benefit the greatest number injured

13. Which is not personal safety measure (protective)?

A. Laboratory coats
B. Face shields
C. Goggles
D. Gloves

Key:

Face shields don't form Personal safety measure

- Respirators and face masks are among oldest devices used to protect workers against air-borne contaminants.
- Other protective devices are earplugs, ear muffs, helmets, safety shoes, aprons, gloves, gum boots, barrier creams, screens and goggles.
- Health care personnel are advised to wear face masks, gloves, goggles and aprons to protect themselves when they are attending potentially infectious patients.

National Health Service Guidelines

- Use face full mask ideally with protective spectacles
- Use of waterproof disposable gowns and drapes
- Avoid clogs and wear boots to prevent sharp injuring leg
- Double glove is needed (Large size inside is more comfortable)
- Allow only essential personnel in theatre
- Avoid unnecessary movement in theatre
- Meticulous technique is needed

Ref: Park 25th Edition Page 278, 875

Ans: (B) Face shields

14. Trench 2 cm for a population of 10000 disposal of waste for this population/year requires:

A. 1 acre
B. 2 acre
C. 3 acre
D. 4 acre

Key:

Trench method: It is estimated that 1 acre of land per year will be required for 10,000 population

- Controlled tipping or sanitary landfill is the most satisfactory method of refuse disposal where suitable land is available.
- Operation where compaction and covering are accomplished once or twice a week is termed as "Modified Sanitary Landfill".

CONTROLLED TIPPING METHODS

- **Trench method**
- **Ramp method**
- **Area method**

- **Trench method:**
  - Trench method is usually chosen, where level ground is available.
  - *Usually 2 to 3 m deep and 4 to 12 m wide.*
  - Where compact refuse is placed in the fill to a depth of 2 m, it is estimated that 1 acre per year land is required for a population of 10,000.
- **Ramp method:** Suited where terrain is moderately sloping.
- **Area method:** Used for filling land depressions, disused quarries and clay pits.

- Controlled tipping operation takes around 7 days to kill the pathogens, 2 to 3 weeks to cool down and 4-6 months for complete decomposition of organic matter.
- *Incineration is the method of choice where suitable land is not available.*
- Composting is a method of combined disposal of refuse and nightsoil or sludge.
- Composting is done in the following methods: Bangalore method (Anaerobic method) and Mechanical composting (Aerobic method).
- *Bangalore method/ Hot fermentation process* takes **4 to 6 months** to complete decomposition whereas *Mechanical composting* takes only **4 to 6 weeks** to complete entire process.
- Environmental Hygiene Committee did not recommend composting by municipalities with a population of over 100,000.

Ref: Park 24th Edition Page 791

Ans: (A) 1 acre

15. Vaccine that needs to be updated every year to protect against strain specific disease is:

A. Influenza
B. Japanese encephalitis
C. Mumps
D. Polio

Key:

Due to antigenic shift and antigenic drift in the influenza virus, new vaccines containing H and N components of prevalent strain are required to keep the vaccines upto date
Major Antigenic variations are seen only with Influenza A

- WHO makes recommendations every year as to what strains to be included in the vaccine.
- Influenza vaccines are highly effective (70-90%) and should be administered at least 2 weeks before the onset of epidemic or 2-3 months before influenza is expected.
- Vaccine is not recommended to control spread of influenza epidemics in the general population but recommended only in certain selected population groups.
- Influenza vaccines are available in the form of killed vaccines and live attenuated vaccine.

Antigenic shift	Antigenic drift
Antigenic change is sudden, complete or major	Antigenic change is gradual over period of time
Result from genetic recombination of human with animal or avian virus	Involves "point mutation" in gene owing to selection pressure by immunity in the host population.
Causes a major epidemic or pandemic.	

Ref: Park 24th Edition Page 165, Harrison 20th Edition Page 1270

Ans: (A) Influenza

16. Concurrent list of Indian Constitution includes which of the following?

A. International immigration rule for quarantine

B. Prevention of extension of communicable disease from one unit to another

C. Mines and oilfield workers rules

D. Establishment and maintenance of drug standards

Key:

Concurrent list of Indian Constitution includes Prevention of extension of communicable disease

Functions of Union Health Ministry are set out in the seventh schedule of Article 246 of Constitution of India under (a) Union list and (b) Concurrent list.

Functions given in the Union list	Functions listed under concurrent list are responsibility of both Union and State governments
• International health relations and administration of port quarantine	• Prevention of extension of communicable diseases from one unit to another

Contd.

Contd.

• Administration of central institutes such as: *All India Institute of Hygiene and Public Health, Kolkata; National Institute for the Control of Communicable Diseases, Delhi.* • Promotion of research through research centres and other bodies • Regulation and development of medical, pharmaceutical, dental and nursing professions • Establishment and maintenance of drug standards • Census, and collection and publication of other statistical data • Immigration and emigration • Regulation of labour in the working of mines and oil fields and • Coordination with States and with other ministries for promotion of health.	• Prevention of adulteration of foodstuffs • Control of drugs and poisons • Vital statistics • Labour welfare • Ports other than major • Economic and social planning • Population control and Family Planning.

Ref: Park 23rd Edition Page 878, Park 24th Edition Page 915

Ans: (B) Prevention of extension of communicable disease from one unit to another

17. End point of reproductive and child health programme is:

A. Sub-centre B. Anganwadi

C. District D. Taluka

Key:

End point of reproductive and child health programme is Sub-centre

RCH

- Phase 1–1997
- Phase 2–2005 (Extended till 2012)
- After 2013 RCH programme is continued as an expanded strategy with NRHM and was renamed as RMNCH-A (Reproductive maternal neonatal child and adolescent health programme)

RCH I

- Includes maternal and child components, Family planning and sexually transmitted infections prevention and control in selected districts.
- Districts are categorized based on crude birth rate and female literacy rate for 3 consecutive years.
- So approach differs from one district to another.

RCH II

- In RCH II work plans for a particular year will ***originate from sub center level*** under each PHC and are subsequently aggregate with appropriate additions at the CHC and district levels.
- Based on district action plans, aggregated state action plans are prepared at state headquarters with appropriate additions.
- Similar reporting system will be followed for the monthly progress reports (Bottom-up, decentralized, Community Needs Assessment Approach)

Goals for RMNCH+A Strategy (As per 12th Five-year Plan)

- Reduction of IMR to 25 per 1,000 live births by 2017.
- Reduction in MMR to 100 per 100,000 live births by 2017.
- Reduction in TFR to 2.1 by 2017.
- *4Ds:* Defects, Deficiencies, Diseases and Disability in children (0–18 years).
- *5×5 Matrix of RMNCH+A: Minimum Essential Commodities.*

Reproductive health	Matern al health	Newborn health	Child	Adolescent health
FP commodities: Tubal rings, CuT 380A, IUCD 375	Injection Oxytocin	Injection Vitamin K	ORS	Tablet Albendazole
OCPs, Mala N, Condoms	Tablet Misoprostol	Mucus extractor	Zinc dispersible tablets	Tablet Dicyclomine
Emergency contraceptive pills (LNG 1.5 mg)	Inj. Magnesium sulphate	Vaccines: BCG, OPV, Hep B	Salbutamol syrup/ nebulising solution	
Pregnancy testing kits–Nischay			Vaccines: DPT, OPV, Measles, Hep-B, JE, Pentavalent vaccine	
Tablet Mifepristone			Syrup Vitamin A	

Ref: Park 24th Edition Page 472, Bhalwar Rajvir Textbook of Public Health and Community Medicine, AFMC, Pune in Collaboration with WHO, India Office New Delhi 2009 Page 503

Ans: (A) Sub-centre

18. Risk of genetic diseases in consanguinous marriage between first cousins:

A. 1-2%
B. 4-8%
C. 8-10%
D. 12-14%

Key:

Risk of genetic diseases in consanguinous marriage between first cousins is approximately 12-14%
Death rate of 116 per 1,000 (11.6%) was found during first 8 years of life amongst offspring of first cousins

- **Trisomy 21:** Mongolism is more frequent in children born of elderly mothers

Age	Risk for Trisomy 21
20	1 : 3000
40	1: 40
40-45	1 : 67
Overall	1 : 800

- Prenatal diagnosis of congenital abnormalities offers parents option of therapeutic abortion.
- Prenatal diagnosis is possible to detect certain congenital anomalies in utero using following techniques: ***AFP, USG, Amniocentesis and Chorionic villi sampling.***
- **Alpha fetoprotein:** Neural tube defects can be detected by measurement of AFP in maternal blood and in amniotic fluid during pregnancy.
- Amniocentesis is possible only in 2nd trimester (i.e., after the completion of 12 weeks).
- Amniocentesis can detect many abnormalities (Down's syndrome, Neural tube defects).
- Chorionic villi sampling technique allows prenatal diagnosis at 9 to 11 weeks of pregnancy. By this test, the chromosome status can be easily determined.

Ref: Park 23rd Edition Page 828

Ans: (D) 12-14%

19. A death certificate is given below. What is the underlying cause of death in this case?

Cause of death		
I hereby certify that to the best of my knowledge and belief, the cause of death was as stated below:		
I	Disease or condition directly leading to death*	(a) MYOCARDIAL INFARCTION due to (or as a consequence of)
	Antecedent causes Morbid conditions, If any, giving rise to the above cause, stating the underlying condition last	(b) METASTASIS TO BONE due to (or as a consequence of) (c) CARCINOMA BREAST due to (or as a consequence of) (d) .... due to (or as a consequence of)
II	Other significant conditions contributing to the death, but not related to the disease or condition causing it	TYPE 2 DIABETES MELLITUS
*This does not mean mode of dying, such as heart or respiratory failure; it means the disease, injury or complication that caused death.		

A. Carcinoma Breast
B. MI
C. Metastasis to lung
D. Type 2 diabetes mellitus

Key:

Death Certificate	
Part 1	*Immediate cause and Underlying cause*
Part 2	*Any associated diseases contributed to death*
(a)	*Condition directly leading to death*
(b)	*Antecedent causes*
(c)	*Underlying cause of death*

- ***Basis of mortality data is the Death Certificate.***
- Part 1 of international death certificate deals with the immediate cause and underlying cause which started the whole trend of events leading to death.
- ***Underlying cause of death is recorded on line (c) i.e., third line.***
- Concept of "underlying cause" is defined as:
    - Disease/injury which initiated train of morbid events leading directly to death or
    - Circumstances of accident or violence which produced fatal injury
- In Part 2 is recorded any significant associated diseases that contributed to death but did not directly lead to it.
- **Death Certificate used in India:** A set of questions related to deaths during pregnancy and infancy, are added to basic structure of international death certificate for use in India.

Ref: Park 24th Edition Page 61

Ans: (A) Carcinoma Breast

20. Vaccine contraindicated in pregnancy is:

A. Hepatitis A
B. Hepatitis B
C. Rabies
D. Varicella

Key:

All Live Vaccines are contraindicated in pregnancy–Varicella

Live Attenuated Vaccines	
• OPV • Yellow fever vaccine • Varicella zoster vaccine	• MMR • Influenza (Attenuated) vaccine

Vaccine	Viral	Bacterial	Rickettsial
Live attenuated	Polio (OPV/Sabin) Yellow fever Measles Mumps Rubella Influenza JE (SA 14-14-2)	BCG Typhoid (oral) Plague	Epidemic typhus
Killed	Police (Salk/IPV) KFD Influenza Hep B JE	Typhoid (IM) Plague Cholera Pertussis Cerebro Spinal Meningitis	–
Toxoid	–	Diphtheria Tetanus	–

Contraindications to Vaccines	
Pregnancy	All live vaccines except Yellow fever vaccine
HIV	Asymptomatic HIV– None Symptomatic HIV– All live vaccines except BCG vaccine
Immunosuppression	All live vaccines
Steroid therapy	All live vaccines
Fever	Typhoid vaccine (Typhoral, Typhium–Vi, TAB)
ARTI/Diarrhoea	None
Contraindicated together	Yellow fever and Cholera vaccine
Preterm *Premature baby with <2 kg weight*	Hepatitis B
Age <1 year (Infants)	Yellow fever, Meningococcal and Pneumococcal vaccine
Age <2 years	Typhoid, Meningococcal and Pneumococcal vaccine
Age >2 years	Pertussis vaccine *(Serious neurological complications)→NIS–given till 5-6 years)*
Progressive neurological disease	Pertussis vaccine *Not contraindicated in epilepsy controlled on medications and Cerebral palsy*
Only Absolute contraindication to Killed vaccine	Severe local reaction/general reaction to previous dose

Specific Side Effects of Vaccines

- **Guillain-Barré syndrome**–Killed Influenza vaccine
- **Vaccine associated paralysis**–OPV (Sabin)
- **Toxic shock syndrome**–Measles vaccine, MMR
- **Shock**–DPT, Pertussis vaccine
- **Hypersensitivity**–Hepatitis B vaccine, DPT, dT and Meningococcal vaccine

AEFI [Adverse Events Following Immunisation]	
Reactions inherent to inoculation	Local [Pain, swelling, redness, tenderness etc. at site of injection] General reactions [Fever, malaise, headache etc]
Reactions due to faulty technique	Faulty production of vaccine (e.g., inadequate inactivation/detoxication of microbe) Improper immunization site or route and dose Incorrect diluents, wrong amount of diluent, drug substituted for vaccine/diluents Vaccine stored incorrectly, vaccine or diluent contaminated

Contd.

Contd.

Reactions due to hypersensitivity	Anaphylactic shock, serum sickness, bronchospasm, dyspnoea, pallor, hypotension and collapse Administration of antisera (e.g., ATS), Viral vaccines with traces of antibiotics or prepared from embryonated eggs (e.g., influenza)
Neurological involvement	Postvaccinial encephalitis and encephalopathy [anti-rabies and smallpox vaccines] Guillain-Barré syndrome in association with swine influenza vaccine
Provocative reactions	A disease totally unconnected with the immunizing agents E.g., provocative polio after APT [Alum precipitated toxoid] or PTAP [Purified Toxoid Preceipitated by Aluminium phosphate] administration against diphtheria Individual is harbouring the infectious agent and administration of vaccine shortens incubation period and produces the disease
Others	Damage to foetus (e.g., with rubella vaccination) Displacement in age-distribution of disease (e.g., Mass vaccination against measles, rubella and mumps).

Immunizations Which Can Be Given During Pregnancy

ACTIVE

- TT and diphtheria toxoid, Rabies (inactivated virus), Hepatitis A and B (inactivated virus)
- Vaccination against pneumococcal, meningococcal and hemophilus (inactivated bacterial)

PASSIVE–Immunoglobulins for post exposure prophylaxis:

- Hepatitis A and B, Tetanus, Rabies and Varicella and Measles

Immunizations Which are Contraindicated in Pregnancy

- Measles (live viral vaccine)
- Mumps (live viral vaccine)
- Varicella zoster (live viral vaccine)
- Smallpox

Immunization Which Require Conditional Consideration

- Japanese encephalitis
- Yellow fever
- Anthrax
- Typhoid (parenteral/oral)

Ref: Park 24th Edition Page 108

Ans: (D) Varicella

21. Which is not an Epidemiological indicator?

A. Annual blood examination rate
B. Annual parasite incidence
C. Annual parasite index
D. Annual falciparum incidence

Key:

API–Sophisticated measure of Malaria Incidence
ABER–Index of Operational efficiency
Most sensitive index of recent malaria transmission–Infant parasite rate

Pre eradication era	Spleen rate, Average enlarged spleen, Parasite rate, Parasite density index Proportional case rate and Infant parasite rate
Eradication era	API, ABER, AFI, SPR and SPF→ ***Microscopic diagnosis method–Main method***

Annual Parasite Incidence (API)

- Sophisticated measure of malaria incidence in a community.
- Areas with API 2 per 1000 population per year are classified as high risk areas, and thereby eligible for vector control.

$$\textbf{Annual parasite incidence (API)} = \frac{\text{Confirmed cases during one year}}{\text{Population under surveillance}} \times 100$$

Annual Blood Examination Rate (ABER)

- Index of **operational efficiency***
- Important vector indices in the malaria survey are: human blood index, sporozoite rate, mosquito density, man-biting rate and inoculation rate.

Annual blood examination rate (ABER) = (Number of slides examined/Population) × 100

- **Slide positivity rate (SPR):** Information on the trend of malaria transmission
- **Slide falciparum rate (SFR):** Information on the trend of malaria transmission

Malaria rates	Definition	Use
Spleen rate	Percentage of children between 2-10 years of age showing enlargement of spleen	Measures malaria endemicity [or prevalence] Hypendemic–Spleen rate <10% Mesoendemic–Spleen rate 11-50% Hyperendemic–Spleen rate > 50%; (Adults over 25%) Holoendemic–Spleen rate in children > 75% (Adult <25%)
Parasite density index	Density of parasite in a sample of well-defined group of population. Only '+'ve slides are included in denominator	Measures average degree of parasitemia
Infant parasite rate	Percentage of infants showing malaria parasites in their blood films	Most sensitive index of recent transmission of malaria in a locality. Used to assess impact of control operations

Contd.

Contd.

Annual parasite incidence (API)	API = (Confirmed cases during one year/ Population under surveillance) × 1000	Measure of malaria incidence in a community
Annual blood examination rate (ABER)	ABER = (Number of slides examined/ Population) × 100	Index of operational efficiency [Minimum prescribed is 10% of the population in a year]
SPR/SFR	Slide positivity rate and slide falciparum rate	Information on trend of malaria transmission
Human blood index	Proportion of freshly-fed female Anopheline mosquitoes whose stomach contains human blood	It indicates the degree of anthrophilism

Vector Indices

Human blood index: The proportion of freshly-fed female Anopheline mosquitoes whose stomach contains human blood. It indicates the degree of anthrophilism

Sporozoite rate: Percentage of female anophelines with sporozoites in their salivary glands

Mosquito density: The number of mosquitoes per man-hour-catch

Man-biting rate (Biting density): Average incidence of anopheline bites per day per person. It is determined by standardised vector catches on human bait

Inoculation rate: Man-biting rate multiplied by the infective sporozoite rate.

Ref: Park 24th Edition Page 278

Ans: (C) Annual parasite index

Chapter 9

ENT

1. **A patient came to ENT OPD with following CT finding. He is on treatment for Allergic rhinitis. On examination of nose, multiple polyps are visible in nasal cavity. What would you name this appearance?**
   A. Double dense
   B. Onion peel
   C. Ground glass
   D. Honey comb

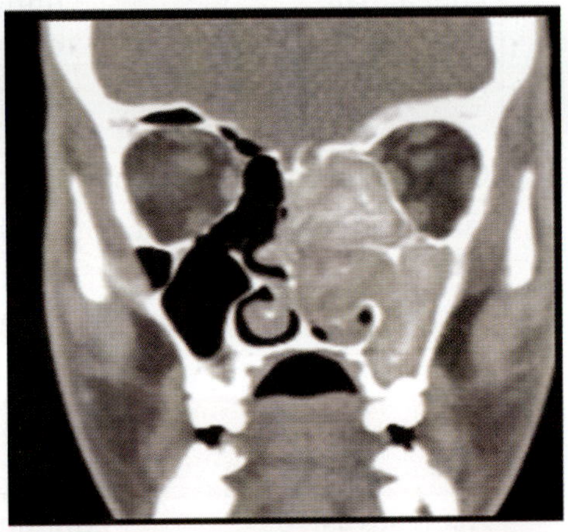

Key:

Patient gives history of treatment taken for allergic rhinitis with nasal polyps on examination. Picture shows Heterogenous opacification (Double dense appearance)

Typical of Allergic Fungal sinusitis

Allergic Fungal Sinusitis

- Allergic reaction to causative fungus and presents with sinunasal polyposis and mucin.
- ***Mucin contains eosinophils, Charcot Leyden crystals and fungal hyphae.***

Bent and Kuhn criteria of allergic sinusitis:

Major criteria and minor criteria for diagnosis of AFRS

Major criteria	*Minor criteria*
Type 1 hypersensitivity to fungus	Asthma
Nasal polyposis	Histopathologic identification of Charcot-Leyden crystals
Characteristic CT scan findings	Eosinophilia
Eosinophilic mucin	Unilateral disease
Positive fungal staining of sinus contents removed during surgery	Osseous erosion
	Positive fungal culture from the nasal cavity

Contd.

Contd.

- CT scanning is preferred initial radiologic modality.
- *CT scan:* AFRS shows heterogeneity of tissue densities within sinuses.

Heterogeneous opacification is noted in multiple sinuses with areas of central hypoattenuation provides a characteristic CT scan of AFRS.

- **Treatment–Surgery, Steroids and Immunotherapy**

Fungal Sinusitis	
Fungal Ball	Implantation of fungus into an otherwise healthy sinus which on CT shows hyperdense area with no evidence of bone erosion/ expansion.
Allergic Fungal sinusitis	Allergic reaction to causative fungus and presents with sinunasal polyposis and mucin. ***Mucin contains eosinophils, Charcot Leyden crystals and fungal hyphae.***
Chronic Invasive Sinusitis	Fungus invades into sinus mucosa and bone erosion by fungus.
Fulminant fungal sinusitis	Acute presentation and mostly seen in immunocompromised or diabetic patients.

Classification of fungal rhinosinusitis

Classification	Immunological status	Treatment	Prognosis
Acute invasive	Immunocompromised	Reversal of immunocompromise; surgery; antifungal agents	Guarded/poor
Chronic invasive	Immunocompetent	Surgery; antifungal agents	Fair/good
Fungus ball (mycetoma)	Immunocompetent	Surgery	Good
Allergic	Atopic	Surgery; steroids; immunotherapy	Excellent
Saprophytic	Immunocompetent	Removal	Excellent

Multiple nasal polyps in nasal cavity suggests ethmoidal polyps. History of allergic rhinitis Both of these suggest allergic fungal sinusitis

Ref: Sataloff Textbook 1st Edition Page 461, Dhingra 7th Edition Page 208, CODT 2nd Edition Page 276, Mohan Bansal Textbook of ENT Page 318, Hazarika Textbook of ENT Page 339

Ans: (A) Double dense

2. **A 2-month-old child who was born by normal delivery to a primi lady presented with hoarseness and below finding on Laryngoscopy. What could be possible diagnosis?**
   A. Laryngomalacia
   B. Recurrent laryngeal papillomatosis
   C. Rienkes edema
   D. Malignancy

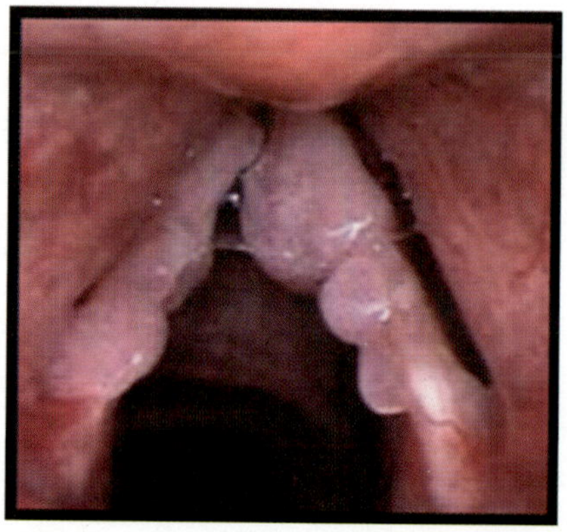

Key:

Picture shows Multiple polyps over free edge of vocal cords–Characteristic of RRP
Children are frequently (75%) the first born, vaginally delivered offspring of teenage mothers in RRP

Laryngomalacia	Inspiratory stridor with Omega shaped epiglottis
Malignancy	Old age, Usually unilateral and Irregular surface
Rienkes edema	Diffuse polyposis of vocal cord Aggravated by Voice abuse, Smoking, Asthma and Hypothyroidism
RRP	Child with multiple polyposis through normal delivery HPV Transmitted from mother to child through birth canal ***Children are frequently (75%) the first born, vaginally delivered offspring of teenage mothers.***

JUVENILE ONSET RECURRENT RESPIRATORY PAPILLOMATOSIS

- Most common benign tumour of the larynx in children is juvenile laryngeal papillomatosis.

Epidemiology

- JORRP patients can present at age of 4 months–13 years.
- Usually seen at 2 to 5 years of age.
  (Adult onset RRP patients usually present at the age of 20–30 years).
- ***Children are frequently (75%) first born, vaginally delivered offspring of teenage mothers.***
- Males and females are equally affected.

Etiology

- Manifestation of human papilloma virus **HPV 6 and 11**
- HPV 11 is associated with more aggressive disease and makes patient more prone for malignant change.

Transmission

- *Exact mode of transmission is not known*
- *Association between genital warts and Recurrent laryngeal papillomatosis has be found*
- Higher risk in those with ***active HPV genital warts***
- *Possible link to cervical papilloma and Vaginal delivery has been found*

Clinical Features

- **Most common site is Vocal fold**

First and most predominant site involved is Vocal fold

- ***Most common symptom of RRP is Hoarseness***
- Children due to small overall size of airway even small lesions can cause significant airway obstruction.
- **Other symptoms:** Husky cry/Dysphonia, Dyspnea, Cough, Failure to thrive, Recurrent pneumonia and Dysphagia.

Prognosis

- *Derkey severity score is used for RRP*
- Adult onset papillomatosis has less severe course than Juvenile
- ***Risk of malignant change 2 to 3%*** (Squamous cell carcinoma)
- *More likely to undergo remission*

TREATMENT

- *Aim of treatment is maintenance of a safe airway and laryngeal function.*
- ***Goal of surgical therapy is to provide symptomatic relief of dysphonia and dyspnea instead of the eradication of HPV.***
- Primary treatment is ***microlaryngoscopic excision***
- Most widely used means of excision being ***CO_2 laser.***
- Chances of recurrence are very high so repeated CO_2 Laser excisions are required to be done.

In severe cases mainstay of therapy is surgical resection

- **Surgical options:** *Cold steel, Phonomicrosurgery, Laser- CO_2, KTP, Pulsed dye.*
- **Adjuvant treatment:** *Criteria for adjuvant methods include >4 procedures per year, rapid recurrence with airway compromise and distant spread of disease.*

Adjuvant therapy	Drug category	Proposed mechanism of action	Route of administration
Cidofovir	Antiretroviral	Prevent viral DNA synthesis	Intralesional injection
Bevacizumab	Anti-vascular endothelial growth factor	Prevent neovascularization	Intralesional injection
Indole-3-carbinol	Estrogen metabolite modulator	Decrease hormone-mediated proliferation	Oral
Interferon α	Cytokine	Increases adaptive immune response	Intravenous
Cimetidine	H_2 Blocker	Inhibits suppressor T cells	Oral
Photodynamic therapy	Chemical sensitizer	Increases cell death from directed laser treatment	Intravenous/ intraoperative
Measles-mumps-rubella	Vaccine	Increases immune response	Subcutaneous/topical
HspE7	Vaccine	Increases immune response	Subcutaneous

- **Most commonly used Adjuvant therapy is recombinant α-interferon**
- Emission rate is high necessitating multiple surgeries if presents at ages 6–10 years and confined to larynx.
- Seeding risk is present if tracheostomy performed

Ref: Sataloff Textbook 1st Edition Page 378

Ans: (B) Recurrent laryngeal papillomatosis

3. **An Unimmunized 2-year-old girl presents with Fever and sore throat. On examination She is toxic in appearance with Bilateral Cervical lymphadenopathy. Throat examination showed below finding. What is the most likely diagnosis?**

A. Diphtheria
B. Candidiasis
C. Acute membraneous tonsillitis
D. Vincents angina

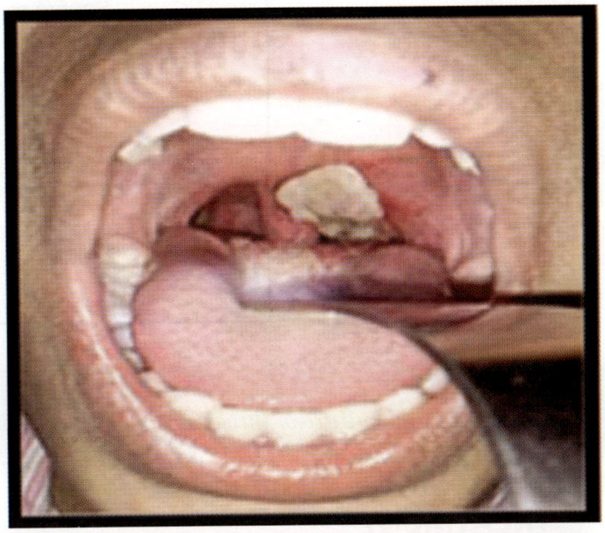

Key:

Toxic unimmunized child with toxic appearance and dirty gray membrane over tonsillar surface along with Bilateral cervical lymphadenopathy suggests Diphtherial infection

DIPHTHERIA

- Acute infection caused by Gram +ve bacillus Corynebacterium diphtheria

Transmission

- Spreads by droplet infection
- Most common source of infection is Carriers
- Nasal carriers are more dangerous than throat carriers–*Mildest form*

Incubation Period: 2 to 6 days

- Infection with slower in onset and Primarily occurs in unimmunized individuals
- Toxin for Diphtheria toxin–Park William strain 8

Clinical Features

- Membrane extends beyond the tonsils on to soft palate and dirty grey in colour.
- Adherent and its removal leaves bleeding surface–***Pseudomembrane***
- ***Most common type–Respiratory diphtheria***
- ***Most severe form is Laryngeal diphtheria***

Pathogenesis

- ***Exotoxin*** produced by C. *diphtheriae* is toxic to heart and nerves.
- *Causes myocarditis, cardiac arrhythmias and acute circulatory failure.*
- *Cutaneous diphtheria- Punched out ulcers*
- ***Bull neck appearance of lymph nodes***

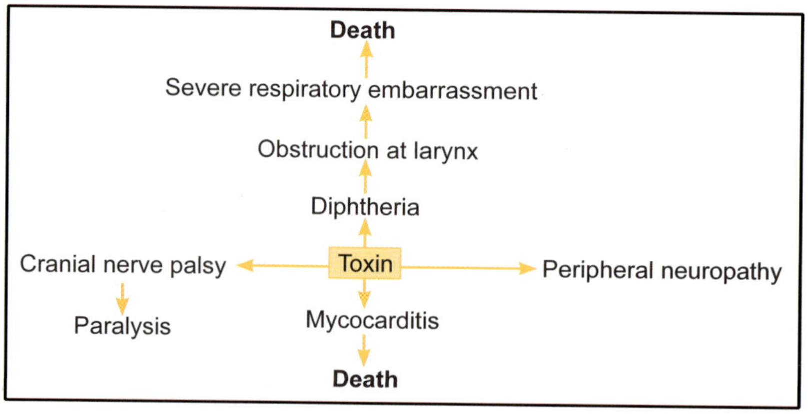

Diagnosis

- *Smear and culture of throat swab will reveal Corynebacterium diphtheria.*
- *Diagnosis is confirmed by culture of pseudomembrane in Loeffler's/Tellurite selective medium.*

TREATMENT

- ***Drug of choice***–Erythromycin/Procaine Pencillin G
- ***Active immunization is by diphtheria toxoid***
- Main stay of treatment is Diphtheria antitoxin

COMPLICATIONS

- Cause of death in Diphtheria infection–**Myocarditis.**
- In the larynx, diphtheritic membrane may cause airway obstruction.
- Neurological complications usually appear few weeks after infection and include *paralysis of soft palate, diaphragm and ocular muscles.*

Causes of White Patch Over Tonsil		
Viral	**Bacterial**	**Autoimmune**
Infectious mononucleosis HSV, HIV	Follicular tonsillitis, Faucial diphtheria, Keratosis,TB Tonsillitis, Secondary syphilis	Lichen planus, Wegener's granulomatosis
Fungal		**Premalignant**
Candidiasis		Leukoplakia, Submucosal fibrosis
Trauma	**Tumors**	**Systemic**
Post tonsillectomy, FB, Thermal injury, Post radiation, Corrosive injury	Tonsillar cyst, Tonsillolith, Papilloma, Fibroma tonsil, Tonsillar malignancy	Leukemia, Agranulocytosis, Aplastic anemia, Blood dyscrasia

Acute follicular tonsillitis	Acute diphtheria
• Children between 6 and 20 years or more	• Children under 10 years usually 2 to 5 years

Contd.

Contd.

• History of attacks of recurrent tonsillitis – Acute onset	• History of exposure to a diphtheria case – Slow onset
• Temperature varies 102°–105°F	• Temperature up to 102°F or less
• Pain is severe	• Pain mild only
• Toxemia not seen	• Toxemia present
• Pulse rate is proportionate to rise of temperature	• Pulse rate out of proportion to fever
• Dirty white pseudomembrane limited to tonsil only, can be easily removed with pillars, palate, uvula separated with no raw areas	• Membrane formation extensive on tonsil, difficulty and leaves a raw bleeding surface and it reforms after removal
• Throat swab shows bacteria such as *Streptococcus, Staphylococcus or Haemophilus influenzae Corynebacterium diptheriae*	• Throat swab shows *Corynebacterium*
• Jugulodigastric glands are enlarged and tender	• Massive lymphadenopathy (Bull's neck)
• Schick test negative	• Schick's test positive
• Albuminuria absent	• Albuminuria present
• Treatment with antibiotics	• Treatment with antidiphtheritic serum (ADS) and antibiotics

Ref: Dhingra 7th Edition Page 395, Tuli 2nd Edition Page 252, CODT 2nd Edition Page 365, Mohan Bansal Textbook of ENT Page 426, Hazarika Textbook of ENT Page 481

Ans: (A) Diphtheria

4. Inspiratory stridor is due to lesion of:

A. Supraglottis B. Subglottis
C. Trachea D. Bronchi

Key:

Inspiratory stridor occurs due to lesions of Supraglottis/Pharynx

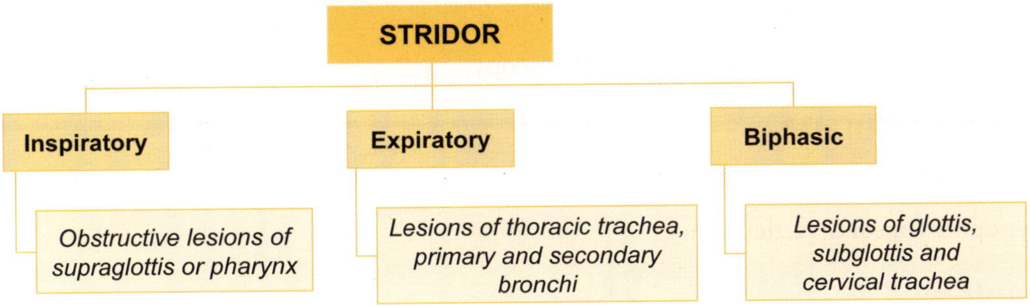

- ***Most common cause of inspiratory stridor in neonates is Laryngomalacia***
- Most common cause of chronic stridor in children is Long term intubation causing laryngotracheal stenosis.
- ***Most common cause stridor in old age group is Carcinoma larynx***

STRIDOR IN CHILDREN

- **Congenital**
  - **Laryngeal causes:** Laryngomalacia, Vocal cord palsy, Subglottic stenosis, Subglottic Hemangioma, Laryngeal web, Laryngocele, Mucocele of ventricle
  - **Extralaryngeal causes:** Tracheomalacia, Cri-du-chat syndrome, Pierre Robin sequence, Lingual thyroid, Vascular ring compressing trachea
- **Acquired**
  - **Infective**
    - Acute epiglottitis
    - Acute LTB
    - Laryngeal diphtheria
    - Edema of larynx
  - **Non infective**
    - Trauma
    - Foreign body
    - Juvenile papilloma
    - Bilateral Vocal cord palsy
    - Neonatal tetany

Ref: Sataloff Textbook 1st Edition Page 465, Dhingra 7th Edition Page 334, CODT 2nd Edition Page 365, Mohan Bansal Textbook of ENT Page 426, Hazarika Textbook of ENT Page 481

Ans: (A) Supraglottis

5. **Dohlman surgery in Zenkers diverticulum is:**

A. Endoscopic stapling of septum
B. Endoscopic suturing of pouch
C. Resection of pouch
D. Laser division of pouch

Key:

Dohlman surgery is Endoscopic diathermy of the partition wall between esophagus and pouch is preferred in poor risk debilitated patients

KILLIAN'S DEHISCENCE

- Site for herniation of pharyngeal mucosa in cases of pharyngeal pouch
- **Thyropharyngeus** with oblique fibres and ***Cricopharyngeus*** with transverse fibres
- Between these two parts exists a potential gap called Killian's dehiscence.
- Also called ***"gateway of tears"***
- Perforation can occur at this site during oesophagoscopy.

ZENKER'S DIVERTICULUM

- Pharyngeal pouch
- Pulsion hypopharyngeal diverticulum

Pathophysiology

- *Exact etiology is not known*
- **Associated with dysmotility**
- ***Patients are usually old adults***

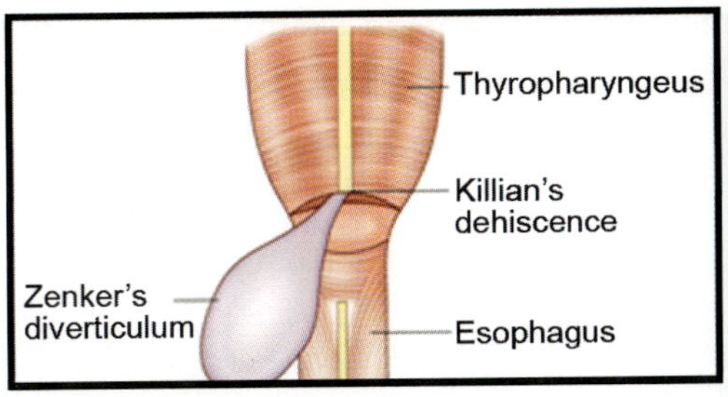

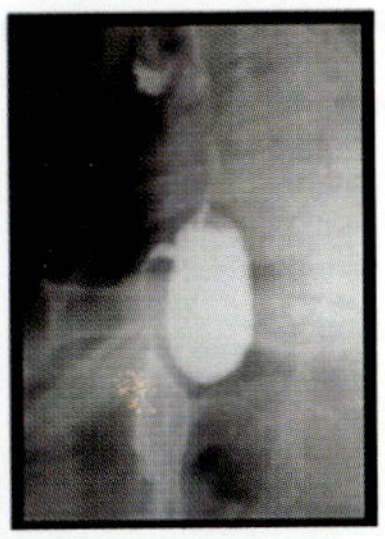

Incoordinated contractions during deglutition

+

Spasm of cricopharyngeal sphincter

→ ***Protrusion of Hypopharyngeal mucosa through weak area (Pharyngeal pouch)***

Clinical Features

Most common symptoms–Halitosis, Transfer dysphagia (difficulty initiating swallowing) and Regurgitation of food days after ingestion.

- *Dysphagia* increase after few swallows
- Pouch gets filled with food slowly and then compresses on esophagus
- ***Gurgling*** sound during swallowing

Boyce sign

Neck shows swelling on left side in anterior triangle. On palpation it is soft and gurgling sound is heard.

- ***Coughing and Choking***→ *Regurgitation of undigested food* at night (recumbency)
- Loss of weight and malnourishment
- Aspiration pneumonia

Diagnosis

- Barium swallow will show the site and size of diverticulum
- Endoscopy and Nasogastric intubation are contraindicated because of risk of perforation of pouch.

Treatment

- Diverticulectomy (Excision of pouch) or cricopharyngeal myotomy or both.
- **DOHLMAN'S PROCEDURE:** Partition wall between oesophagus and pouch is divided by *diathermy* through an endoscope. Done in poor risk debilitated patients.
- Endoscopic injection of botulinum toxin into cricopharyngeus is used for small diverticula.

Ref: Dhingra 7th Edition Page 311, CODT 2nd Edition Page 512, Mohan Bansal Textbook of ENT Page 463, Hazarika Textbook of ENT Page 537, Tuli 2nd Edition Page 348

Ans: (A) Endoscopic stapling of septum

6. **A 60-year-old patient presented with Hoarseness of voice. On examination following finding is seen (See picture). What could be the diagnosis?**
   A. Multinodular goiter
   B. Secondaries neck
   C. TB lymphadenitis
   D. Sternomastoid tumor

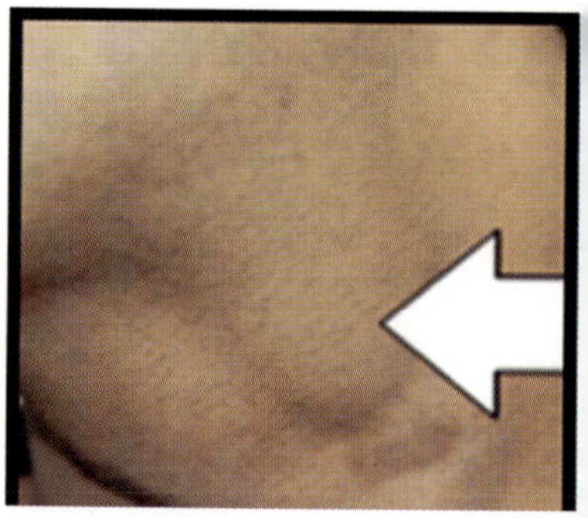

Key:

Picture shows neck mass anterior to Sternocleidomastoid
Most probable diagnosis would be Secondaries Neck

TB Lymphadenitis	*Usually affects Jugular chain nodes* ***(Multiple and Matted)*** *Frequent cold abscess* ***TB Larynx rarely results in Vocal cord palsy and Cricoarytenoid joint fixation***
Sternomastoid tumor	*Involves region of muscle not anterior to it*
Multinodular goiter	*Usually involve ½ of thyroid lobe and diffuse growth in front of neck*

In children congenital lesions are most common cause of Hoarseness
In younger age group hoarseness can be mostly due to acute or chronic infections
In elderly malignancy should be ruled out

HOARSENESS OF VOICE

LARYNGEAL CAUSES

Congenital
Laryngeal web, Stenosis, Hemangioma, Laryngomalacia

Inflammatory
Acute laryngitis, Acute laryngotracheobronchitis, Diphtheria, Herpes zoster, Polio, Chronic laryngitis, TB, Lupus, Syphilis, Leprosy

Traumatic
Birth trauma, laryngotracheal trauma, surgery (laryngeal, thyroid), corrosive inhalation, prolonged intubation, radiation

Neoplastic
Benign: Papilloma, chondroma, Cyst, vocal polyp, granuloma, angioma or fibroma
Malignant: Carcinoma larynx, Carcinoma thyroid, esophagus, trachea or nasopharynx

Miscellaneous
Vocal nodule, FB, laryngocele, amyloidosis, myesthenia gravis, dysphonia plica ventricularis, vocal cord paralysis, leukoplakia, Reinke's edema, angioneurotic edema, pachydermia vocal cords, hysteria, contact ulcers, vocal cords fixation due to arthritis, DM and Cardiac disease

EXTRALARYNGEAL CAUSES
Myxedema
Multiple sclerosis
Peripheral neuritis
Mercury and lead poisoning
Aneurysms of arch of aorta
Pharyngeal diverticulae
Diabetes
Mitral stenosis
Metastatic lymph nodes in mediastinum

Sudden onset Hoarseness–Vocal abuse, URTI

Insidious onset Hoarseness–Chronic laryngeal disease

Occupation:

- Teachers, hawkers and singers are supposed to be voice abusers and prone to hoarseness.
- Workers in factories who are exposed to chemical fumes and dust may be candidates for hoarseness/malignancy.

Hoarseness following surgery–RLN Paralysis

History of long duration disease with rapidly progressive hoarseness and dyspnea along with stridor suggests *Cancer larynx*

Sudden onset of Hoarseness of voice with improvement over a period of time–*Suspect Vocal cord palsy (Compensation of healthy cord)*

Ref: Dhingra 7th Edition Page 355, Mohan Bansal Textbook of ENT Page 496, Hazarika Textbook of ENT Page 585, Tuli 2nd Edition Page 305

Ans: (B) Secondaries neck

7. **A patient presented after RTA with left sided epistaxis and diplopia. On performing CT following finding is noted. What would be the cause for Diplopia?**
   - A. Fracture zygoma
   - B. Blow out fracture
   - C. Lefort fracture
   - D. Fracture ethmoid bone

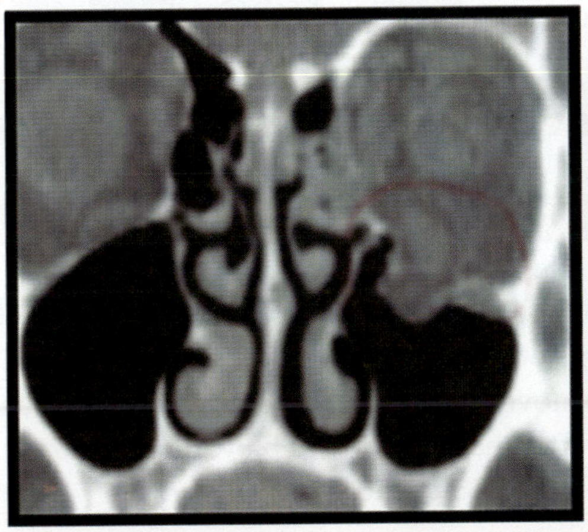

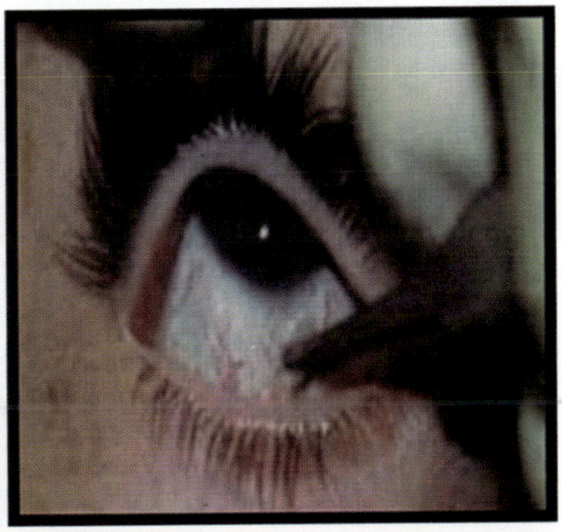

Key:

Picture shows CT scan with Tear drop sign (seen in Blow out fracture)

Second picture shows forced duction test which is also done for blow out fracture

BLOW OUT FRACTURE

- Caused typically by sudden increase in pressure by impacting object which is greater in diameter than orbital aperture
- Occurs when nonpenetrating blunt object *(ball, fist, hockey puck and cork)* strikes globe
- Bones of lateral wall and Roof usually withstand trauma
- Increase in intraorbital pressure→ Blows out weak walls of orbit
- So most commonly fractured wall is floor of orbit along infraorbital canal ***(Floor > Medial wall)***
- ***No damage to Orbital rim***

Clinical Features	
• Ecchymosis • Infraorbital anesthesia–Lower lid, cheek, side of nose, upper lip and upper teeth • Periorbital edema • Diplopia–Entrapped inferior rectus	• Enophthalmos • Mechanical ptosis • Ipsilateral epistaxis–Bleeding from maxillary sinus into nose • Subcutaneous emphysema

INVESTIGATIONS

- **X-ray water's view:** ***Hanging drop sign****–Herniation of orbital contents into maxillary antrum.* ***(Tear drop sign)***
- ***Loss of double cortical lines (Orbital rim and floor)***
- Confirmed by CT scan

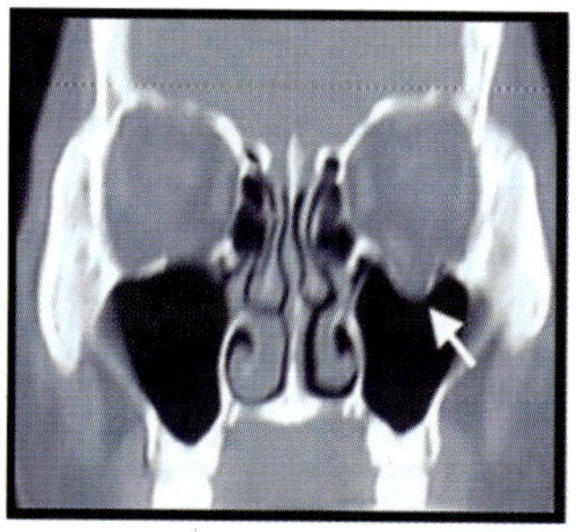

Forced Duction Test

- Done after topical conjunctival anesthesia.
- Episcleral tissue in the region of inferior oblique insertion is grasped with fine toothed forceps.
- By passively rotating, restrictions of the eyeball movements are checked.
- Complete restriction of passive movements indicates entrapment of muscle.
- Test is done in operation room after the reduction of blow out fracture.
- Free passive movements of eyeball indicate success of surgery.

Simple forced duction testing detects extraocular muscle entrapment.

- **TREATMENT:** Main stay of treatment is Orbital floor reconstruction.

Ref: Dhingra 7th Edition Page 206, Mohan Bansal Textbook of ENT Page 307, Hazarika Textbook of ENT Page 360, Tuli 2nd Edition Page 208

Ans: (B) Blow out fracture

8. **Potts puffy' tumor is:**

A. Osteomyelitis of ethmoid bone
B. Osteomyelitis of frontal bone
C. Allergic fungal sinusitis
D. Sinusitis of dental origin

Key:

Potts puffy tumor is Subperiosteal abscess formed as a result of osteomyelitis of frontal bone

POTT'S PUFFY TUMOR

- Subperiosteal abscess formed as a result of osteomyelitis of frontal bone.
- More common in adults (Frontal sinus is not developed in infants and children).

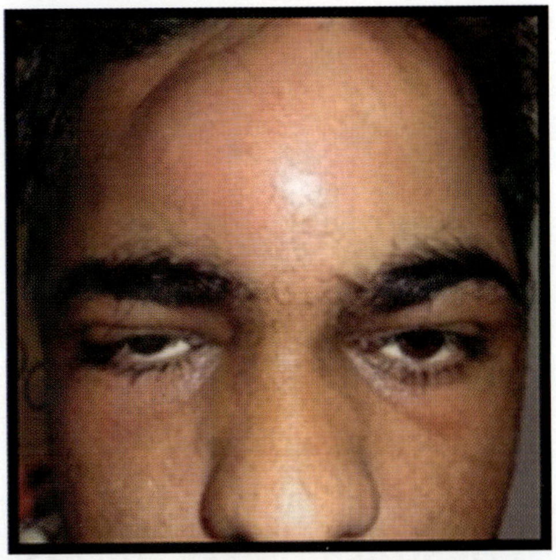

Etiology

- Usually results from acute infection of frontal sinus→direct spread/thrombophlebitis
- Trauma and surgery
- **Pott's puffy tumor:** *Subperiosteal abscess develops over anterior surface of frontal sinus and results in swelling of overlying soft tissue* ***(soft doughy swelling)***
- ***Patient presents with past history of sinusitis along with purulent nasal discharge.***

Treatment

- Large doses of antibiotics, Drainage of abscess and Trephining along floor of frontal sinus
- Removal of sequestra and necrotic bone with osteoplastic flap.

OSTEOMYELITIS OF MAXILLA

- More common in infants and children than adults (Spongy bone in anterior wall of maxilla).
- Infection usually starts in the dental sac and spreads to the maxilla.
- ***Clinical features:*** Erythema, swelling of cheek, edema of lower lid, purulent nasal discharge and fever.
- Subperiosteal abscess and fistulae form in infraorbital region, alveolus/palate/zygoma.
- ***Treatment:*** Large doses of antibiotics, drainage of abscess and removal of sequestra.

COMPLICATIONS OF SINUSITIS

ACUTE LOCAL
Orbital, Intracranial, Bony, Dental

ACUTE DISTANT
Toxic shock syndrome

CHRONIC
Mucocele
Pyocele

A. Local	• Mucocele/Mucopyocele • Mucous retention cyst • Osteomyelitis o Frontal bone (more common) o Maxilla
B. Orbital	• Preseptal inflammatory oedema of lids • Orbital cellulitis

Contd.

Contd.

	• Orbital abscess • Superior orbital fissure syndrome • Orbital apex syndrome
C. Intracranial	• Meningitis • Extradural abscess • Subdural abscess • Brain abscess • Cavernous sinus thrombosis
D. Descending infections	
E. Focal infections	

ORBITAL COMPLICATIONS

- Route of spread: Lamina papyracea, infraorbital canal.
- Associated thrombophlebitis.
- In children the orbital complication of sinusitis are due to ethmoiditis.
- In adults it is due to frontal sinusitis.

Inflammatory edema	Lid edema present, normal visual acuity and extraocular movements
Orbital cellulitis	Diffuse edema of orbital contents but no discrete abscess formation
Subperiosteal abscess	Pus collection along lamina papyracea; inferior and lateral eyeball shift
Orbital abscess	Pus within orbit, proptosis, chemosis, ophthalmoplegia, dim vision
Cavernous sinus thrombosis	Bilateral involvement of eyes, toxic look and findings of meningismus

Inflammatory edema of lids→Preseptal cellulitis→Subperiosteal abscess→Orbital cellulitis→ Orbital abscess

Superior Orbital Fissure Syndrome

- Subsequent to sphenoiditis
- **Clinical features**–Deep orbital pain, Frontal headache, Progressive paralysis of 3rd, 4th and 6th Cranial Nerves

Orbital Apex Syndrome

- **Superior orbital fissure syndrome** with involvement of optic nerve and maxillary division of trigeminal nerve (II, III, IV, V2, VI).

Mucocele

- Mucocele is either a retention cyst of mucous glands of sinus or may be due to blockage of sinus ostium, resulting in thinning and expansion of sinus wall.
- Frontal and ethmoidal sinuses are the usual sinuses involved.
- If infection is superadded, it is called pyocele.

Contd.

Contd.

Clinical Features

- Dull headache.
- Swelling in the floor of frontal sinus above the inner canthus.
- Eye is displaced downwards and laterally.
- Swelling has tense cystic consistency or like egg-shell crackling.
- Ultimately may result in fistula formation near supraorbital margin.

Radiology

- Enlargement of sinus, floor of frontal sinus will be flattened and then bulges into orbit.
- Loss of scalloping of the superior border of frontal sinus.

Treatment

- Howarth incision and exploration of frontal sinus, removing mucocele and establishing drainage into the nose from affected sinus.

Ref: Dhingra 7th Edition Page 224, CODT 2nd Edition Page 300, Mohan Bansal Textbook of ENT Page 307, Hazarika Textbook of ENT Page 336, Tuli 2nd Edition Page 205

Ans: (B) Osteomyelitis of frontal bone

9. **What is the maneuver shown below:**

A. Lempert
B. Semont
C. Brandt
D. Epley

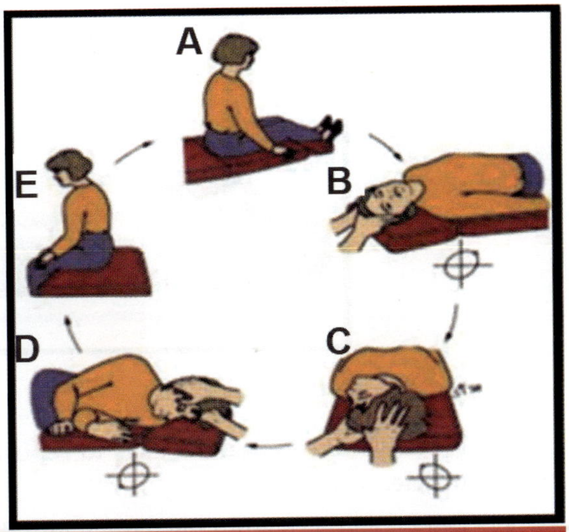

Key:

Picture shown is about Epley Maneuver which is used for Management of BPPV

BPPV (Benign Positional Paroxysmal Vertigo)

- **Most common cause of Peripheral vertigo**
- Occurs usually in 4th to 5th decade
- **Pediatric BPPV is associated with Migraine**
- More common in females
- **Etiology:** Head trauma, Infections, Old age, Surgery (Stapedectomy), Prolonged bed rest and Inactivity

PATHOGENESIS

- Usually caused by disorder of posterior semicircular canal.
- Otoconial debris, consisting of crystals of calcium carbonate, is released from degenerating macula of utricle and floats freely in endolymph.

- *When it settles on the cupula of posterior semicircular canal in a critical head position→ Causes displacement of cupula→ Vertigo.*

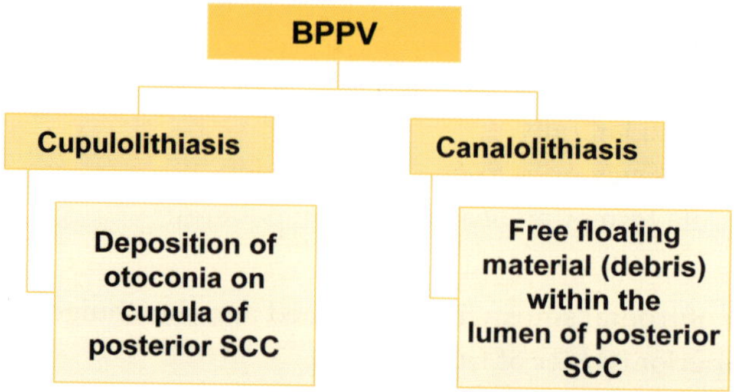

DIAGNOSTIC TEST

- *Careful history taking aids in diagnosis in most of cases (Positional variation)*
- **Dix hallpike Positional test–*Best diagnostic test***

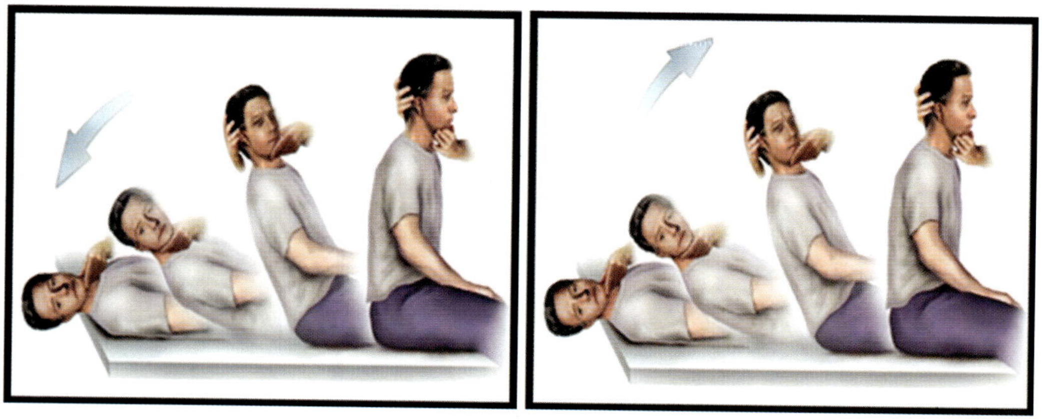

EPLEY MANEUVER

- Principle of this maneuver is to reposition otoconial debris from the posterior semicircular canal back into the utricle.
- Doctor stands behind the patient and the assistant on the side.
- Patient is made to sit on table so that when he is made to lie down, his head is beyond the edge of the table as is done in Dix-Hallpike maneuver.
- His face is turned 45° to the affected side.

Maneuver Consists of Five Positions

- ***Position 1:*** With head turned 45°, the patient is made to lie down in head-hanging position (Dix-Hallpike maneuver). It will cause vertigo and nystagmus. Wait till vertigo and nystagmus subside.
- ***Position 2:*** Head is now turned so that affected ear is up.
- ***Position 3:*** Whole body and head are now rotated away from the affected ear to a lateral recumbent position in a face-down position.
- ***Position 4:*** Patient is now brought to a sitting position with head still turned to unaffected side by 45°.
- ***Position 5:*** The head is now turned forward and chin brought down 20°.

Contd.

Contd.

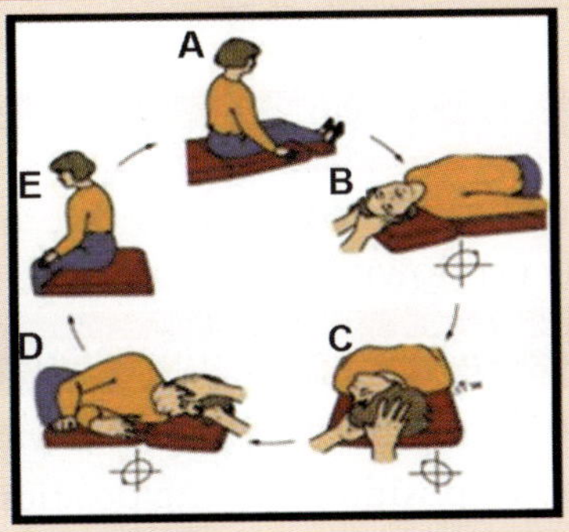

If Epley's Maneuver Fails

- Repeat Epley's maneuver after 1 month
- Try Semont's maneuver
- Advice home exercises–***Brandt Daroff Exercises***

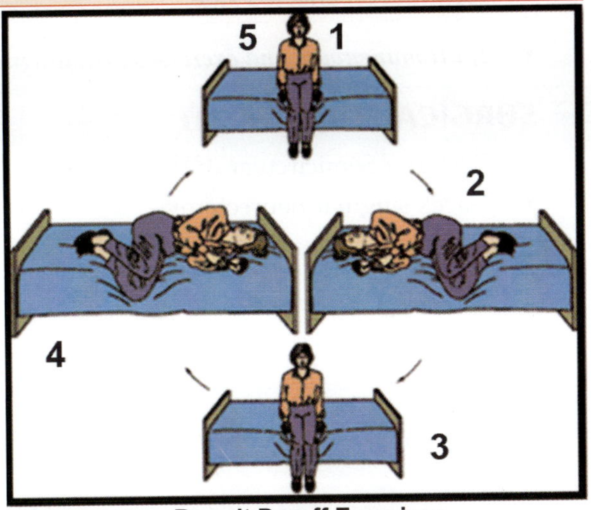

Brandt Daroff Exercises

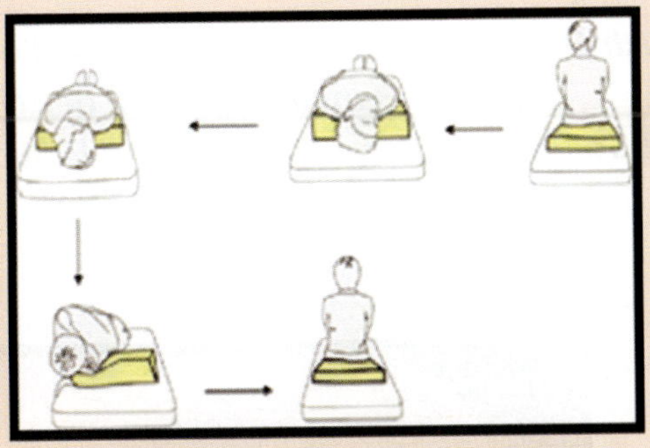

Modified Epley's Maneuver
Posterior canal cupulolithiasis

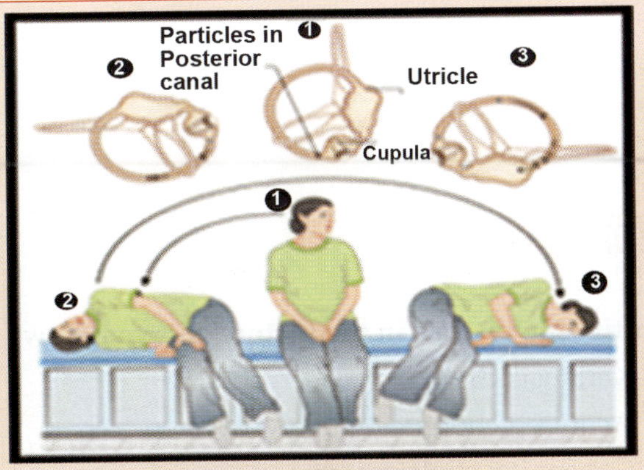

Semont Maneuver
Posterior canal cupulolithiasis

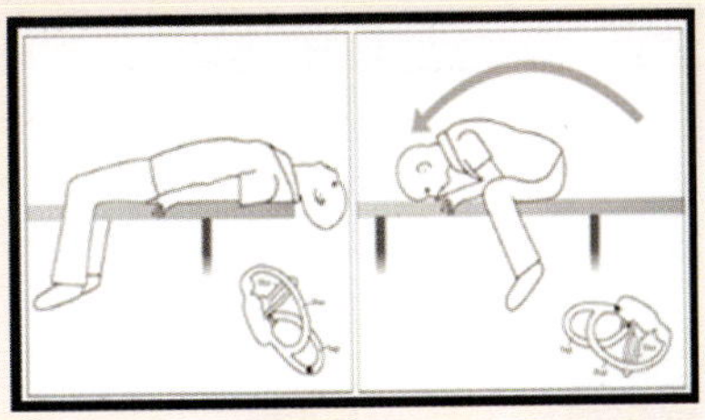

Li Maneuver
Superior canal cupulolithiasis

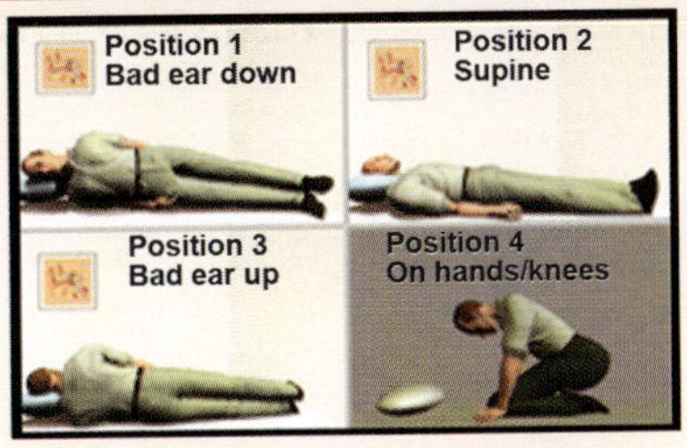

Log Roll/Barbecue Maneuver
Lateral canal cupulolithiasis

Vanucchi Maneuver
• Forced prolonged position of head on healthy side • Sleep in lateral position with healthy ear down for 12 hours.
360° Yaw Rotation Maneuver
• Patient head and body is rotated 360° in rapid 90° steps and towards unaffected ear • Lying position on affected side→ Supine position→ Lying position on unaffected side→ Supine position→ Lying position on affected side

- ***If all maneuvers and exercises fail, diagnosis is clear and symptoms are intolerable: Surgical Therapy***

SURGICAL TREATMENT

- Posterior Semicircular canal plugging
- Gacek singular neurectomy

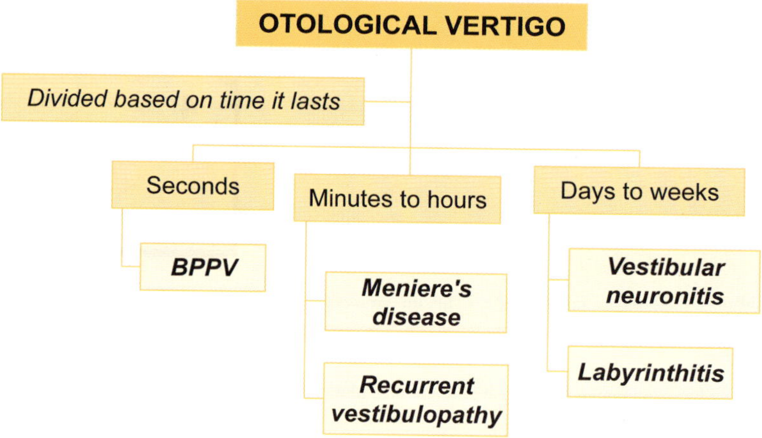

Ref: Dhingra 7th Edition Page 47, CODT 2nd Edition Page 730, Mohan Bansal Textbook of ENT Page 238, Hazarika Textbook of ENT Page 108, Tuli 2nd Edition Page 118

Ans: (D) Epley

10. Identify the disease in the picture shown below:

A. Keratosis Obturans
B. Acquired cholesteatoma
C. Congenital cholesteatoma
D. Osteoma

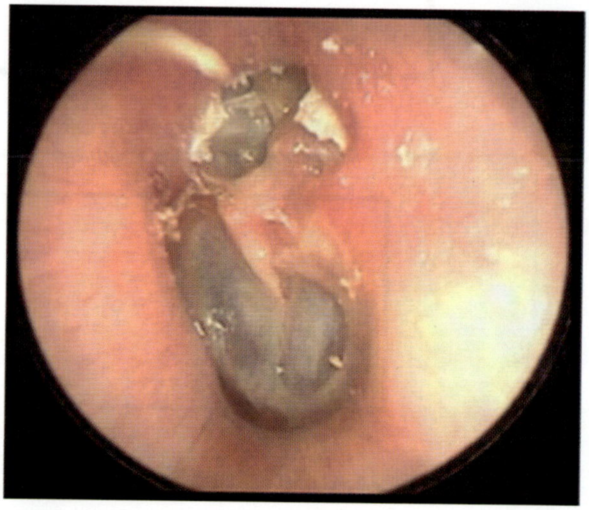

Key:

Picture shows Perforation in Attic/Pars flaccida region that suggests Attic cholesteatoma/Unsafe type of CSOM–Acquired cholesteatoma

Keratosis Obturans 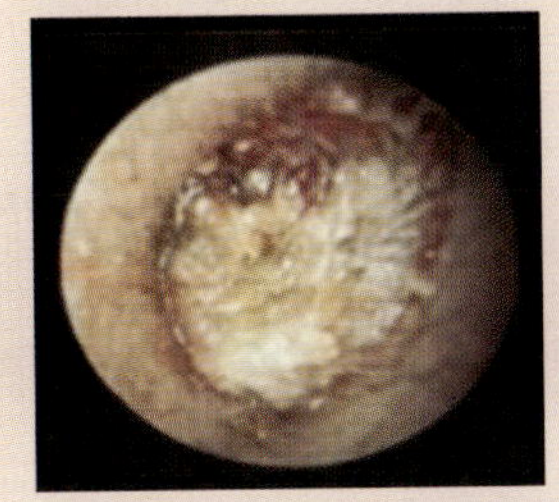	***Firm mass*** consisting of wax, desquamated keratinized epithelium and cholesterol granules.
Congenital cholesteatoma 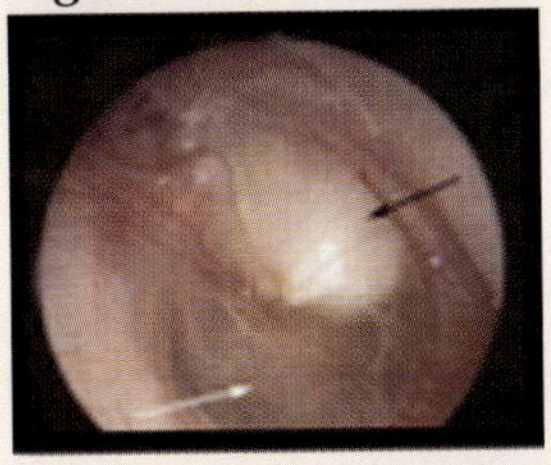	Ruled out because cholesteatoma is ***behind intact TM.***
Osteoma 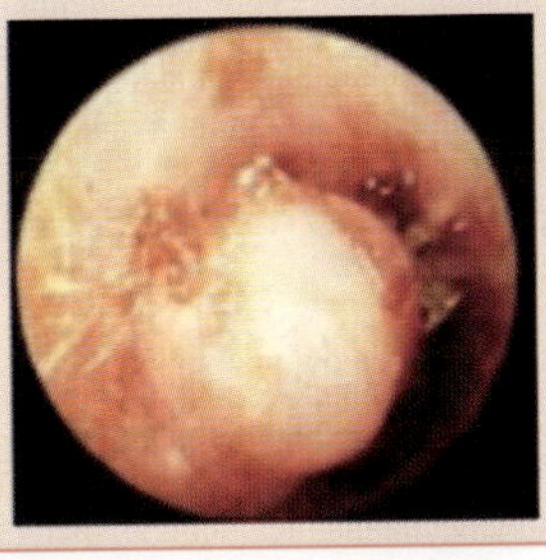	Single and occurs **at junction of bony and cartilaginous meatus.**

CHOLESTEATOMA

TYPES

- **Congenital**
  - Arises from epidermal cell rests (keratinizing epithelium) entrapped in middle ear cleft / temporal bone.
  - 3 Important sites–Middle ear, Petrous apex and CP angle.
  - **Clinical features:** Middle ear congenital cholesteatoma presents with conductive hearing loss and white mass that can be seen behind an intact tympanic membrane.
- **Acquired**
  - **Primary**: No history of previous Otorrhea/perforation
  - **Secondary**: Cholesteatoma occurs in pre-existing perforation of pars tensa

Theories of Cholesteatoma	
Wittmaack theory	Invagination/Retraction pocket theory
Habermann theory	Migration/Epithelial invasion
Reudi's theory	Basal cell hyperplasia
Sade's theory	Metaplasia

CLINICAL FEATURES

- Cholesteatoma has property of expansion with destruction of underlying structures.

Primary acquired cholesteatoma: Defect in attic or posterosuperior region containing keratin debris. ***Most common sites are attic and posterosuperior region.***

Secondary acquired cholesteatoma: Keratinizing epithelium migrating through pre-existing perforation into middle ear.

- *Discharge*→Foul smelling, Blood stained, **Continuous,** Scanty, purulent discharge not associated with URTI and not relieved by medication
- *Hearing loss*→Destruction of ossicles–Conductive hearing loss, Destruction of labyrinth–Sensorineural hearing loss
- Pearly white flakes of cholesteatoma can be seen in the retraction pockets.
- Fleshy polyps with granulations occur
- Granulation tissues surround area of osteitis especially attic and posterosuperior region

Treatment

- Surgical treatment is the treatment of choice
- Ideal surgery is Modified radical mastoidectomy (MRM)/Canal wall down mastoidectomy.
- Canal wall up procedures are advocated by few surgeons to avoid cavity problems that occur with canal wall down but clearance of disease is accurate with canal wall down only.

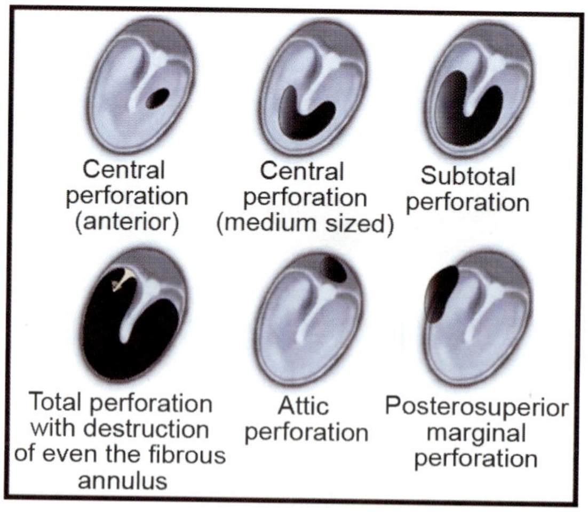

Posterosuperior marginal perforation/Total perforation can lead to Secondary Acquired cholesteatoma

Ref: Dhingra 7th Edition Page 74, CODT 2nd Edition Page 682, Mohan Bansal Textbook of ENT Page 212, Hazarika Textbook of ENT Page 155, Tuli 2nd Edition Page 69

Ans: (B) Acquired cholesteatoma

Chapter 10

OPHTHALMOLOGY

1. Topical ocular hypotensive causing apnea in child and infants:

A. Non-selective Beta blocker
B. Carbonic anhydrase inhibitors
C. Cholinergic agonists
D. Prostaglandins PGE1

Key:

Non-selective beta blockers used as ocular hypotensive agents can cause apnea in children and infants

- Beta blockers are effective topical agents, with mean peak IOP lowered by 25%.
- Non-selective agents like timolol lower IOP in a much more than beta 1 selective agents like betaxolol.
- Contraindications to beta blocker use include asthma, COPD, pulmonary disease, bradycardia, second- or third-degree heart block, and congestive heart failure.
- Use of beta blocker is avoided in neonates because of risk of apnea.

Antiglaucoma Agents

Drug	Mode of Action	Side Effects	Contraindications
Beta blocker	*Decrease aqueous production*	*Allergic blepharon conjunctivitis, Superficial punctate keratitis, Ocular cicatricial pemphigoid* ***Metipranolol-granulomatous anterior uveitis***	*Asthma, COPD, Pulmonary disease and Bradycardia* *Second or third-degree heart block, Caution in Diabetes patients*
PG analogs	*Increase uveoscleral outflow*	*Conjunctival hyperemia, Hyperchromic heterochromia iridis, Hypertrichosis, hyperpigmentation, Uveitis, Reactivation of herpetic keratitis and **Iris cysts***	*Contraindicated in hypertensive uveitis*
Alpha adrenergic agonists	*Decrease aqueous outflow* *Increase trabecular outflow*	*Follicular conjunctivitis, Mydriasis, Ocular allergies* *Upper lid retraction-more common with Apraclonidine* *Black conjunctival pigmentation- seen with Dipivefrin*	*Can cause drowsiness and CNS depression by acting on CNS. So, contraindicated in children*
Carbonic anhydrase inhibitor	*Decreases aqueous outflow by acting on CA 2 isoform enzyme*	*Metabolic acidosis, Hypokalaemia, Paraesthesia, Myopic shift and Idiosyncratic bone marrow suppression* *Can cause cornea decompensation in patients with corneal endothelial dysfunction*	*Patients allergic to sulfonamide drugs* *Kidney stones, Aplastic anemia and Sickle cell disease*
Cholinergic agonists	*Increase trabecular and uveoscleral outflow*	*Local side effects–miosis, brow ache, myopic shift, exaggerating symptoms of cataract, retinal detachment, nasolacrimal duct obstruction* *Systemic side effects–confusion, bradycardia, bronchospasm, GI symptoms and urinary frequency*	–

Ref: Yanoff 4th Edition Page 1094, A K Khurana 7th Edition Page 469, Kanski 7th Edition Page 345, Nema 4th Edition Page 204, Parson 22nd Edition Page 288

Ans: (A) Non-selective Beta blocker

2. **Possible cause for subnormal vision in patient with given condition shown below is:**
   A. Astigmatism
   B. Involvement of visual axis
   C. Cataract
   D. Glaucoma

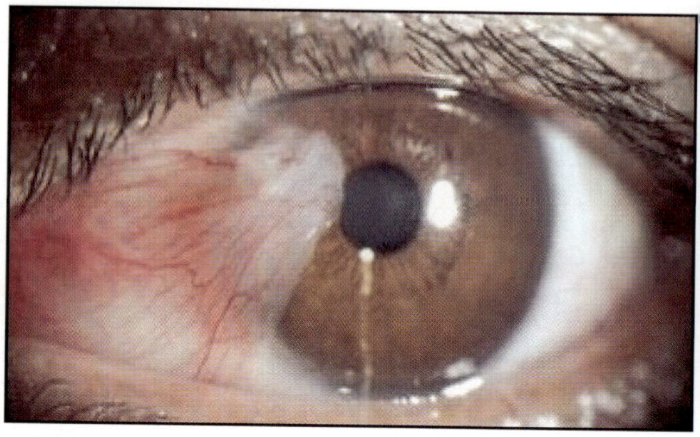

Key:

Image depicts presence of a triangular fibrovascular subepithelial ingrowth of degenerative bulbar conjunctiva over the limbus on to cornea-indicating Ptergium as diagnosis

In picture, Pterygium is not encroaching on to visual axis as we can clearly see pupillary margin here. So cause of subnormal vision is Astigmatism

PTERYGIUM (WING LIKE)

- Non malignant growth of conjunctiva, proliferation of subconjuctival fibrovascular tissue that encroaches upon cornea.
- **Pterygium** is a triangular fibrovascular subepithelial ingrowth of degenerative bulbar conjunctiva over the limbus on to cornea.

Etiology

- UV rays exposure, Dry heat, High wind and dust.
- *Typically develops in patients living in hot climate.*

Parts of Pterygium

Made up of three parts:

- **Head**–Rests on cornea
- **Neck**–Constricted portion seen at limbus
- **Body**–Remaining bulk of mass
- **Cap–Semilunar infiltrating portion in front of head showing opaque spots suggestive of progression–FUCH SPOTS** *(Avascular halo-like zone at the advancing edge)*

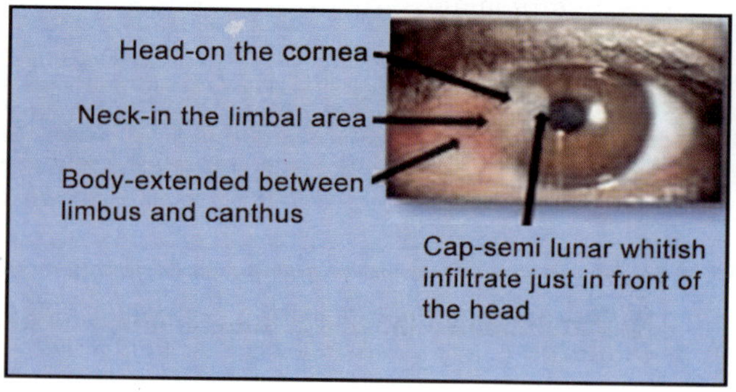

Pathogenesis

- Elastotic degeneration of subconjuctival tissue along with fibrovascular proliferation
- Results in destruction of epithelial and Bowman's layer–*Causes Scarring*

Clinical Features

- *Most of the small lesions are asymptomatic and they don't lead to decrease in vision.*

- Usually asymptomatic at initial stages
- Later foreign body sensation and growth may occur

CAUSES OF SUBNORMAL VISION

- **Astigmatism (Fibrosis)**
  Fibrovascular tissue contracts–Flattening of cornea in horizontal axis (With the rule)
- **Pupillary axis encroachment**
- **Severe tear film disturbances**

- ***Diplopia***–Restricted Ocular movement

Progressive Pterygium	Atrophic Pterygium (Stationary)
Thick and Fleshy	Thin and Pale
Highly vascularized	No vascularization
Cap present	No cap

- Linear iron deposition seen in corneal epithelium anterior to head of pterygium (**Stockers line**)–Typically seen in Atrophic ptergium
- Histologically shows ***Elastotic degenerative changes*** in vascularized subepithelial stromal collagen.
- Can undergo cystic degeneration and very rarely malignant change

Treatment

- ***Pterygium excision with conjunctival autograft is the preferred technique***

Indications for surgical intervention

- Proximity to the visual axis resulting in diminution of vision
- Encroachment of visual axis
- Significant amount of astigmatism
- Restriction of ocular movements
- Atypical appearance such as dysplasia
- Symptomatic growth
- Cosmetic concerns

Simple excision ('Bare sclera' technique/Mc Gravics method)

- ***Excise pterygium and conjunctival defect left as it is***
- Associated with a high rate of recurrence (around 80%) that may be more aggressive than initial lesion.
- High incidence of Granuloma formation

Mac Reynolds operation

- Head is dissected and sutured to fornix

Latest Methods

- Surgical excision with amniotic membrane graft
- Surgical excision with Mitomycin C (Large pterygium)
- Surgical excision with lamellar keratectomy and lamellar keratoplasty (Recurrent pterygium)
- Subconjunctival anti VEGF–Used to prevent recurrences

COMPLICATIONS OF PTERYGIUM SURGERY

- Recurrence–*Most common*
- Residual/Induced astigmatism
- Residual corneal opacity
- Rarely diplopia–Damage to medial rectus

Pseudopterygium

- Appears similarly like pterygium
- Caused by band of conjunctiva adhering to an area of compromised cornea at its apex.
- Forms as a response to inflammatory episodes such as a chemical burn, marginal corneal ulcer, trauma and cicatrizing conjunctivitis.

	Pterygium	Pseudopterygium
Pathogenesis	Degenerative process	Inflammatory process
Etiology	UV rays, Dry heat	Chemical injury
Age	Elderly	At any age
Site	Always situated in palpebral aperture (Nasal and Temporal)	At any site around limbus
Stages	Progressive/Regressive/Stationary	Always stationary
Recurrence after excision	Common	No recurrence usually
Probe test	Can be passed underneath (-ve)	Can be passed under neck (+ve)

Ref: Kanski's Clinical Ophthalmology 8th Edition Chapter 5 Page 162, Parson 22nd Edition Page 184, Nema 6th Edition Page 140, Kanski 7th Edition Page 438, Yanoff 4th Edition Page 197

Ans: (A) Astigmatism

3. **Esotropia is most commonly caused by:**

A. Myopia
B. Hypermetropia
C. Aphakia
D. Presbyopia

Key:

Esotropia is most commonly caused by Hypermetropia

Esotropia

- In young individuals with moderate hypermetropia, patient uses accommodation to see near and distant objects as there is intact accommodation. **Along with accommodation, convergence also occurs as patient accommodates or focuses** the eyes, the eyes converge.
- This phenomenon is called *ESOTROPIA*
- This results in Apparent divert squint→ *PSEUDOEXOTROPIA*
- Over–convergence associated with the accommodation to overcome a hyperopic refractive error can cause a loss of binocular control and development of esotropia.

Contd.

Contd.

Hypermetropia
• Refractive state in where parallel rays of light coming from infinity are focused behind retina with accommodation being at rest.

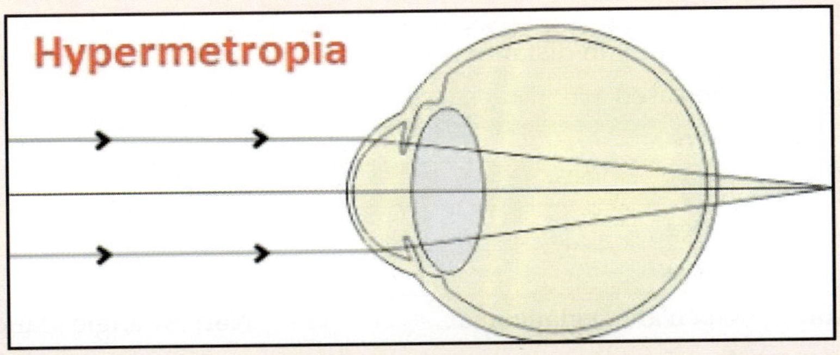

CLASSIFICATION

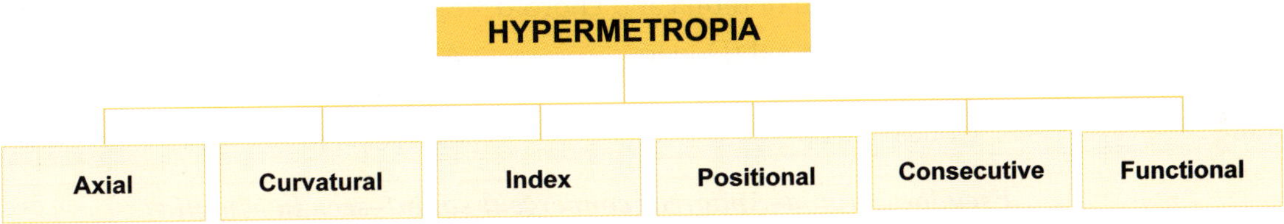

- **Axial**–Decreased length of eye ball–***Most common cause (1 mm decrease→ 3D)***
- **Curvatural**–Flattened cornea ***(1 mm flattening of cornea→ 6D)***
- **Index**–Increase in refractive index of cortex
- **Positional**–Backward displacement of lens
- **Consecutive**–Overcorrection of myopia and under correction of pseudophakia
- **Functional**–Paralysis of accommodation following 3rd nerve palsy
- **Facultative hyperopia**–*Overcome by an effort of accommodation*
- **Absolute hyperopia**–*Can't overcome by effort of accommodation*
- **Latent hyperopia**–Corrcted by tone of ciliary muscle
- **Manifest hyperopia**–Has 2 components–Facultative and Absolute
- **Total hyperopia**–***Latent and Manifest***→After complete cycloplegia with atropine

- **Symptoms:** Difficulty in near vision tasks and aestheniopia
- **Signs:** Small eyeball, Shallow anterior chamber, Pseudopapillitis and Shot silk appearance of retina
- **Complications:** *Recurrent stye, Blepharitis, Chalazion, Accommodative esotropia, Amblyopia and Primary acute angle closure glaucoma*
- **Treatment:** Convex spherical lens/+ve lens

Cornea based procedures	Lens based procedures
Thermal laser keratoplasty	Phakic refractive lens corrects more than +4D
Hyperopic PRK	Refractive lens exchange
Hyperopic LASIK upto +4D	
Conductive keratoplasty upto +3D	

Feature		Myopia (Short Sightedness)	Hypermetropia/Hyperopia (Long Sightedness)
Pathology		Difficulty in distant vision	Difficulty in near and distant vision
Axial length of globe		Increased	Decreased
Power		More	Less
Topography	*Eyeball*	*Large*	***Small***
	Pupil	*Large*	***Small***
	Angle of AC	*Large*	***Shallow***
Predisposition to squint		Open angle glaucoma	Narrow angle glaucoma
		Exophoria	***Esophoria***
Fundus examination	*Optic disk*	Myopic crescent	Small, more vascular, ill defined margins
	Retina	Degeneration of retina and choroid	Shines due to greater brilliance of light reflection
Investigations		ERG–Subnormal (Due to chorioretinal atrophy)	A scan biometry–Short AP length of eyeball
Correction		Concave lens	Convex lens

Pseudoesotropia–Apparent convergent squint–seen in Myopia

Ref: Parson 22nd Edition Page 246, Kanski 7th Edition Page 748, Yanoff 4th Edition Page 38, Nema 6th Edition Page 287, Agarwal 2nd Edition Page 422

Ans: (B) Hypermetropia

4. **Drug used for chemotherapy of retinoblastoma:**
   A. Etoposide + Vincristine + Carboplatin
   B. Etoposide + Vincristine + Cyclophosphamide
   C. Etoposide + Vincristine + 5FU
   D. Carboplatin + Vincristine + Cyclophosphamide

Key:

Combination of vincristine, etoposide and carboplatin (VEC) is employed, generally given four weeklies for 6 cycles for Intravenous chemotherapy

RETINOBLASTOMA/GLIOMA RETINAE

- **Most common intraocular tumor of childhood**
- Incidence 1 in 20,000 live births
- Usually seen between 1-2 years
- No sex prediction
- Common in Whites than Negroes
- **Bilateral–25%**
- 15% of heritable cases are Unilateral
- RB gene located on 13q14 (Tumor suppressor gene)
- Deletion/Inactivation of this gene by 2 mutations
- ***Most common–Sporadic (90%),*** 10% Familial
- **Trilateral Retinoblastoma:** Bilateral retinoblastoma and Pinealoblastoma
- **HPE: *Flexner wintersteiner rosettes (Highly specific),*** *Homer wright rosettes, Pseudorosettes, Fleurettes*
- Raised LDH level in aqueous (relative to serum level)

Clinical Presentation

- **Most common feature–Leukocoria (60%)**

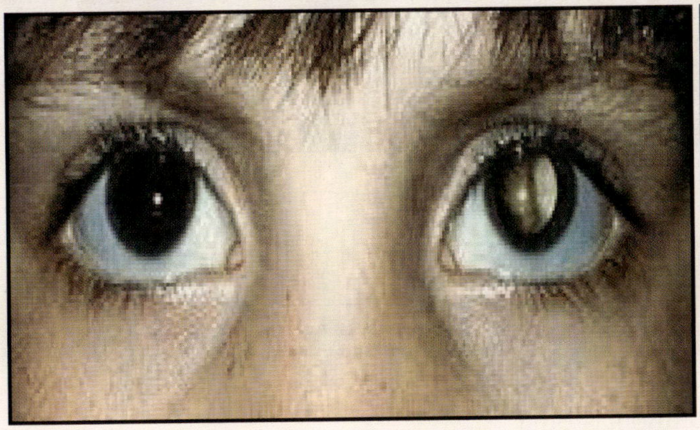

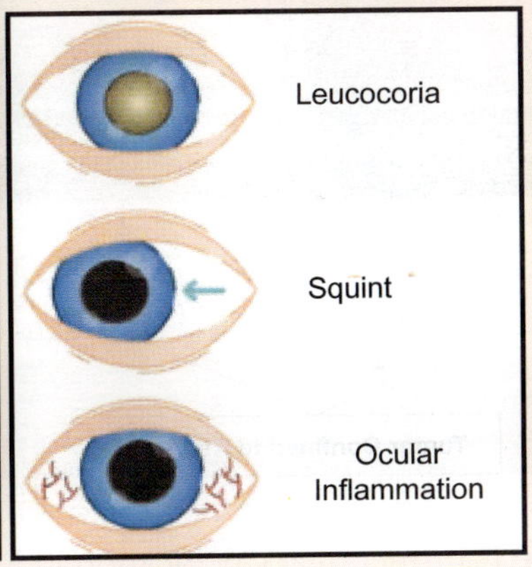

- Squint (20%), ***Orbital cellulitis***, Nystagmus, Red eye, Excessive tearing, Corneal clouding, Iris discoloration, Defective vision and Proptosis
- **Most common sign:**
  - ***Small lesions***–Simulates endophthalmitis (Endophytic)
  - ***Large lesions***–Simulates Coats disease (Exophytic)

Reese Ellsworth Classification (Prognosis)

Predicts Survival of Eye

Group I: Very favourable for sight
- *Smaller tumor, <4DD in size at/behind equator*
- *Multiple tumors none larger than 4DD in size all at/behind equator*

Group II: Favourable for sight
- *Smaller tumor, 4-10DD in size at/behind equator*
- *Multiple tumors none larger than 4DD in size all at/behind equator*

Group III: Possible for sight
- *Any lesion anterior to equator*
- *Solitary tumor >10DD in size behind equator*

Group IV: Unfavourable for sight
- *Multiple tumors some larger 10DD in size*
- *Any lesion extending anteriorly to ora serrata*

Group V: Highly unfavourable for sight
- *Massive tumors more than ½ of retina*
- *Vitreous seeding*

Clinical Staging

- Quiescent stage
- Glaucomatous stage
- Extraocular extension
- Distant metastasis

Contd.

Contd.

International Intraocular Retinoblastoma Classification

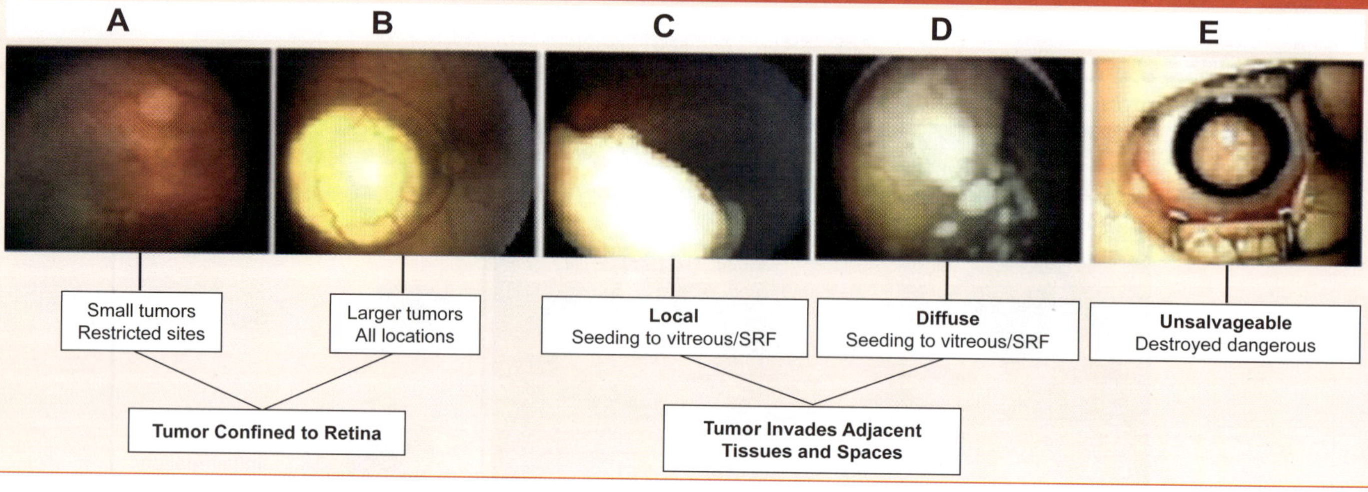

- *X-ray/CT*–Intracranial calcification in Retinoblastoma
- *USG*–Useful for diagnosis and monitoring treatment
- *MRI*–Used only to differentiate tumors from other exudative detachments

Treatment

- Tumor involves ***less than half of retina and optic nerve not involved***–Sequential aggressive local therapy (Salt) is recommended.
- Small tumors (<4DD size)–Cryotherapy for anterior tumors
- More than half of retina, Optic nerve and Anterior chamber involved–*ENUCLEATION*
- Orbital/Intracranial extension/Extensive metastasis–Palliative therapy
- ***Primary treatment for Bilateral RB***–Chemotherapy
- ***Poor prognosis***–*Optic nerve involvement, Undifferentiated tumor cells and Massive choroidal invasion*
- ***Grabowski Abramson classification***–Extraocular retinoblastoma
- *Osteosarcoma–Most common secondary tumors in Retinoblastoma patients*

Enucleation–*Removal of eyeball (Adjacent eye socket and lids intact)*→ **Intraocular tumor**
Evisceration–*Removal of internal eye contents (Sclera left behind with Extraocular muscles still attached)*
Exenteration–*Removal of contents of eye socket (orbit) including eyeball, fat, muscles and other adjacent eye structures (Eye lids) removed in cutaneous cancers and unrelenting infection*
Evisceration–Contraindicated in Malignant intraocular tumor

Chemotherapy

- Intravenous chemotherapy causes reduction in tumor volume, this is known as chemo reduction.
- ***Most commonly, combination of three drugs vincristine, etoposide and carboplatin (VEC) is employed, generally given four weeklies for 6 cycles.***
- Drugs used for intra-arterial chemotherapy are–melphalan, topotecan, carboplatin
- Drugs used for intra-vitreal chemotherapy are–melphalan, topotecan

Ref: Parson 22nd Edition Page 380, Yanoff 4th Edition Page 1009
Kanski 6th Edition Page 111, Basak 2nd Edition Page 359, Nema 4th Edition Page 290
Recent Developments in Retinoblastoma Article by Santosh Honaver

Ans: (A) Etoposide + Vincristine + Carboplatin

5. **Operation using glaucoma valve implant shunt is:**

A. Seton operation
B. Deep sclerotomy
C. Trabeculotomy
D. Trabeculotomy

Key:

Seton operation is glaucoma valve implant shunt operation for Glaucoma surgery

GLAUCOMA TUBE SHUNT SURGERIES

- Tube-shunt surgery (Seton glaucoma surgery) involves placing a flexible plastic tube with an attached silicone drainage pouch in the eye to
- Helps to drain fluid (aqueous humor) from the eye.
- ***Creates alternate communication between Anterior chamber and Sub-Tenon's space***
- This type of surgery is usually done after a trabeculectomy has failed.
- If a person already has/likely to form scar tissue in eye, this type of surgery may be done at start.

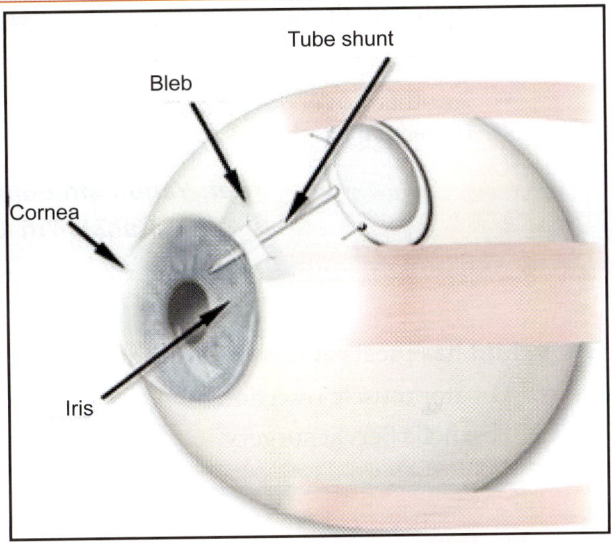

Indications of Drainage Implants

- Refractory glaucoma
- Aphakic, pseudophakic glaucoma
- Uveitic glaucoma
- Neovascular glaucoma
- Congenital glaucoma with iridocorneal dysgenesis
- ICE syndrome
- Glaucoma that follows corneal transplantation
- Previously failed trabeculectomy

Tube Implants are of Two Types

- **Valved implants**–Molteno implants, Baerveldt implants, Krupin implant
- **Nonvalved implants**–Ahmed glaucoma implant

Complications of Drainage Surgery

- Excessive drainage may occur due to leakage around or down tube if occluding suture is loose and result in hypotony and shallow anterior chamber
- Malposition that may result in endothelial or lenticular touch
- Tube erosion through the sclera and conjunctiva
- Early drainage failure may occur as a result of blockage of end of tube by vitreous, blood/iris

Mini Shunts

1. Ex-Press Glaucoma Implant:

- Small stainless steel device now implanted under partial-thickness sclera flap as a modification of trabeculectomy.
- Provides more favorable safety and postop recovery profile.
- So, it is now alternative to glaucoma drainage valves like Ahmed glaucoma valve.

2. iSTENT:

- Another novel device consisting of tiny titanium hooked tube inserted ***ab interno*** into Schlemm canal via the trabecular meshwork, and shows promise for moderate IOP reduction.

Ref: Yanoff 4th Edition Part 10 Section 4 Page 1159, AK Khurana 7th Edition Page 263, Kanski 7th Edition Page 399, Postgraduate Ophthalmology Volume 1 Page 947

Ans: (A) Seton operation

6. A child has ptosis and poor levator function. What surgery will you do?

A. Levator muscle resection
B. Mullerectomy
C. Fasanella Servat surgery
D. Frontalis suspension surgery

Key:

Mild ptosis with good levator action is treated by Fasanella servat surgery
Ptosis with Poor levator function is treated by Frontalis suspension surgery

PTOSIS

- *Drooping of upper eyelid to level that covers more than 2 mm of superior cornea*

Grading of Ptosis

- **Mild**–2 mm
- **Moderate**–3 mm
- **Severe**–4 mm and above

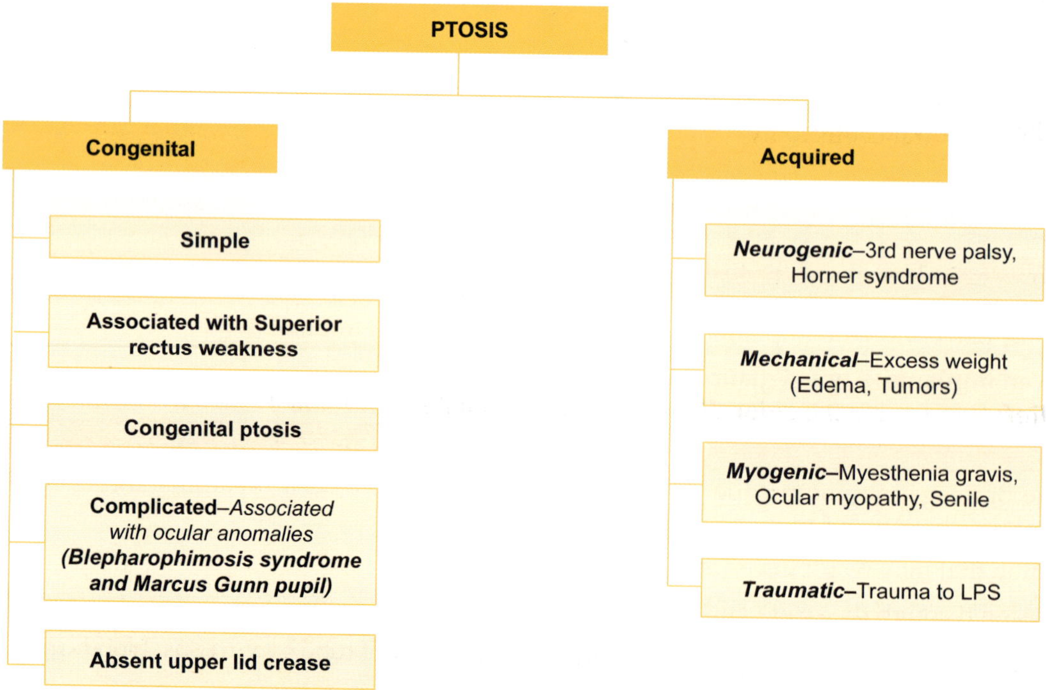

Bilateral Ptosis–Myasthenia gravis, Myotonic dystrophy, Kearns Sayre syndrome, Fisher syndrome, CPEO and Botulism

- **Acquired aponeurotic ptosis–***Treated by aponeurotic reattachment*
- **Ptosis associated with Mysthenia gravis–**Neostigmine, Pyridostigmine and Crutch glass
- **Ptosis due to CPEO–**Crutch glass
- **Ptosis in Horner syndrome–***Fasanella servat surgery*

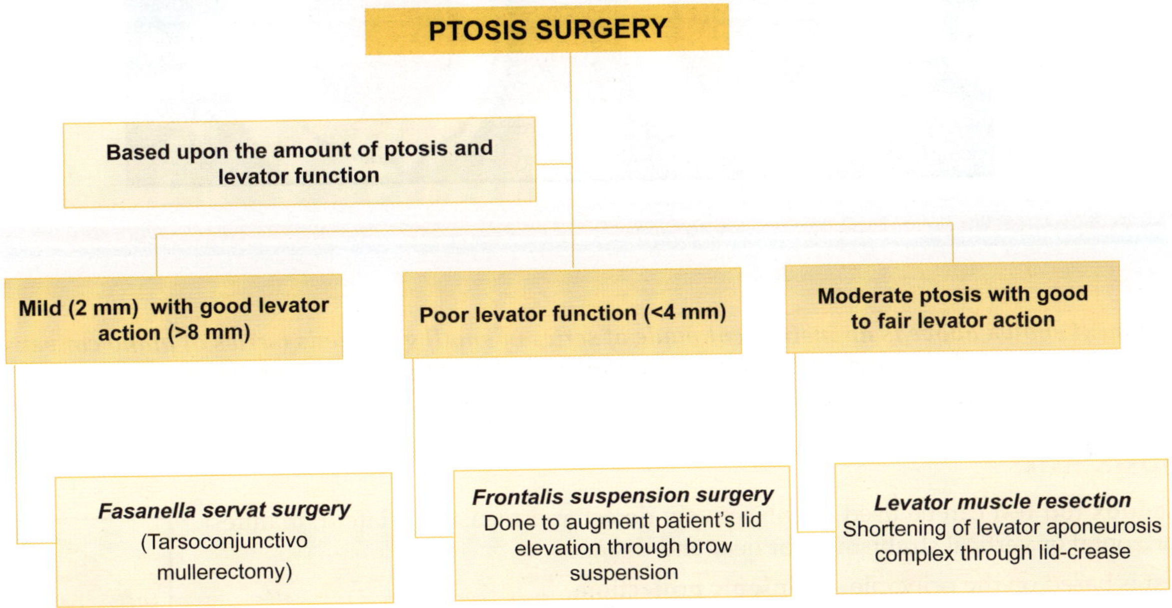

Marcus Gunn jaw winking syndrome
Retraction of ptotic lid in conjunction with stimulation of Ipsilateral Pterygoid muscles (Chewing, Sucking or Opening mouth). **Treatment**–Levator disinsertion and frontalis sling surgery
Horner syndrome
MAPE→ Miosis, Anhydrosis, Ptosis and Enophthalmos with Loss of ciliospinal reflex. Heterochromia is seen in congenital horner's syndrome **Treatment**–Fasanella servat surgery
CPEO: Chronic progressive external ophthalmoplegia
Bilateral symmetrical progressive ptosis, progressive external ophthalmoplegia. Associated with cardiac conduction defect, pigmentary retinopathy and dysphagia **Treatment**–Crutch glass

Ref: Parson 22nd Edition Page 460, Yanoff 4th Edition Page 1272, AK Khurana 7th Edition Page 395, Kanski 7th Edition Page 850, Agarwal 2nd Edition Page 592

Ans: (D) Frontalis suspension surgery

7. **Identify instrument shown below:**

A. Maddox rod
B. Maddox wing
C. Maddox glass
D. Red glass

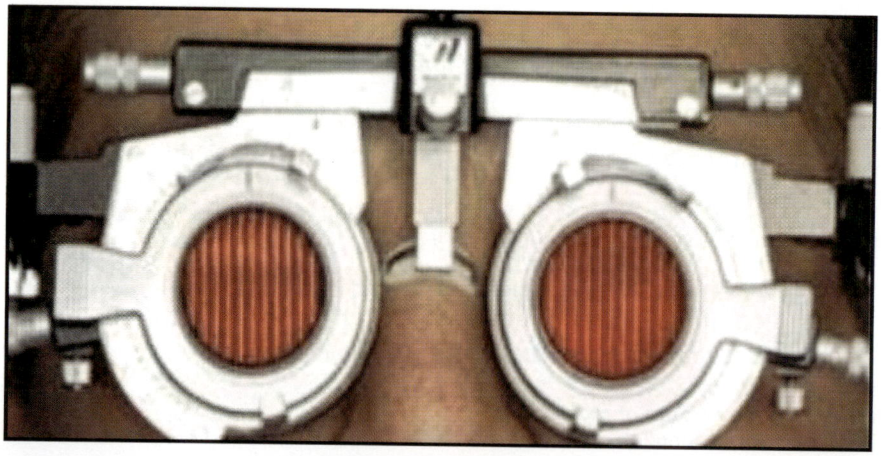

Key:

Instrument shown above is an instrument made of series of small glass rods (series of plano convex cylinders in red/white)–Causes Astigmatic elongation of fixation light

Produces vertical/horizontal streak to measure horizontal and vertical deviation

MADDOX ROD

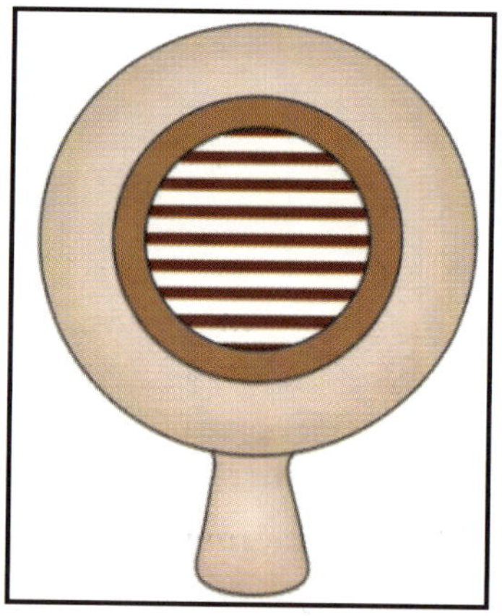

- **Maddox rod test** can be used to subjectively detect and measure a latent, manifest, horizontal or vertical strabismus for near and distance.
- Test is based on the principle of **diplopic projection.**
- Maddox rod test uses a specially constructed device consisting of a series of parallel cylinders that converts a point source of light into a line image.
- Optical properties of the cylinders cause the streak of light to be situated 90° to the orientation of the parallel cylinders.
- Because fusion is precluded by Maddox rod, heterophorias and heterotropias can't be differentiated.
- Maddox rod can be used to test for **horizontal and vertical deviations**, and, when used in conjunction with another Maddox rod, for **cyclodeviations**.

*Double Maddox rod test is used to determine cyclodeviations***

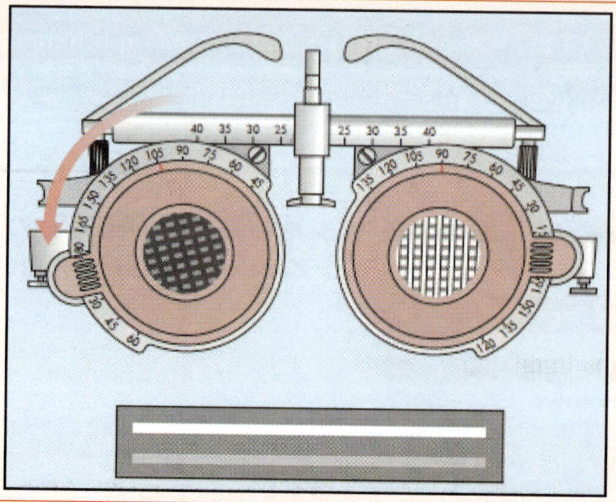

Uses of Maddox Rod

- **Evaluation of Squint**
- **Macular function test**–To assess macula in case of dense cataract

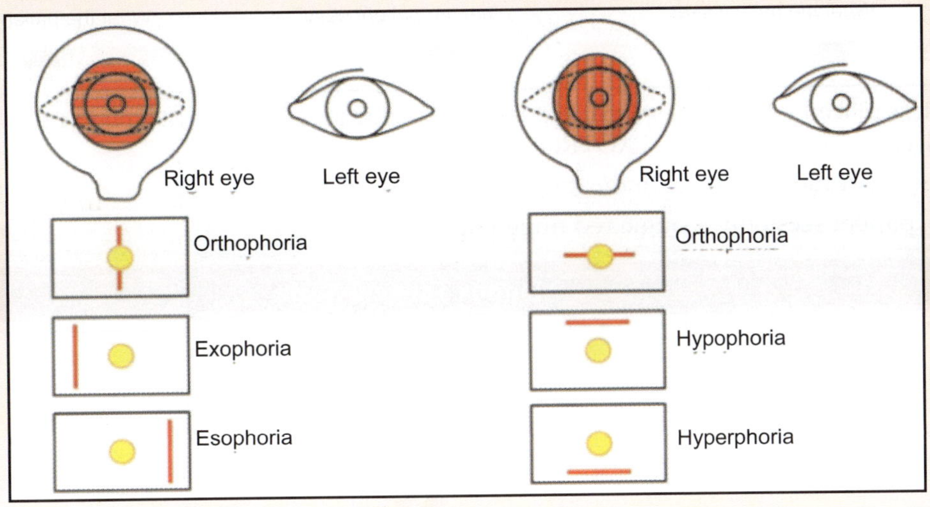

Maddox rod test for Horizontal and Vertical Heterophorias

Maddox Wing

- **Instrument by which amount of phoria for near at (33 cm) can be measured.**
- Maddox wing dissociates eyes for near fixation (1/3 m) and measures heterophoria.
- Instrument is constructed in such a way that right eye sees only a white vertical arrow and red horizontal arrow, whereas the left eye sees only horizontal and vertical rows of numbers.
- **Measurements are made as follows:**
  - *Horizontal deviation*–Measured by asking patient to which number white arrow points.
  - *Vertical deviation*–Measured by asking patient which number red arrow intersects.
  - *Amount of cyclophoria*–Determined by asking patient to move red arrow so that it is parallel with the horizontal row of numbers.

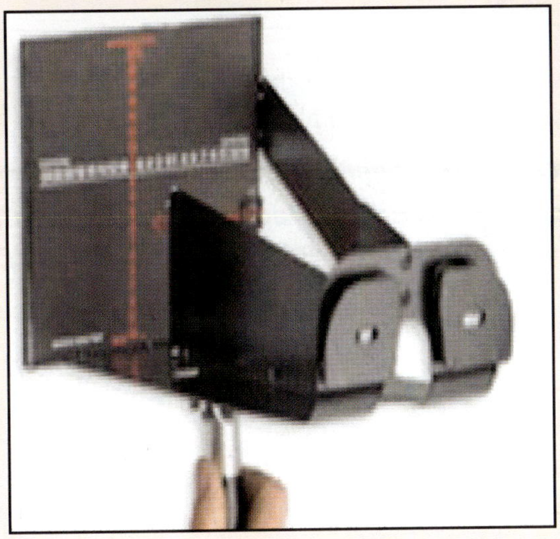

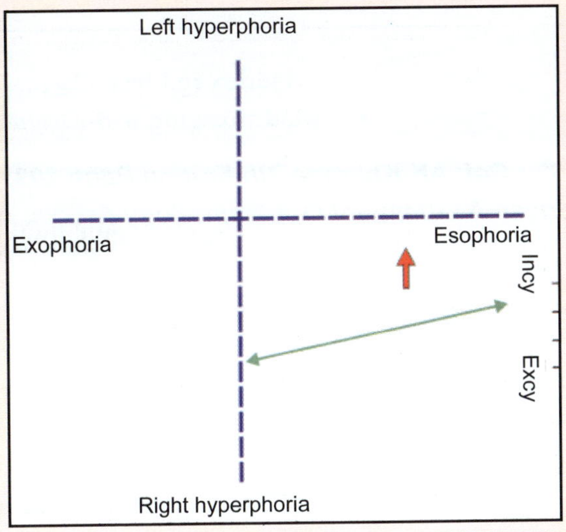

Red Glass Test

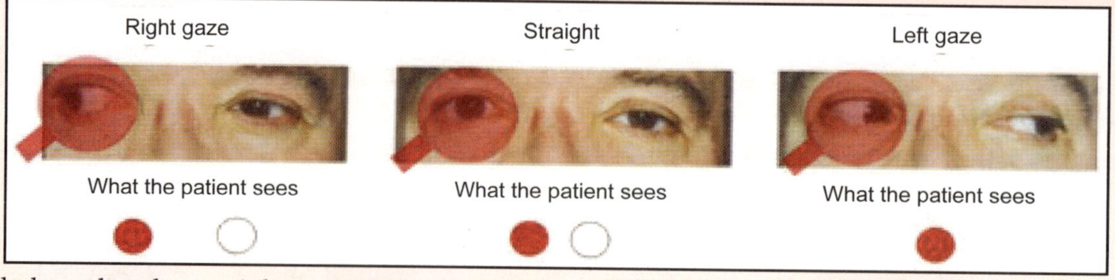

- With red glass placed over right eye, patient reports that he sees. In straight a head gaze, red light appears to left and while light to right indicating EXOTROPIA.
- In right gaze separation increases, indicating greater exotropia in right gaze.
- In left gaze, patient sees only a single red tinged light.

Maddox Tangent Scale

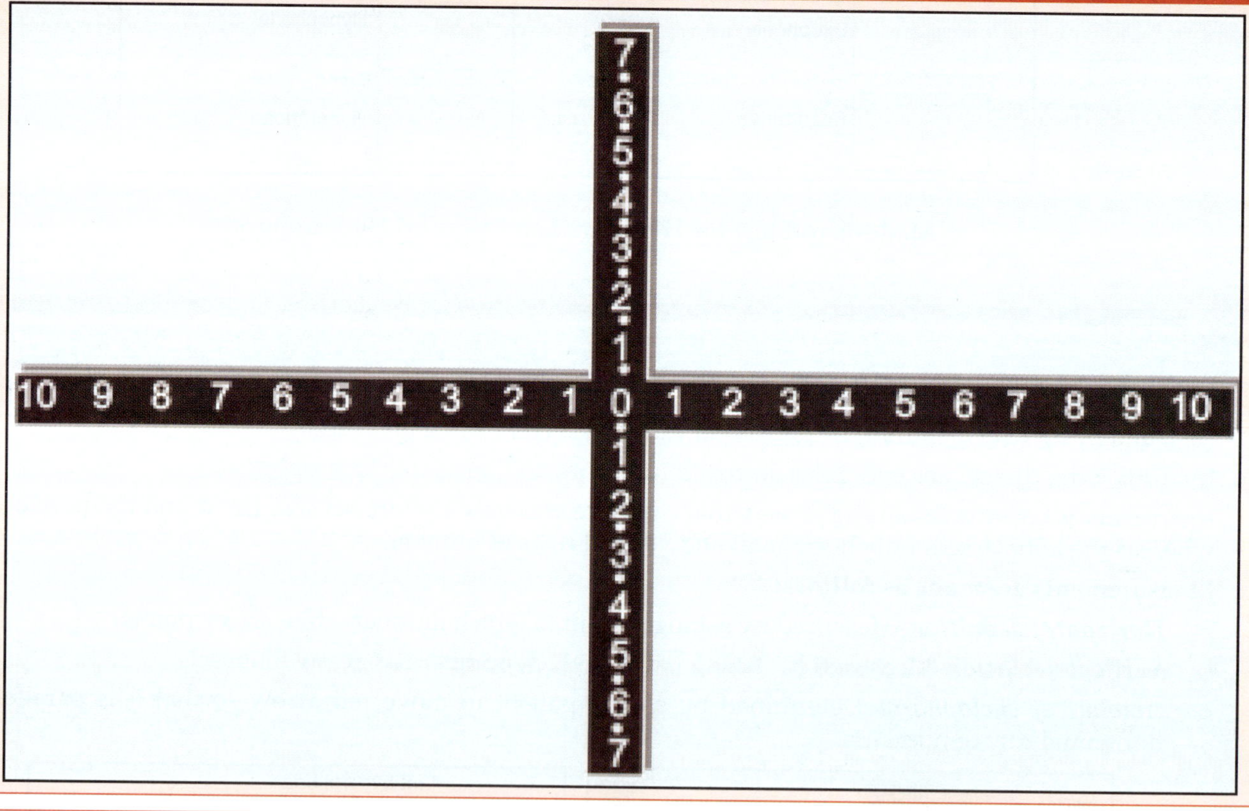

- **Maddox rod test**–*Diagnosis of latent squint in Distant vision (6 m)*
- **Maddox wing test**–*Diagnosis of latent squint in Near vision (33 cm)*

Ref: AK Khurana 7th Edition Page 203, Kanski 7th Edition Page 857, Yanoff 4th Edition Page 11.3, American Academy of Ophthalmology Article, Agarwal 2nd Edition Page 591, Basak 2nd Edition Page 319, Nema 4th Edition Page 316, Vaughan 15th Edition Page 272

Ans: (A) Maddox rod

8. **Most common ocular manifestation of myasthenia gravis:**

A. Ptosis
B. Proptosis
C. Enophthalmos
D. Lagophthalmos

Key:

Most common ocular manifestation of myasthenia gravis–Ptosis (Weakness of muscles)
(Insidious, Bilateral and frequently Asymmetrical ptosis worse at tend of the day)

Myasthaenia Gravis

- Autoimmune disorder
- Women > Men
- Involves 20–30 years usually
- Antibodies against Ach Receptor

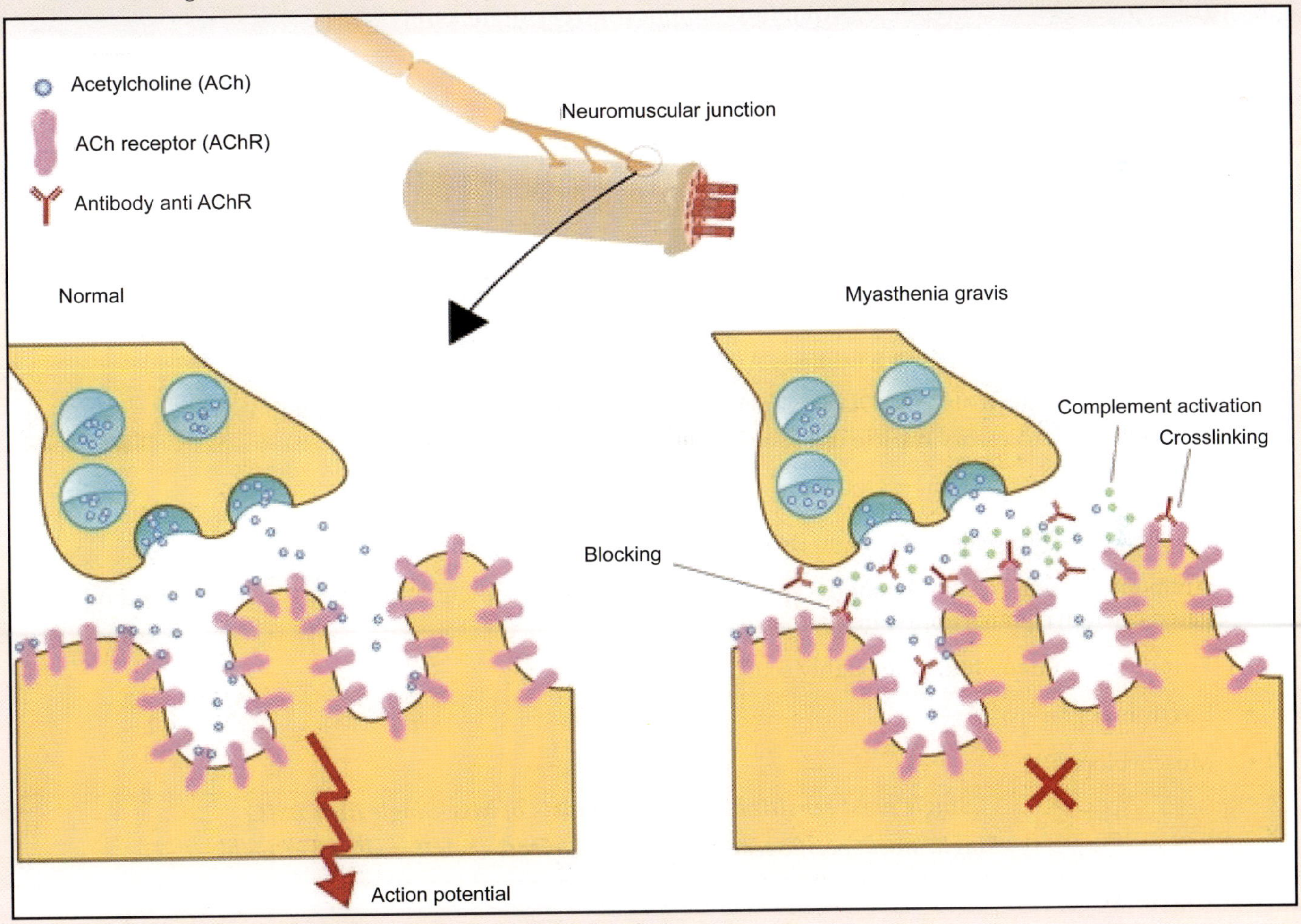

- **Cardinal Features**–Weakness and Fatigability of muscles
  - *Lid and Extraocular muscles are often involved in early course*
  - *Diplopia and ptosis are initial common complaints*
  - *Weakness in chewing, Snarling expression on attempt to smile is present*
  - *Limb Weakness–Proximal and Asymmetrical (85% of patients)*
  - *Deep tendon reflexes are preserved*
  - *Sensations are normal*

Contd.

Contd.

- Ocular involvement occurs in 90% cases and it is the presenting feature in 60%.
- Two-third of patients have both ptosis and diplopia.
- Ptosis–insidious, bilateral and frequently asymmetrical. Typically, worse at tend of the day.

***Cogan twitch sign**–Brief upshot of eyelid as eye saccade from depression to primary position*

- Fluctuating ophthalmoparesis, Ptosis, Diplopia (Frequently vertical) and Pseudo internuclear ophthalmoplegia
- Diplopia is frequently vertical, although all extraocular muscles can be affected.
- Nystagmoid movements–at extremes of gaze
- Associated with ***Thymoma and Thymic abnormalities along with Rheumatoid arthritis, SLE, Pernicious anemia, Hyperthyroidism, Ulcerative colitis, Polymyositis***

Major Symptoms of Myasthenia Gravis	
Ocular	Ptosis–Most common Diplopia Weakness of eye closure
Bulbar	Dysarthria with nasal speech Dysphagia with nasal regurgitation Facial weakness
Cervical	Neck flexor weakness causing head lag upon lifting up from lying down Neck extensor weakness manifesting as posterior head pain and head drop
Limb	Proximal limb weakness, Arm more than leg, Finger extensor weakness
Respiratory	Intercostal and Diaphragm muscle weakness causing respiratory failure, Accessory muscle usage

Investigations

- **Ice pack test**–Improvement after an ice pack is placed on the ptotic eyelid
- Antibody testing–Acetyl choline receptor antibodies, MuSK protein antibodies, striational antibodies, voltage gated calcium channel antibodies
- **Edrophonium (tensilon) test**–Highly sensitive test
- Electromyography
- Muscle biopsy

Single most sensitive test for diagnosis of MG–Single fiber EMG

Single most specific test for diagnosis of MG–Ach Receptor Antibody

Treatment

- Acetylcholine esterase inhibitors–*Pyridostigmine, Neostigmine*
- Immunosuppression–Steroids, Azathioprine, Cyclosporine A, Methotrexate, Cyclophosphamide
- Symptomatic treatment of ocular abnormality
- Avoidance of substances that worsen neuromuscular transmission
- Thymectomy
- Plasmapheresis and IVIG

Contd.

Contd.

Myasthenia Gravis Subgroups			
Subgroup	**Antibody**	**Age at onset**	**Thymus**
Early onset	Ach Receptor	<50 years	Hyperplasia
Late onset	Ach Receptor	>50 years	Atrophy
Thymoma	Ach Receptor	Any age	Lymphoepithelioma
Muscle specific kinase	Muscle specific kinase	Any age	Normal
LRP 4	LRP 4	Any age	Normal
Seronegative	None	Any age	Variable
Ocular	Variable	Any age	Variable

Ref: Kanski's Clinical Ophthalmology 8th Edition Chapter 19 Page 838, Parson 22nd Edition Page 460, Yanoff 4th Edition Page 1272, AK Khurana 7th Edition Page 395, Agarwal 2nd Edition Page 592

Ans: (A) Ptosis

9. Which of following is against the rule of astigmatism?

A. 1D Cylindrical 90°
B. 1D Cylindrical 180°
C. 1.25D, -4D Cylindrical 180°
D. 2D Cylindrical 90°

Key:

WTR astigmatism*–concave cylinder at 180 degree* ***OR*** *convex cylinder at 90 degree*
ATR astigmatism*–concave cylinder at 90 degree* ***OR*** *convex cylinder at 180 degree*

With the rule: +Power 90° or –Power at 180°

Astigmatism

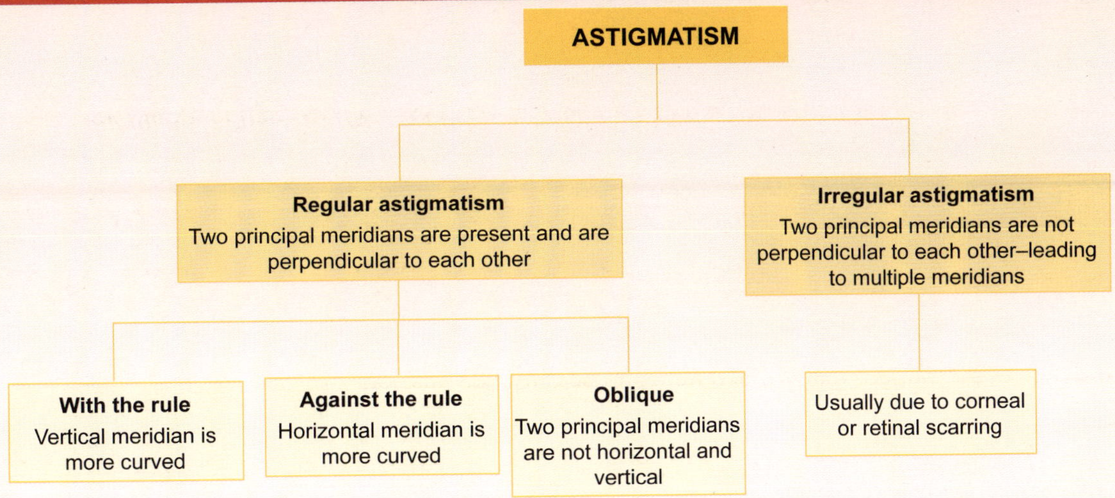

Contd.

Contd.

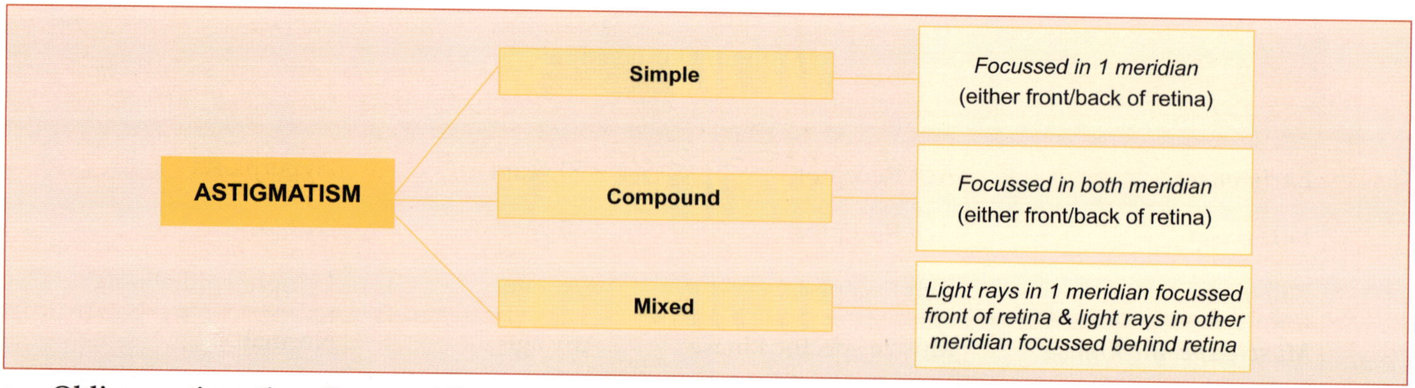

- **Oblique astigmatism**–Two meridians are at right angles to each other, but do not lie at or near 90 or 180 degree meridian.
- **Bioblique astigmatism**–Both meridians can be made out, they are neither at right angles to each other, nor are they near 90 or 180 degree meridian.

Refraction through Cylindrical/Toric surface is called STRUM OF CONOID
Placido disc is used to detect Corneal astigmatism

Clinical Features

Blurring of vision, Asthenopic symptoms, Tilting of head and squinting

Treatment

- **Regular Astigmatism**–*Bicylindrical lens LASIK is used upto +6D astigmatism*
- **Irregular Astigmatism**–*Best corrected by Hard contact lens*

***Ref:** Yanoff 4th Edition Page 38, Parson 22nd Edition Page 53, A.K. Khurana 5th Edition Page 35, Nema 5th Edition Page 31, Postgraduate Ophthalmology Volume 1 Page 48, Kanski 7th Edition Page 640, Agarwal 2nd Edition Page 422*

Ans: (B) 1D Cylindrical 180°

Chapter 11

MEDICINE

1. A 45 years old HIV patient presents with fever, cough, chest pain and dyspnea for 3 weeks. His chest X-ray shows diffuse interstitial and alveolar infiltrates. Most common diagnosis:

A. Streptococcus pneumonia
B. Pneumocystis jirovecii
C. Staphylococci
D. Klebsiella

Key:

Bilateral Diffuse air space involvement mainly perihilar region with peripheral sparing in HIV patient is characteristic feature of Pneumocystis jiroveci pneumonia

- Three of 10 most common AIDS-defining illnesses are:
    - Recurrent **bacterial pneumonia**
    - **Tuberculosis** and
    - Pneumonia due to unicellular fungus **P. jirovecii**

PATHOGENESIS

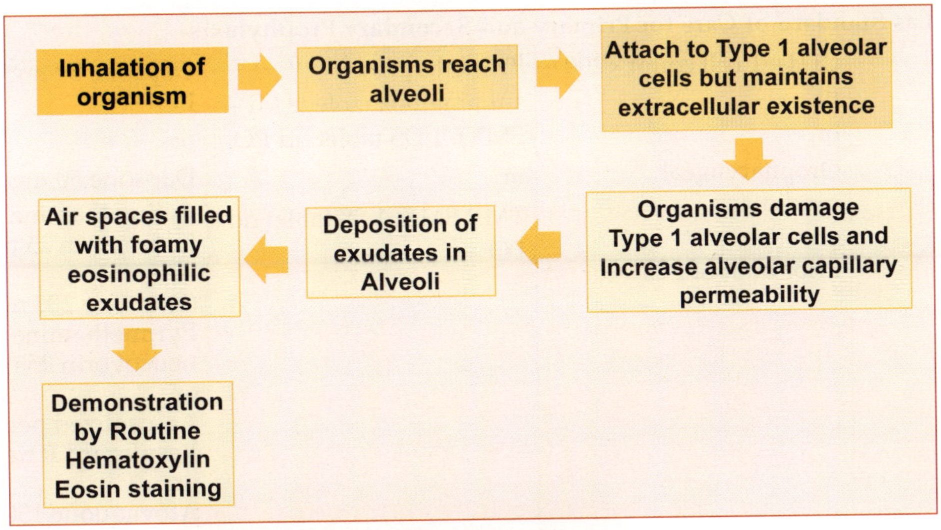

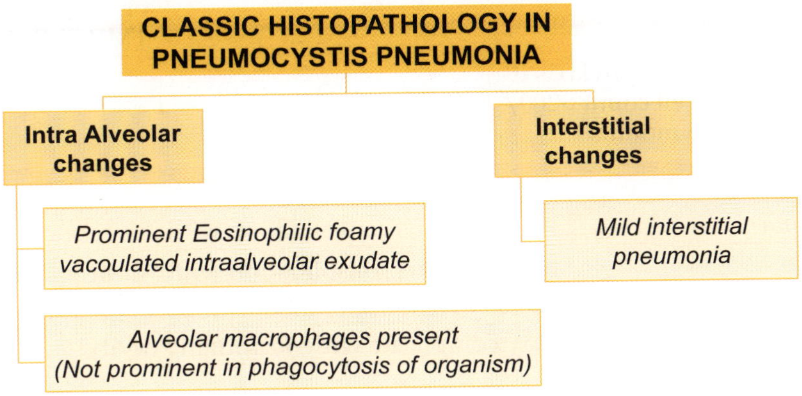

- Patients with PCP generally present with **fever and cough** that is usually **nonproductive** or productive of only scant amounts of white sputum.
- Affected parts of lung are consolidated, dry and grey.

Risk for Pneumocystis Pneumonia
• HIV with CD4 count <200/ml • Patients receiving Immunosuppressive therapy • Organ transplantation • Children with primary immunodeficiency • Premature malnourished children

- Definitive diagnosis of PCP requires demonstration of organism in samples obtained from induced sputum, bronchoalveolar lavage, transbronchial biopsy, or open-lung biopsy.
- Mainstay of diagnosis of pneumocystis pneumonia–***Bronchoalveolar lavage.***
- Most sensitive test–DNA Amplification by PCR.
- Fibreoptic bronchoscopy with Bronchoalveolar lavage is more sensitive than sputum examination and remains mainstay of diagnosis of PCP.
- *Treatment of choice*–Trimethoprim + Sulphamethoxazole.

NIH/CDC/IDSA 2013 Guidelines for the Prevention of Opportunistic Infections in Persons Infected with HIV

Pathogen	Indications	First Choice(s)	Alternatives
Recommended as Standard of Care for Primary and Secondary Prophylaxis			
Pneumocystis jirovecii	CD4+ T cell count <200/ µL or Oropharyngeal candidiasis or Prior bout of PCP	Trimethoprim sulfamethoxazole (TMP-SMX), 1 DS tablet qd PO or TMP-SMX, 1 SS tablet qd PO	Dapsone 50 mg bid PO or 100 mg/d PO or Dapsone 50 mg/d PO + Pyrimethamine 50 mg/week PO + Leucovorin 25 mg/week PO or (Dapsone 200 mg PO + Pyrimethamine 75 mg PO + Leucovorin 25 mg weekly PO) or Aerosolized pentamidine, 300 mg via Respirgard II nebulizer every month or Atovaquone 1500 mg/d PO or TMP-SMX 1 DS tablet 3x/week PO
	May stop prophylaxis if CD4+ T cell count >200/ pL for >3 months		

Pneumonia	
Streptococcus pneumonia	Homogenous consolidation with Air bronchogram
Klebsiella pneumonia	Homogenous consolidation with Air bronchogram Usually right upper lobe with Bulging fissure May complicate with necrotizing cavity

Contd.

Contd.

Gram –ve bacilli and Mixed anerobes	Unilateral/Bilateral extensive alveolar consolidation
Pneumocystis carinii	Bilateral diffuse air space involvement mainly perihilar region with peripheral sparing
Staphylococcus	Pneumatocele (Younger age), Bronchopneumonia
Mycoplasma, P. carinii, Sarcoidosis, Bleomycin and Methotrexate toxicity, Post radiation	Interstitial pneumonia (Peribronchovascular infiltrates) Diffuse and Bilateral alveolar opacities
Cavity	TB, Staphylococcus aureus, Aspergillosis, Histoplasmosis, Septic emboli, Granulomatosis with polyangitis
Lung abscess	Necrotizing pneumonia, Complicated aspiration pneumonia
Nodular infiltrates round pneumonia size >1 cm	Random, Centrilobular (Tree in bud), Perilymphatic

Risk Factor	Etiology
Alcoholism	Streptococcus pneumonia
Alcoholic with red currant jelly sputum	Klebsiella pneumoniae
Structural lung disease	Pseudomonas aeuroginosa
Dementia, Stroke	Oral anaerobes
Lung abscess	Community acquired MRSA, Oral anaerobes
Ventilator associated pneumonia	**Non MDR**–Streptococcus pneumoniae **MDR**–Pseudomonas
COPD/Smoking	Haemophilus influenza
Bird Handler's Pneumonia	Chlamydia psittaci

Ref: Harrison 20th Edition Page 1430

Ans: (B) Pneumocystis jirovecii

2. A person with chest pain, palpitation with BP of 80/60 mm of Hg. ECG shows PSVT. What is the treatment of this condition?

A. IV adenosine

B. DC cardioversion

C. Propranolol

D. Lignocaine

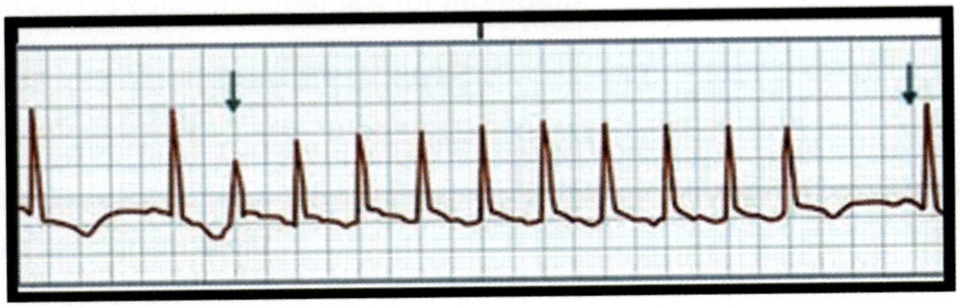

Key:

ECG shown above is consistent with findings of PSVT

PSVT

- Most common form of paroxysmal supraventricular tachycardia (PSVT) is due to AV nodal re-entry with dual AV nodal pathways.
- Identification of P waves is difficult or impossible because atrial and ventricular depolarisations occur simultaneously.
- Occasionally, abnormal P waves may follow QRS complexes.
- Ventricular rate varies from 170 to 250/min.
- Rhythm is absolutely regular, i.e., the RR interval is constant.
- QRS morphology is usually normal.
- ST segment may be depressed, and T wave may be inverted.
- PSVT most commonly occurs in individuals with structurally normal hearts.
- It is precipitated by an atrial premature beat.
- Occasionally PSVT occurs in association with Wolff-Parkinson-White or LownGanong-Levine syndrome.

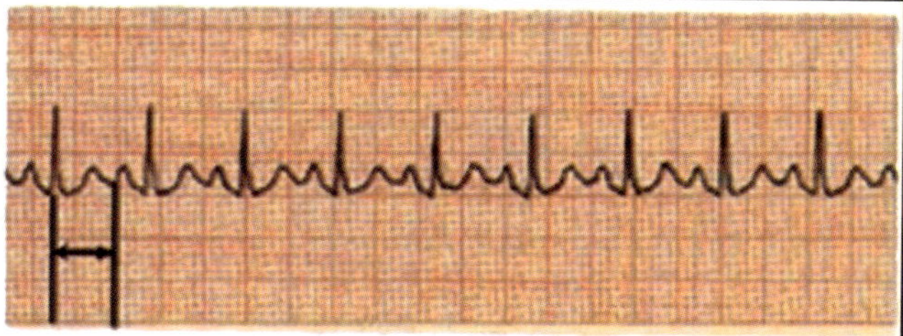

Long R-P tachycardia

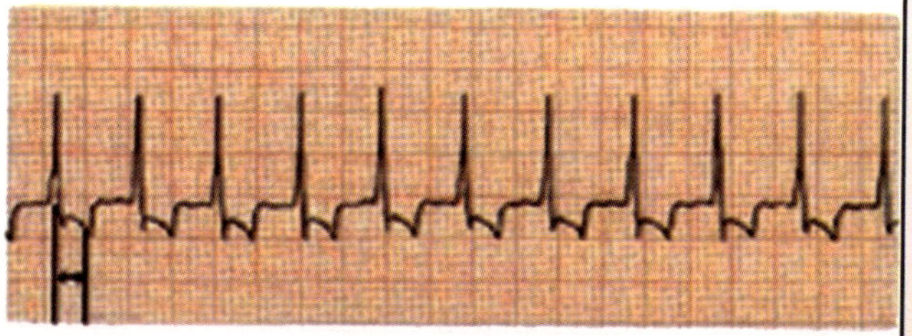

Short R-P tachycardia

Algorithm for Hemodynamically stable paroxysmal supraventricular tachycardia

HEMODYNAMICALLY STABLE REGULAR, NARROW QRS TACHYCARDIA

↓

Vagal maneuvers, IV adenosine, IV verapamil/diltiazem → Termination

↓

No termination

↓

IV ibutilide + AV nodal-blocking agent, IV procainamide + AV nodal-blocking agent
Cardioversion

Tachycardia

1 TACHYCARDIA
With Pulses and Poor Perfusion
- Assess and support ABCs as needed
- Give oxygen
- Attach monitor/defibrillator

Symptoms Persist

2 Evaluate QRS duration

Narrow QRS (≤0.008 sec) → **3 Evaluate rhythm with 12-lead ECG or monitor**

Wide QRS (>0.08 sec) → **9 Possible ventricular Tachycardia**

4 Probable Sinus Tachycardia
- Compatible history consistent with known cause
- P waves present/normal
- Variable R-R; constant P-R
- Infants: Rate usually < 220 bpm
- Children: Rate usually <180

6 Search for and treat cause

5 Probable Supraventricular Tachycardia
- Compatible history (vague, nonspecific)
- P waves absent/abnormal
- HR not variable
- History of abrupt rate changes
- Infants: rate usually ≥ 220 bpm
- Children rate usually ≥ 180 bpm

7 Consider vagal maneuvers (no delays)

8
- If IV access readily available:
  Give adenosine 0.1 mg/mg (maximum first dose 6 mg) by rapid bolus
  May double first dose and give once (maximum second dose 12 mg)
  or
- Synchronized cardioversion: 0.5 to 1 J/kg; If not effective, increase to 2 J/kg
  Sedate if possible but don't delay cardiovesion

10
- Synchronized cardioversion: 0.5 to 1 J/kg; if not effective; increase to 2 J/kg
  Sedate if possible but don't delay cardioversion
- May attempt adenosine if it does not delay electrical cardioversion

11 Expert consultation advised
- Amiodarone 5 mg/kg IV over 20 to 60 minutes
  or
- Procainamide 15 mg/kg IV over 30 to 60 minutes

Do not routinely administer amiodarone and procainamide together

During Evaluation
- Secure, verify airway and vascular access when possible
- Consider expert consultation
- Prepare for cardioversion

Treat possible contributing factors:
- Hypovolemia
- Hypoxia
- Hydrogen ion (acidosis)
- Hypo-/hyperkalemia
- Hypoglycemia
- Hypothermia
- Toxins
- Tamponade, cardiac
- Tension pneumothorax
- Thrombosis (coronary or pulmonary)
- Trauma (hypovolemia)

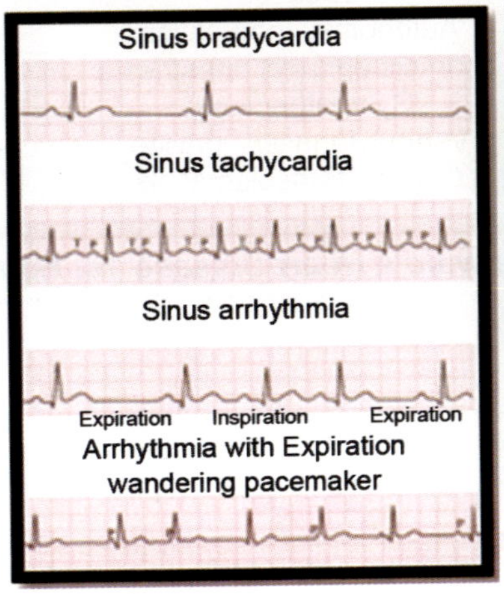

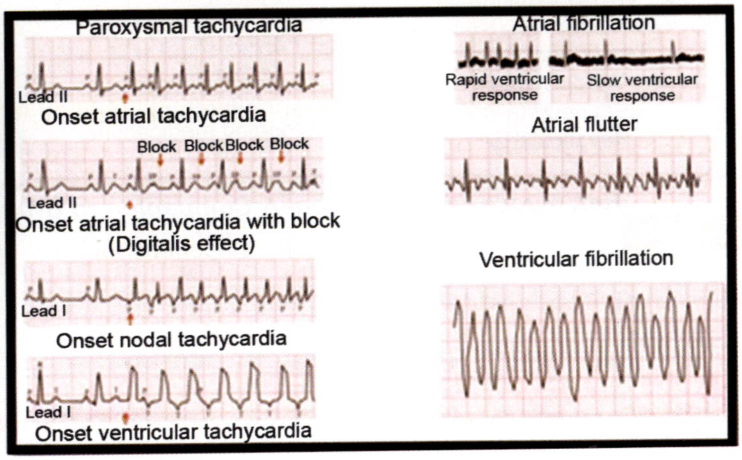

Ref: Harrison 20th Edition Page 1743

Ans: (B) DC cardioversion

3. **Drug of choice for ventricular tachycardia with myocardial ischemia:**

A. Propanolol
B. Lignocaine
C. Diltiazem
D. Adenosine

Key:

Class 1C antiarrhythmics are contraindicated in setting of myocardial ischemia owing to their proarrhythmic potential

Antiarrhythmics such as Amiodarone or Lidocaine may be considered in acute phase

- **Class 1C antiarrhythmics** are **contraindicated** in setting of MI owing to their **proarrhythmic potential.**
- **Sustained VT and VF** in setting of **myocardial infarction** result from complex interaction of multiple factors, including myocardial ischemia (with resulting local electrolyte abnormalities), necrosis, reperfusion, healing, and scar formation. In addition, there are autonomic changes (especially activation of the sympathetic nervous system and elevated levels of catecholamines) resulting from infarction that have an important impact. These events produce mechanisms that initiate arrhythmias and substrate for arrhythmia perpetuation. Arrhythmia pathogenesis varies at different stages in this process. For ventricular arrhythmias occurring more than 48 to 72 hours after an acute MI, scar formation is of primary importance.
- **Ventricular arrhythmias** during acute MI are typically classified based upon their time of onset. This scheme is useful clinically because **VT & VF** occurring early (≤24 to 48 hours) have been thought to be epiphenomena of MI and do not require long-term therapy because they are not associated with ***worse prognosis after hospital discharge.*** In contrast, VT or VF occurring later is generally thought to reflect development of arrhythmic substrate, and require chronic therapy because of an increased risk of sudden cardiac death.

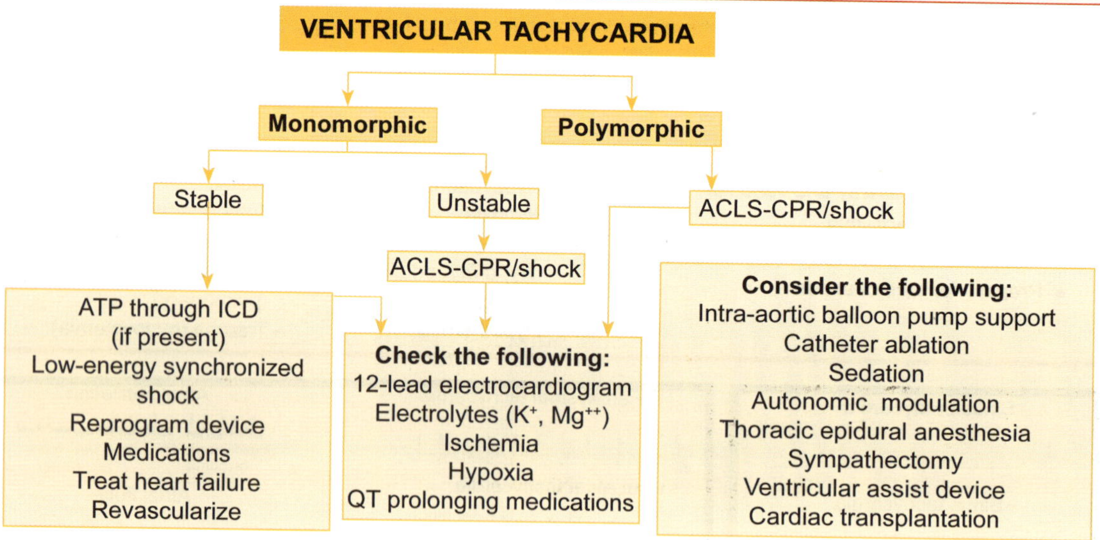

Ref: Myocardial Infarction–A Companion to Braunwald's Heart Disease 1st Edition Page 349

Ans: (B) Lignocaine

4. **Which wall is involved in post MI aneurysm formation?**

A. Posteroinferior
B. Anteroinferior
C. Lateral
D. Medial

Key:

Ventricular aneurysms may develop in few patients following Especially Anterior wall MI (Large MI)

- True LV Aneurysm is defined as well delineated, thin, scarred, or fibrotic wall, devoid of muscle or containing necrotic muscle, that is a result of healed transmural myocardial infarction.
- Involved wall segment is either akinetic (without movement) or dyskinetic (with paradoxical ballooning) during systole, and collapses inward when ventricle is fully vented during surgery.
- Aneurysms of apex and anterior wall are more than four times as common as those of **inferior/inferoposterior walls.**
- Although size of an aneurysm varies widely, ***most are between 1 and 8 cm in diameter.***
- There may be persistent elevation of ST segment; however, this finding is usually result of large area of scar and does not necessarily imply an aneurysm.
- American College of Cardiology/American Heart Association (ACC/AHA) guidelines on ST elevation MI concluded that it is reasonable (class IIa recommendation) to consider aneurysmectomy, accompanied by CABG, in patients with an LVA who have intractable ventricular arrhythmias and/or heart failure unresponsive to medical and catheter-based therapy.

Features	Anterior MI	Inferior MI
1. Extent of necrosis	Large	Small
2. Extent of coronary atherosclerosis	Small	Large
3. Complications		
a. Ventricular septal rupture	Apical, easily repaired	Basal, difficult to repair
b. Aneurysm	Common	Uncommon
c. Free wall rupture	Uncommon	Rare
d. Mural thrombus	Common	Uncommon
e. Heart block	Uncommon	Common
f. Bundle branch blocks	Common	Uncommon
4. Prognosis	Worse than that of inferior MI	Better than that of anterior MI
5. Diagnosis		
a. Symptoms	Gastrointestinal symptoms unusual	Gastrointestinal symptoms (nausea, vomiting, hiccough) common
b. Physical examination	Tachycardia; hypotension uncommon, Jugular venous distention less common than with inferior MI 50% have S_3	Bradycardia; hypotension common, Jugular venous distention common, 20% have S_3
c. ECG	Features of anterior wall MI	Features of inferior wall MI
d. Echocardiogram	Abnormal left ventricular wall motion is anterior in location. No abnormal right ventricular wall motion	Abnormal left ventricular wall motion is inferior in location. Right ventricular abnormal wall motion present in approximately one-third of patients

Ref: Myocardial Infarction–Companion to Braunwald's Heart Disease 1st Edition Page 415, Friedman Clinical Cardiology Page 507

Ans: (B) Anteroinferior

5. **True regarding decerebrate posturing:**
   A. Abnormal extension of upper and lower extremities
   B. Abnormal flexion of upper and lower extremities
   C. Abnormal extension of upper and flexion of lower extremities
   D. Abnormal flexion of upper and extension of lower extremities

Version 2

Which of the following is false in decerebrate rigidity?

A. Upper limb flexed lower limb extended
B. Both upper and lower limbs extended
C. Lesion between the superior and inferior colliculi produces this rigidity
D. Cutting dorsal root abolishes the rigidity

Ans: (A) Upper limb flexed lower limb extended

Key:

Abnormal Extension of upper and lower extremities occurs in Decerebrate rigidity
Lesion lies between superior and inferior colliculus
Cutting dorsal root abolishes rigidity

Flexion of upper limbs at elbow and extension of lower limbs occurs in Decorticate rigidity

DECEREBRATE RIGIDITY

- Decerebrate rigidity (DR) in humans results from a **midbrain lesion** and is manifested by an **exaggerated extensor posture of all extremities.**
- Characterized by shortening and lengthening reactions and can be modified by tonic neck, labyrinthine (Magnus-de Kleijn), and phasic spinal reflexes.
- Factor in the best motor response of the GCS and should be assigned major importance in the prognosis of comatose head-injured patients.
- Describes involuntary extension of upper extremities in response to external stimuli.
- Hallmark of decerebrate posturing is **extended elbows*.**
- ***Arms and legs are extended and rotated internally.***
- Patient is rigid, with teeth clenched.
- **Decerebration reveals tonic, static postural reflex mechanisms maintained by:**
  - Brainstem reticular formation
  - Facilitates gamma motor neuron activity (gamma rigidity)
  - Vestibulospinal system
  - Facilitates alpha motor neuron activity (alpha rigidity)
- Complete pattern of decerebrate rigidity is extension in all four limbs, although the complete decerebration pattern is rarely observed in humans.
- No phenomena akin to spinal shock, as rigidity occurs as soon as the brainstem stops functioning.
- Progression from decorticate to decerebrate rigidity is an ominous sign, as it indicates that lesion is progressing from cortex to brainstem and decerebration is usually fatal.
- ***Final step in this progression would be elimination of brainstem and vestibulospinal inputs, which causes muscles to become flaccid (as patient dies).***

Decerebrate Rigidity	Decorticate Rigidity
Extensive extensor posture (All arms extended)	Flexor posturing (Arms flexed and adducted)
Jaws clenched and Neck retracted	Legs and often trunk extended
Righting reflexes absent	Righting reflexes present

Contd.

Contd.

Temperature regulation absent	Temperature regulation Normal
Only standing posture can be maintained	Can stand and walk reflexly, placing and hopping.

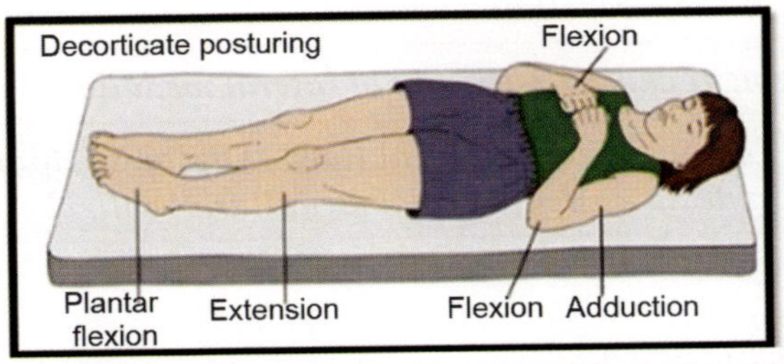

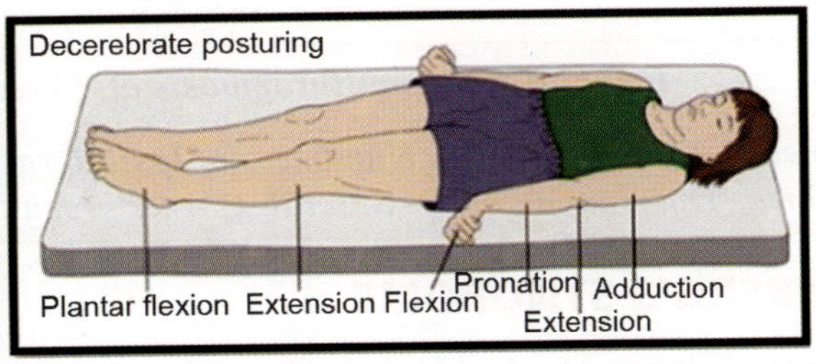

Decorticate rigidity Upper midbrain damage 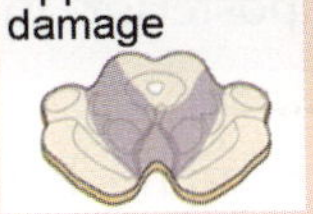	• Removal of **cerebral cortex (decortication)** • Characterized by **flexion of the upper limbs** at **elbow and extension of lower limbs.** • **Flexion of Upper limbs is due to rubrospinal excitation of flexor muscles.** • **Extension** of **lower limbs** occurs due to excitation from **reticulospinal pathways.**
Decerebrate rigidity Upper pontine damage 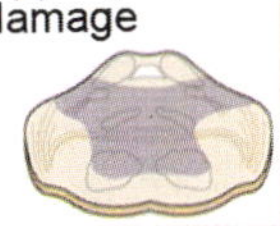	• Complete transection at **midcollicular level (midcollicular decerebration).** • In this lesion, **corticospinal, corticobulbar tracts and rubrospinal tract** that innervate primarily to **distal muscles** of extremities are interrupted. **Reticulospinal pathways** that innervate **postural extensor muscles** remain **intact.** • Dominance of drive from ascending sensory pathways to the excitatory reticulospinal pathway leads to **hyperactivity in extensor muscles** in all four extremities which is called **decerebrate rigidity.** • Decerebrate rigidity is due to excitatory input from the **reticulospinal pathway** that activates **γ-motor neurons** which further activates **α-motor neurons (Gamma Loop).**

Ans : (A) Abnormal extension of upper and lower extremities

Another Version

True about decorticate rigidity:

A. Extension of lower limbs and Flexion of upper limbs

B. Flexion of lower limbs and Extension of upper limbs

C. Flexion of both upper and lower limbs

D. Extension of both upper and lower limbs

Flexion of upper limbs at elbow and extension of lower limbs occurs in Decorticate rigidity

Ans: (A) Extension of lower limbs and Flexion of upper limbs

Ref: Harrison 20th Edition Page 2071, Ganong's Review of Medical Physiology 26th Edition Page 238, Comprehensive Textbook of Physiology by GK Pal Page 1075, Textbook of Medical Physiology by Indu Khurana 2nd Edition Page 529

6. **Thrombosis of posterior inferior cerebellar artery leads to:**

A. Wallenberg syndrome
B. Medial medullary syndrome
C. Median Pontine syndrome
D. Lateral Pontine syndrome

Key:

Posterior inferior cerebellar artery in its proximal segment supplies lateral medulla and in its distal branches, inferior surface of the cerebellum
Embolic occlusion/thrombosis of V4 segment causes ischemia of lateral medulla
Constellation of Vertigo, Numbness of Ipsilateral Face and Contralateral limbs, Diplopia, Hoarseness, Dysarthria, Dysphagia and Ipsilateral Horner's syndrome is called Lateral medullary/Wallenberg syndrome

WALLENBERG'S SYNDROME

- Hemiparesis is not a typical feature of vertebral artery occlusion; however, quadriparesis may result from occlusion of anterior spinal artery
- Lateral medullary syndrome (occlusion of any of 5 vessels may be responsible—vertebral, posterior inferior cerebellar, superior, middle, or inferior lateral medullary arteries)
- **On side of lesion:** Pain, numbness, impaired sensation over one-half the face: Descending tract and nucleus fifth nerve
- **Ataxia of limbs, falling to side of lesion:** Uncertain—restiform body, cerebellar hemisphere, cerebellar fibers, spinocerebellar tract
- Nystagmus, diplopia, oscillopsia, vertigo, nausea, vomiting: Vestibular nucleus Horner's syndrome–***Descending sympathetic tract***
- Dysphagia, hoarseness, paralysis of palate, paralysis of vocal cord, diminished gag reflex: Issuing fibers ninth and tenth nerves Loss of taste: ***Nucleus tractus solitarius***
- Numbness of ipsilateral arm, trunk, or leg: ***Cuneate and gracile nuclei***
- Weakness of lower face: Genu flected upper motor neuron fibers to I/L facial nucleus
- **On side opposite lesion:** Impaired pain and thermal sense over half the body, sometimes face: Spinothalamic tract

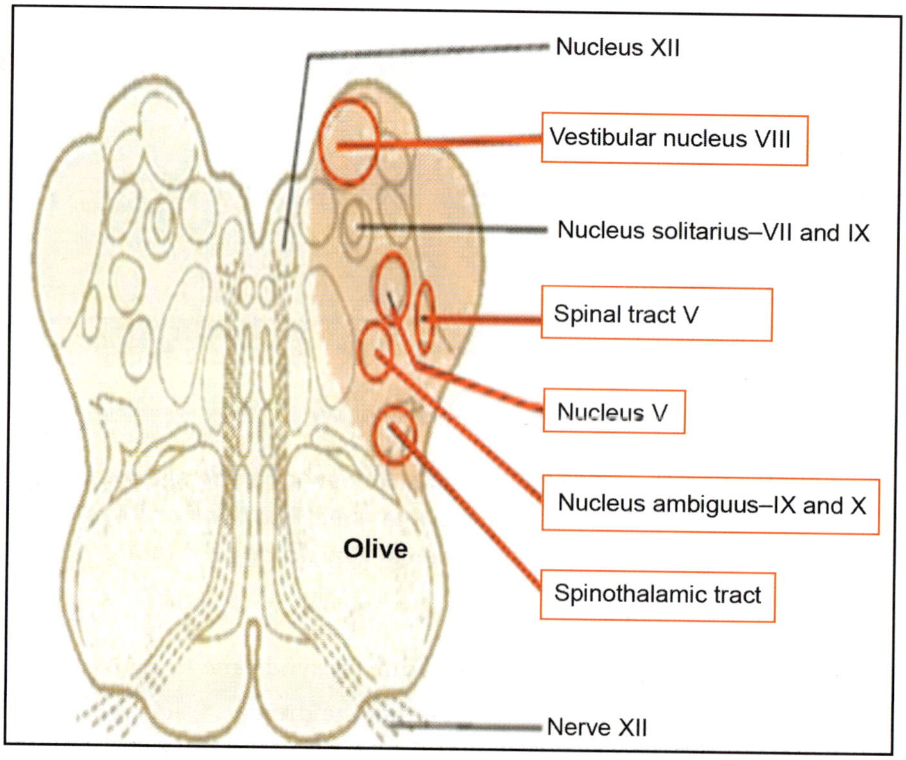

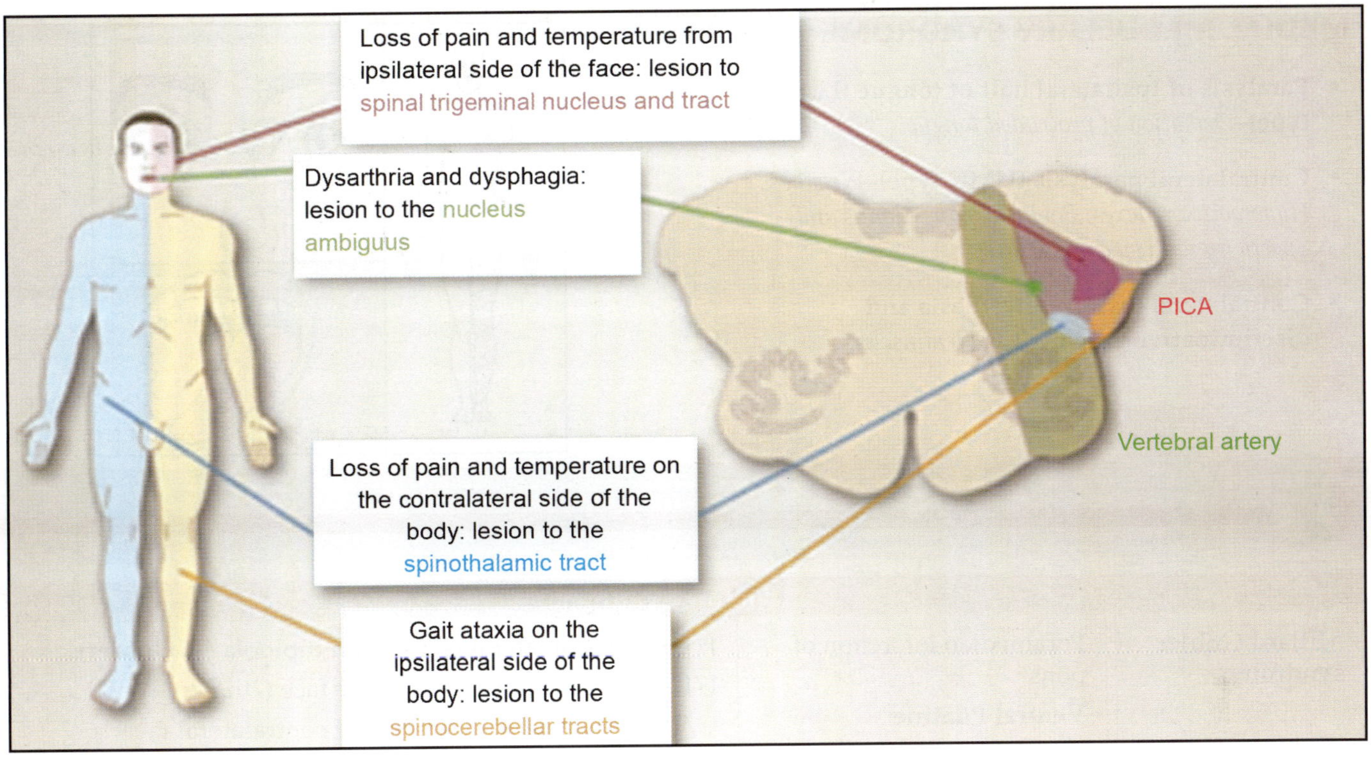

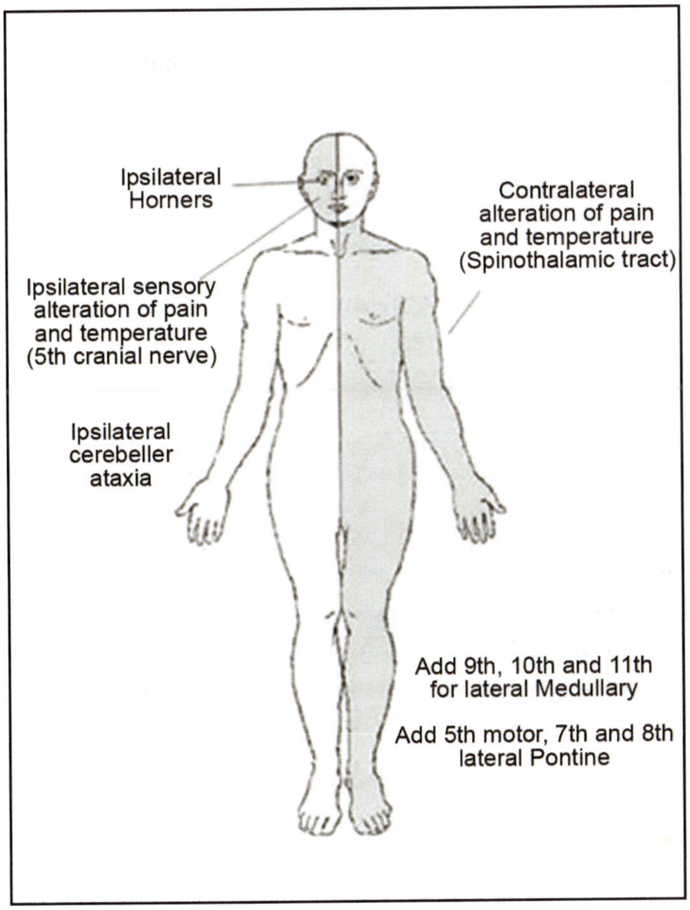

Anatomical location	Presenting symptoms
Spinothalamic tract	Contralateral loss of pain and temperature sensation
Spinal trigeminal nucleus	Ipsilateral facial loss of pain and temperature
Nucleus ambiguus	Supplies vagus and glossopharyngeal nerves; dysphagia/dysphonia/ diminished gag reflex
Inferior vestibular nucleus	Vertigo/diplopia/nystagmus/ vomiting
Sympathetic fibres	Ipsilateral Horners syndrome
Central trigeminal tract	Palatal clonus
Inferior cerebellar peduncle	Ataxia

MEDIAL MEDULLARY SYNDROME

- **Paralysis of Ipsilateral half of tongue (LMN type)**–*Deviation of protruded tongue*
- **Contralateral paralysis (UMN type)**–*Weakness, Hyperactive reflexes, Babinski sign, Clonus and Spasticity with sparing of face*
- **Contralateral loss of kinesthesia and discriminative touch**–*Medial lemniscus*

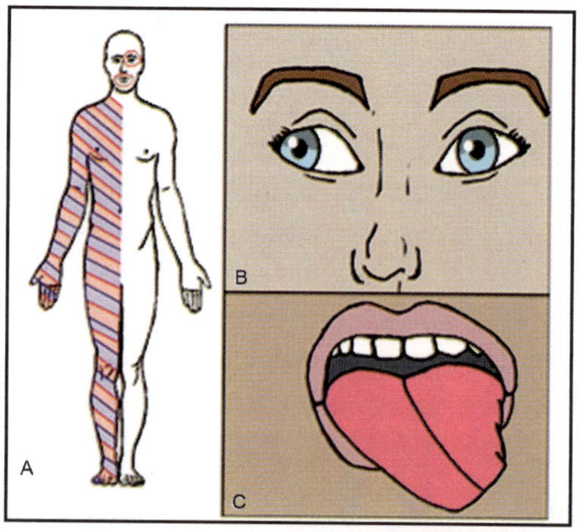

Pontine Syndrome		
Millard Gubler syndrome	Paramedian infarction of pons **Ventral Pontine**	I/L paresis of lateral rectus with diplopia (Abducent) I/L damage of upper and lower face (7th nerve) C/L hemiplegia with sparing of contralateral face
Fovelli syndrome	Lesion in dorsal tegmentum of lower pons **Lower Dorsal Pontine**	I/L horizontal gaze palsy (Abducent nerve and PPRF) I/L paresis of whole face (7th Nerve fibers) C/L hemiplegia with sparing of contralateral face (Corticospinal tract)
Raymond Ceston syndrome	Obstruction of Long circumferential branches of basilar artery **Upper Dorsal Pontine**	I/L ataxia and coarse intention tremor (Superior and Middle cerebellar peduncle) I/L Paralysis of muscles of mastication and Sensory loss in face (5th Nerve) C/L Loss of sensory modalities in body (Spinothalamic and Medial leminiscus) C/L Hemiparesis of face and body Horizontal gaze palsy
Locked in syndrome	Most common cause of pontine infarction **Bilateral Ventral Pontine Lesion**	Quadriplegic (B/L damage to corticospinal tract in ventral pons) Unable to speak and Incapable of facial movements (Corticobulbar tracts) Limited horizontal eye movements Intact vertical eye movements and blinking Preserved consciousness

Mid Brain Syndromes				
Syndrome	Site	Nerve	Tract	Features
Weber syndrome	Base of brain	III	Corticospinal tract	Ipsilateral 3rd nerve palsy Contralateral hemiplegia including face

Contd.

Contd.

Claude syndrome	Tegmentum of midbrain	**III**	Red nucleus and Brachium conjunctivum	Ipsilateral 3rd nerve palsy Contralateral hemiataxia and hemiasynergia
Benedikt syndrome	Tegmentum of midbrain	**III**	Red nucleus, Corticospinal tract and Brachium conjuctivum	Ipsilateral 3rd nerve palsy Contralateral hemiparesis including face Contralateral intention tremor
Parinaud syndrome	Dorsal midbrain	–	Superior colliculus	Bilateral vertical palsy (Upward gaze palsy) Bilateral convergence paralysis, Fixed pupil
Nothnagel syndrome	Tectum of midbrain	**U/L or B/L III**	Superior cerebellar peduncle	Ocular palsy, Gaze paralysis and Cerebellar ataxia

Ref: Harrison 20th Edition Page 3074

Ans: (A) Wallenberg syndrome

7. Conjunctival injection with jaundice is characteristic of:

A. Malaria
B. Enteric fever
C. Leptospirosis
D. Hepatitis B

Key:

Conjunctival injection with jaundice is characteristic of Leptospirosis

Leptospirosis/Weil's Disease

- Leptospira–Actively mobile spirochete with hooked end
- Zoonotic disease

Mode of transmission:

- Indirect contact with water, Moist soil and wet surfaces contaminated with animal urine
- Direct contact with urine and products of parturition, placenta of infected animals

Direct human to human transmission doesn't occur

- **Sources of infection**–Rats, Dogs, Cattle and Pigs

Rodents, Rainfall and Ricefield–Epidemiological determinants for Leptospirosis

Clinical Features

- **Incubation period:** Around 5-14 days
- High grade fever
- Jaundice and Raised Liver enzymes
- ***Pulmonary–Most common*** (Hemorrhages)
- Kidney–Raised serum urea and creatinine

Contd.

Contd.

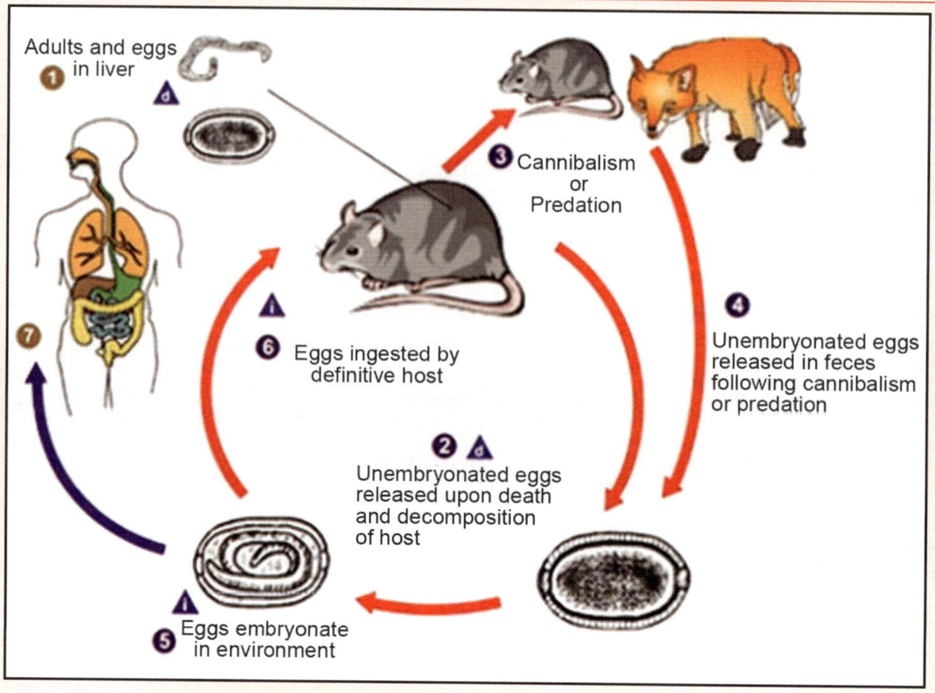

LEPTOSPIROSIS

- Anicteric febrile illness
  - *Most common (90%)*
    Mild form
    Most common finding–Fever with conjunctival suffusion
- Weil's disease
  - *Hepatorenal form (5-10%)*
    High grade fever, Jaundice and Raised Liver enzymes
    Hemorrhagic diathesis,
    Hepatosplenomegaly

Lab Diagnosis

- ***Gold Standard serodiagnostic method–Microscopic agglutination test***
- It is specific but has inherent complexity (Alternative screening tests–ELISA, IHA and Macroscopic slide agglutination test)
- ***Definite diagnosis is based on either isolation of organism from patient or on seroconversion or rise in antibody titer in MAT***

Diagnostic test	Method	Test accuracy
Microscopy	Gram stain	Organisms too thin to be detected
	Darkfield examination	Insensitive, nonspecific
	Silver impregnation stain	Insensitive, specific
	Direct fluorescent antibody	Insensitive, specific
Culture	Blood	Positive during first 10 days
	Cerebrospinal fluid	Positive during first 10 days
	Urine	Positive after first week

Contd.

Contd.

Serology	Indirect hemagglutination	Insensitive, nonspecific
	Slide agglutination	Insensitive, nonspecific
	ELISA	Insensitive, nonspecific
	Microscopic agglutination test	Sensitive, specific serovar specific
Molecular methods	Direct hybridization	Insensitive, specific
	Polymerase chain reaction	Sensitive, specific

Treatment

- **Mild cases**–Doxycycline/Ampicillin/Amoxicillin
- **Moderate to severe cases**–Pencillin G/Ampicillin/Amoxicillin/Erythromycin
- *Doxycycline–Drug of choice for chemoprophylaxis*
- **Vasculitis**–*Most important manifestation of Kidney and Liver disease*
- *When antibodies are formed, Leptospira gets eliminated from all sites except Eye, Proximal renal tubules and Brain.*

Classical features	Infections
Fever, Jaundice and Conjuctivitis	***Leptospirosis***
Fever and Splenomegaly	***Enteric fever***
Fever and Eschar	***Scrub typhus***
Fever with chills (Intermittent), Splenomegaly	***Malaria***
Fever, Arthralgia and Rash	***Dengue***

Ref: Harrison 20th Edition Page 1290

Ans: (C) Leptospirosis

8. **Patient who is a known case of Acute pancreatitis presents with Breathlessness and Basal crepitations on day 4. Chest X-ray is shown below. Most probable diagnosis is:**

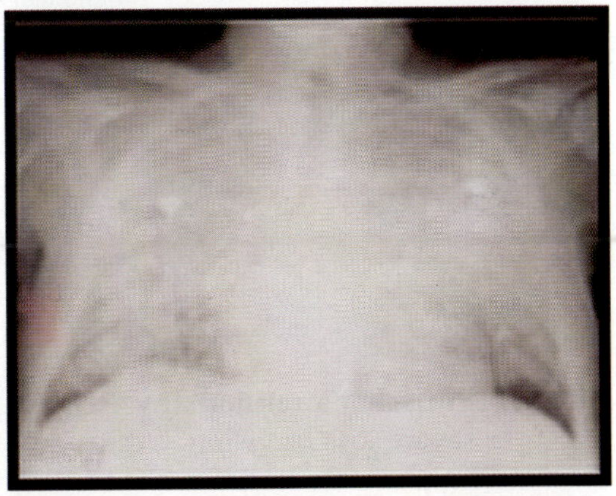

A. Lung collapse
B. ARDS
C. Pleural effusion
D. Aspiration pneumonia

Key:

Given Image of Chest X-ray shows Diffuse alveolar interstitial shadowing in Acute pancreatitis. ARDS is a dangerous complication of Acute pancreatitis

- **Acute lung injury and Acute respiratory distress syndrome** in **acute pancreatitis** still represents a substantial problem, with mortality rate of **30%-40%.**
- ALI is a consequence of a pronounced systemic inflammatory response with increased endothelial and epithelial barrier permeability, with leakage of protein-rich exudate into alveolar space and interstitial tissues, thus compromising oxygenation and gas exchange.
- Acute respiratory failure, including ALI and more severe form, ARDS, has radiological findings with bilateral pulmonary infiltrates.

- **Acute pancreatitis-associated acute lung injury (ALI)**–Potential mechanisms including endothelial barrier dysfunction. Several adhesion molecules [selectins, intercellular adhesion molecule-1 (ICAM-1), platelet endothelial cell adhesion molecule-1 (PECAM-1) among others] involved in the extravasation of not at least polymorphonuclear neutrophils (PMNs). Tissue injury by not at least these PMNs.

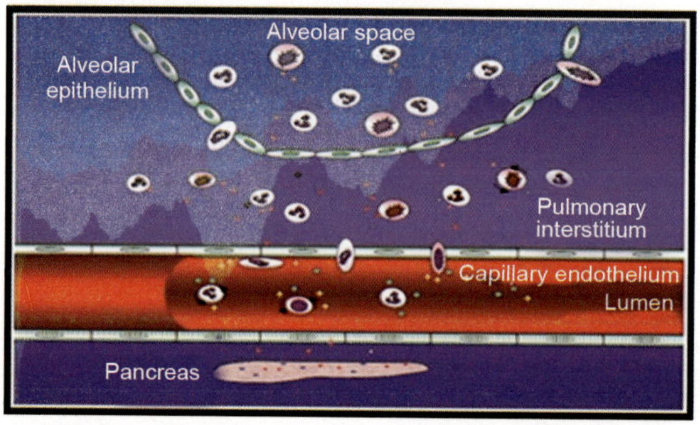

Complications

- Acute–Necrosis and Infected necrotic fluid collections
- Chronic–Diabetes mellitus
- Miscellaneous–Splanchnic vein thrombosis, Pseudoaneurysm, Abdominal compartment syndrome

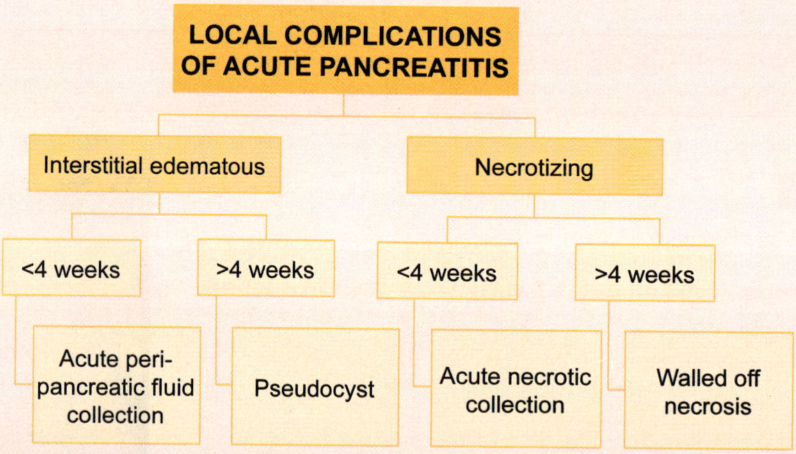

- **Purtscher's retinopathy**–Relatively unusual complication of acute pancreatitis. Manifested by sudden and severe loss of vision. Occlusion of posterior retinal artery with aggregated granuocytes→Cottonwool spots and haemorrhages confined to optic disc and macula.

Ref: Harrison 20th Edition Page 2441

Ans: (B) ARDS

9. **Drug used in treatment of Hypertension and pulmonary edema caused by Scorpion sting is:**

A. Prazosin B. Clonidine
C. Furosemide D. Mannitol

Key:

Drug used in treatment of Hypertension and pulmonary edema caused by Scorpion sting is Prazosin

Scorpion Bite

- More venomous black widow spiders ***(Latrodectus mactans)*** causes generalized muscular pains, muscle spasms and rigidity.
- Brown recluse spider ***(Loxosceles reclusa)*** causes progressive local necrosis as well as hemolytic reactions.
- Stings by more toxic ***Centruroides species*** may cause muscle cramps, twitching and jerking, and occasionally hypertension, convulsions and pulmonary edema.

Management of Lethal Scorpion Sting

- Hospitalization in Emergency unit
- Sedate and control of involuntary movements (Monitored IV Midazolam infusion)
- Hypertension and Pulmonary edema–Prazosin and Nifedipine, Nitroprusside or Hydralazine
- Administrate antivenom

Prazosin

- An α-1 adrenergic receptor blocker **reduces preload, left ventricular impedance** without causing **tachycardia.**
- Reverses metabolic syndrome evoked due to excessive catecholamines release.
- **Prazosin is a pharmacological and physiological antidote to scorpion venom actions–** *Also inhibits sympathetic outflow in CNS.*
- Inhibits **phosphodiesterase,** thereby enhancing **cGMP level** which is one of the mediators of nitric oxide synthesis.
- ***Enhances insulin secretion*** which is inhibited by venom.
- Thus, its pharmacological properties can antagonise the haemodynamic, hormonal and metabolic effects of scorpion venom.
- It can be administered orally in a dose of **250 to 500 µg/Kg in children** and **500 to 1000 µg/kg in adults** and should be repeated **every 3 hourly** until the signs of clinical improvement appear or till dry and cool extremities persist.

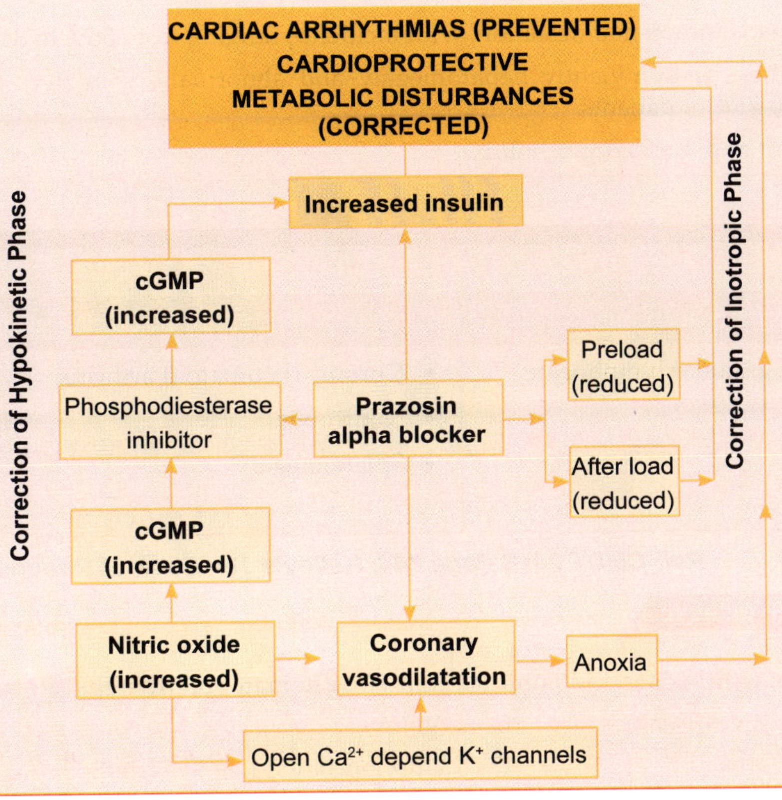

Ref: Harrison 20th Edition Page 3329, API Textbook of Medicine 9th Edition Page 1963, CMDT 2018 Page 1618

Ans: (A) Prazosin

10. Condition with Arthritis, Lymphadenopathy with Hepatomegaly is seen in:

A. Reactive arthritis
B. Adult onset still disease
C. Ritter syndrome
D. Psoriatic arthritis

Key:

AOSD typically manifests as a triad of symptoms that include High-spiking fevers, Characteristic rash and Arthritis/arthralgias
Diagnosis of adult Still disease is strongly suggested by quotidian fever pattern, sore throat and classic rash but requires exclusion of other causes of fever

Adult Onset Still Disease

- Fever transient, lasting typically under 4 hours, generally exceeds 39°C and is most commonly **quotidian/double quotidian** in pattern, with highest temperatures seen in **late afternoon or early evening.**
- Typical rash is an evanescent, salmon-pink, maculopapular eruption, predominantly found on proximal limbs and trunk, with rare involvement of face and distal limbs.
- Arthralgia and arthritis are found in the majority of patients with AOSD, with incidences ranging from 64% to 100%.
- Joints affected most frequently are the knees, wrists and ankles, although involvement of the elbow, shoulder, proximal and distal interphalangeal joints, metacarpophalangeal and metatarsophalangeal joints, temporomandibular joints.
- Myalgia is another common manifestation, with incidence ranging from 56% to 84%.
- Liver abnormalities, predominantly hepatomegaly and abnormalities in liver biochemistry, are present in approximately 50-75% of patients.
- AOSD can present as pseudo-angiocholitis.

Pseudofelty's Syndrome	Felty's Syndrome
• Circulating large granular lymphocyte • Neutropenia • Splenomegaly • Frequent infection	• Chronic rheumatoid arthritis • Neutropenia • Splenomegaly

Ref: CMDT 2018 Page 846, Kelley's Textbook of Rheumatology 9th Edition Page 602

Ans: (B) Adult onset still disease

11. Painful hepatomegaly with ascites and jaundice following hematopoietic stem cell transplantation is seen in:

A. Hepatic veno-occlusive disease
B. GVHD
C. Hepatorenal syndrome
D. Lymphoproliferative disorder

Key:

Painful hepatomegaly with ascites and jaundice following hematopoietic stem cell transplantation is seen in Graft-versus-Host disease

Graft-Versus-Host Disease

- Acute GVHD usually occurs within the first 3 months after allogeneic transplant with peak onset around 4 weeks.
- Characterized by an erythematous **maculopapular rash;** by persistent **anorexia** or **diarrhea**, or both; and by **liver disease** with increased serum levels of **bilirubin, alanine** and **aspartate aminotransferase**, and **alkaline phosphatase.**

Clinical Staging and Grading of Acute Graft-versus-Host Disease

Clinical Stage	Skin	Liver-Bilirubin, μmol/L (mg/dL)	GUT
1	Rash <25% body surface	34-51 (2-3)	Diarrhea 500-1000 mL/d
2	Rash 25-50% body surface	51-103 (3-6)	Diarrhea 1000-1500 mL/d
3	Generalized erythroderma	103-257 (6-15)	Diarrhea >1500 mL/d
4	Desquamation and bullae	>257 (>15)	lleus
Overall Clinical Grade	**Skin Stage**	**Liver Stage**	**Gut Stage**
I	1-2	0	0
II	1-3	1	1
III	1-3	2-3	2-3
IV	2-4	2-4	2-4

Hepatorenal Syndrome

Hepatorenal syndrome occurs in up to 10% of patients with advanced cirrhosis and ascites.

Characterized by

- Azotemia (increase in serum creatinine level of greater than 0.3 mg/dL within 48 hours or increase by 50% or more from baseline within the previous 7 days in the absence of current or recent nephrotoxic drug use.
- Macroscopic signs of structural kidney injury.
- Shock, and
- Failure of kidney function to improve following 2 days of diuretic withdrawal and volume expansion with albumin, 1 g/kg up to maximum of 100 g/day.

Type I hepatorenal syndrome is typically associated with at least doubling of serum creatinine to level >2.5 mg/dL or by halving of the creatinine clearance to <20 mL/min in less than 2 weeks– ***Often irreversible in patients with a systemic infection.***

Type II hepatorenal syndrome is more slowly progressive and chronic. Acute decrease in cardiac output is often precipitating event.

Hepatic Veno- Occlusive Disorder

- Sinusoidal obstruction syndrome.
- This disorder may result from treatment with antineoplastic agents (pre-bone marrow transplant, oxaliplatin) and pyrrolizidine alkaloids.
- Clinical manifestations generally include tender, painful hepatic enlargement, jaundice, splenomegaly and ascites.
- With chronic disease, bleeding varices and hepatic encephalopathy may be evident; hepatopulmonary syndrome may occur.
- ***Screening test of choice is contrast-enhanced, color, or pulsed-Doppler ultrasonography*** (Sensitivity of 85% for detecting evidence of hepatic venous/IVC thrombosis).
- Direct venography can delineate caval webs and occluded hepatic veins ***("spider-web" pattern)*** most precisely.

Post-transplantation Lymphoproliferative Disorders

- Especially B cell lymphoma, are recognized complication associated with immunosuppressive drugs such as azathioprine, tacrolimus and cyclosporine.
- EBV has been shown to play contributory role in these tumors, that may regress when immunosuppressive therapy is reduced.
- De novo neoplasms appear at increased frequency liver transplantation, ***particularly SCC skin.***
- Routine screening should be performed.

Ref: Harrison 20th Edition Page 819

Ans: (B) GVHD

12. Which of the following satisfies major criteria for diagnosing infective endocarditis?

A. 3 cultures positive Streptococcus viridans
B. Single culture positive HACEK
C. Single culture positive Borrelia vincenti
D. Culture positive Enterococci

Key:

Single culture positive Borrelia vincenti satisfies criteria of Diagnosing Infective Endocarditis

The Modified Duke Criteria for the Clinical Diagnosis of Infective Endocarditis[a]

Major Criteria

1. Positive blood culture

Typical microorganism for infective endocarditis from two separate blood cultures

- Viridans streptococci, Streptococcus gallolyticus, HACEK group organisms, Staphylococcus aureus, ***or***
- Community-acquired enterococci in the absence of a primary focus,

or

Peristently positive blood culture, defined as recovery of a microorganism consistent with infective endocarditis from:

- Blood cultures drawn $\geq$ 12 hours apart, or

Contd.

Contd.

- All of 3 or a majority of ≥4 separate blood cultures, with first and last drawn at least 1 hour apart

  or

Single positive blood culture for Coxiella burnetii or phase 1 IgG antibody titer of ≥1:800

2. **Evidence of endocardial involvement**

Positive endocardiogram[b]

- Oscillating intracardiac mass on valve or supporting structures or in the path of regurgitant jets or in implanted material, in the absence of an alternative anatomic explanation, *or*
- Abscess, *or*
- New partial dehiscence of prosthetic valve,

  or

New valvular regurgitation (increase or change in pre-existing murmur not sufficient)

Minor Criteria

1. **Predisposition:** Predisposing heart conditions[c] or injection drug use
2. Fever > 38.0°C (≥100.4°F)
3. **Vascular phenomena:** Major arterial emboli, septic pulmonary infarcts, mycotic aneurysm, intracranial hemorrhage, conjunctival hemorrhages, Janeway lesions
4. **Immunologic phenomena:** Glomerulonephritis, Osler's nodes, Roth's spots, rheumatoid factor
5. **Microbiologic evidence:** Positive blood culture but not meeting major criterion, as noted previously,[d] or serologic evidence of active infection with an organism consistent with infective endocarditis

a Definite endocarditis is defined by documentation of two major criteria, of one major criterion and three minor criteria, or of five minor criteria.

b Transesophageal echocardiography is required by optimal assessment of possible prosthetic valve endocarditis or complicated endocarditis.

c Valvular disease with stenosis or regurgitation, presence of a prosthetic valve, congenital heart disease including corrected or partially corrected conditions (except isolated atrial septal defect, repaired ventricular septal defect, or closed patent ductus arteriosus), prior endocarditis, or hypertrophic cardiomyopathy.

d Excluding single positive cultures for coagulase-negative staphylococci and diphtheroids, which are common culture contaminants, or for organisms that do not cause endocarditis frequently, such as gram negative bacilli.

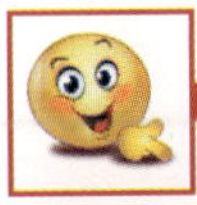

Features of Infective Endocarditis

Clinical features	Lab features
Fever (Most common) Chills and sweats, Anorexia, weight loss, malaise, Myalgias, Arthralgias, Back pain, Heart murmur, New/Worsened regurgitant murmur, Arterial emboli, Splenomegaly, Clubbing, Petechiae, Neurological manifestations **Peripheral manifestations–**Osler nodes, Subungual hemorrhages, Janeway lesions, Roth spots	**Anemia (Most common)** Leukocytosis, Microscopic hematuria, Raised ESR, Raised CRP, Rheumatoid factor, Circulating immune complexes, Reduced serum complement

Ref: Harrison 20th Edition Page 926

Ans: (C) Single culture positive Borrelia vincenti

13. A 40 years lady has unilateral facial pain during eating, 3-4 episodes per week, each episode lasting for 40 to 60 seconds. What is the probable diagnosis?

A. Atypical neuralgia
B. SUNCT
C. Frey's syndrome
D. Trigeminal neuralgia

Key:

Trigeminal Neuralgia

- Characterized by excruciating paroxysms of pain in **lips, gums, cheek, or chin** and very rarely, in distribution of **ophthalmic division of the fifth nerve**.
- Pain seldom lasts more than a few seconds or a minute or two but may be so intense that the patient winces, hence the term tic.
- Paroxysms, experienced as single jabs or clusters, tend to recur frequently, both day and night for several weeks at a time.
- May occur spontaneously or with movements of affected areas evoked by speaking, chewing, or smiling.
- An essential feature of trigeminal neuralgia is that objective signs of sensory loss cannot be demonstrated on examination.

Treatment

- **Carbamazepine** should be started as a single daily dose of 100 mg taken with food and increased gradually (by 100 mg daily in divided doses every 1–2 days) until substantial (>50%) pain relief is achieved.
- **Oxcarbazepine** (300–1200 mg bid) is an alternative to carbamazepine that has less bone marrow toxicity and probably is equally efficacious.

Sites of Headache

Frontal region	Sinusitis > Raised ICT
Temporal region	Giant cell arteritis
Occipital region	Hypertension > Basilar headache

Trigeminal Autonomic Cephalalgia

Character	Cluster headache	SUNCT	Paroxysmal hemicrania
Type and Severity	Stabbing/Boring Excruciating	Burning/Stabbing Severe to Excruciating	Throbbing/Boring, Stabbing Excruciating
Site of pain	Orbit, Temple	Periorbital	Orbit, Temple
Autonomic features	+	++ *(Conjunctival injection and Lacrimation)*	+
Migrainous features	+	+	+
Treatment	Sumatriptan and Oxygen Inhalation	IV Lidocaine	No effective treatment

Ref: Harrison 20th Edition Page 3167

Ans: (D) Trigeminal neuralgia

14. A 14-year-old child with Naïve Rheumatoid arthritis with deformity as shown below. What is treatment if the patient has been awaiting for DMARD therapy?

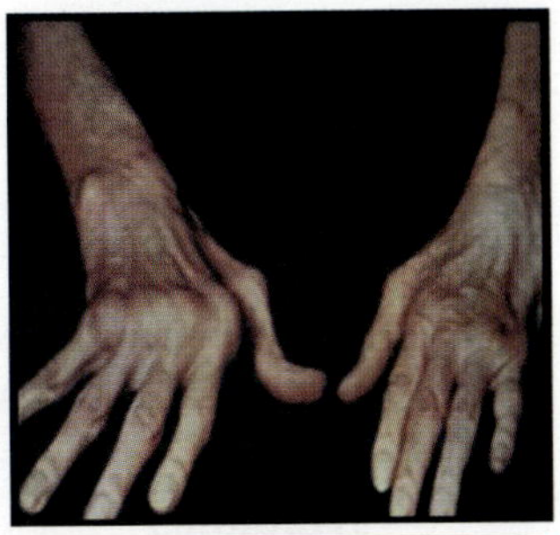

A. DMARDs after initial 3 months NSAIDS

B. Only NSAIDS

C. Monotherapy with TNF drugs

D. DMARDs with short course steroids

Key:

Currently glucocorticoids are most often and most appropriately used along with DMARD's as part of initial "induction" therapy to get RA patients under control rapidly and then aggressively tapered as slower acting DMARD's start to kick in.

Importantly, glucocorticoids should almost never be used in RA without DMARDs.

NSAIDS–Used as an adjunctive therapy for symptomatic management

Role of Steroids in RA

- **Bridging therapy:** Low to moderate doses to achieve rapid disease control before onset of fully effective DMARD therapy which takes several weeks or even months
- **Acute disease flares:** 1 to 2 weeks burst of glucocorticoids may be prescribed for acute disease flare management
- **Inadequate response to DMARD's:** Chronic low dose administration may also be warranted

  Intra articular injections

Rheumatoid Arthritis

- Chronic inflammatory disease of unknown etiology marked by *Symmetric bilateral peripheral polyarthritis*
- Most common form of chronic inflammatory arthritis and often results in joint damage and physical disability
- Women affected 3 times more commonly than men
- Potential for synovial inflammation to cause cartilage damage and bone erosions along with subsequent changes in joint integrity is Hallmark of disease
- HLA DRB1 is associated with pathogenesis of Rheumatoid arthritis
- Most common age group affected between 25 and 55 years
- Earliest involvement occurs in small joints of hands and feet
- Most frequent joints involved–Wrist, MCP and PIP
- DIP is typically spared

Classification Criteria for Rheumatoid Arthritis

		Score
Joint Involvement	1 large joint (shoulder, elbow, hip, knee, ankle)	0
	2-10 large joints	1
	1-3 small joints (MCP, PIP, thumb IP, MTP, wrists)	2
	4-10 small joints	3
	>10 joints (at least 1 small joint)	5

Contd.

Contd.

Serology	Negative RF and negative ACPA Low-positive RF or low-pssitive anti-CCP antibodies (≤ 3 times U/LN) High-positve RF of high-positive anti-CCP antibodies (> 3 times U/LN)	0 2 3
Acute phase reactants	Normal CRP and normal ESR Abnormal CRP or abnormal ESR	0 1
Duration of symptoms	<6 weeks ≥6 weeks	0 1
Note: These criteria are aimed at classification of newly presenting patients who have at least one joint with definite clinical synovitis that is not better explained by another disease. **A score of ≥6 fulfills requirements for definite RA.**		

- ***Flexor tendon tenosynovitis***–Frequent Hallmark of Rheumatoid arthritis
- Irreversible deformities:
  - Piano key movement of Ulnar styloid–Subluxation of Distal ulna
  - ***Boutonniere deformity***–Flexion at PIP and ***Hyperextension at DIP*** **(Code: BD- HD)**
  - Swan neck deformity–Flexion at MCP, Flexion at DIP and Hyperextension at PIP
  - Z line deformity–Subluxation of 1st IP joint
- Axial skeleton involvement is usually limited to cervical spine
- Extra articular manifestations – 40%
- **Most common Extra articular manifestation**–Subcutaneous nodules (20%)
- **Secondary Sjögren's syndrome**–10%
- **Most common pulmonary manifestation**–*Pleuritis*
- **Most common haematological feature**–*Normocytic Normochromic Anemia*
- **Most frequent site of cardiac involvement**–*Pericardium*
- **Most common cause of death**–CVS disease (Coronary artery disease)
- **CAPLAN SYNDROME**–Rheumatoid arthritis associated with Pulmonary nodules and Silica pneumoconiosis ***(Coal workers pneumoconiosis)***

Extra articular manifestations of rheumatoid arthritis

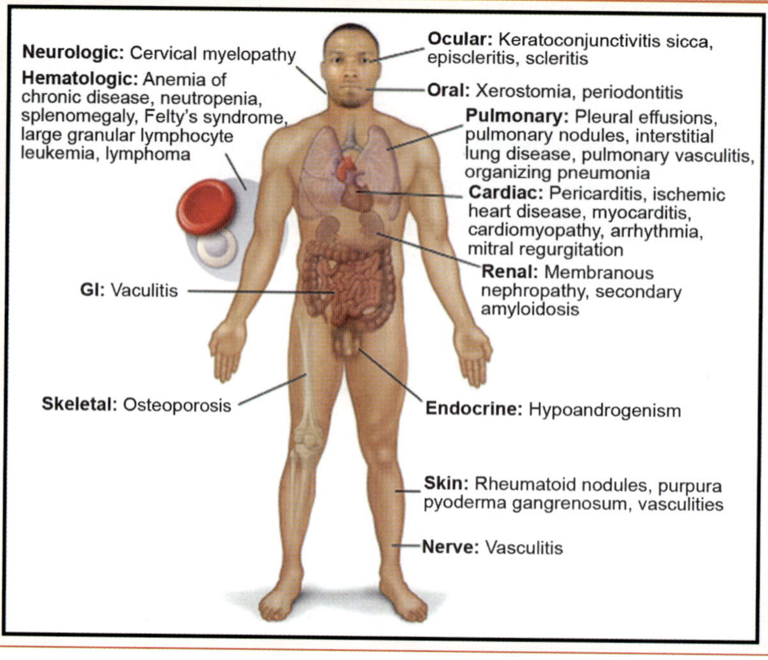

Contd.

Contd.

- **Screening test:** RA factor (Ig M linked to Ig G)
- **Investigation of choice:** Anti cyclic citrulline phospholipid antibody (Anti CCP)
- **Most specific blood test for Rheumatoid arthritis:** Anti CCP Antibody

Treatment

Disease Modifying Anti-Rheumatic Drugs (DMARDs): Standard DMARDs and Biological DMARDs			
Synthetic small molecules empirically found to be effective in the treatment of RA (Standard DMARDs)			**Mechanism-based molecules produced biotechnologically for targeted modification of biological response (Biological DMARDs)**
DMARDs presently used widely	**DMARDs presently used sparingly**	**DMARDs not widely used now**	**Inhibitors of tumour necrosis factor-α (iTNF-α):** Infliximab, etanercept, adlimumab*, certolizumab pegol*
Low-dose methotrexate (LD-MTX), Sulphasalazine, Hydroxychloroquine, Leflunomide	Minocycline, Cyclosporine, Tacrolimus	Organic-gold compounds D-Penicillamine Chloroquine **Cytotoxic drugs:** Azathioprine, cyclophosphamide, chlorambucil, others	**B-cell depletion therapies:** **Rituximab** **Others:** Tocilizumab (inhibitor of IL-6), abatacept (co-stimulation blocker), large number of other molecules in the 'pipeline'

- ***DMARD of choice- Methotrexate***
- Other DMARD's–Methotrexate, Gold compounds, D Pencillamine, Chloroquine, Sulfasalazine
- **Tofacitinib-** Inhibitor of Janus Kinase 3→Used to manage rheumatoid arthritis refractory to methotrexate.

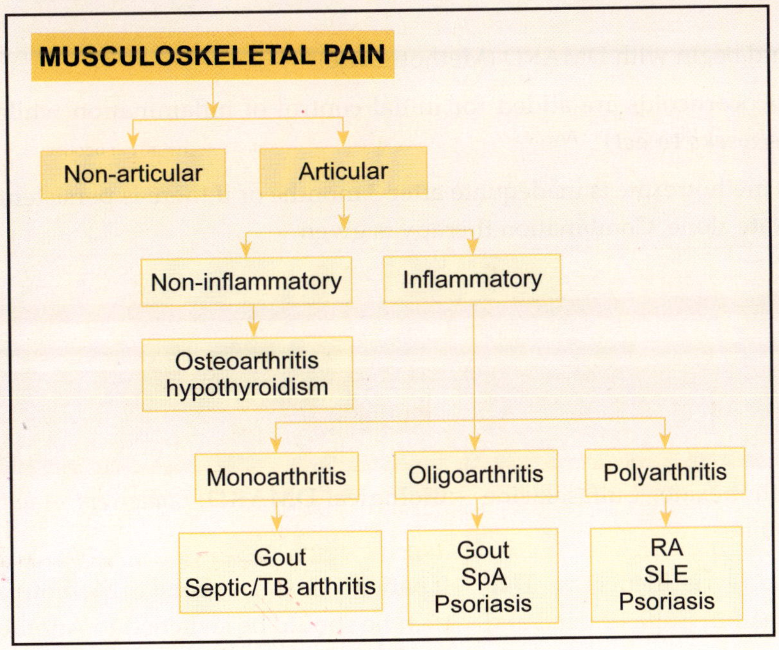

Contd.

Contd.

Differentiating Inflammatory from Non-Inflammatory Rheumatic Diseases		
	Inflammatory rheumatic diseases	**Non-inflammatory rheumatic diseases**
Examples	RA, SpA, SLE	OA, trauma, hypothyoidism
Morning stiffness	> 30 minutes	< 30 minutes
Pain aggravation	On resting the joint	On moving the joint
Spontaneous flares	Common	Uncommon
Acute phase reactants like ESR, CRP	Increased	Normal

Ref: Harrison 20th Edition Page 2538, Kelley's Textbook of Rheumatology 9th Edition Page 1144

Ans: (D) DMARDs with short course steroids

15. A known case of Rheumatoid arthritis on NSAIDs and methotrexate for more than 6 months but continues to have pain. What is the next line of management?

A. Start on leflunomide and stop methotrexate

B. Start on sulfasalazine and continue methotrexate

C. Continue NSAIDs and start steroids if no response

D. Start steroids immediately

Key:

Steps
Step 1: Therapy should begin with DMARD (Methotrexate)
Step 2: NSAIDS/Glucocorticoids are added for initial control of inflammation while awaiting DMARD response ***(DMARD's take days/weeks to act)***
Step 3: If response to methotrexate is inadequate after 3 months or if there is persistently high level of disease activity on methotrexate alone, Combination therapy is given

Combination Therapy	
Non-biological DMARD triple therapy	**Methotrexate plus Biological DMARD**
Triple therapy: Methotrexate, Sulfasalazine and Hydroxychloroquine	**Biological DMARD:** *Etanercept, Adalimumab, Infliximab*
If DMARD triple therapy is ineffective TNF inhibitor is used instead of Sulfasalazine and Hydroxychloroquine	If patient doesn't respond to Methotrexate plus initial TNF inhibitor, then he should be switched to Another TNF inhibitor

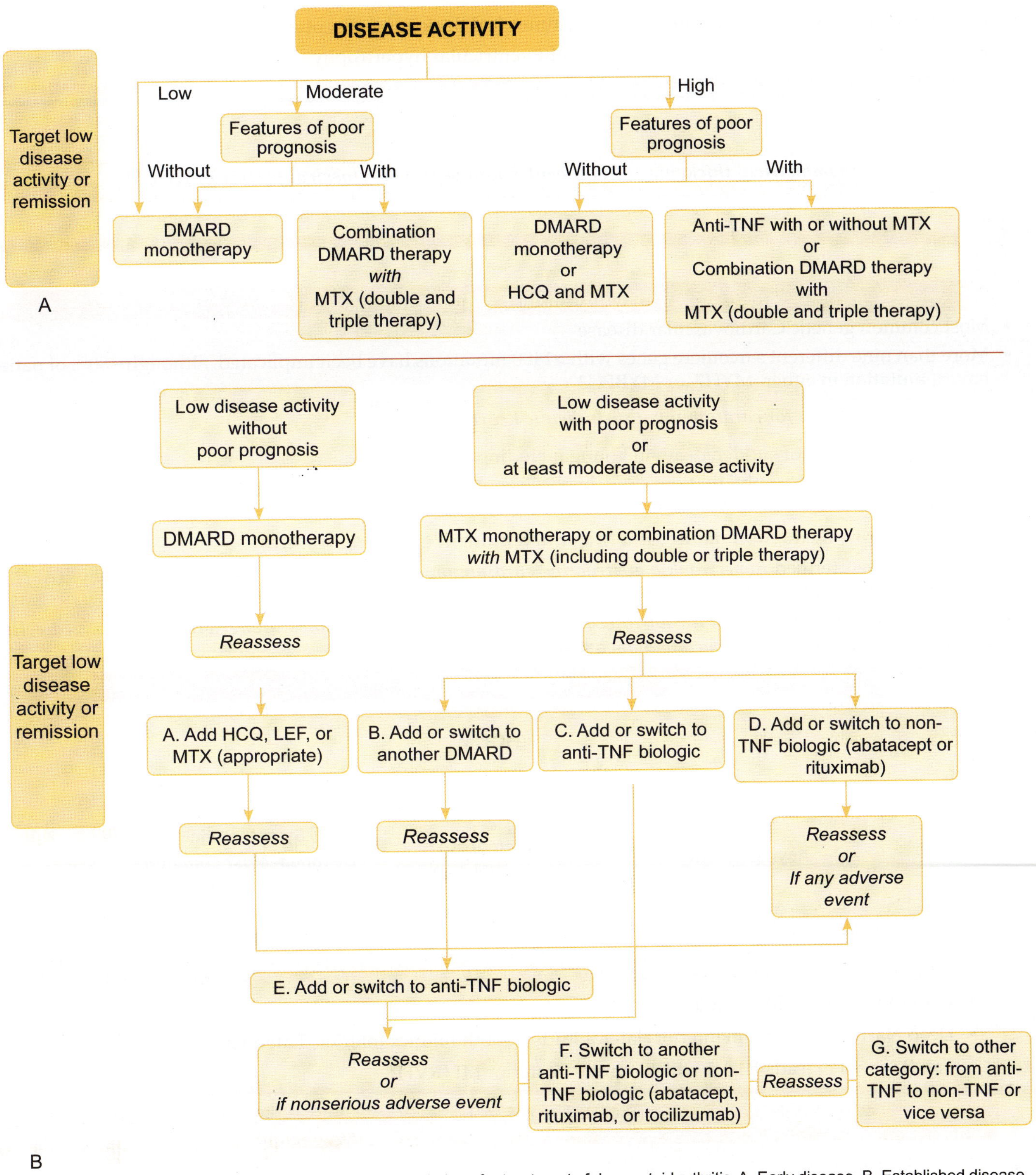

Figure: American College of Rheumatology recommendations for treatment of rheumatoid arthritis. A. Early disease. B. Established disease. DMARD, disease-modifying antirheumatic drug; HCQ, hydroxycholoroquine; LEF, leflunomide, MTX, methotrexate; TNF, tumor necrosis factor.

Ref: Harrison 20th Edition Page 2538, Kelley's Textbook of Rheumatology, 9th Edition Page 1144

Ans: (A) Start on leflunomide and stop methotrexate

16. Features of HOCM include:

A. Asymmetrical thickening of septum
B. Symmetrical thickening of septum
C. RVOT
D. Right ventricular hypertrophy

Key:

Asymmetrical thickening of Left ventricular septum is classical feature of HOCM

Hypertrophic Cardiomyopathy

- Most common genetic Cardiovascular disease
- More than nine different sarcomere genes with >1400 mutations have been implicated, although ~80% of patients have a mutation in either MYH7 or MYBPC3
- ***Most common cause for cardiomyopathy-Ischemic heart disease***
- Most common cause of sudden death in young including athletes
- Left ventricular hypertrophy that develops in absence of causative hemodynamic factors, such as hypertension, aortic valve disease, or systemic infiltrative or storage diseases
- **LVH–Both gross anatomical marker and Major determinant of clinical features**
- Previously been termed ***hypertrophic obstructive cardiomyopathy, Asymmetric septal hypertrophy (ASH and idiopathic hypertrophic subaortic stenosis)***
- ***Cardiac muscle hypertrophy with narrowed intramural coronary arterioles along with disorganized cellular architecture, microvascular ischemia and cardiac fibrosis***

Clinical Features

HOCM

- **Asymptomatic**
- **Sudden death** (Young athletes)
- **Symptomatic** ***Dyspnea–Most common,*** Angina pectoris, Syncope

ECG Findings

- Large amplitude QRS complex
- Deep Narrow Q waves in inferior/lateral leads or both mimics Inferior/Lateral MI
- Tall R waves in leads V1-V2 which mimics Posterior MI/RVH

Ausculatation

- Normal S1, Normally Split S2, S3 gallop is common
- S4 is frequently heard and results from atrial systole against highly non complaint left ventricle
- Double/Triple precardial impulse
- Brisk carotid upstroke
- Harsh diamond shaped Murmur *(Best heard at lower sternal border as well as at apex)*

Contd.

Contd.

JVP
• Reveals ***prominent "a" wave*** *(Diminished RV compliance, Secondary to massive Ventricular septum hypertrophy)*

Effect of Maneuvers on Hypertrophic Cardiomyopathy		
	Physiologic effect	**Change in murmur intensity**
Valsalva (straining phase)		
Abrupt standing from sitting or supine position)	↓ Preload	↑
Nitroglycerin administration		
Sustained hand grip	↑ Afterload	
Squatting (from standing position)	↑ Afterload and preload	↓
Passive leg raise	↑ Preload	

- Patients may be diagnosed after undergoing evaluations triggered by the abnormal physical findings (murmur) or symptoms of exertional dyspnea, angina or syncope.
- Biopsy is not needed to diagnose hypertrophic cardiomyopathy but can be used to exclude infiltrative and metabolic diseases.

Differentiating Hypertrophic Cardiomyopathy from Athlete's Heart		
	HCM	**Athlete's Heart**
Family history of HCM	+	–
Marked LVH or unusual patterns of hypertrophy	+	–
LV cavity dilatation	–	+
LA enlargement	+	–
Abnormal ECG patterns	+	–
Doppler interrogation of mitral inflow velocities	+	–
Female gender	+	–
Thickness with deconditioning	–	+

Risk Factors for Sudden Death in Hypertrophic Cardiomyopathy		
Major Risk Factor		**Screening Technique**
History of cardiac arrest or spontaneous sustained ventricular tachycardia		History

Contd.

Contd.

Syncope	Non-vagal, often with or after exertion	History
Family history of sudden cardiac death		Family history
Spontaneous non-sustained ventricular tachycardia	>3 beats at rate >120	Exercise or 24- to 48-hour ambulatory recording
LV thickness > 30 mm	Present in <10% of patients	Echocardiography
Abnormal blood pressure response to exercise	Systolic blood pressure fall or failure to increase at peak exercise	Maximal upright exercise testing

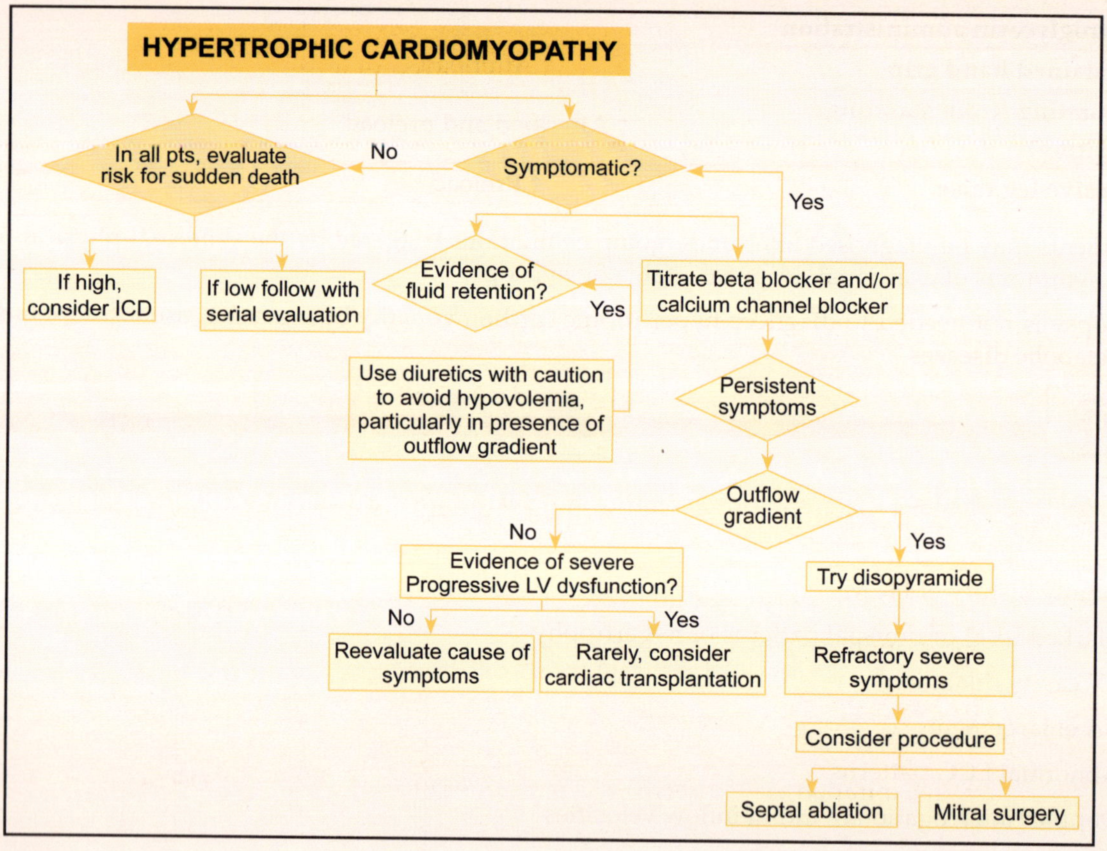

Management

- Avoid strenuous physical activity
- Beta blockers–Initial drug in symptomatic patients→***Reduces HR, BP, Stiffness of left ventricle, Fatal arrhythmias***
- Calcium channel blockers–Reduces stiffness of ventricle and Elevated Diastolic Pressure
- Amiodarone–Reduce arrhythmias
- Surgical myomectomy

Ref: Braunwald Heart Disease 10th Edition Page 104, Harrison 20th Edition Page 1793

Ans: (A) Asymmetrical thickening of septum

17. Intensity of murmur increases on standing in:

A. TOF B. VSD C. HOCM D. AS

Key:

Intensity of murmur increases on standing in HOCM

	Venous Return/Preload		Afterload		Drugs	
	Increase (Leg raise/ Squat)	Decrease (Valsalva/ Standing)	Increase (Handgrip)	Decrease (Amy/Nitrate)	Diuretic	ACEIs
MS, AS	↑	↓	↓(AS) Negligible Effect in (MS)	↑(AS)	Yes, but better As (Replace) MS (Balloon)	×
MR, AR	↑	↓	↑	↓	✓	✓
VSD	↑	↓	↑	↓	✓	✓
HOCM	↓	↑	↓	↑	×	×
MVP	↓	↑	↓	↑	×	×

Murmurs	Inspiration and Expiration	Increased Preload (Rapid squatting, Passive leg raising)	Decreased Preload (Valsalva, Standing)	Increased Afterload (Handgrip)	Decreased Afterload (Amyl nitrite)
Most murmurs	↑ Right-sided murmurs on inspiration; ↑ Left-sided murmurs on expiration	↑ Increase	↓ Decrease	Stenotic murmurs (except MS):↓ Regurgitant murmurs: ↑	Stenotic murmurs (except MS):↑ Regurgitant murmurs: ↓
AS	↑ on expiration	↑ Increase	↓ Decrease	↓ Decrease	↑ Increase
MVP	No effect	↓ Decrease with later onset click	↑ Increase with early onset click	↓ Decrease with later onset click	↑ Increase with early onset click
HOCM	No effect	↓ Decrease	↑ Increase	↓ Decrease	↑ Increase

Ref: Braunwald Heart Disease 10th Edition Page 104, Harrison 20th Edition Page 1793

Ans: (C) HOCM

18. Ascending areflexic paralysis without sphincter involvement is seen in:

A. GBS
B. Kearns Sayre syndrome
C. Snake bite
D. Botulism

Key:

Ascending areflexic paralysis without sphincter involvement is seen in Guillain-Barré syndrome

Guillain-Barré Syndrome

- Acute, frequently severe and fulminant polyradiculoneuropathy
- Autoimmune in origin

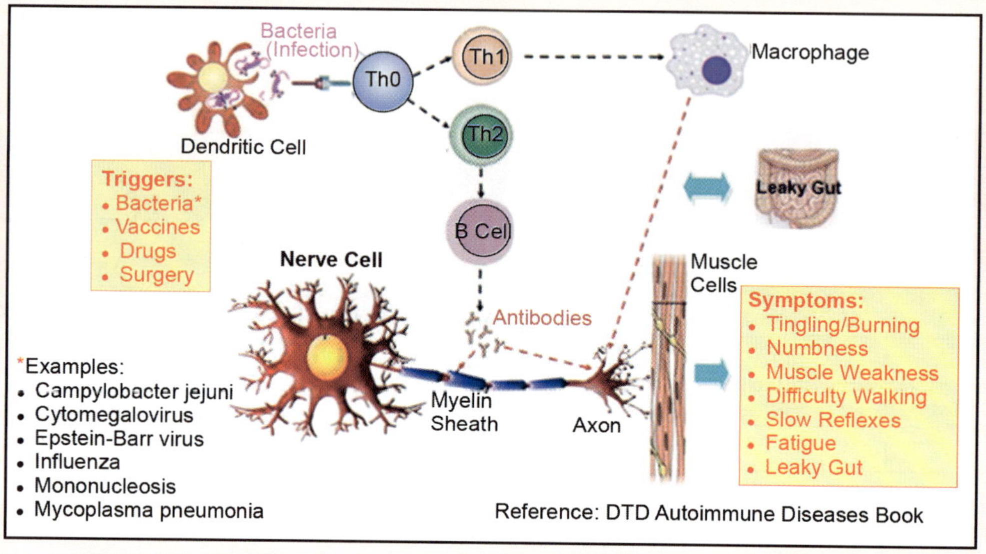

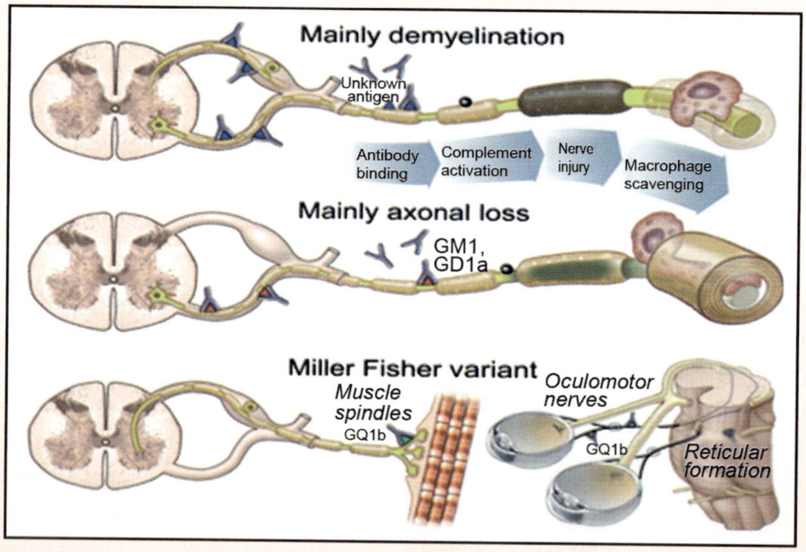

Clinical Manifestations

- Manifests as a **rapidly evolving areflexic motor paralysis** with or without sensory disturbance.
- Usual pattern is an **ascending paralysis** that may be first noticed as **rubbery legs.**
- Typically evolves over hours to few days and is frequently accompanied by tingling dysesthesias in extremities.
- Legs are usually more affected than arms.
- Facial diparesis is present in 50% of affected individuals.
- Lower cranial nerves are also frequently involved, causing bulbar weakness with difficulty handling secretions and maintaining an airway.
- **Cutaneous sensory deficits** (e.g., loss of pain and temperature sensation) are usually relatively **mild**, but functions subserved by large sensory fibers, such as deep tendon reflexes and proprioception, are more severely affected.
- Approximately 70% of cases of GBS occur **1–3 weeks** after an **acute infectious** process, usually **respiratory** or **gastrointestinal.**

Contd.

Contd.

- **Campylobacter jejuni human herpes virus infection, often CMV or Epstein-Barr virus.** Other viruses (e.g., HIV, hepatitis E, Zika) and also **Mycoplasma pneumoniae** have been identified as agents involved in antecedent infections, as have recent immunizations.

Diagnosis

- CSF findings are distinctive, consisting of an **elevated CSF protein level (1–10 g/L [100–1000 mg/dL]) without accompanying pleocytosis (Cytoalbuminologic dissociation).**
- CSF is often normal when symptoms have been present for ≤48 hours; by end of 1st week, protein level is usually elevated.
- In AIDP, the earliest features are **prolonged F-wave latencies, prolonged distal latencies, and reduced amplitudes of compound muscle action potentials (CMAPs),** probably owing to the predilection for involvement of nerve roots and distal motor nerve terminals early in course.
- Later, slowing of conduction velocity, conduction block and temporal dispersion may be appreciated.

Treatment

- **IVIG** is administered as five daily infusions for a total dose of 2 g/kg body weight.
- Course of **plasmapheresis** usually consists of ~40–50 mL/kg PE 4–5 times over 7–10 days.

Subtypes of Guillain-Barré Syndrome

Subtype	Features	Electrodiagnosis	Pathology
Acute inflammatory demyelinating polyneuropathy (AIDP)	Adults affected more than children 90% cases in western world Recovery rapid Anti GM1 Antibody (<50%)	***Demyelinating***	First attack on Schwann cell surface, widespread myelin damage, macrophage activation and lymphocytic infiltration, Secondary axonal damage
Acute motor axonal neuropathy (AMAN)	Children and Young adults Prevalent in China and Mexico Recovery rapid, Anti GD1a Antibody	***Axonal***	First attack at motor nodes of Ranvier, Macrophage activation, Few lymphocytes, Frequent Peri-axonal macrophages, Extent of Axonal damage highly variable
Acute motor sensory axonal neuropathy (AMSAN)	Mostly adults, Recovery slow, Often incomplete, Closely related to AMAN	***Axonal***	Same as AMAN, but also affects sensory nerves and roots Axonal damage usually severe
Miller Fisher syndrome	Adults and children Ophthalmoplegia, Ataxia and Areflexia Anti GQ1b antibodies (90%)	Axonal/ Demyelinating	Resembles AIDP

Ref: Harrison 20th Edition Page 3225

Ans: (A) GBS

19. Compression of Esophagus in mitral stenosis occurs due to:

A. Enlarged LA   B. Enlarged LV
C. Enlarged RV   D. Enlarged RA

Key:

Compression of Esophagus in Mitral stenosis occurs due to Enlarged Left atrium

Dysphagia Megalatriensis

- Also known as **Cardiovascular dysphagia/Cardiac dysphagia,** is an impairment of **swallowing** due to esophageal compression from a **dilated left atrium.**
- Presentation is generally with mild dysphagia, although minority of patients will have dysphagia severe enough to develop weight loss and nutritional imbalances.

Most serious complication is development of Atrio-esophageal fistula resulting in fatal hematemesis

- When atrium enlarges, it grows posterior, occupying the space between the aorta and esophagus in which esophagus was totally impinged by the giant atrium.
- Chest radiographs demonstrate features consistent with left atrial enlargement.
- Treatment is necessary only if symptomatic, and generally patients will require a nasogastric tube for enteric feeding

Ortner's Syndrome

- **Vocal cord paralysis** results from impingement of **Left recurrent laryngeal nerve** by **Giant left atrium** as nerve passes around the aortic arch
- Most important differential diagnoses of Ortner syndrome includes all space-occupying thoracic lesion tumors, which can compress Recurrent laryngeal nerve such as lymphomas, lung cancer and mediastinal infections.

Dysphagia Lusoria: *Results from esophageal compression by aberrant aortic arch vessels.*

Ref: Harrison 20th Edition Page 1814

Ans: (A) Enlarged LA

20. In ECG, J wave (Osborn wave) is seen in:

A. Hypocalcemia
B. Hypothermia
C. Hypernatremia
D. Hypomagnesemia

Key:

Osborn wave is typically seen in Hypothermia

Hypothermia

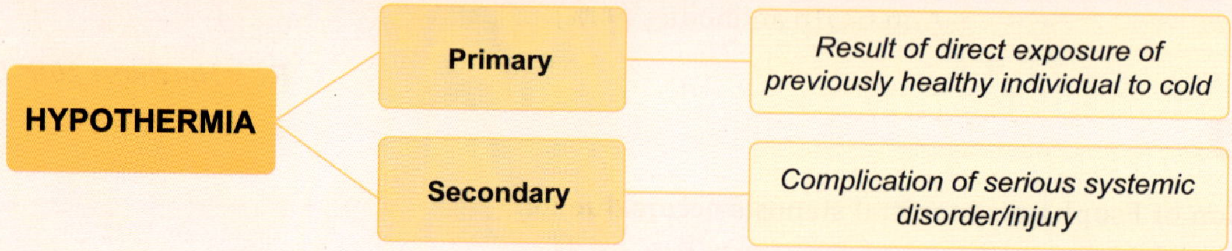

Contd.

Contd.

Mild: *32.2 to 35°C*
Moderate: *28 to <32.2°C*
Severe: *<28°C*

- Patients with systemic **hypothermia** may develop a distinctive ECG pattern in which a humplike elevation is usually localized to the junction of the end of the QRS complex and the beginning of the ST segment **(J point).**
- These pathologic **J waves** are sometimes called Osborn **waves.**
- This pattern disappears with rewarming.
- Basic mechanism of prominent J waves appears to be related to the differential effects of systemic cooling on repolarization of different layers of ventricles.

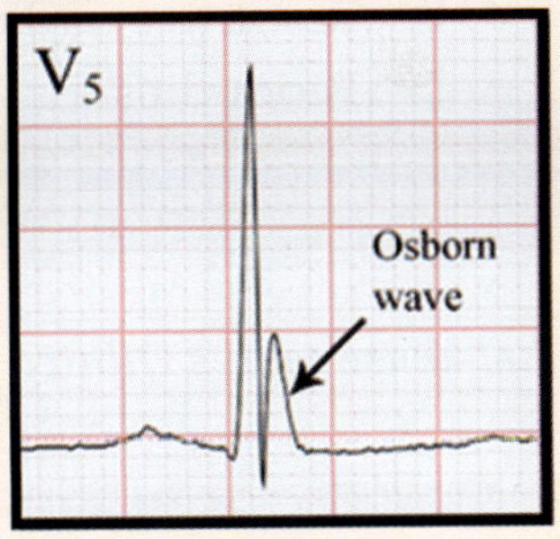

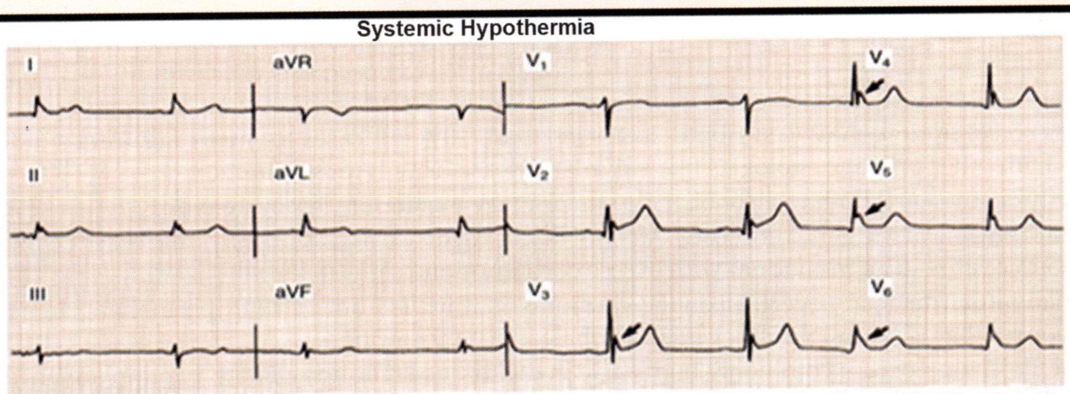

Systemic hypothermia is associated with a distinctive bulging of the J point (the very beginning of the ST segment). The prominent J waves (arrows) with hypothermia are referred to as Osborn waves

Abnormal venous wave	Clinical significance
Absent A wave	**Atrial fibrillation**
Fused A wave (with C wave)	**Supraventricular tachycardia**
Giant A wave	**Right atrial contraction against increased resistance**–Tricuspid stenosis, Tricuspid atresia, Right atrial tumor **Abnormal RV Compliance**–Pulmonary stenosis, Pulmonary hypertension, Restrictive cardiomyopathy
Cannon wave	Regular–Normal heart rate→ ***Nodal rhythm*** Regular–Rapid heart rate→***Junctional Tachycardia*** Irregular–Slow heart rate→ ***Complete heart block*** Irregular–Rapid heart rate→ ***Ventricular tachycardia, Ventricular Ectopic beats***
Absent X wave	Tricuspid regurgitation
Prominent X wave	Constrictive pericarditis, Restrictive cardiomyopathy, ASD

Contd.

Contd.

Large V wave (Fused with C wave)	Tricuspid regurgitation
Slow Y descent	Tricuspid stenosis
Prominent rapid Y descent	Tricuspid regurgitation
Deep Y descent	Constrictive pericarditis, Restrictive cardiomyopathy, Severe heart failure

Ref: Harrison 20th Edition Page 3338,
Goldberger's Clinical Electrocardiography–Simplified Approach 8th Edition Page 98

Ans: (B) Hypothermia

21. Alcohol abuse causes:

A. Dilated cardiomyopathy
B. Restrictive cardiomyopathy
C. HOCM
D. Pericarditis

Key:

Alcohol abuse causes Dilated cardiomyopathy

Dilated Cardiomyopathy

- **Alcohol** is the most common toxin implicated in ***Chronic DCM.***
- Excess consumption may contribute to more than 10% of cases of **heart failure,** including exacerbation of cases with other primary etiologies like valvular disease or previous infarction.
- Toxicity is attributed both to alcohol and to its primary metabolite, **acetaldehyde.**
- Polymorphisms of the genes encoding Alcohol dehydrogenase and ACE may influence the likelihood of alcoholic cardiomyopathy in an individual with excess consumption.
- Cardiac impairment in severe alcoholic cardiomyopathy is sum of both permanent damage and substantial component that is reversible after cessation of alcohol consumption.
- Atrial fibrillation occurs commonly both early in the disease **("holiday heart")** and in advanced stages.

Major Causes of Dilated Cardiomyopathy (with Common Examples)

Inflammatory Myocarditis

Infective

- Viral (coxsackie,[a] adenovirus,[a] HIV, hepatitis C)
- Parasitic (*T. cruzi*–Chagas' disease, trypanosomiasis, toxoplasmosis)
- Bacterial (diphtheria)
- Spirochetal (*Borrelia burgdorferi*–Lyme disease)
- Rickettsial (Q fever)
- Fungal (with systemic infection

Noninfective

- Granulomatous inflammatory disease
  - Sarcoidosis
  - Giant cell myocarditis
- Eosinophilic myocarditis
- Polymyositis, dermatomyositis
- Collagen vascular disease
- Checkpoint inhibitor chemotherapy
- Transplant rejection

Contd.

Contd.

Toxic
Alcohol Catecholamines: Amphetamines, cocaine Chemotherapeutic agents (anthracyclines, trastuzumab) Interferon Other therapeutic agents (hydroxychloroquine, chloroquine) Drugs of misuse (emetine, anabolic steroids) Heavy metals: Lead, mercry Occupational exposure: Hydrocarbons, arsenicals
Metabolic
Nutritional deficiencies: Thiamine, selenium, carnitine Electrolyte deficiencies: Calcium, phosphate, magnesium Endocrinopathy • Thyroid disease • Pheochromocytoma • Diabetes Obesity Hemochromatosis
Inherited Metabolic Pathway Defects
Familial
Skeletal and cardiac myopathy Dystrophin-related dystrophy (Duchenne's, Becker's) Mitochondrial myopathies (e.g., Kearns-Sayre syndrome) Arrhythmogenic ventricular cardiomyopathy Hemochromatosis Associated with other systemic diseases Susceptibility to immune-mediated myocarditis
Overlap with Nondilated Cardiomyopathy
"Minimally dilated cardiomyopathy" Hemochromatosis Amyloidosis Hypertrophic cardiomyopathy ("burned-out")
"Idiopathic"[a]
Miscellaneous (Shared Elements of Above Etiologies)
Peripartum cardiomyopathy Left ventricular non-compaction Tachycardia-related cardiomyopathy • Supraventricular arrhythmias with uncontrolled rate • Very frequent nonsustained ventricular tachycardia or high premature ventricular complex burden

	Dilated	Restrictive	Hypertrophic
Ejection fraction (normal >55%)	Usually < 30% when symptoms severe	25-50%	>60%
Left ventricular diastolic dimension (normal <55 mm)	≥ 60 mm	<60 mm (may be decreased)	Often decreased
Left ventricular wall thickness	Normal or decreased	Normal or increased	Markedly increased
Atrial size	Increased, may also be primarily affected	Increased; may be massive	Increased; related to elevated filling pressures
Valvular regurgitation	Related to annular dilation; mitral appears earlier during decompensation; tricuspid regurgitation with right ventricular dysfunction	Related to endocardial involvement; frequent mitral and tricuspid regurgitation, rarely severe	Related to valve-septum interaction; mitral regurgitation
Common first symptoms	Exertional intolerance	Exertional intolerance, fluid retention early, may have dominant right-sided symptoms	Exertional intolerance; may have chest pain
Congestive symptoms	Left before right, except right prominent in young adults	Right often dominates	Left-sided congestion at rest may develop late
Arrhythmias	Ventricular tachyarrhythmia; conduction block in Chagas' disease, and some families. Atrial fibrillation	Ventricular uncommon except in sarcoidosis, conduction block in sarcoidosis and amyloidosis. Atrial fibrillation	Ventricular tachyarrhythmias; atrial fibrillation

[a]"Left-sided symptoms of pulmonary congestion; dyspnea on exertion, orthopnea, paroxysmal nocturnal dyspnea. Right-sided symptoms of systemic venous congestion; hepatic and abdominal distention, discomfort on bending, peripheral edema.

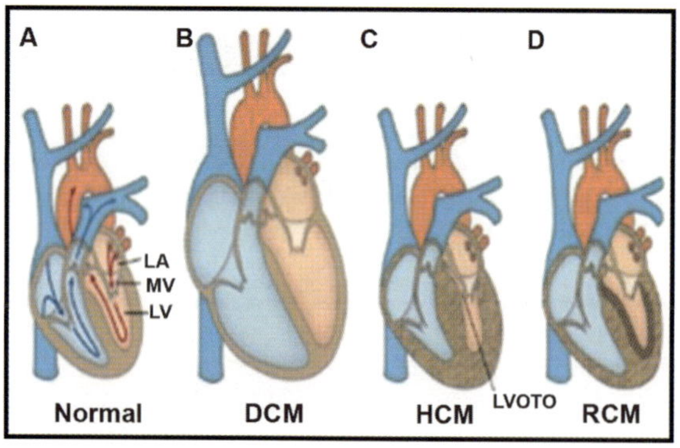

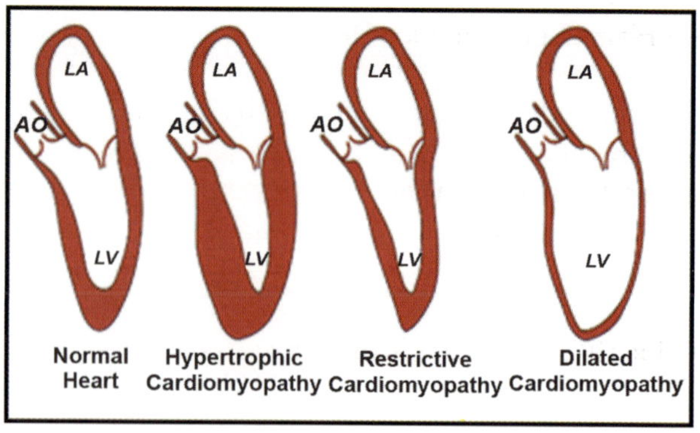

Ref: Harrison 20th Edition Page 1779

Ans: (A) Dilated cardiomyopathy

22. Which of the following is not an AIDS defining illness?

A. Pulmonary tuberculosis
B. Tertiary syphilis
C. Disseminated salmonellosis
D. Primary CNS lymphoma

Key:

Tertiary syphilis is not an AIDS Defining Illness

WHO Clinical Staging in Adults, Adolescents and Children	
Adults and adolescents	**Children**
Clinical stage 1	
• Asymptomatic • Persistent generalized lymphadenopathy	• Asymptomatic • Persistent generalized lymphadenopathy
Clinical stage 2	
• Moderate unexplained weight loss (<10% of presumed or measured body weight) • Recurrent respiratory tract infections (Sinusitis, Tonsillitis, Otitis Media, Pharyngitis) • Herpes Zoster • Angular Cheilitis • Recurrent Cheilities • Recurrent oral ulceration • Papular Pruritic Eruption • Fungal nail infections • Seborrhoeic Dermatitis	• Unexplained persistent hepatosplenomegaly • Recurrent or chronic upper respiratory tract infections (Otitis Media, Otorrhoea, Sinusitis, Tonsillitis) • Herpes Zoster • Lineal gingival erythema • Recurrent oral ulceration • Papular Pruritic Eruption • Fungal nail infections • Extensive wart virus infection • Extensive Molluscum Contagiosum • Unexplained persistent parotid enlargement
Clinical stage 3	
• Unexplained severe weight loss (>10% of the presumed or measured body weight) • Unexplained chronic diarrhoea for more than 1 month • Unexplained persistent fever (intermittent or constant for longer than 1 month) • Persistent Oral Candidiasis • Oral Hairy Leucoplakia (OHL) • Pulmonary Tuberculosis • Severe bacterial infections (such as Pneumonia, Empyema, Pyomyositis, bone or joint infection, Meningitis, bacteraemia) • Acute necrotizing ulcerative stomatitis, Gingivitis or Periodontitis • Unexplained anemia (<8 g/dL), neutropenia (<0.5 × 10^9/L) and or chronic thrombocytopenia (<50 × 10^9/L)	• Unexplained moderate malnutrition not adequately responding to standard therapy • Unexplained persistent diarrhoea (14 days or more) • Unexplained persistent fever (above 37.5°C, intermittent or constant, for longer than one 1 month) • Persistent Oral Candidiasis (after the first 6 weeks of life) • Oral Hairy Leucoplakia (OHL) • Lymph node Tuberculosis • Pulmonary tuberculosis • Severe recurrent bacterial Pneumonia • Acute necrotizing ulcerative gingivitis or Periodontitis • Unexplained anemia (<8 g/dL), neutropenia (<0.5 × 10^9/L) or chronic thrombocytopaenia (<50 × 10^9/L) • Symptomatic Lymphoid Interstitial Pneumonitis • Chronic HIV-associated lung disease, including Bronchiectasis

Contd.

Contd.

Clinical stage 4	
• HIV wasting syndrome • Pneumocystis (jirovecii) Pneumonia • Recurrent severe bacterial Pneumonia • Chronic Herpes Simplex infection (orolabial, genital or anorectal of more than 1 month duration or visceral at any site) • Oesophageal Candidiasis (or Candidiasis of trachea, bronchi or lungs) • Extra pulmonary Tuberculosis • Kaposi sarcoma • Cytomegalovirus infection (retinitis or infection of other organs) • Central nervous system Toxoplasmosis • HIV encephalopathy • Extra pulmonary Cryptococcosis, including Meningitis • Disseminated non-tuberculous mycobacterial infection (NTM) • Progressive Multifocal Leukoencephalopathy (PML) • Chronic Cryptosporidiosis • Chronic Isosporiasis • Disseminated mycosis (extra pulmonary Histoplasmosis, Coccidioidomycosis) • Lymphoma (cerebral or B-cell non-Hodgkin) • Symptomatic HIV-associated nephropathy of cardiomyopathy • Recurrent septicaemia (including non-typhoidal Salmonella) • Invasive cervical carcinoma • Atypical disseminated leishmaniasis	• Unexplained severe wasting, shunting or severe malnutrition not responding to standard therapy • Pneumocystis (jiroveci) Pneumonia • Recurrent severe bacterial infections (such as Empyema, Pyomyositis, bone or joint infection, Meningitis, but excluding Pneumonia) • Chronic Herpes Simplex infection (orolabial or cutaneous of more than 1 month duration of visceral at any site) • Oesophageal Candidiasis (or Candidiasis of trachea, bronchi or lungs) • Extra pulmonary Tuberculosis • Kaposi sarcoma • Cytomegalovirus infection (retinitis or infection of other organs with onset at age more than 1 month) • Central nervous system Toxoplasmosis (after the neonatal period) • HIV encephalopathy • Extra pulmonary Cryptococcosis, including Meningitis • Disseminated nontuberculous mycobacterial infection (NTM) • Progressive Multifocal Leukoencephalopathy (PML) • Chronic Cryptosporidiosis (with diarrhoea) • Chronic Isosporiasis • Disseminated endemic mycosis (extra pulmonary Histoplasmosis, Coccidioidomycosis, Penicilliosis) • Cerebral or B-Cell non-Hodgkin Lymphoma • HIV-associated nephropathy or cardiomyopathy

(a) In the development of this table, adolescents were defined as 15 years or older. For those aged less than 15 years, the clinical staging for children should be used.

(b) For children younger than 5 years, moderate malnutrition is defined as weight-for-height <-2 z-score or mid-upper arm circumference ≥ 115 mm to < 125 mm.

(c) Some additional specific conditions can be included in regional classifications, such as penicilliosis in Asia, HIV-associated rectovaginal fistula in southern Africa and reactivation of trypanosomiasis in Latin America.

(d) For children younger than 5 years of age, severe wasting is defined as weight-for-height <-3 z-score; stunting is defined as length-for-age height-for-age <-2 z-score; and severe acute malnutrition is either weight for height <-3 z-score or mid-upper arm circumference <115 mm or the presence of oedema.

Ref: NACO Guidelines 2018

Ans: (B) Tertiary syphilis

23. Prophylactic Anti-diphtheria toxin dose to be used in suspected cases:

A. 5000–10000
B. 10000–20000
C. 1000–2000
D. 20000–40000

Key:

Prophylactic Anti-diphtheria toxin dose in suspected cases is 5000-10,000 Units

Prophylactic Regimen

- Prophylactic treatment with DAT can be considered for contacts but is recommended only in exceptional circumstances.
- If it is concluded that close contact may benefit from receiving DAT, DAT can be administered in addition to antimicrobial prophylaxis and immunization with diphtheria toxoid.
- **Before administering DAT:**
  - Perform appropriate sensitivity tests.
  - If sensitivity testing is negative, give 10,000 units IM.
  - ***If sensitivity testing is positive, proceed with desensitization and then administer 10,000 units of DAT IM.***

Antitoxin

- Dose of anti-toxin to be administered is empirically based on site of infection, duration of illness and severity of manifestations as follows:
  - **Mild nasal or pharyngeal diphtheria:** 20,000 to 40,000 units.
  - **Nasopharyngeal lesions:** 40,000 to 60,000 units.
  - **Moderately severe pharyngeal diphtheria:** 80,000 to 100,000 units.
  - **Severe pharyngeal or laryngeal diphtheria, symptoms involving multiple sites, presence of brawny oedema or illness over 48 hours:** 120,000 units.
- Antitoxin should be administered as an I.V. infusion over 60 minutes to ensure rapid inactivation. (Fatality rate increases with delay in starting anti-toxic therapy).
- Intravenous immunoglobulin (IVIG) preparations are not recommended for the treatment of diphtheria, as they contain only low-titres of anti-diphtheria antibodies.
- Antibiotic treatment only supplements and doesn't replace Anti-toxic therapy.

Ref: Park 24th Edition Page 851, Ananthanarayan and Paniker 10th Edition Page 245, Manson's Tropical Diseases 23rd Edition Page 419

Ans: (A) 5000 - 10000

24. Rapid diagnostic methods to diagnose UTI includes all except:

A. Dipstick nitrities
B. Catalase test
C. Dipstick leukocyte estrase
D. Dipstick culture

Key:

Dipstick culture is not a Rapid diagnostic method to diagnose UTI

- **UTI may be asymptomatic** (subclinical infection) or symptomatic (disease). Thus, the term urinary tract infection encompasses a variety of clinical entities, including asymptomatic bacteriuria (ASB), cystitis, prostatitis and pyelonephritis.
- Urine collected in a normal individual by suprapubic aspiration of the bladder is sterile and does not contain leukocytes. This method represents the gold standard in the diagnosis of urinary tract infection.

Urine Culture–Indications

- Role of pretreatment urine culture in the evaluation of suspected UTI is to confirm the presence of bacteriuria and to identify and provide antibiotic susceptibility information on the causative organism (often retrospectively, if treatment is empirically given).
- Culture of a clean-catch voided urine specimen is warranted for these purposes among most patients with suspected UTI, except for healthy non-pregnant young women with typical symptoms of non-febrile cystitis, that is, of uncomplicated UTI.

Dipsticks to Evaluate for Urine Leukocyte Esterase and Nitrite

- Can be used as a screening tool for the diagnosis of UTI.
- Dipsticks are generally performed whenever UTI is suspected.
- However, we don't routinely collect urine for dipstick in young non-pregnant women with a history clearly suggestive of a UTI (i.e., typical symptoms without vaginal discharge or irritation), as dipstick generally does not provide additional useful information.

Clinical Presentation	Patient Characteristics	Diagnostic and Mangaement Considerations
Acute onset of urinary symptoms • Dysuria • Frequency • Urgency	Otherwise healthy woman who is not pregnant, low risk for multidrug resistance	Consider uncomplicated cystitis • No urine culture needed • Consider telephone management
	Woman with a history of or risk factors for STD	Consider uncomplicated cystitis or STD • Urinalysis, culture • STD evaluation, pelvic exam
	Male with perineal, pelvic, or prostatic pain	Consider acute prostatitis • Urinalysis and culture • Consider urology evaluation
	Patient with indwelling urinary catheter	Consider CAUTI • Exchange or remove catheter • Urinalysis and culture • Blood cultures if fever
	All other patients	Consider complicated UTI • Urinalysis and culture • Address any modifiable anatomic or functional abnormalities
Acute onset of back pain, nausea/vomiting, or fever with or without cystitis symptoms	Otherwise healthy woman who is not pregnant	Consider uncomplicated pyelonephritis • Urine and culture • Consider outpatient management
	All other patients	Consider pyelonephritis or acute prostatitis (male) • Urine culture • Blood cultures
Systemic symptoms • Fever • Altered mental status • Leukocytosis	Elderly patient; patients with spinal cord injury, immunocompromise, no alternate diagnosis	Consider complicated UTI • Consider other etiologies • Urine culture • Blood cultures
No urinary symptoms	Positive urine culture in patient who is pregnant, renal transplant recipient, or patient undergoing invasive urological procedure	Consider ASB • Screening and treatment warranted
	Positive urine culture in all other patients	Consider ASB • No additional workup or treatment needed
	Positive urine culture in patient with indwelling catheter	Consider CA-ASB • No additional workup or treatment needed • Remove unnecessary catheters
Recurrent acute urinary symptoms	Otherwise healthy woman who is not pregnant	Consider recurrent cystitis • Urine culture to establish diagnosis • Consider prophylaxis or patient-initiated management (see text)
	Male patient	Consider chronic bacterial prostatitis • Consider urology consult

Diagnostic approach to urinary tract infection (UTI). ASB, asymptomatic bacteriuria; CA-ASB, catheter-associated ASB; CAUTI, catheter-associated UTI; STD, sexually transmitted disease.

Ref: Harrison 20th Edition Page 968

Ans: (D) Dipstick culture

25. Which gives long lasting remission in ITP?

A. Corticosteroids
B. IVIG
C. Splenectomy
D. Anti-D

Key:

IVIG is used for Long lasting remission in ITP

Immune Thrombocytopenia

- IWG definition proposed use of the term "immune thrombocytopenia" instead of "idiopathic thrombocytopenic purpura" as the basis for the ITP acronym, because the immune nature of ITP is clear but most ITP patients do not have purpura.
- Platelet count of 100 × 109/L was proposed as threshold level to entertain ITP diagnosis.
- ITP is classified based on the absence or presence of other diseases as **"primary" or "secondary".**

Pathogenesis

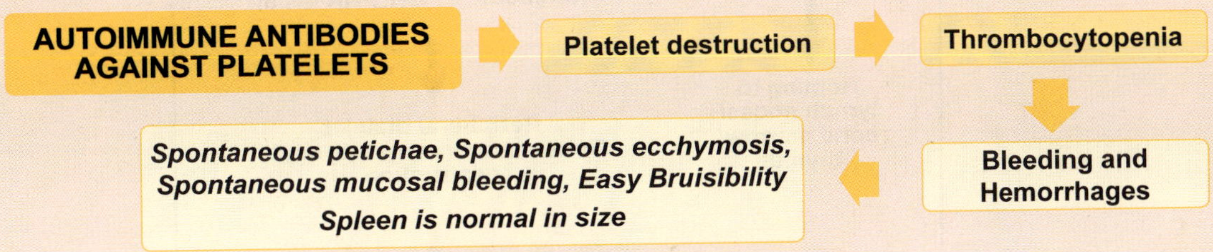

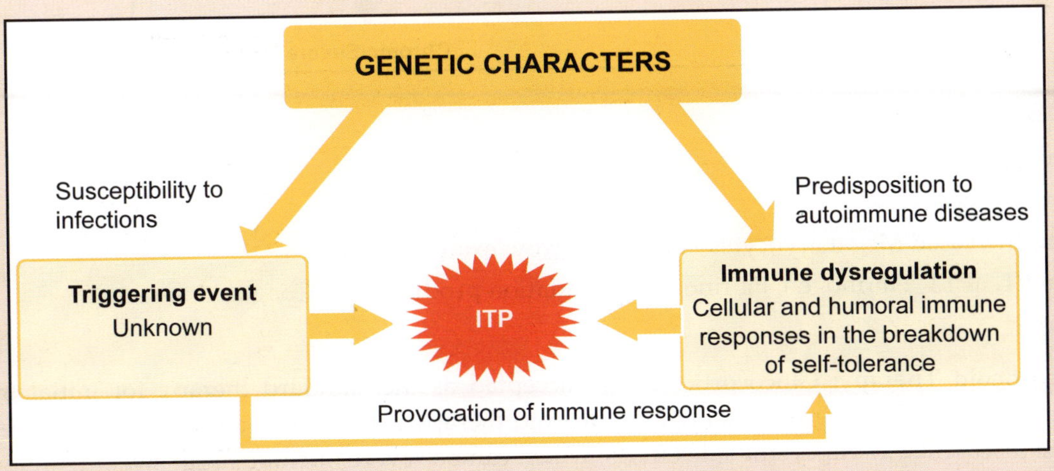

- Common bleeding signs include purpura (ecchymoses and petechiae), epistaxis, menorrhagia, and gingival bleeding.
- Purpuric lesions seen in ITP are not palpable, do not blanch with pressure, and often develop on distal regions of the extremities and on skin areas exposed to pressure.
- Fatigue is one of common, but often neglected, complaints of patients with primary ITP.

Contd.

Contd.

Phases of ITP

- Newly diagnosed ITP (within 3 months of diagnosis).
- Persistent ITP (patients who do not achieve a stable remission between 3 and 12 months after diagnosis); and
- Chronic ITP (continuing for more than 12 months).

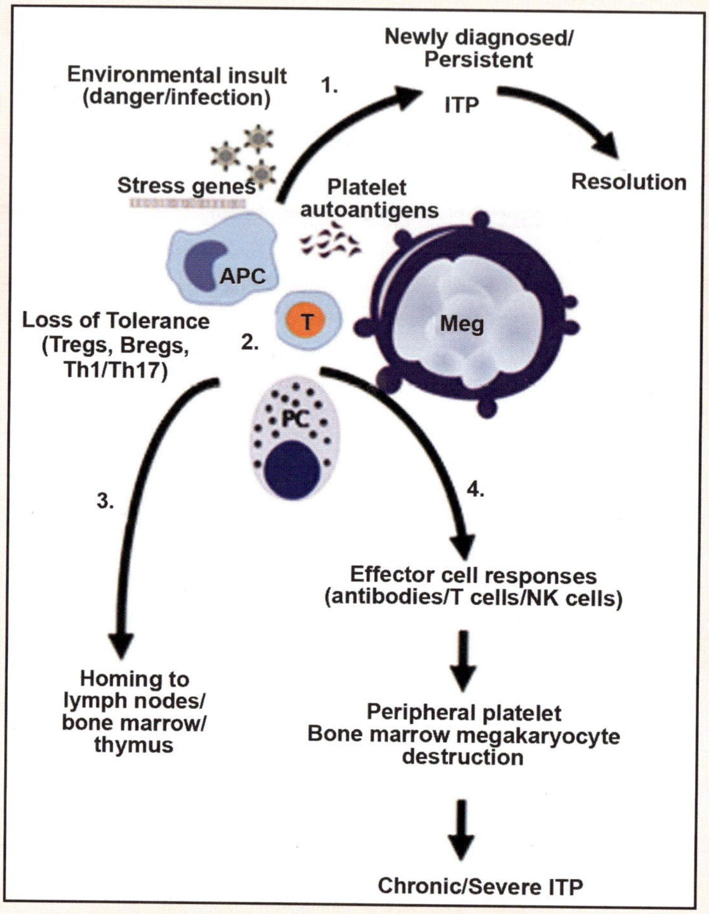

Lab Diagnosis

- Isolated thrombocytopenia
- Platelet antibodies
- Normal/Increased Megakaryocytes on Bone marrow examination
- Normal PT. aPTT, Fibrinogen, Fibrinogen degradation products and Coagulation factors

Treatment

- **Glucocorticoid Therapy:** Glucocorticoids are accepted as the standard therapy for initial treatment in adult patients with ITP. Major drawback of glucocorticoid therapy is that often adverse effects of treatment are worse than the disease itself. Important side effects, which can be severe, include facial swelling (chipmunk or moon facies), weight gain, folliculitis, hyperglycemia, hypertension, cataracts, osteoporosis, aseptic bone necrosis, opportunistic infections and behavioral disturbances.
- **Splenectomy:** Splenectomy is standard second-line therapy. Splenectomy will decrease antibody production and platelet destruction, and will be effective in patients in whom antibody-mediated platelet destruction rather than platelet production is the major cause of thrombocytopenia.

Contd.

Contd.

- **Intravenous Immunoglobulin:** IVIG rapidly increases platelet count in more than 75 percent of patients with chronic ITP and normalizes platelet count in approximately 50% patients. Recommended total dose of IVIG is 2 g/kg administered either as 0.4 g/kg per day on 5 consecutive days or as 1 g/kg per day on 2 consecutive days. If need to increase platelet count is urgent, preferred dosing is 1 g/kg per day for 2 days combined with glucocorticoids.
- **Anti (Rh) D:** Polyclonal γ-globulin containing high titers of antibodies against Rho(D) antigen of erythrocytes. It is administered intravenously for treatment of ITP. Anti-(Rh)D binds Rh-positive erythrocytes and leads to their destruction in the spleen. Because splenic Fc receptors are blocked, more antibody-coated platelets survive in the circulation. Recommended that anti-(Rh)D be given as a single dose of 50 to 100 mcg/kg by intravenous infusion over 3 to 5 minutes.
- **Rituximab: B** lymphocytes play many roles in the pathophysiology of ITP, including producing antibodies, presenting antigens, and regulating the functions of T cells and dendritic cells. B cells are targeted therapeutically with rituximab, chimeric monoclonal antibody against CD20, which binds B cells and causes Fc-mediated lysis, thereby depleting these cells from blood, lymph nodes and marrow. Rapidly depletes B cells in patients with autoimmune diseases, with effect usually lasting 6 to 12 months.Usual rituximab doses are in the range of 100 to 375 mg/m^2.

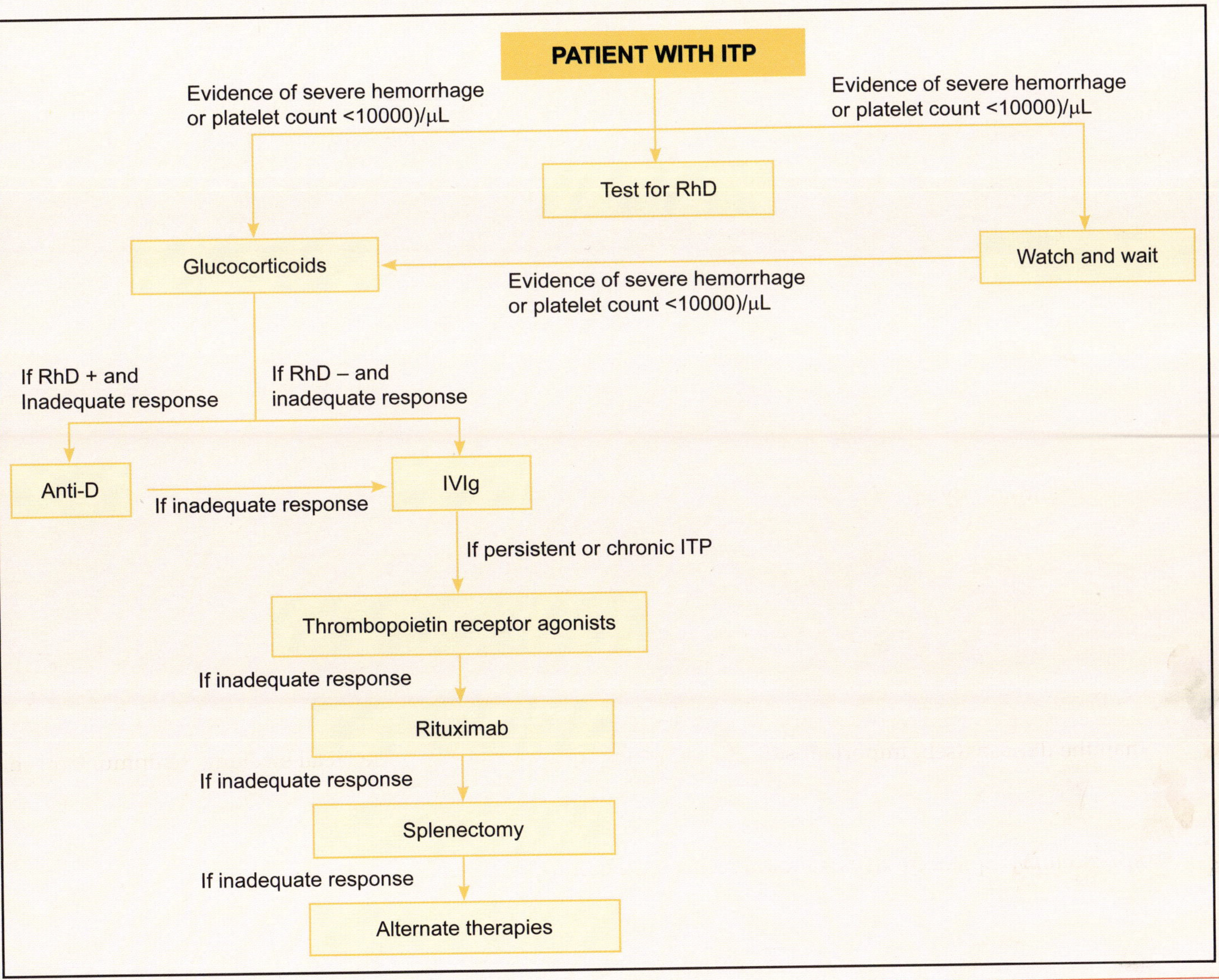

Contd.

Contd.

Treatment	Typical Use in ITP
Platelet transfusion	Low platelet emergency, rescue treatment
Corticosteroids	First-line treatment, rescue treatment
IVIG	First-line treatment, rescue treatment
Anti-D	Alternative to IVIG
Rituximab	Second-line treatment
Older agents	Alternative or supplementary to other ITP treatments
Other treatments	Experimental/supplementary
Splenectomy	Long-term treatment in patients with refractory/chronic disease

Ref: Williams Hematology 9th Edition Page 2004, Harrison 18th Edition Page 986

Ans: (B) IVIG

Chapter 12

SURGERY

1. Most common indication for liver transplant in children:

A. Wilson's disease
B. Primary biliary cirrhosis
C. Biliary atresia
D. Hemochromatosis

Key:

Most common indication of Liver transplant in children is Biliary atresia
Most common indication of Liver transplant in Adults is HCV Associated Cirrhosis
Most common indication for Liver transplant following Acute liver failure is Acetaminophen toxicity
Most common metabolic disorder indication for Liver transplantation–Alpha 1 Antitrypsin deficiency

Liver Transplantation

- First Liver transplantation was done by Starzl
- First Split liver transplant was done by Pichlmayr
- First live donor liver transplant was done by Tanaka

Indications for Liver Transplantation	
Adults	**Noncholestatic cirrhosis–HCV (Most common), HBV, Alcoholic and Cryptogenic** **Cholestatic**–Primary Biliary Cirrhosis, Primary sclerosing cholangitis Autoimmune, Malignant neoplasms, Miscellaneous
Children	**Biliary atresia (Most common)** Primary sclerosing cholangitis, Alagille syndrome Inbron errors of metabolism, Autoimmune, Viral hepatitis, Miscellaneous

Types of Liver Transplantation	
Live	*Right lobe segments 5 to 8 are used in Adult to Adult liver transplantation* *Left lobe segments 2-3 are used in Pediatric liver transplantation*
OLT- Orthotopic	*Graft is placed at normal position after recipient hepatectomy*

Contd.

Contd.

HLT- Heterotopic	*Graft is placed at an alternative site different normal anatomical position*
ALT- Auxiliary	*Native liver remains in situ and whole or partial transplant is added*
APOLT	*Left lobe of recipient liver is excised and donor liver occupies vacant space*
Auxiliary Heterotopic	*Whole liver or lobe is placed in sub hepatic space (Without disturbing original liver)*
Piggyback	*Orthotopic transplant that preserves recipient IVC*
Split	*Cadaveric donor liver is divided and given to 2 recipients*
Reduced	*Graft is reduced to a functional unit of appropriate size for recipient*
Domino	*Explanted liver graft from recipient can be reused for transplantation (Maple Syrup Urine Disease and Familial Amyloid Polyneuropathy)*

Contraindications to Liver Transplantation	
Absolute	**Relative**
Advanced cardiopulmonary disease	Age >70 years
Active untreated sepsis	Obesity (BMI >40 kg/m^2)
Metastatic malignancy to Liver	Cholangiocarcinoma
Active Alcohol abuse	Chronic or Refractory active infections
Severe intractable depression	Ongoing tobacco use or Illegal drug use
Excessive venous thrombosis	

- *Combined Heart and Lung transplantation is done in* ***Cystic fibrosis***
- *Combined Liver and Heart transplantation is done in* ***Amyloidosis***
- *Common cause of death in Liver transplantation–**Sepsis***

Ref: Bailey 27th Edition Page 1533, Sabiston 20th Edition Page 638, Schwartz 11th Edition Page 379, Blumgart 6th Edition Page 1775, Shackelford 7th Edition Page 1529

Ans: (C) Biliary atresia

2. **Name the knot shown below:**
   A. Reef knot
   B. Granny knot
   C. Surgeon's knot
   D. Half in Half knot

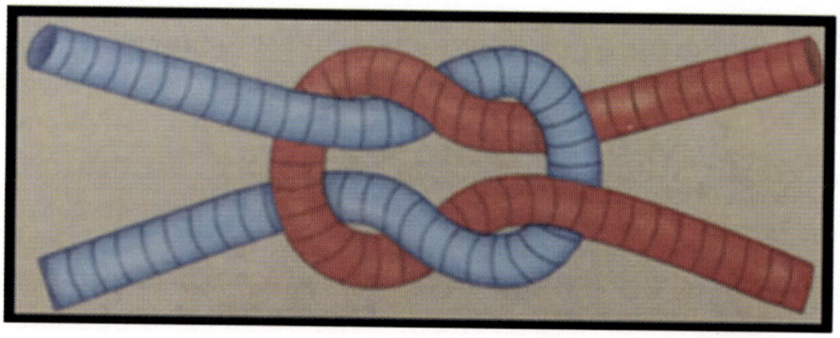

Key:

Granny knot is differentiated from Reef Knot by simple precision that in Square knot each loop passes completely over or completely under neck of other

Type of Knot	Features
Granny knot *(Slip knot/Pseudosquare knot)*	Consists of 2 throws *Crossing doesn't occur in any throw→* ***Binding Knot*** Not secured knot→***Tendency to slip when subjected to increasing pressure→ Inferior to Reef knot*** 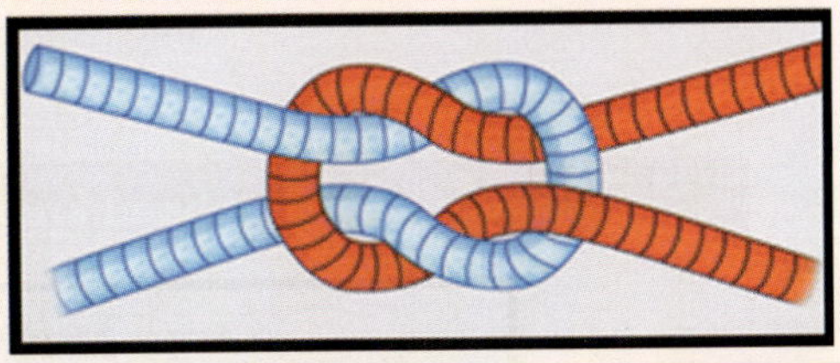
Reef knot *(Square knot)*	Consists of 2 rows ***Crossing is done in each throw→Secured knot*** Performed for tissues that are not under tension 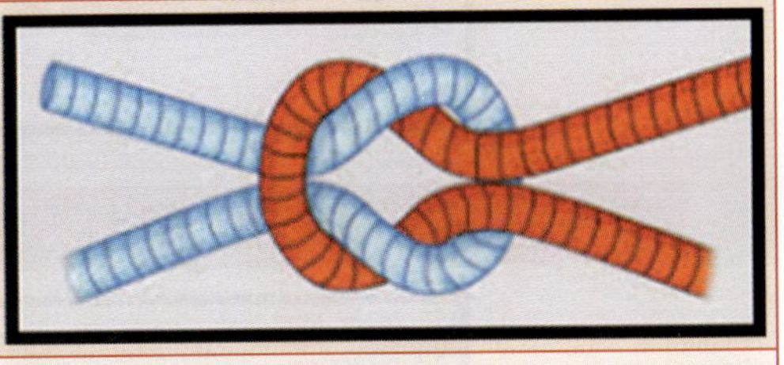
Surgeon's knot *(Friction knot)*	Consists of 2 throws ***Crossing occur in each throw*** Two wraps in first throw Simple modification to reef knot Adds extra twist when tying first throw forming a double overhand knot Additional throw provides more friction and can reduce loosening while 2nd half of knot is tied Knot is used to maintain tension on a suture 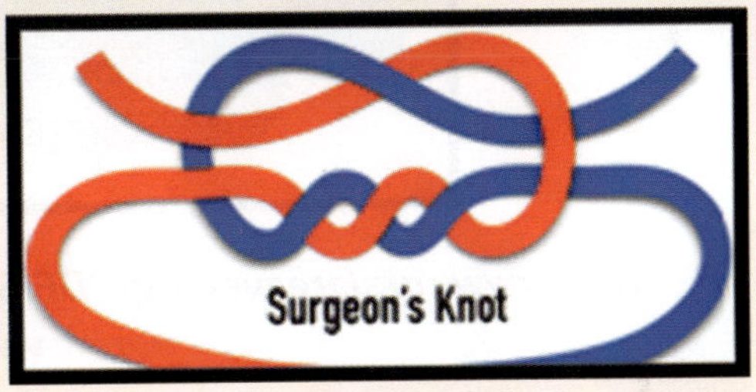

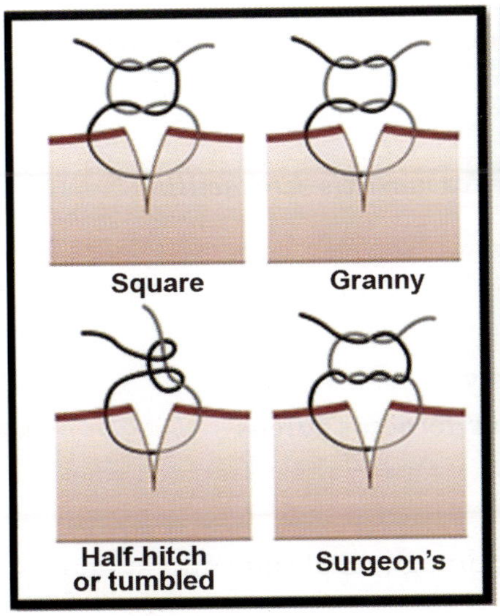

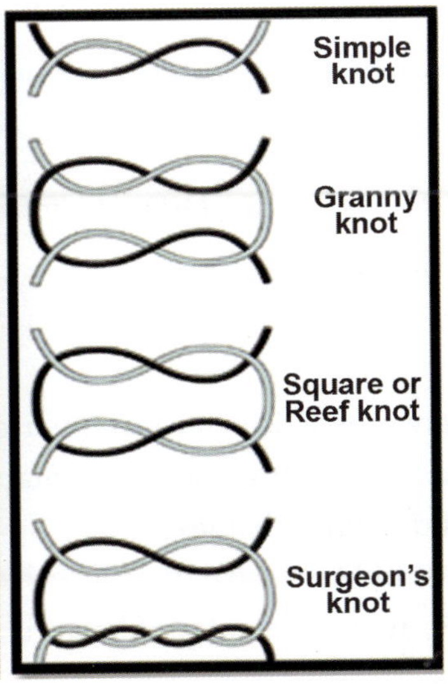

Granny Knot	Reef Knot
Two half hitches in same direction	Two half hitches in opposite direction
Slipping knot–Not tight	*Secure and Tight knot*

Contd.

Contd.

Less stable ***Less area of contact***	More stable
Half hitch: *Single Index or middle finger knot (either right over left/Left over right)* *Threads must CROSS in order to get stable knot*	

Over hand knot	Prusik knot
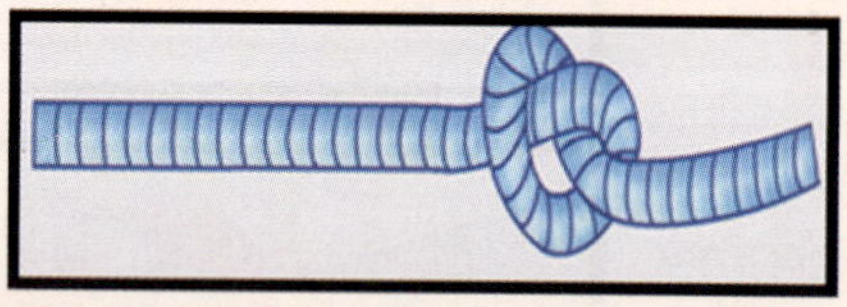	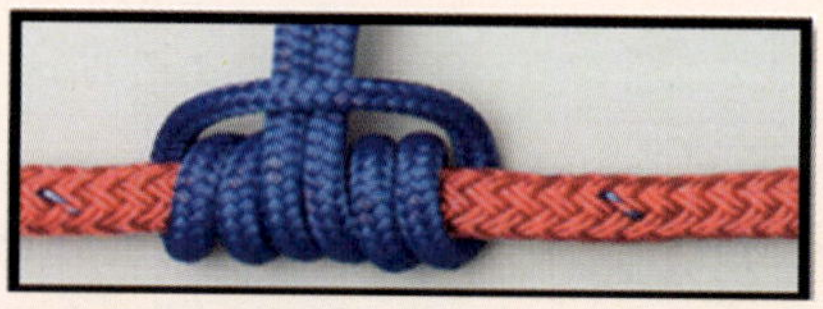
Figure of 8 bend	**Half knot**
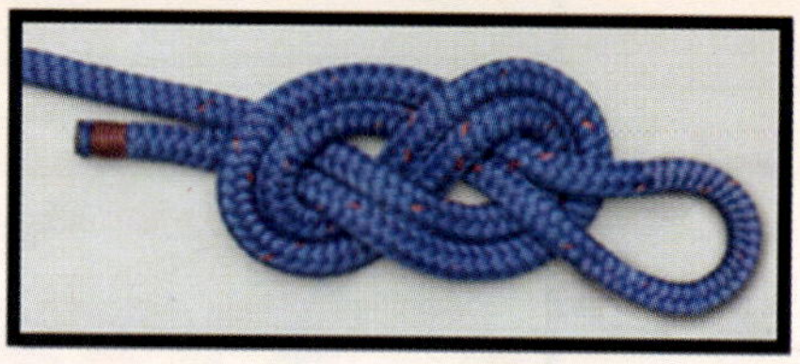	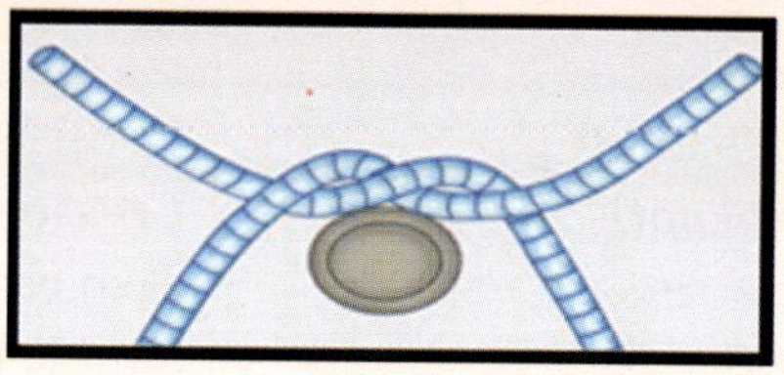

Ref: www.ruralareavet.org/PDF/Surgery-Knot_Tying.pdf, Principles and Techniques of Tying Surgical Knots, www.veteriankey.com/suturing-techniques-and-common-surgical-procedures

Ans: (B) Granny knot

3. **First line drug of choice for mastitis is:**
   A. Cefazolin
   B. Metronidazole
   C. Amoxicillin
   D. Cloxacillin

Key:

Drug of choice for mastitis–Cloxacillin

ACUTE MASTITIS

Etiology

- **Most common variety of mastitis–Bacterial variety**
- **Most common organism causing mastitis is Staphylococcus aureus**
- Infected breast should not feed babies
- Presents after 2nd day of life
- Lactational infections arise from entry of bacteria through nipple into duct system.

Features

- Can affect whole breast or usually segment of it.
- Presents with classical signs of acute inflammation.
- *Characterized by fever, leukocytosis, erythema and tenderness*
- This generalised cellulitis later can form an abscess.

Treatment

- Frequent emptying is advocated using breast pump.

- Analgesic and breast support should be given.
- ***Drug of choice for mastitis–Cloxacillin.***
- If hospital acquired infection is more likely to be pencillin resistant.
- If an antibiotic is used in presence of undrained pus→***'Antibioma'*** is formed

(Antibioma appears as large, sterile, brawny oedematous swelling that takes many weeks to resolve)

- **Incision and Drainage:** Recommended within 48 hours if infection doesn't resolve within 48 hours or tense induration or abscess after emptying of milk.

Puerperial /Non Endemic/Sporadic Mastitis

- Involvement of ***Interlobular connective tissue*** of breast by infectious process.
- Patient develops nipple fissuring and milk stasis→this further initiates retrograde infection.
- Emptying of breasts by pumps shortens duration of symptoms and reduces incidence of recurrence.
- Addition of antibiotic therapy→Successful outcome in >95% of cases.

Epidemic Puerperial Mastitis

- Initiated by highly ***virulent strains of MRSA.***
- Transmitted via suckling neonate.
- May result in substantial morbidity and occasional mortality.
- Purulent fluid is expressed from the nipple.
- Stop breastfeeding, antibiotics are started and surgical therapy is initiated.

Ref: Sabiston 20th Edition Page 836, Bailey 27th Edition Page 866, Schwartz 11th Edition Page 550

Ans: (D) Cloxacillin

4. Following blade is used for Incision and Drainage. Find out what number blade is it?

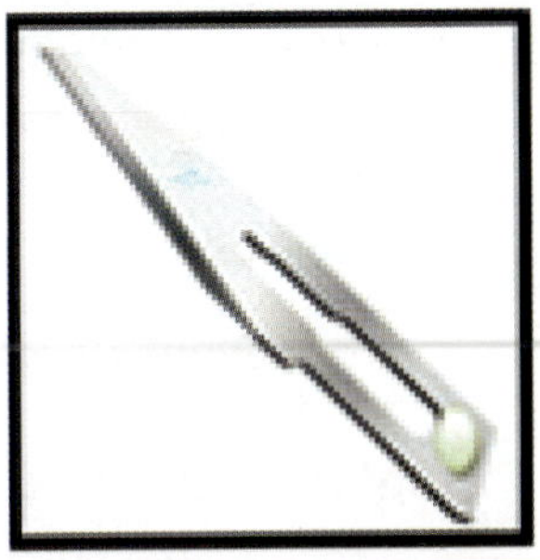

A. 15 Size
B. 22 Size
C. 11 Size
D. 13 Size

Key:

No. 11 blade is used for Arteriotomy and Incision and Drainage. *It is also used for other small incisions for example when inserting a laparoscopic port, vein and artery central lines, opening the aorta and removing calcifications in the aortic or mitral valves*

Elongated, triangular blade *sharpened along the hypotenuse edge with a pointed tip*

Scalpel Blades and Sizes

Blade Size	Purpose	Distinguishing Feature
10	*Used to open skin/Give skin incision*	*Large curved cutting edge*

Contd.

Contd.

11	***Used for Arteriotomy and Incision and Drainage***	***Elongated, triangular blade*** sharpened along the hypotenuse edge with a pointed tip
15	Used for minor surgical procedures, plastic and pediatric procedures	Small, curved cutting edge ideal for making short, precise incisions
22	Used for Abdominal Incisions	***Larger version of the number 10 blade*** with a curved cutting edge
23	Used for very thick skin	Flat, unsharpened back edge

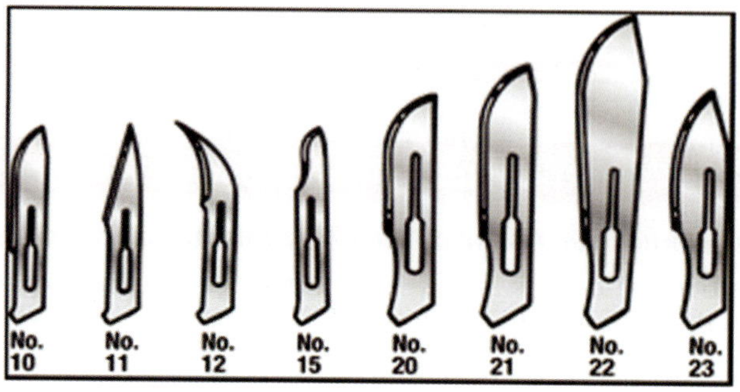

Most common type of scalpel blade used in surgery–Non-attached, replaceable blade

Ref: www.usamedicalsurgical.com/surgical-blades

Ans: (C) 11 Size

5. **Omphalocele is result of:**
   A. Duplicated Intestinal loops
   B. Failure of GIT to return to body cavity from its physiological herniation site
   C. Abnormal rotation of Intestinal loop
   D. Reversed rotation of Intestinal loop

Key:

Omphalocele is result of failure of GIT to return to body cavity from its physiological herniation site

OMPHALOCELE

- Congenital abnormality in anterior abdominal wall.
- ***Incidence: 1 in 5000 live births.***
- Bowel and solid viscera are covered by peritoneum and amniotic membrane.
- Umbilical cord inserts into sac.

TYPES

EXOMPHALOS MAJOR

Defect <5 cm
Only small bowel protrudes
Umbilical cord attached to summit
Strapping–Treatment
Good prognosis

EXOMPHALOS MINOR

Defect >5 cm
Small bowel and liver protrudes
Umbilical cord attached to side
Needs staged treatment
Bad prognosis

Moore's Classification of Omphalocele	
Type	**Diameter of Defect**
Type 1	< 2.5 cm
Type 2	2.5 to 5 cm
Type 3	>5 cm

- Intestine is freely mobile within intact sac with no inflammation/adhesions.
- Liver has dense adhesions into sac.
- *Small:* Single loop of intestine may not be obvious.
- *Large:* Liver, spleen, stomach, pancreas, colon or bladder may be seen through membrane.
- *Associated with cardiac anomalies and chromosomal anomalies.*

Gastroschisis	Omphalocele
Normal umbilical cord	Umbilical cord goes to defect
No protective membrane	Membrane (thin) covering present
Bowel contents protrude, may be	Normal bowel
Urgent surgical treatment to protect exposed intestine	Repaired electively
Good prognosis	Poor prognosis
Associated anomalies are rare (10-15% associated with intestinal atresia)	Higher incidence of congenital anomalies and Pulmonary hypoplasia
Lower mobidity and mortality	Higher morbidity and mortality

Ref: Bailey and Love 27th Edition Page 135, Schwartz 11th Edition Page 1554, Sabiston 20th Edition Page 1071

Ans: (B) Failure of GIT to return to body cavity from its physiological herniation site

6. **Frey's syndrome nerve occurs due to aberrant misdirection of fibers from salivary glands to sweat glands. These fibers come from which of the following?**

A. Facial
B. Trigeminal
C. Vagus
D. Glossopharyngeal

Key:

Frey syndrome occurs due to misdirected fibers of auriculotemporal nerve due to damage of nerve fibers after parotidectomy

FREY SYNDROME
Auriculotemporal nerve syndrome/Ballainger syndrome/Gustatory sweating

Etiology

- **Occurs usually as a complication of parotid surgery**
- **Others:** Mandibular surgery, drainage of parotid abscess, neck dissection
- Manifests 2-3 months after surgery

(May occur 2 weeks to 2 years after surgery→Latency in regeneration of parasympathetic fibers)

- Can also be caused by severe trauma–Penetrating trauma parotid region, Closed mandibular fractures.
- Nerve responsible for this is Cutaneous branch of Auriculotemporal nerve (Postganglionic parasympathetic fiber).

Pathogenesis

- Parasympathetic fibers supplying parotid gland are misdirected after parotidectomy and innervate sweat glands of the parotid area.
- **Aberrant regeneration of cut *parasympathetic fibers* between otic ganglion and parotid tissue**
- ***These aberrant fibers unite with fibers of superior cervical ganglion which innervates sweat glands and subcutaneous vessels.***

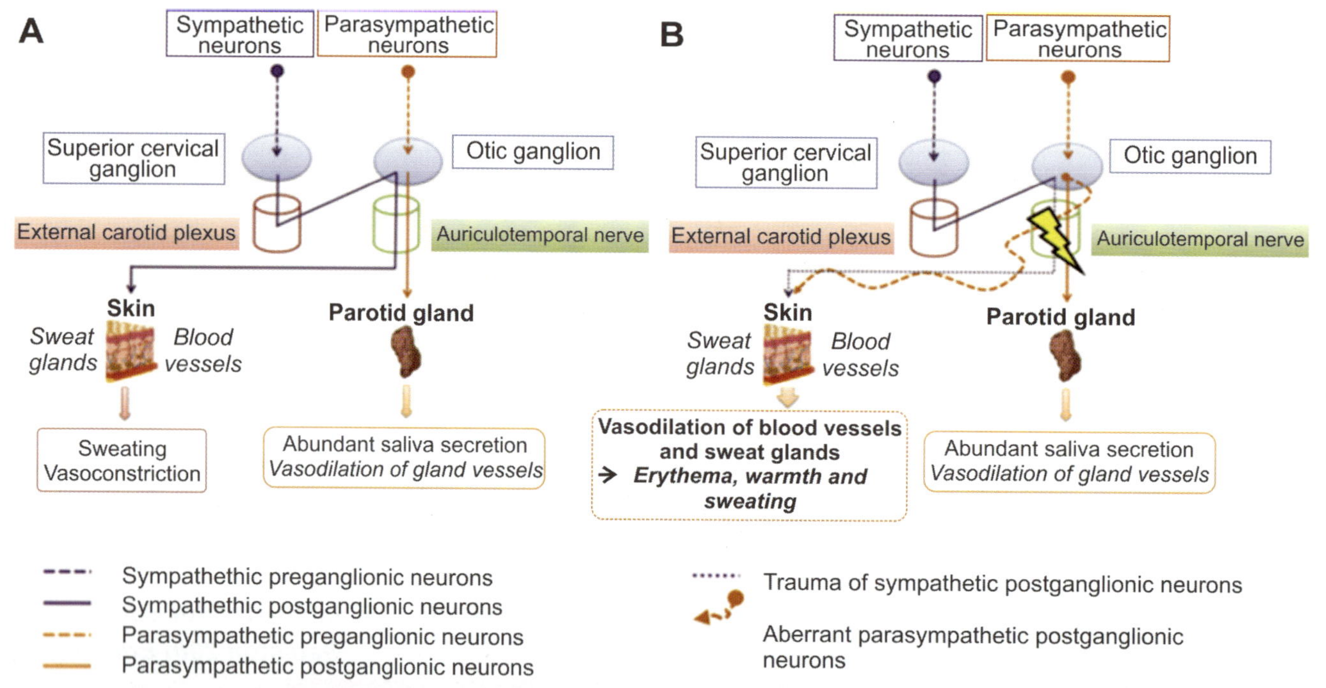

Pathophysiology hypothesis. **A.** Normal physiology of auriculotemporal nerve, and **B.** Pathophysiology hypothesis in case of injury of the auriculotemporal nerve.

Clinical Features

- Characterized by Flushing and sweating of skin of parotid region and neck during mastication/smell of food.
- ***Minor's Starch iodine test:*** Paint the affected area with iodine, allow it to dry then apply starch. In the presence of sweat starch turns blue.

Prevention

- Place a sheet of fascia lata between the skin and the underlying fat to prevent secretomotor fibers reaching the sweat glands–*Sternomastoid muscle flap, Temporalis fascial flap and Insertion of Artificial membrane.*

Generally No treatment is required in most of these patients
(Reassurance is best policy)→Self limiting disease

Treatment of Frey's Syndrome

Antiperspirant–*Aluminium chloride*

Administration of oral anticholinergic–reduces salivary secretion

Tympanic neurectomy: *Section of tympanic branch of CN IX will interrupt these fibers and give relief (Jacobson's nerve)–Indicated for Non-responding patients*

Surgical division of tympanic branch of glossopharyngeal nerve below round window of middle ear

Botulinum toxin–Injection into affected skin subcutaneously–Indicated for patients who can tolerate better, having long lasting symptoms/Recurrent symptoms→*Most effective*

With extracapsular dissection Frey's syndrome is almost zero percent (Less chance if tumor alone is enucleated).
With Traditional superficial parotidectomy, Frey's syndrome can be nearly 60%
Only 10% have symptomatic Frey's syndrome

Why you have to cut IXth nerve when auriculotemporal nerve (5th nerve branch) is damaged

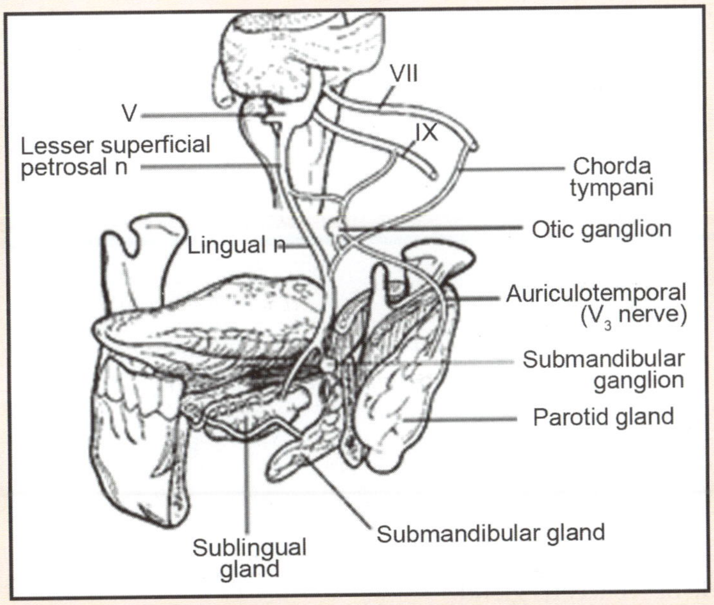

Preganglionic fibers of otic ganglion include tympanic branch of 9th Nerve–To reduce stimulus tympanic neurectomy is done

Version 2

All of the following statements are true about Frey's Syndrome except:

(a) Gustatory sweating

(b) Aberrant misdirection of sympathetic fibers of auriculotemporal nerve

(c) Botulinum toxin is one of the treatment suggested

(d) Less chances with enucleation than parotidectomy

Contd.

Contd.

Options	Statement	T/F
OPTION A	*Gustatory sweating* *(Perspiration on mastication)*	**True**
OPTION B	Aberrant misdirection of sympathetic fibers of auriculotemporal nerve *(Parasympathetic not sympathetic)*	**False**
OPTION C	Botulinum toxin is one of the treatment suggested *(Effective, Non-responders, Recurrent symptoms)*	**True**
OPTION D	Less chances with enucleation than parotidectomy *(Limited if tumor alone is removed by enucleation)*	**True**

Ans: (B) Aberrant misdirection of sympathetic fibers of auriculotemporal nerve

Ref: Bailey and Love 27th Edition Page 795, Myer's Cancer of Head and Neck 4th Edition Page 498

Ans: (B) Trigeminal

7. **Cystic lesion over scalp as shown below. What could be most probable diagnosis?**
   A. Meningioma
   B. Dermoid cyst
   C. Neural tumor
   D. Sebaceous cyst

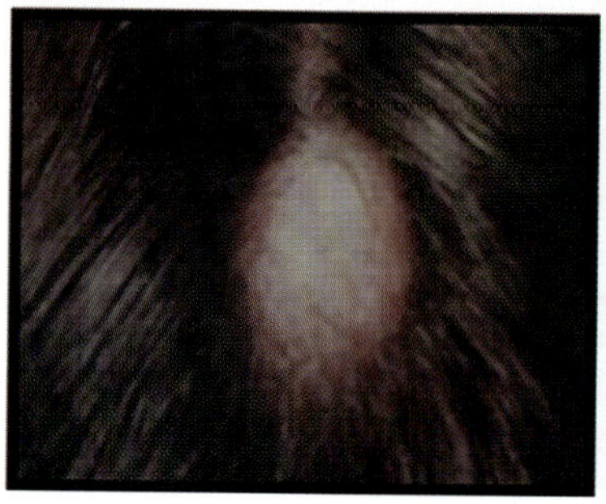

Key:

Given picture shows cystic swelling arising from scalp
Sebaceous cyst is implicated as one of the cause of Hair loss due to constant pressure

SEBACEOUS CYSTS/EPIDERMOID CYST/WEN

- Cysts are lined with true, stratified-squamous epithelium.
- Derived from hair follicle infundibuli or traumatic inclusion.
- Occurs due to blockade of sebaceous gland.
- Common in face scalp and scrotum.
- It has putty like consistency.
- Causative parasite implicated lies within the wall of sebaceous cyst–Demodex folliculorum.
- Fixed to the underlying skin.
- ***Usually have a central punctum (30% of cases have no punctum).***
- Usually scrotal sebaceous cysts are small and multiple.
- Hair loss over surface is common due to constant pressure over roots of hair follicles.

Smooth, soft, nontender, freely mobile, adherent to skin, fluctuant (positive Paget's test), non-transilluminating with punctum over summit.

- ***Treatment depends on clinical state of cyst.***
- ***Inflamed and Infected cyst***–Incised and drained initially→Removed after inflammation subsides.
- Excise cyst completely–If not recurrence can occur.

COMPLICATIONS

- **Infection and Abscess**
- **Cock's peculiar tumor** — Surface gets ulcerated and results in painful mass with discharge
- **Sebaceous horn** — Keratin deposition

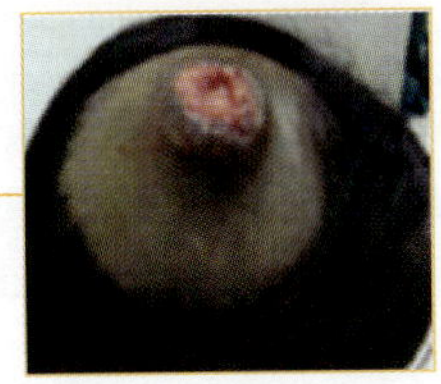

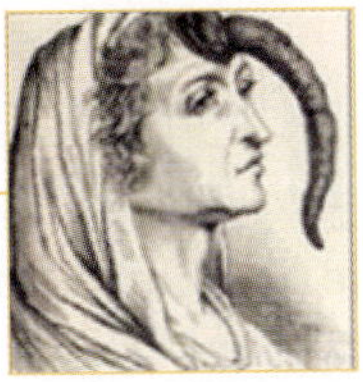

Ref: Schwartz 11th Edition Page 527, Sabiston 20th Edition Page 1913, Bailey 27th Edition Page 1511, SRB Manual of Surgery Page 75

Ans: (D) Sebaceous cyst

8. **A patient presented with gradually progressive painless mass since 10 years. It is firm to nodular and variable in consistency at each site. Most probable diagnosis is:**
   - A. Dermoid cyst
   - B. Sebaceous cyst
   - C. Pleomorphic adenoma
   - D. Malignancy

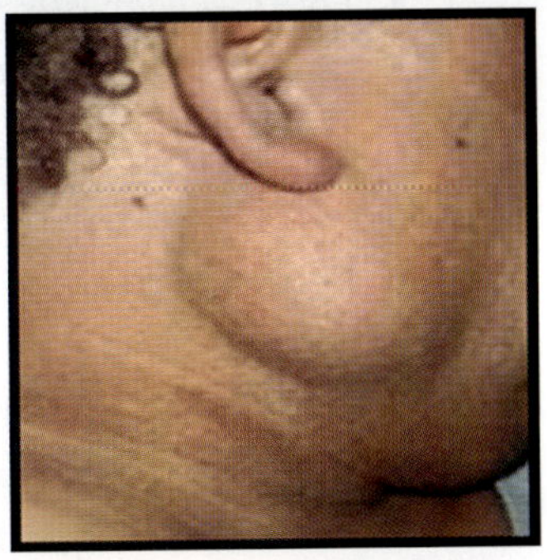

Key:

Picture depicts mass involving parotid region with elevation of ear lobule–Typically depicts Parotid tumor
Most common tumor of parotid gland–Pleomorphic adenoma

Dermoid cyst usually involve preauricular area–Not firm to nodular but cystic in consistency
Sebaceous cyst usually occur in post auricular area with a punctum
Gradually progressive growth since 10 years–Indicate benign nature of swelling (Malignancy ruled out)
So most likely diagnosis is Pleomorphic adenoma

Pleomorphic Adenoma

- Most common of all salivary gland neoplasms
- Most common major salivary gland tumor
- Most common benign salivary gland tumor
- Also called mixed tumor
- *Contains Epithelial and Mesenchymal elements*
- Well defined capsule is present
- Tumor extends pseudopods into normal tissue
- Usually involves females
- Most common age group involved is 40 years age

Contd.

Contd.

Clinical Features

- ***Most common site–Tail of parotid gland (Superficial lobe)***
- *Slow growing typically painless swelling below/in front/behind ear lobule*
- Lifts ear lobule
- Obliterates retromandibular groove
- *Dumbbell tumor*–Involves deep lobe pushes tonsil and pillars of fauces towards midline
- ***Curtain sign: +ve*** (Inability to move gland above zygomatic bone due to deep fascia attachment to bone
- ***Usually unicentric***
- ***Recurrence occur in multicentric fashion***

Investigations

- *FNAC–Diagnostic*
- ***Imaging investigation of choice***–*MRI (Most sensitive study to determine soft tissue extension and involvement of adjacent structures)→Can't differentiate between benign and malignant neoplasms*

Treatment

- *Involving superficial lobe→Superficial parotidectomy (PATEY'S OPERATION)*
- Involves deep lobe→Total parotidectomy with preservation of facial nerve
- Lazy S/Modified blair–Given for parotidectomy
- *If arising from submandibular gland–Excise whole gland*
- *Enucleation–High risk of recurrence* (Removes Tumor directly at capsule without normal tissue.

Extracapsular dissection (Bailey 27th Edition Update): Total excision of benign tumor with surrounding healthy parotid tissue, Meticulous dissection immediately outside tumor capsule with facial nerve preservation.

Indications for radiotherapy in salivary gland tumors: *Large primary tumors, High grade tumors, Bone invasion, Perineural invasion, Cervical lymph node metastasis and +ve surgical margins.*

COMPLICATIONS

- **Malignancy**
  - Occurs in 3-5% of patients **_Known as Carcinoma Ex pleomorphic adenoma_**
  - Rapid growth, pain, paraesthesia, enlarged cervical lymph nodes and restricted jaw movements, facial weakness or skin invasion and fixation of mastoid tip
  - *Histological findings suggestive of malignant change–Microscopic foci of necrosis, hemorrhage, calcification and excessive hyalinization*
- **Recurrence**
  - ***Usually after Enucleation***

Ref: Bailey 27th Edition Page 792, Sabiston 20th Edition Page 807, Schwartz 11th Edition Page 650

Ans: (C) Pleomorphic adenoma

9. **Degloving injury includes:**

A. Separation of skin only

B. Separation of skin and subcutaneous tissue with fascia intact

C. Separation of skin, subcutaneous tissue and fascia exposing tendons
D. Separation upto tendons exposing bone

Key:

Degloving injury occurs when skin and subcutaneous tissues are separated/stripped by avulsion from its underlying fascia leaving neurovascular structures, tendons and bone exposed

DEGLOVING INJURY

- Degloving injury occurs when skin and subcutaneous tissues are separated/stripped by avulsion from its underlying fascia.
- It leaves neurovascular structures, tendons and bone exposed.
- Result from shearing forces that cause parallel tissue planes to move against each other.
- Large areas of apparently intact skin may be deprived of their blood supply by rupture of feeding vessels.
- *Example–When hand is caught between rollers or in moving machinery.*

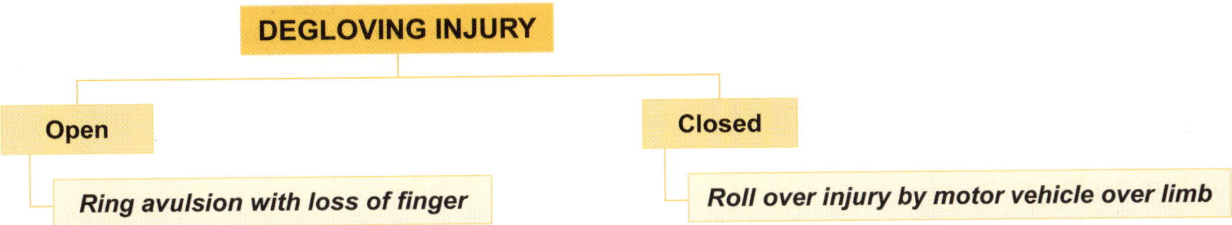

- Fascia is intact.
- Blood supply is severed.
- This injury is analogous to process of removing glove.
- Typically involves head or torso–which is more likely to be lethal.
- *Examination under anaesthetic is required with radical excision of all non-bleeding skin, as judged by bleeding dermis.*

FLUOROSCEIN TEST

- Patient is anaesthetized and Fluorescein can be administered in intravenous route.
- Viable/Perfused skin shows fluorescent yellowish green colour under UV light.
- Non-viable skin is cleary mapped out and Excision can be planned.
- *Possible anaphylactic shock due to fluorescein sensitivity–Main objection.*
- *Serial excision until punctate dermal bleeding is obvious–Reliable factor.*
- Split skin grafts can be harvested from degloved non-viable skin and meshed to cover raw areas resulting from debridement.

Morel Lavallee lesions–Degloving injury after blunt trauma
Morel-Lavallée lesion–Ecchymotic lesion over greater trochanter that represents subcutaneous degloving injury and frequently associated with acetabular fractures.

Midfacial degloving procedure allows excellent bilateral exposure of the maxillae, paranasal sinuses, and nasopharynx without facial incisions for tumors of nose and nasopharynx
Coronal scalp degloving approach–Indicated when Zygomatic arch component of transverse buttress is communuted (Establishes facial projection)

Ref: Bailey and Love 27th Edition Page 27, Sabiston 20th Edition Page 423, SRB Manual of Surgery 5th Edition Page 12, Principle and Practice of Surgery 7th Edition Page 302

Ans: (B) Separation of skin and subcutaneous tissue with fascia intact

10. Cushing ulcers are:

A. Stress ulcers in burns
B. Stress ulcers in head injury
C. Stress ulcers in hiatus hernia
D. Stress ulcers in analgesic drug abuse

Key:

CUSHING ULCER: Stress ulcers associated with Intracranial injury/Increase in Intracranial pressure. Cushing's ulcers are more prone to perforate than other stress ulcers

CUSHING ULCER: *Ulcer usually occurs after Head trauma*
CURLING ULCER: *Ulcer usually occurs after burn injury and any kind of shock (>30% BSA)*

STRESS ULCERS

- **Early**
  - *Appears within first 24 hours*
  - *Typically multiple and shallow*
  - *Discrete araes of erythema along with focal hemorrhage/adherent clot*
  - *Erodes submucosa–Bleeding*
- **Late**
  - *Tissue reaction/Organization around clot/ Inflammatory exudate*

- Stress ulcers usually occurs after physical trauma, shock, sepsis, hemorrhage, or respiratory failure and may lead to life-threatening gastric bleeding.
- Stress gastritis develops within 1 to 2 days after traumatic event in >50% patients.
- Presence of luminal acid appears to be prerequisite for stress gastritis to evolve.
- ***Only clinical sign of delayed onset***→ Painless upper GI bleeding (Usually slow and Intermittent-detected by flecks of blood in NG tube/unexplained decrease in hemoglobin level.
- Stool is frequently guaiac-positive.
- Endoscopy is required to confirm diagnosis.

Treatment

- Fluid resuscitation and coagulation correction
- Treat underlying sepsis
- More than 80% stop bleeding with supportive care
- Selective infusion of vasopressin into left gastric artery
- Embolization of left gastric artery
- *Bleeding that recurs or persists, requires >6U of blood (3000 mL)→Indication for surgery*
- Figure of 8 stitches deep in gastric wall
- Anterior gastrotomy and truncal vagotomy along with pyloroplasty has been tried
- Total gastrectomy should be performed only in patients with life-threatening hemorrhage refractory to other forms of therapy.

Peptic Ulcer
(Usually occur in following sites in descending order)
• ***Duodenum 1st portion–Most common site OVERALL***
• Antrum

Contd.

Contd.

- At Gastroesophageal junction→ GERD/Barrett's esophagus
- Within margins of Gastrojejunostomy
- Duodenum, Stomach/Jejunum occurs in patients of ZES
- Within or adjacent to Meckel's diverticulum (Ectopic gastric mucosa)

ETIOLOGY OF ACUTE PEPTIC ULCER

- **NSAID ingestion**
- **Stress**
  - **Cushing**–*Head trauma*
  - **Curling**–*Burn injury*
- **Sepsis**
- **Steroids**

ETIOLOGY OF CHRONIC PEPTIC ULCER

- **Gastric ulcer**
  - NSAIDS, Helicobacter pylori
    Pyloroduodenal reflux, Cirrhosis,
    Mucosal trauma,
    Low socio-economic status, Irregular diet, Spicy food, Excessive coffee and tea drinking, Cigarette smoking,
    Anxiety and stress
- **Duodenal ulcer**
  - Helicobacter pylori, NSAIDS
    Acid hypersecretion, Blood group O, ZES,
    Hyperparathyroidism, Multiple adenoma syndrome (MEN 1), Cushing syndrome, Cirrhosis, Chronic lung disease, Chronic pancreatitis, Reduced bicarbonate production, Alcohol, Smoking, Vitamin deficiency,
    Stress and Anxiety

- ***Most common site of Gastric ulcer***–Lesser curvature along Incisura angularis (Type I)
- ***Most common site of duodenal ulcer***–1st part of duodenum
- ***Most common cause of death in Peptic ulcer disease***–*Bleeding*
- Most common complication of Gastric ulcer–Perforation
- Most common complication of duodenal ulcer–Bleeding (Gastroduodenal artery)
- Most common complication that requires surgery in peptic ulcer–Bleeding
- Complication associated with Highest mortality–Perforation
- Incidence of malignancy in Gastric ulcer–0.5 to 5%
- Incidence of malignancy in Duodenal ulcer→ Almost zero (Never turns Malignant)

Ref: Bailey and Love 27th Edition Page 1115,
Sabiston 20th Edition Page 1211

Ans: (B) Stress ulcers in head injury

11. Maintenance level of Mixed Venous Oxygen Saturation in Shock must be:

A. >70%   B. 50-70%
C. 40-50%   D. <40%

Key:

Maintenance level of Mixed Venous Oxygen Saturation in Shock must be 50-70%

MIXED VENOUS OXYGEN SATURATION (MVOS)

- Percentage saturation of oxygen returning to heart from body.

- **Normal MVOS→ 50-70%.**
- True mixed venous sample (called SvO_2) is drawn from the tip of pulmonary artery catheter and includes all of venous blood returning from head and arms (via SVC), gut and lower extremities (via IVC) and coronary veins (via coronary sinus).
- Measure of oxygen delivery and extraction by tissues.

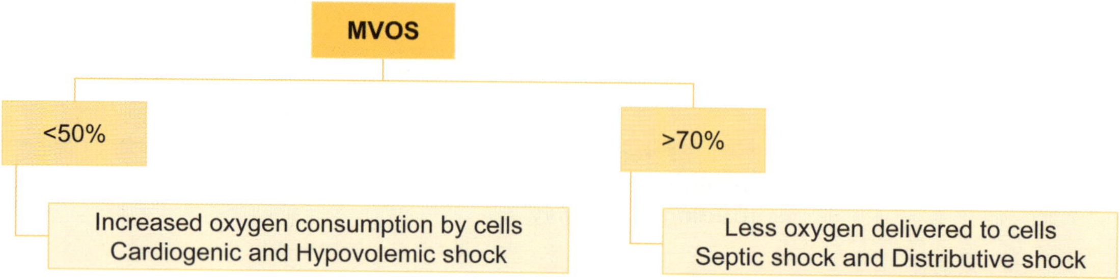

Septic Shock

- At cellular level in sepsis, there is disordered utilisation of oxygen.
- At microvascular level, there is AV shunting of blood.
- ***Therefore, less oxygen is presented to cells, and those cells cannot utilise what little oxygen is presented.***
- Venous blood has a higher oxygen concentration than normal.
- Hypovolaemia should be corrected with fluid therapy, and low cardiac output due to myocardial depression or failure should be treated with dobutamine, to achieve a mixed venous saturation greater than 70% (normal for the septic state).

Hemodynamic Responses to Different Types of Shock

Type of Shock	Cardiac Index	SVR	Venous Capacitance	CVP/ PCWP	SVO_2	Cellular/Metabolic Effects
Hypovolemic	↓	↑	↓	↓	↓	Effect
Septic	↑↑	↓	↑	↑↓	↑↓	Cause
Cardiogenic	↓↓	↑↑	→	↑	↓	Effect
Neurogenic	↑	↓	→	↓	↓	Effect

Ref: Bailey and Love 27th Edition Page 17, Schwartz 11th Edition Page 135

Ans: (B) 50-70%

12. Histological difference between Crohn's disease and ulcerative colitis is:

A. Crypt abscess
B. Diffuse distribution of pseudopolyps
C. Mucosal edema
D. Lymphoid aggregates in mucosa

Key:

Crypt abscess can be seen in both Crohn's disease and Ulcerative colitis
But it is most common in Ulcerative colitis than Crohn's disease

Only distinctive feature in Crohn's disease is noncaseating granuloma (Not given in options)

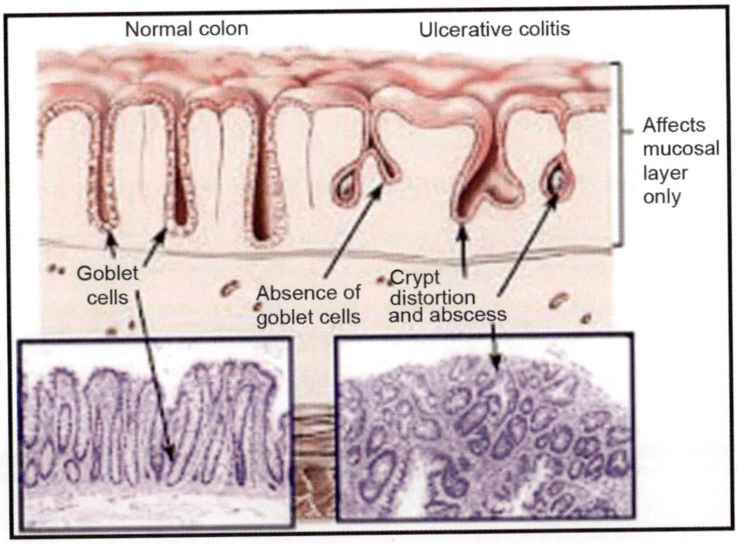

Differences Between Crohn's Disease and Ulcerative Colitis		
	Crohn's Disease	**Ulcerative Colitis**
Site	Any where	Colon/Rectum
Distribution of lesion	Skip lesions	Continuous
Layers involved	Full thickness	Mucosa/Submucosa
Mucosal appearance	Cobblestone appearance	Friable, Diffusely involved
Rectum	Often spared (>50%)	Always involved (>90%)
Associated ileal	50% have combined ileal and colonic involvement	10% mild, Terminal ileal inflammation
Perianal disease	Common	Rare
Fistula formation	Common	Rare
Stricture	Common	Rare
Granulomas	Common	No
Fissures	Common	No
Crypt abscess	*Rare*	*Common*
Toxic megacolon	Very rare	Rare (more than Crohn's disease)
Sclerosing cholangitis	Rare	Common
Uveitis and arthritis	Common	Common
Pyoderma gangrenosum	Rare	Common
Creeping mesenteric fat	Common	Not seen
Pseudopolyps	Rare	Common
Dysplasia	Rare	Common

Contd.

Contd.

Carcinoma	Rare	10%
Surgery	Palliative	Curative

Ref: Schwartz 10th Edition Page 1198, Bailey and Love 27th Edition Page 1242, Sabiston 20th Edition Page 1339

Ans: (A) Crypt abscess

13. On Endoscopy Serpigenous ulcers in distal esophagus with otherwise normal mucosa is seen with:

A. Pill induced Esophagitis
B. CMV Esophagitis
C. Herpes Esophagitis
D. Corrosive Esophagitis

Key:

Characteristic appearance of Geographical Serpentine ulcer border is seen on Endoscopy of CMV Esophagitis
CMV classically causes serpiginous ulcers in distal esophagus that may coalesce to form giant ulcers
Characteristic Universal Symptom of Infectious Esophagitis–Odynophagia

INFECTIOUS ESOPHAGITIS
- Immunocompromised
  - Candida, Herpes and CMV
- Non-immunocompromised
  - Herpes and Candida

CMV ESOPHAGITIS

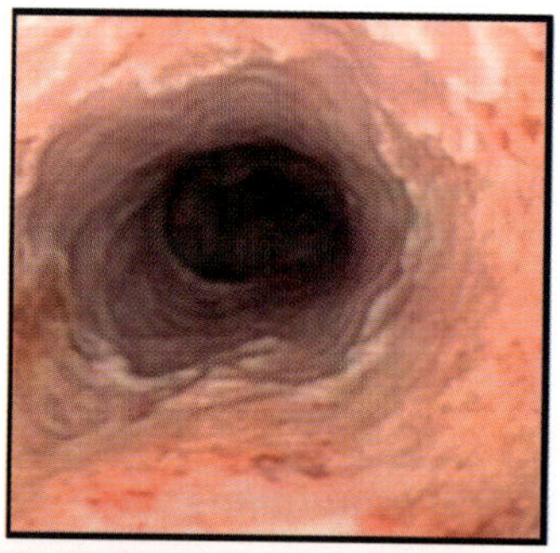

- Primarily occur in Organ transplant recipients
- Seen in Graft versus host disease following Bone marrow transplantation
- *Endoscopy and Biopsy–Diagnostic*
- **ENDOSCOPY**–Geographical serpentine ulcers
- **Usually involves Distal esophagus**
- Ganciclovir–Drug of choice

Candida Esophagitis

- Candida albicans is most common pathogen
- Most common fungal esophagitis–Candidal Esophagitis
- Usually occurs in Immunocompromised conditions (Steroids inducers, Transplant recipients, Chemotherapy patients and Uncontrolled DM
- Can also occur in patients with Esophageal stasis secondary to motility disorders and diverticula
- Strongly associated with Oropharyngeal candidiasis
- *Endoscopy shows characteristic numerous friable white plaques which can't be moved (Unlike food residues)*

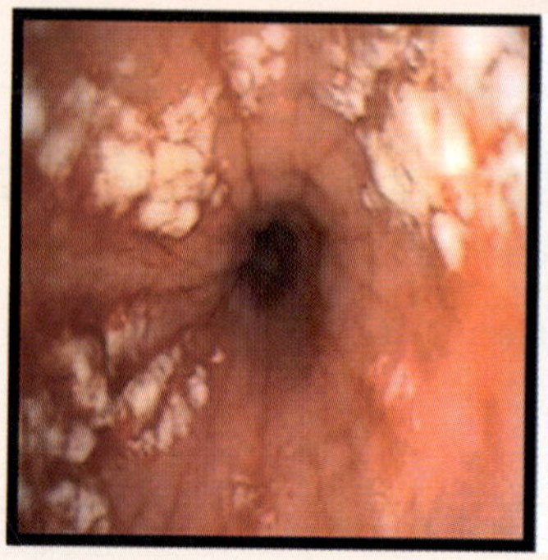

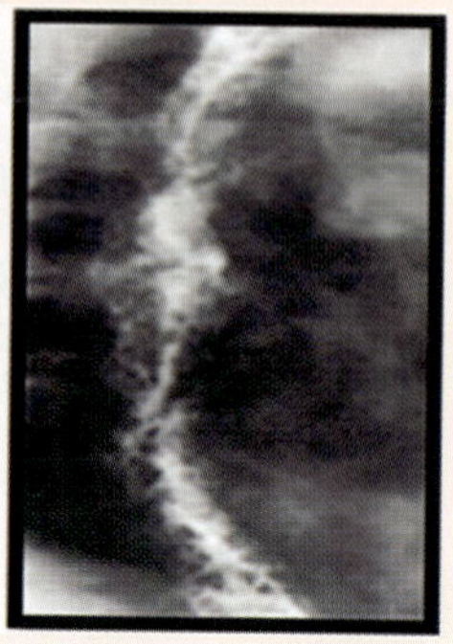

Contd.

Contd.

- ***Barium swallow→Dramatic irregular mucosal ulceration that looks like esophageal varices (SHAGGY APPEARANCE)***
- **Treatment–***Topical Antifungal agent (Azoles)→If resistant Intravenous Echinocandin*
- **During pregnancy–Amphotericin B is drug of choice**

HSV Esophagitis

- HSV 1 and 2 can cause Esophagitis
- May have co existing vesicles on nose and lips
- **Endoscopy–***Vesicles and small punched out ulcers with raised margins usually seen in upper half of esophagus*
- ***Endoscopy and Biopsy–Investigation of choice***→Reveals characteristic ground-glass nuclei, Eosinophilic Cowdry's type A inclusion bodies and giant cells
- **Acyclovir–Drug of choice**

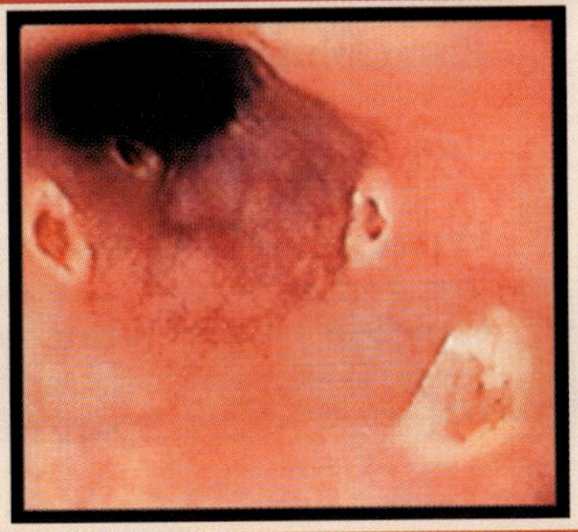

Pill Induced Esophagitis

- Direct esophageal injury by drug taken
- Most commonly invoved drugs include bisphosphonates, NSAIDs, Tetracyclines, Vitamin C, and potassium chloride tablets
- Ulcers with occasional bleeding is noticed
- No specific histological features
- Removal of cause resolves condition without any complications–*Self limiting*

With AIDS, Infectious esophagitis is common if CD4 count is less than 100

HIV itself is associated with a self-limited syndrome of acute esophageal ulceration with oral ulcers and maculopapular skin rash at seroconversion time.

VZV–Chickenpox causes Esophagitis in children, Zoster causes Esophagitis in Adults

Ref: Bailey and Love 27th Edition Page 1104, Robbins Pathology 9th Edition Page 755, Harrison 20th Edition Page 2218, Shackelford 8th Edition Page 486

Ans: (B) CMV Esophagitis

14. Small punched out lesions on Endoscopy in lower esophagus in Immunocompromised patients is seen in:

A. Pill induced Esophagitis
B. CMV Esophagitis
C. Herpes Esophagitis
D. Corrosive Esophagitis

Key:

Herpes ulcers	***Punched out with nuclear viral inclusions within a rim of degenerating epithelial cells at ulcer margin***
CMV ulcers	Shallow ulcers with nuclear and cytoplasmic inclusions within capillary endothelium and stromal cells
Pill induced ulcers	Usually occurs at site of strictures often accompanied by superficial necrosis with Granulation tissue and Fibrosis
Corrosive ulcers	No neutrophils with strictures

Esophagitis	Appearance
CMV	Serpiginous ulcers at distal esophagus
HSV	Volcano ulcer, punched out, small, vesicle type, lower esophagus
Eosinophilic	Circular rings, linear furrow, whitish papules and plaques (Feline esophagus)
Infectious	Involves proximal and diffuse ulceration
Peptic	Single and Distal esophagus
Candida	White-yellow friable plaques giving cottage-cheese appearance
Pill	Spare distal esophagus, singular and deep at point of luminal narrowing

(Refer above question for Explanation)

Ref: Bailey and Love 27th Edition Page 1104, Robbins Pathology 9th Edition Page 755, Harrison 20th Edition Page 2218, Shackelford 8th Edition Page 486

Ans: (C) Herpes Esophagitis

15. Cholesterol gallstones are made up of:

A. Amorphous cholesterol monohydrate B. Amorphous cholesterol dehydrate
C. Crystalline cholesterol monohydrate D. Crystalline cholesterol dehydrate

Key:

Cholesterol stones are made up of Crystalline cholesterol monohydrate

GALLSTONES

- Risk factors–Obesity, Rapid weight loss, Multiparity, Child bearing, Female sex, 1st degree relatives, Ileal resection/bypass, Native Americans, Drugs–Estrogens, Ceftriaxone and TPN

GALL-STONES

- **CHOLESTEROL STONES** *Most common (75%)*
  - Formed by Nucleation of ***cholesterol monohydrate crystals*** from multilamellar vesicles
  - ***Most common type of gallstone in Western*** countries
- **PIGMENT STONES** *Contains <30% cholesterol*
  - **BROWN PIGMENT STONE**
    - *Composed of calcium bilirubinate, palmitate and stearate along with cholesterol*
    - *Most common organism–E.coli*
    - *Most common recurrent stone type*
    - **Infection in CBD, Clonorchis and Ascariasis**
  - **BLACK PIGMENT STONES**
    - Composed of largely insoluble bilirubin pigmeny polymer mixed with calcium phosphate and bicarbonate
    - ***Sickle cell disease and Hereditary spherocytosis, Cystic fibrosis, Prosthetic heart valves, Cirrhosis, Gilbert syndrome, Ileal disease/resection***

Mechanism of Cholesterol Gallstone Formation

NORMAL MIXED MISCELLE (CHOLESTEROL, LECITHIN AND BILE ACIDS)

↓

Lithogenic Bile

↓

Supersaturation of bile ***(Reduced bile acid pool, Increased cholic acid)***

↓

CHOLESTEROL NUCLEATION
Increased pro nucleating factors (Mucin, Non mucin glycoproteins
Reduced antinucleating factors (Apolipoproteins AI and AII)

↓

Gallbladder hypomotility
TPN, Pregnancy, Fasting, Octreotide, OCP and Massive Burns

↓

Biliary sludge

↓

Gallstones

LITHOGENIC BILE

- **Increased biliary cholesterol**–Obesity, Cholesterol rich diet and Clofibrate therapy
- **Reduced bile acids**–Primary biliary cirrhosis, OCP, Mutation of CYP7A1, Impaired enterohepatic circulation of bile acids–Ileal disease/resection, Cholestyramine/Colestipol
- **Decreased Biliary lecithin**–MDR 3 mutation.

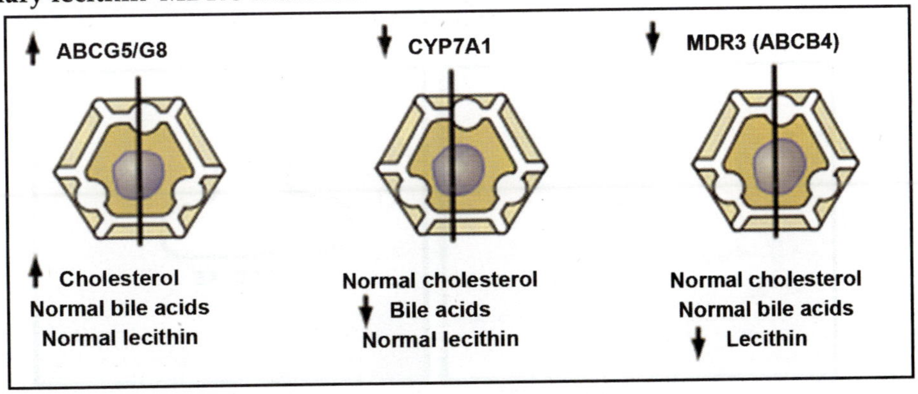

- If there is an excess of cholesterol in relation to phospholipids and bile acids, unstable, cholesterol-rich vesicles remain, which aggregate into large multilamellar vesicles from which ***cholesterol crystals*** precipitate→Cholesterol gallstones

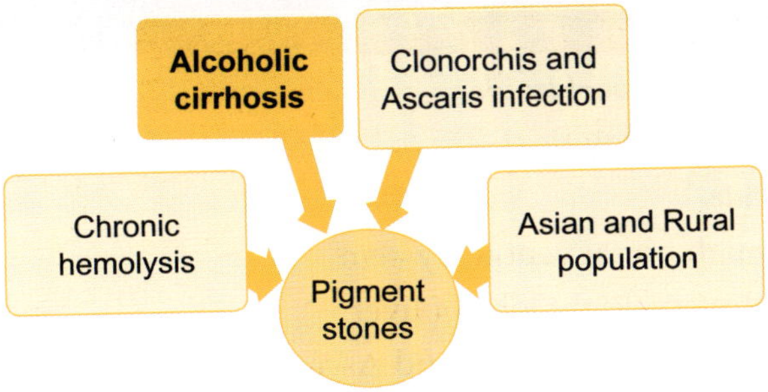

- ***Most common type of stone–Mixed stone***
- ***Most common stone in Asia–Pigment stone***
- ***90% of Gallstones are radiolucent***
- Investigation of choice for diagnosing Acute cholecystitis–***USG***
- Gold standard for diagnosing Acute cholecystitis–***HIDA Scan***
- Investigation of choice for Chronic cholecystitis–***USG***
- ***Laparoscopic cholecystectomy–Gold standard for Gallstone treatment***
- ***Indications for cholecystectomy***–All symptomatic gallstones, Gallstones of size >2.5 cm, associated with polyp/ Anomalies of gallbladder, Family history of gallbladder stones or carcinoma, Acalculous cholecystitis, Gallstone pancreatitis and as a part Prophylactic treatment.

Ref: Bailey and Love 27th Edition Page 1200, Sabiston 20th Edition Page 1491, Schwartz 11th Edition Page 1401, Robbins Pathology 9th Edition Page 640, Harrison 20th Edition Page 2426

Ans: (D) Crystalline cholesterol dehydrate

16. Flask shaped ulcers in colon is caused by:

A. Giardia lamblia

B. Entamoeba Histolytica

C. H. pylori

D. Enterobius vermicularis

Key:

Flask shaped ulcers typically on colonoscopy involving Cecum and Ascending colon–Broad base and Narrow neck Typically seen with Amoebic colitis

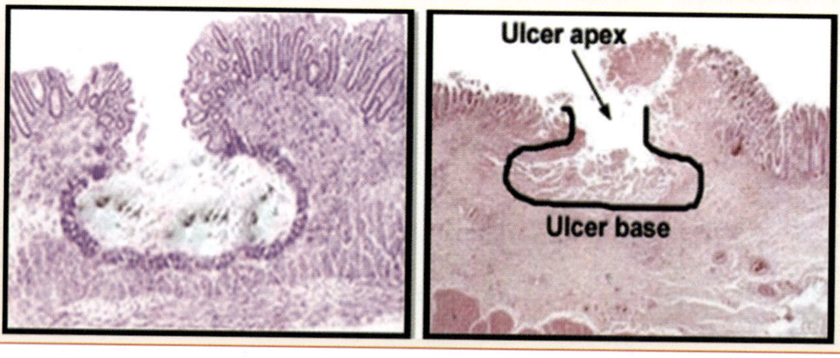

Amoebiasis

- ***Most common type of liver abscess worldwide***
- **Causative organism**–Entamoeba histolytica
- **Route of spread**– *Feco oral route*
- Trophozoites reach liver through portal venous system
- **Most common site of liver abscess**–Right lobe of liver
- **Most common site of infection in GIT**–Cecum and Ascending colon

Contd.

Contd.

Clinical Features

- Young age of 20-40 years
- Males > Females (10:1)
- Most common symptom–Abdominal pain
- **Recent history of diarrhea is not common**

Anchovy sauce pus is a feature of Amoebic liver abscess (Liquefactive necrosis of liver)

- Jaundice–Result of large abscess compressing biliary tree
- Pleuritic/Right shoulder pain–Irritation of right hemidiaphragm
- ***1/3rd of Active amoebic colitis*→ synchronous liver abscess**

Investigations

- **LFT**–Mild abnormalities
  (Most common abnormality–Elevated PT)
- **USG**–Hypoechoic and Non-homogenous rounded lesion abutting liver capsule without significant rim echoes.

*Diagnosis–**Confirmed** by Serological tests (EIA) for antiamoebic antibodies→High sensitivity and specificity*

- *CT–Mainstay investigation*
  Well defined border with absent peripheral rim enhancement along with peripheral edema
  Abscess limited to glisson capsule→Characteristic feature

Treatment

- **Metronidazole–Drug of choice**
- Curative in >90% of patients
- **Therapeutic needle aspiration–Avoided**
- ***Indications of needle aspiration***–Diagnostic uncertainty, Fails to respond to metronidazole in 3 to 5 days, High risk of rupture (> 5 cm, left lobe), Abscess secondary to pyogenic organism, Pregnancy.

Complications

- Rupture into peritoneum, pleura or pericardium

Most common complication of amoebic liver abscess–Rupture

- Most common site of rupture–***Peritoneum***
- Size of abscess is most important factor for rupture
- Rupture into bronchus–***Self limiting (Bronchodilator and postural drainage)***→Thoracocentesis
- ***Laparotomy***–Doubtful cases, Hollow viscus perforation, Fistula formation and failure of conservative therapy.

Ulcers in GIT	
Stress induced ulcer in Trauma	Cushing ulcer
Stress induced ulcer in Burns	*Curling ulcer*
Hiatus hernia (Proximal stomach)	Cameron ulcer
Tuberculosis	Transverse ulcer in small intestine

Contd.

Contd.

Typhoid	Longitudinal ulcers in small intestine
Amoebiasis	Flask shaped ulcers of colon on microscopy (Bottleneck ulcers)
HSV	Punched out ulcers on esophageal endoscopy
CMV	Serpentine ulcers on esophageal endoscopy
Crohn's disease	Serpentine ulcers in small intestine
Ulcerative colitis	Collar button ulcers in large intestine
Syphilis	Snail track ulcers of oral cavity

Ref: Bailey and Love 27th Edition Page 711

Ans: (B) Entamoeba Histolytica

17. Mother donating kidney to her son. This is an example of:

A. Autograft
B. Allograft
C. Isograft
D. Xenograft

Key:

Mother donates kidney to her son–Imples Organ transplanted to another individual of same species→Allograft

Autograft	Tissue transplanted from one part of body to another in same individual/ Autotransplant
Isograft	Graft tissue between 2 individuals who are genetically identical ***(Monozygotic twins)*** Transplant rejection between 2 such individuals never occurs
Allograft/Homograft	Organ/Tissue transplanted from one individual to another ***(same species)*** ***Alloantigen: transplant antigen*** ***Alloantibody: transplant antibodies***
Xenograft/Heterograft	Transplant performed between different species
Orthotopic graft	Graft placed in its normal anatomical site
Heterotopic graft	Graft placed in a site different from that where organs are normally located

Transplant History (There are a lot of mistakes regarding this topic in many surgery guide books–Entirely updated from Bailey 27th Edition)		
1st successful kidney transplant	1954	Murray

Contd.

Contd.

1st successful liver transplant	1963	Starzl
1st liver donor liver transplant	***1991***	***Tanaka***
1st split donor liver transplant	***1988***	***Pichlmayr***
1st Heart transplant	1967	Bernard
1st Human lung transplant	1968	Derom
1st Small intestinal transplant	1967	Lillehei
1st Pancreatic islet cell transplant	1974	Sutherland and Najarin
1st Successful heart lung transplant	1981	Reitz and Shumway
1st Corneal transplant	1905	Eduard Zinn
Multivisceral transplant	1989	Starzl
Transplantation of Human Organs Act was passed in 1994		

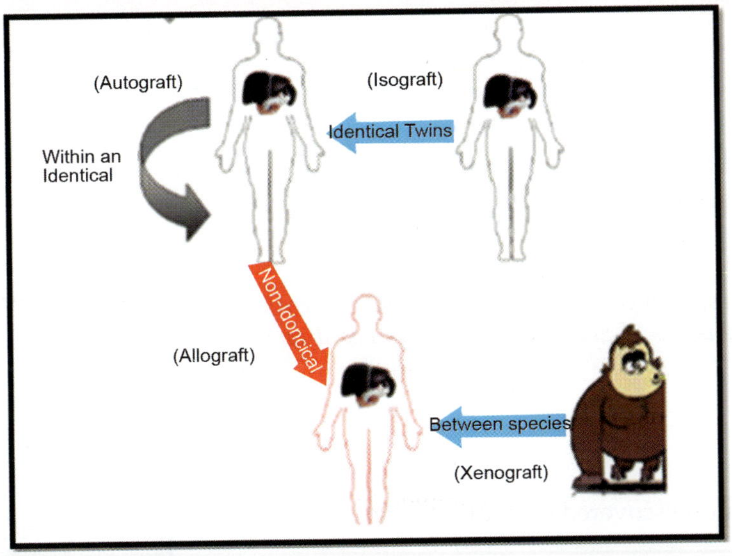

Ref: Sabiston 20th Edition Page 599, Bailey and Love 27th Edition Page 1533, Schwartz 11th Edition Page 358

Ans: (B) Allograft

18. Most commonly used approach for Retrosternal goiter is:

A. Transthoracic via 2nd Intercostal space

B. Transthoracic via 4th Intercostal space

C. Trans sternal through Anterior mediastinum

D. Transcervical

Key:

More than 95% of retrosternal goiters are removed transcervically

RETROSTERNAL GOITRE

- Common in short neck males with strong pretracheal muscles

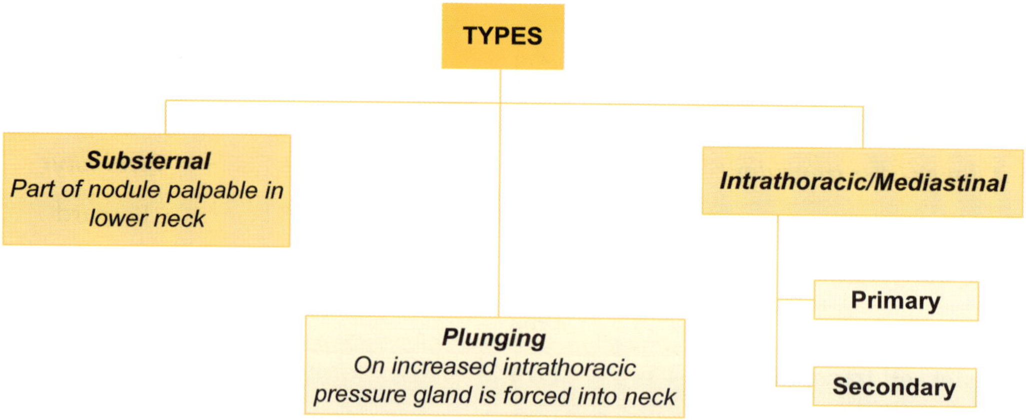

Primary Mediastinal	Secondary Mediastinal
• **Only <1%** • Arises from accessory/ectopic thyroid tissue in chest • Supplied by Intrathoracic blood vessels • Don't have any connection to thyroid tissue in neck	• **Constitute Majority of mediastinal goiters** • Arises from downward extension of cervical thyroid tissue along fascial planes of neck • *Derives blood supply from superior inferior thyroid arteries*

- *Most intrathoracic or substernal goiters are termed secondary because they are enlargements or extensions of multinodular goiters based on inferior thyroid vessels.*

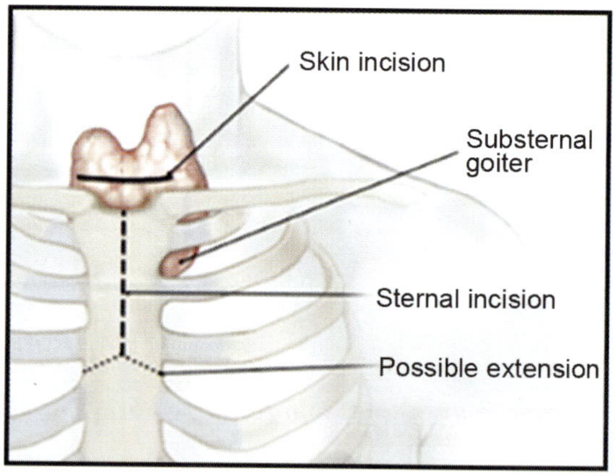

Clinical Features

- Often asymptomatic and Discovered on routine X-ray
- Dysphagia, Dyspnea
- Recurrent laryngeal nerve palsy
- Enlarged neck veins–Compression of major veins (Chest and Neck)
- Can lead to tracheal deviation and scabbard trachea *(Flattening of trachea caused by compression)*
- **Pemberton test +ve→** *Symptoms of faintness with evidence of facial congestion and external jugular venous obstruction when arms are raised above the head.*

Investigations

- X-ray shows widened mediastinum
- CT scans are helpful to evaluate extent of retrosternal extension and airway compression

Treatment

- Mediastinal goiter can be removed by neck incision ***(Transcervical incision)***
- ***More than 95% of retrosternal goiters are removed transcervically***
- ***Tobaggan technique:*** *Maneuver of removal of goiter through neck using finger and hooking out gland*

Classification and Approach for Retrosternal Goitre		
Grade	**Anatomical location**	**Approach**
1	*Above Aortic arch (Above T4)*	*Cervical*
2	*Aortic arch to pericardium*	*Manubriotomy*
3	*Below right atrium*	*Full Sternotomy*

Indications for Median Sternotomy

- *Primary mediastinal goiters with no thyroid tissue in neck*
- *Posterior mediastinal goiters*
- *Invasive thyroid cancers/Malignancy*
- *Immobile substernal goiters*
- *Previous thyroid operations and developed parasitic mediastinal vessels*
- *Rarely Hashimoto's and Graves' disease*

Ref: Bailey and Love 27th Edition Page 810, Sabiston 20th Edition Page 894, Schwartz 11th Edition Page 1642

Ans: (D) Transcervical

19. Cholecystocaval line separates:

A. Gallbladder from portal vein
B. Right and Left hepatic lobes
C. Right anterior and Right posterior sectors
D. Left medial and Left lateral sectors

Key:

Imaginary line that runs from Gallbladder fossa to IVC and divides Right and Left lobes

CHOLECYSTOCAVAL LINE/CANTLE'S LINE/CHOLECYSTOVENOCAVAL LINE

- **Physiological Right and Left lobes of the liver are demarcated by an imaginary line called as the Cholecystovenocaval line.**
- Line extends along the floor of fossa from gallbladder to groove for inferior vena cava.
- **Cantle line is described as Main portal fissure.**
- ***It is described to be at 75° angle with horizontal plane.***
- **This plane passes through Middle hepatic vein and IVC.**
- On Anterosuperior surface of liver line passes little to right of falciform ligament.
- Physiological right and left lobes are supplied respectively by right and left branches of portal vein and hepatic artery, bile of these lobes is conveyed by corresponding hepatic ducts.

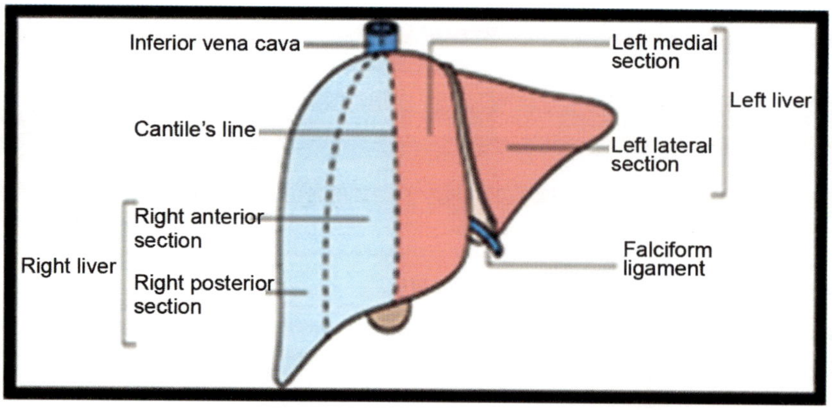

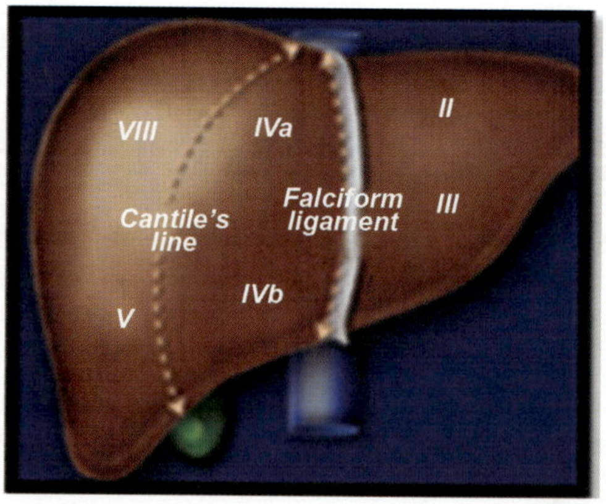

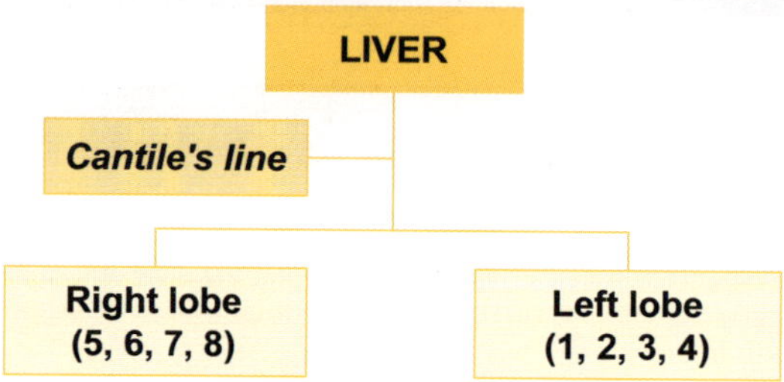

- ***Caudate lobe–Segment I.***
- Reidel lobe–Tongue like extension from right liver inferiorly.
- ***Quadrate lobe–Segment IV.***
- ***Caudate lobe***–Lobe that is not affected in Budd chiari syndrome and cirrhosis of liver because of its direct drainage into IVC.
- ***Right portal fissure*** divides right lobe into anteromedial and posterolateral sector.
  - Right hepatic vein courses along this fissure.
- ***Left portal fissure*** divides left lobe into anterior and posterior sector.
  - Left hepatic vein courses along this fissure.

Right Lobe	Left Lobe
Anteromedial sector–Segment V and VIII	***Anterior Sector***–Divided by Umbilical fissure into Segment IV and III
Posteromedial sector–Segment VI and VII	***Posterior Sector***–Comprised only one segment II

Ref: Bailey 27th Edition Page 161, Sabiston 20th Edition Page 1421, Schwartz 11th Edition Page 1347, AK Dutta Essentials of Human Anatomy 9th Edition Page 243

Ans: (B) Right and Left hepatic lobes

20. Elderly male Bus conductor by occupation has 1 mm dilated tortuous vein in posterior part of right calf along with heaviness of leg. What is the stage as per CEAP grading?

A. C0
B. C1
C. C2
D. C3

Key:

C1 refers to small veins like Telangiectasias (<1 mm) and reticular veins (<3 mm)

- Revised CEAP classification was introduced in 2004 that included a Venous Disability Score to document a patient's ability to perform activities of daily living.

Classification of Varicose Veins	
C- Clinical **E-Etiological**	**A- Anatomical** **P- Pathological**

Clinical Classification
• **C0**–No signs of Venous ulcers • **C1**–Telangiectasia (<1 mm diameter)/Reticular veins (1-2.9 mm diameter) • **C2**–Varicose veins (>3 mm diameter) • **C3**–Edema • **C4**–Pigmentation, Eczema, Lipodermatosclerosis • **C5**–Healed venous ulcer • **C6**–Active venous ulcer ***Add S for Symptomatic and Add A for Asymptomatic***

Aetiological Classification	Anatomical Classification	Pathophysiological Classification
• Ec: congenital; • Ep: primary; • Es: secondary (post-thrombotic); • En: no venous cause identified.	• As: superficial veins; • Ap: perforator veins; • Ad: deep veins; • An: no venous location identified.	• Pr: reflux; • Po: obstruction; • Pr,o: reflux and obstruction; • Pn: no venous pathophysiology identifiable.

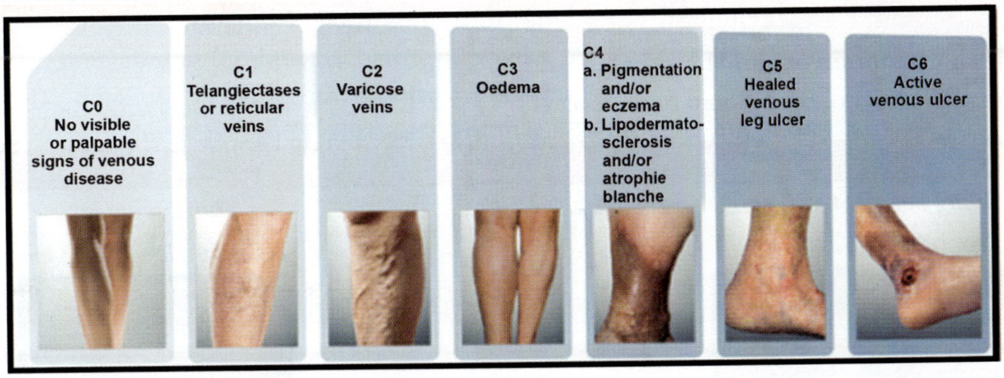

Ref: Sabiston 20th Edition Page 1833, Bailey and Love 27th Edition Page 974

Ans: (B) C1

21. All are true about Barrett's esophagus except:

A. Columnar to squamous metaplasia

B. Hyperplastic change in lining mucosa of esophagus

C. Associated with GERD

D. Predisposes to Adenocarcinoma

Key:

Barrett's esophagus is Intestinal metaplasia of squamous epithelium of Esophagus

BARRETT'S ESOPHAGUS

- When columnar mucosa extends at least 3 cm into esophagus or when it shows intestinal metaplasia, it is described as Barrett's esophagus
- Repeated reflux results in shifting of esophago-gastric junction upwards
- This further increases reflux resulting in intestinal metaplasia of **lower esophagus**
- 40 times more prone to adenocarcinoma of lower esophagus
- ***Most common site–Within 2 cm from junction of squamocolumnar epithelium***
- It is important to screen these patients regularly with **repeat endoscopies and multiple biopsies to find dysplasia**
- ***Increased incidence in white obese males***
- **Hallmark of Intestinal metaplasia**–*Intestinal Goblet cells on histology*
- **Investigation of choice**–Endoscopy and Biopsy
- **Endoscopy**–Red velevety GI mucosa between pale squamous mucosa of lower esophagus and lush pink gastric mucosa.

Pathological Types		
Gastric Type	**Intestinal Type**	**Junctional Type**
Chief and parietal cells	Goblet cells is a marker of intestinal metaplasia. Mucosa is smooth	Mucus glands and resembles gastric cardia.

Prague Criteria→ Grading for Barret's Esophagitis

- Prague C–Circumferential metaplasia
- Prague M–Most Proximal extent of metaplasia

Clinical Types	
Long segment (Classic)	***Short segment***
Involving more than 3 cm 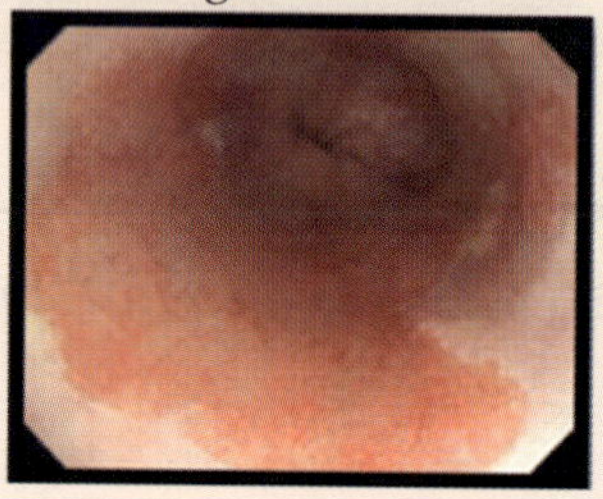	*Involving less than 3 cm* 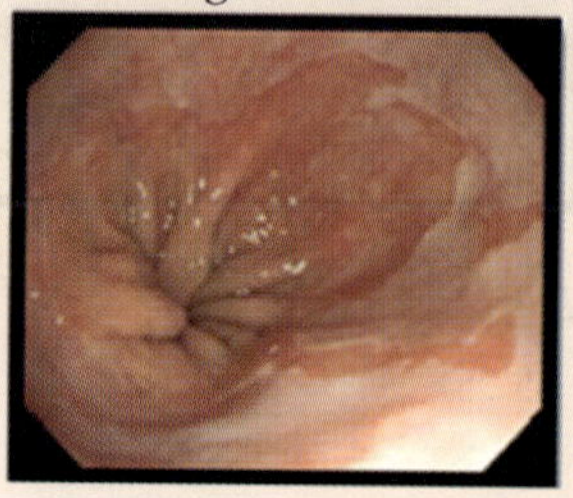

Treatment

- High dose proton pump inhibitors for 8 weeks.
- Laser photodynamic therapy and Argon beam plasma coagulation.
- ***Asymptomatic Barrett's esophagus responds well to laparoscopic antireflux surgery***

- Antireflux surgery–Also prevents progression to high-grade dysplasia or adenocarcinoma.
- Endoscopic mucosal resection for Barrett's esophagus with low-grade dysplasia.
- Oesophagectomy in cases of high-grade dysplasia.

Nondysplastic Barrett

- Repeat Esophagogastroscopy with surveillance biopsies in 1-2 years

Indefinite for Dysplasia

- Maximize acid suppression therapy (High dose PPI plus a Nocturnal H_2 blocker)
- Repeat Esophagogastroscopy with surveillance biopsies after period for healing (weeks to months)

Low Grade Dysplasia

- Aggressive reflux control with recommendation for anti reflux surgery in appropriate candidates and second opinion from expert GI pathologist
- Repeat Esophagogastroscopy with ***surveillance biopsies in 6 months***
- Regression on two consecutive exams → De-escalate to non-dysplastic Barrett
- Persistent or high-risk features → Ablative therapy to reduce progression risk

High-Grade Dysplasia or Intramucosal Adenocarcinoma

- Second opinion from expert GI pathologist
- ***Endoscopic resection of visible lesions***
- Ablation of Barrett mucosa
- ***Consider esophagectomy in patients with ultra-long*** (8 cm or more Barrett), when multifocal disease present, or in patients with difficult to control or severe GERD especially in poor esophageal motility and large hiatal hernia

Complications

- **Esophageal ulcers:** Barrett's ulcer–Pain, bleeding and perforation
- **Esophageal stricture:** Usually located in the middle or upper esophagus
- **Peptic stricture** occurs in the distal oesophagus
- **Dysplasia and adenocarcinoma**

Carcinoma in Barrett's Esophagus

Invasive, More proximal, Poor prognosis

Risk Factors for Carcinoma

- *Columnar lined Esophagus > 8 cm*
- Smoking is a risk factor
- Reflux due to previous gastric surgery
- High-grade dysplasia—indications for esophagectomy
- *Incidence of cancer is 0.5% per patient per year*

Ref: Sabiston 20th Edition Page 1032, Bailey 27th Edition Page 1081, Schwartz 11th Edition Page 1035

Ans: (B) Hyperplastic change in lining mucosa of esophagus

22. A resident while doing Scalp suture accidentally got injured his index finger. All the following are done about needle stick injury except:

A. Inform Higher authorities
B. Injury is more common in Non-dominant Index finger
C. Wash finger in Running water
D. HIV transmission is high in surgeons handling patients

Key:

Surgeons have comparatively low risk of HIV transmission than Nurses and Non-surgical physicians

NEEDLE STICK INJURY

- **Most common site of needle stick injury during surgery**–*Non-dominant index finger*
- *Hollow needles have high risk than surgical needles*
- ***Injured part is washed under running water***
- Report incident to authorities
- Role of HIV transmission from patient to surgeon is Low
- Surgeons have comparatively low risk than Nurses and Non-surgical physicians

Estimated risk of transmission from needle stick from source with HIV-infected blood is 0.3% for percutaneous exposure and 0.09% for mucous membrane exposure.

Post Exposure Prophylaxis of HIV

- Local policies dictate to start ART treatment or not.
- Occupational health advice is required for high risk exposure along with HIV/Hepatitis B testing.
- Post exposure prophylaxis for HIV has significantly decreased the risk of seroconversion for health care workers with occupational exposure to HIV.
- For effective preventive therapy, steps to initiate post exposure prophylaxis should be initiated within hours.
- Post exposure prophylaxis with a three-drug regimen should be initiated for health care workers with significant exposure to patients with an HIV-positive status.
- ***If patient's HIV status is unknown, it may be advisable to begin post exposure prophylaxis while testing is carried out***→*Particularly Consider this if the patient is at high risk for infection due to HIV (e.g., has had a history of intravenous drug use).*
- Post exposure prophylaxis is **NOT NEEDED** for exposure to sources with unknown status (Deceased persons or needles from a sharps container).

Transmission route	%
Sexual intercourse	**70-80**
Mother-to-child-transmission	5-10
Blood transfusion	3-5
Injecting drug use	5-10
Health care–e.g., needle stick injury	<0.01

HCV is not transmitted efficiently through occupational exposures to blood, with seroconversion rate after accidental needle stick approximately 1.8%

Ref: Bailey 27th Edition Page 52, Schwartz 11th Edition Page 177

Ans: (D) HIV transmission is high in surgeons handling patients

23. All of the following statements are correct about Deep vein thrombosis except:

A. Clinical assessment is highly reliable
B. Can occur bilaterally
C. Most common clinical presentation is pain & tenderness in calf
D. Some cases may directly present as pulmonary thromboembolism

Key:

Clinical assessment in DVT is unreliable

CLINICAL PICTURE OF DEEP VEIN THROMBOSIS

- **Most common presentation of DVT**–*Pain (Tenderness) and swelling especially in calf*
- Usually involves one leg only
- ***Bilaterality is seen with 30%***→*Should be differentiated from hypoproteinaemia, renal and heart failure.*
- Some cases may directly present as pulmonary thromboembolism with chest pain, hemoptysis and shortness of breath.
- Clinical examination is unreliable.
- No physical signs are present.
- **Leg pain occurs in 50% of patients with DVT and is not specific.**
- Tenderness occurs in 75% of patients.
  It is also found in 50% of patients without objectively confirmed DVT.
- ***Pain and tenderness associated with DVT doesn't usually correlate with size, location or extent of thrombus.***
- Clinically pulmonary embolus signs and symptoms can occur in about 10% of patients with confirmed DVT.

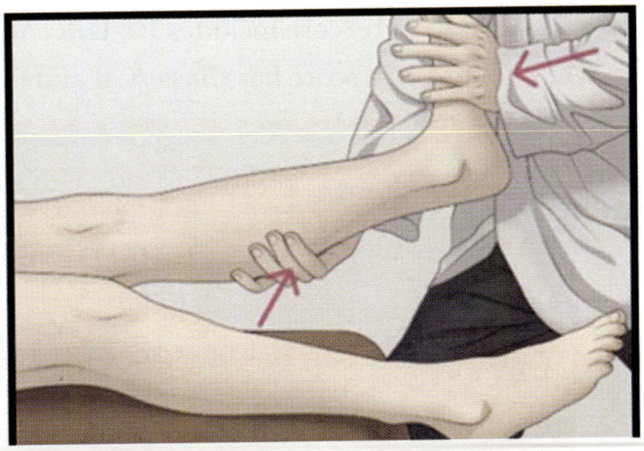

Homans' sign – resistance of calf muscles to forcible dorsiflexion – not specific and should not be elicited.

Post Thrombotic Syndrome

- Post thrombotic syndrome–Common and Unfortunate manifestation of DVT
- Occurs in 20% to 50% of patients after documented episode of DVT

Risk factors for development

- Persistent leg symptoms for months after acute episode of DVT, an anatomically extensive DVT involving iliofemoral system, recurrent ipsilateral DVT and prolonged state of subtherapeutic anticoagulation for DVT.

Supportive and compressive therapy remains mainstay of treatment
Early use of thrombolysis prevents PTS

- ***Most common site of DVT–Calf veins (Soleal)***
- ***Most common site of thrombosis for pulmonary thromboembolism–Femoropopliteal veins***
- Most dangerous complication–Pulmonary embolism
- ***Investigation of choice for diagnosis–Duplex ultrasound***

Contd.

Contd.

• Plegmasia alba dolens–Painful white leg→***Obstruction of major deep veins*** • Plegmasia cerulean dolens–Painful blue leg→***Obstruction of both collaterals and deep veins***
Signs of DVT
• ***Homan's sign:*** Resistance of calf muscles to forcible dorsiflexion (Not pain) • ***Pratt's sign:*** Calf tenderness on squeezing of calf from sides • ***Perthes test:*** Elastocrepe bandage is applied and patient is asked to walk. In case of DVT there will be severe pain on walking • ***Moses sign:*** Calf tenderness on direct pressure over calf (Bancroft's sign) • **Virchow triad:** *Hypercoagulability, Endothelial injury and Stasis of blood flow* • Most important predisposing factor–Hospital admission (For medical/surgical treatment) • ***Earliest sign of DVT–Calf tenderness*** • Palma operation–Surgical treatment of DVT

Ref: Bailey 27th Edition Page 987, Sabiston 20th Edition Page 1843, Schwartz 11th Edition Page 986

Ans: (A) Clinical assessment is highly reliable

24. All of the following statements are true regarding liver disease parameters except:

A. MELD score is used frequently to see who needs transplant early

B. MELD score includes Serum albumin, Serum creatinine and INR

C. Child Pugh Score includes PT-INR, Albumin and Bilirubin

D. Child Pugh score has Class A, B and C

Key:

MELD score include Serum creatinine, Bilirubin and INR

Meld Score
• **Priority for liver transplant is based on MELD Score** • Model for end stage liver disease–Chronic liver disease severity scoring system to predict 3 months survival of patient • Values range from 6 to 40

Model for End Stage Liver Disease (MELD) Score
MELD = 3.78 × log, serum bilirubin (mg/dL)+ 11.20 × log, INR + 9/57 × log, serum creatinine (mg/dL)+ 6.43 (constant for liver disease etiology)

• High MELD score is seen with sicker patient

• Cirrhosis patients are candidates for transplantation typically once their MELD scrore is greater than or equal to 15

• ***Minimum MELD score of 18 is necessary to have a survival benefit post-transplant.***

• A MELD score between 15 and 18 does not confer a survival advantage, but transplant is justified if patient has significant morbidity from cirrhosis.

Contd.

Contd.

Uses
• Primary use is prioritizing patients on waitlist for deceased donor liver transplantation based on liver disease severity and short term mortality risk • It can predict mortality after TIPS placement • It has predictive value for outcomes in cirrhosis patients undergoing nontransplant surgical procedure
"MELD exceptions" are used for diseases like amyloidosis, portopulmonary hypertension, and hepatopulmonary syndrome.
PELD (Pediatric end stage liver disease *Bilirubin levels, INR, Albumin levels, Age and Growth failure*

Child Turcotte Pugh Score			
Measurements	**Score**		
	1	**2**	**3**
Encephalopathy	None	Mild	Moderate
Ascites	None	Sight	Moderate
Bilirubin (md/dL)	1-2	2-3	>3
Albumin (mg/dL)	>3.5	2.8-3.5	<2.8
PT (Prolonged–Seconds)	<4	4-6	>6
Stage A, 5-6 Points, Stage B, 7-9 points, Stage C, 10-15 points			

Liver Transplantation Criteria		
Milan's Criteria	**UCSF Criteria**	**Silva *et al.***
Single tumor ≤ 5 cm	Single tumor ≤ 6.5 cm	
Or up to 3 tumors ≤ 3 cm	Or up to 3 tumors ≤ 4.5 cm, and total sum is ≤ 8 cm	Up to 3 tumors ≤ 5 cm, and total sum is ≤ 10 cm
All Three Criteria Lists–No vascular invasion, No regional nodal/distant metastasis		

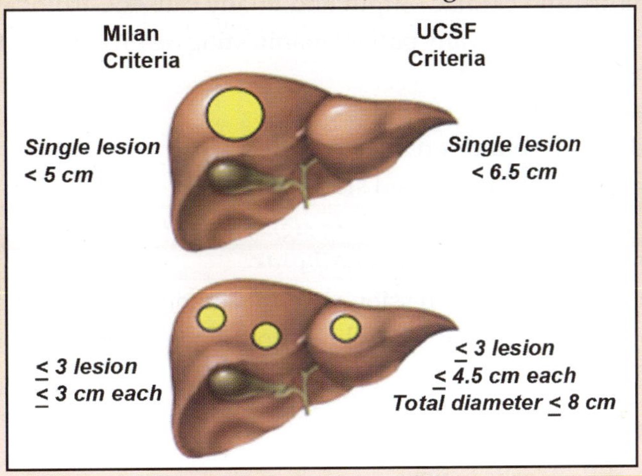

Ref: Bailey 27th Edition Page 1157, Sabiston 20th Edition Page 640, Schwartz 11th Edition Page 381

Ans: (B) MELD score includes Serum albumin, Serum creatinine and INR

25. A 40-year-old patient complains of Breathlessness following trauma, Trachea is shifted to opposite side. On percussion Resonant note is found and Absent Breath sounds. Which of the following statement is not true about ICD insertion?

A. Done in upper part of lower rib to avoid nerve and vessel injury
B. Inserted into 4th/5th Intercostal space along scapular line
C. Insertion area need to be palpated digitally to confirm position
D. Direction of Insertion is Posterior and Superior

Key:

Given Clinical picture points out that patient developed Tension pneumothorax
Immediate rapid needle insertion of large bore needle in 2nd ICS in midclavicular line
This is immediately followed by insertion of ICD chest tube in 5th intercostal space in Mid axillary line

TENSION PNEUMOTHORAX

- ***Parenchymal tear in lung acts as a one-way valve, with each inhalation allowing additional air to accumulate in the pleural space.***
- Normally negative intrapleural pressure becomes positive, which depresses ipsilateral hemidiaphragm and shifts mediastinal structures into contralateral chest.
- ***Subsequently, contralateral lung is compressed and heart rotates about superior and inferior vena cava.***

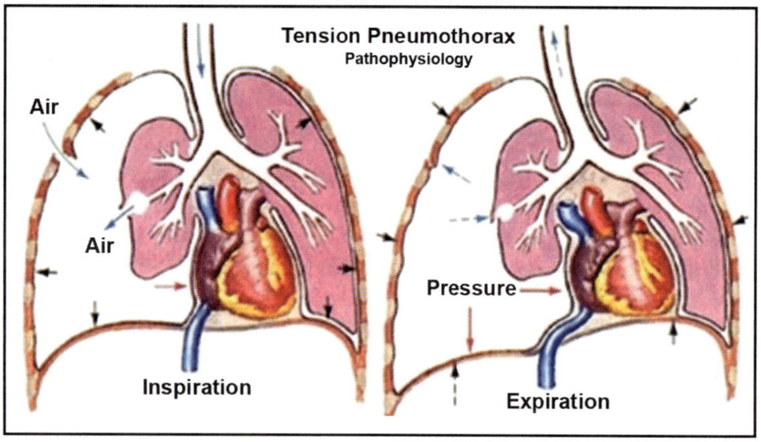

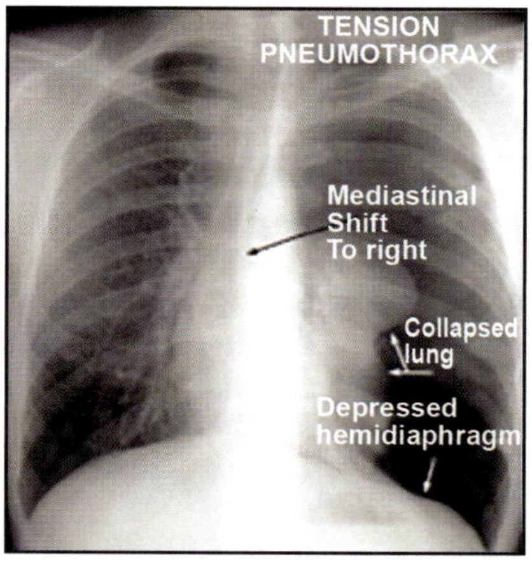

- This decreases venous return and cardiac output and finally causes Cardiovascular collapse.
- Tension pneumothorax is diagnosed in any patient manifesting **respiratory distress** and **hypotension** in combination with any of the following physical signs:
  - Tracheal deviation away from affected side.
  - Lack of or decreased breath sounds on affected side.
  - Subcutaneous emphysema on the affected side.
- ***Tension and simple pneumothorax have similar signs, symptoms and examination findings, but hypotension qualifies the pneumothorax as a tension pneumothorax.***
- Immediate needle thoracostomy decompression with 14G angiocatheter is indicated.
- Followed by tube thoracostomy in midaxillary line should be performed immediately in Emergency department before a chest radiograph is obtained.

TRIANGLE OF SAFETY

- Anteriorly–Lateral edge of Pectoralis major
- Posteriorly–Mid axillary line
- Inferiorly–Horizontal line drawn at nipple level to meet mid axillary line

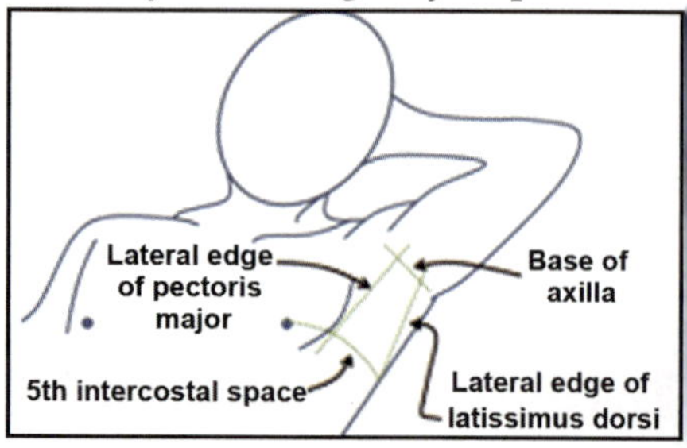

Indications for Tube Thoracostomy in Thoracic Injury
• Hemothorax >1500 ml (Blunt trauma) and >1000 ml (Penetrating trauma) in ICD • Hourly collection of ICD >200 ml/hr for 3 hours • Hemopericardium and Cardiac tamponade • Massive air leak, Tracheal or main bronchus injury • Esophageal and thoracic duct injury, Diaphragmatic injury, Descending aorta injury • Associated liver and spleen injury, Bronchial and branchial vessel injury • Open pneumothorax and Air embolism

Ref: Bailey 27th Edition Page 367, Sabiston 20th Edition Page 428, Schwartz 11th Edition Page 186

Ans: (B) Inserted into 4th/5th Intercostal space along scapular line

26. Name the triangle shown below:

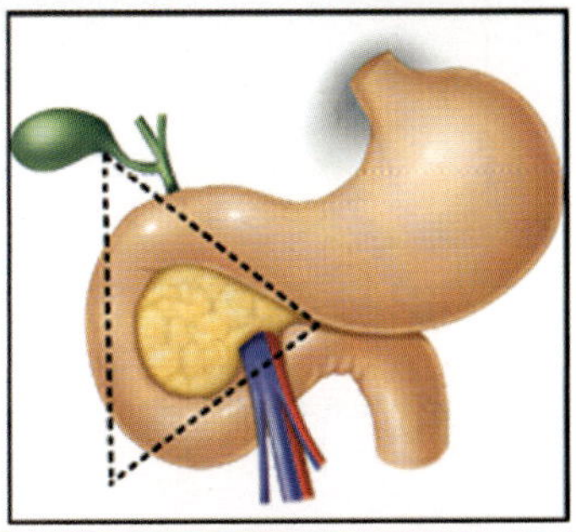

A. Calot's triangle
B. Gastrinoma triangle
C. Triangle of Doom
D. Cholecystohepatic triangle

Key:

Given picture shows Triangle Formed by Junction of cystic duct and CBD, Junction of 2nd and 3rd part of duodenum and Junction of neck and body of pancreas–Gastrinoma triangle

GASTRINOMA TRIANGLE/TRIANGLE OF PASSARO

- **About 70-90% of Gastrinomas occur in this triangle**

Triangle is formed by joining following three points
• ***Superiorly:*** Confluence of the cystic and common bile ducts • ***Inferiorly:*** Junction of the second and third portions of the duodenum • ***Medially:*** Junction of the neck and body of the pancreas

Triangles	Boundaries	
Joll's triangle	Laterally by Upper pole of thyroid and superior thyroid vessels, Superiorly by Attachment of strap muscles and deep investing layer of fascia to hyoid, Medially by midline and Floor is by Cricothyroid muscle	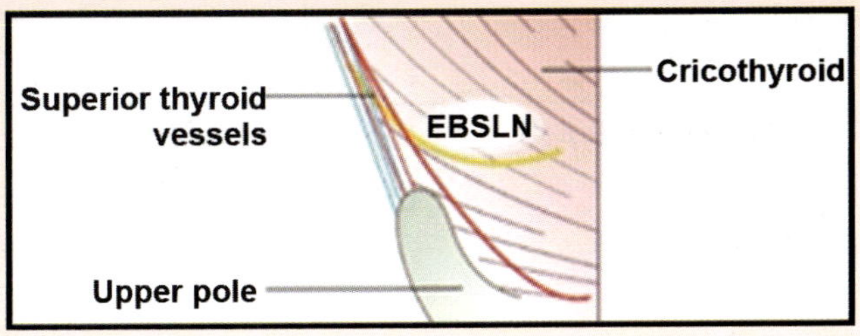

Contd.

Contd.

Femoral triangle	Superiorly by Inguinal ligament, Medially by Medial border of adductor longus and Laterally by medial border of Sartorius 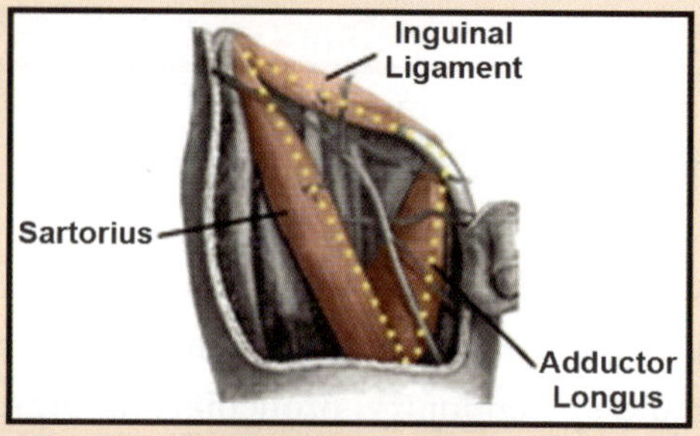
Hesselbach triangle	Laterally by epigastric artery, Medially by Lateral border of rectus abdominus and Inferiorly by Inguinal ligament 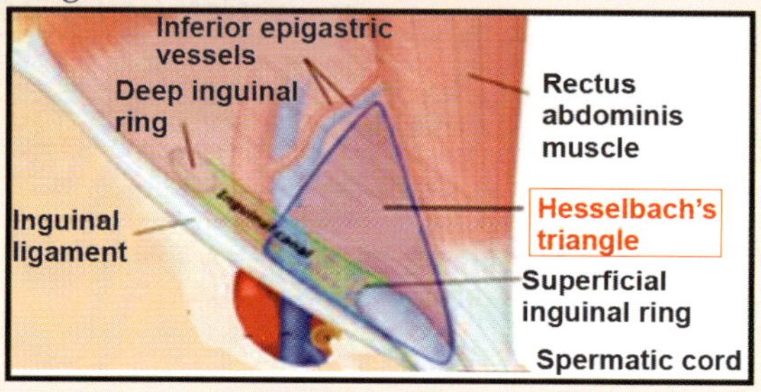
Calot's triangle	Superiorly by Cystic artery, Medially by Common hepatic duct and Laterally by Cystic duct 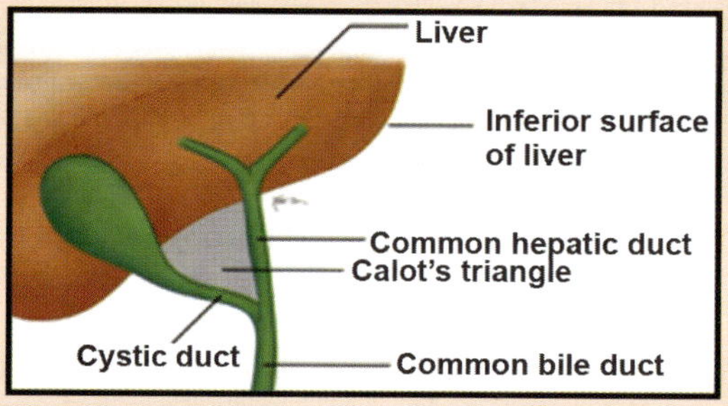
Inferior triangle of Petit	Inferiorly by Iliac crest, Medially by Latissimus dorsi and Laterally by External oblique 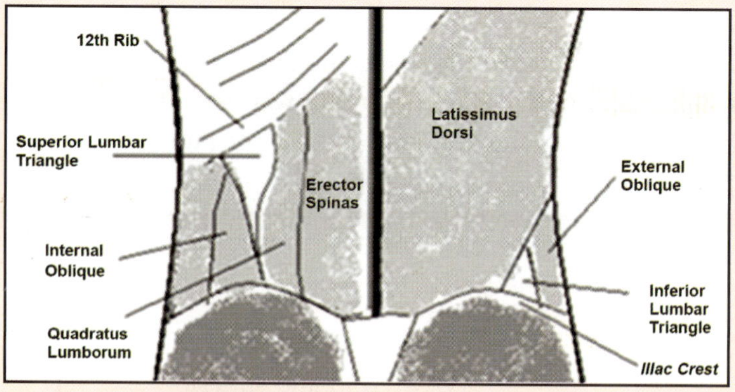
Shereen's triangle	Bounded by ASIS, Pubic tubercle and Umbilicus–Area of hyperesthesia in Acute appendicitis
Triangle of Koch	Ring of tricuspid valve, Sinus venosus and Todaro tendon

Ref: Bailey 27th Edition Page 1141, Sabiston 20th Edition Page 1210, Schwartz 11th Edition Page 1117

Ans: (B) Gastrinoma triangle

27. Lady primigravida and lactating mother developed fluctuant Shiny painful mass of breast along with fever after 14 days of delivery. Preferred treatment option is:

A. Stop lactation
B. Analgesics and continue breastfeeding
C. Antipyretics
D. Incision and drainage

Key:

Lactating mother, Tender swelling, Pyrexia, Fluctuant shiny mass favour diagnosis of Breast abscess
Best treatment for Breast abscess would be Incision and Drainage

BREAST ABSCESS

- Typically seen in Lactating males
- ***Most common organism associated with Breast abscess–Staphylococcus aureus***
  Staphylococcus gets transmitted via neonate who is breast fed
- Tenderness, erythema along with fever and tense shiny skin is present
- **Diagnosis: USG** *(Delineates extent of drainage needed)*

Treatment

- Local wound care by applying warm compressors
- Intravenous antibiotics
- 1st line drug–Cloxacillin (Cellulitic stage)
- Drainage is best done by Circumareolar incision (parallel to langer lines)

Best and Preferred treatment of Breast abscess–Incision and Drainage

Intramammary Abscess
• Initial treatment is Needle aspiration • Radial incision is done on opposite side • All loculi must be broken and dependent drainage is kept
Retromammary Abscess
• Extension of breast abscess, empyema thoracis and Osteomyelitis of ribs • No need to drain–*Only conservative treatment is done*

Ref: Sabiston 20th Edition Page 836, Bailey 27th Edition Page 866, Schwartz 11th Edition Page 550

Ans: (D) Incision and drainage

28. A 30-year-old lady presented with cystic neck swelling as shown in below picture. What could be possible diagnosis?

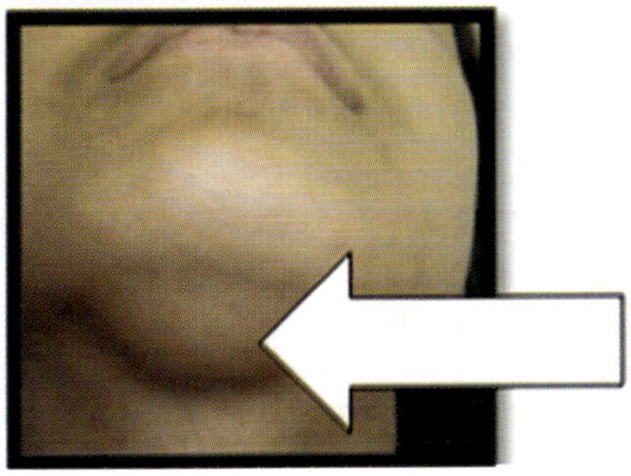

A. Dermoid cyst
B. Sebaceous cyst
C. Branchial cyst
D. Secondaries neck

Key:

Midline swelling in floor of mouth points towards diagnosis of Dermoid cyst most probably

Branchial cyst	**Lateral neck swelling**
Sebaceous cyst	**Punctum present (Rare in submental region)**
Secondaries	**Elderly age group** **History of malignancy at some other site** **Usually lateral neck swelling**

SUBMENTAL DERMOID

- **Thin walled cyst lined by Squamous epithelium**
- Contains cheesy material
- ***Almost always midline***
- Usually 10-15 years age
- Involves both sexes equally
- Clinical features–Painless swelling in midline of neck

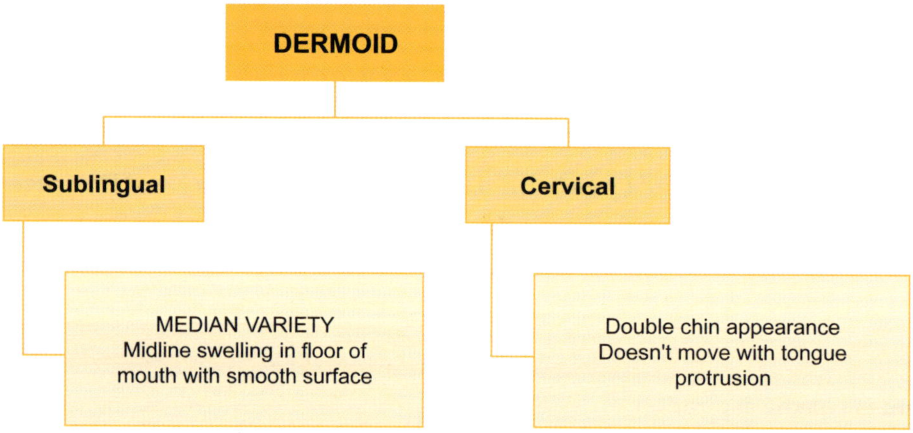

- Excision is treatment of choice–*Cervical incision*

Dermoid cysts are benign congenital choristomas that originate from fetal bone suture lines during development
Occurs most commonly between forehead and nose tip *Most frequent site is eyebrow (Most commonly the frontozygomatic suture)*

Ref: Schwartz 11th Edition Page 527, Hazarika Textbook of ENT 4th Edition Page 560, SRB Manual of Surgery Page 78

Ans: (A) Dermoid cyst

29. Parathyroid gland accidentally removed and found after surgery is autotransplanted to which of the following structure?

A. Brachioradialis
B. Biceps
C. Sartorius
D. Triceps

Key:

Parathyroid autografts are placed in Heterotopic site like Brachioradialis or Sternocleidomastoid

PARATHYROID AUTOTRANSPLANTATION

Identification of Parathyroid

- Nearly 85% of parathyroid glands are located within 1 cm of junction of Inferior thyroid artery and RLN
- Normal parathyroids are brown in colour compared to adjacent fat
- Upper parathyroids–Superior to junction of Inferior thyroid artery and RLN (Dorsal to RLN)
- Lower parathyroids–Inferior to junction of Inferior thyroid artery and RLN (Ventral to RLN)
- Most common site of Ectopic parathyroid–Paraesophageal

Methods

- ***Incise fascia over fat lobule if parathyroid gland, it pops out***
- **Float sign**–Suggests abnormal parathyroid gland→ Blunt peanut sponge dissection between carotid sheath and the thyroid gland
- **Resected parathyroid tissue is confirmed by frozen section or PTH assay**

- Involves complete parathyroid tissue resection from its normal location and heterotopic implantation into muscle bed either in Brachioradialis or sternocleidomastoid
- Forearm of nondominant arm is used for Brachioradialis pocket
- Parathyroid tissue is usually cut into 1-2 mm fragments and placed in separate small pockets within muscle
- Gland develops new blood supply and typically starts functioning within 4-6 weeks

If gland is identified during surgery, it can be implanted directly into Sternocleidomastoid muscle

Ref: Schwartz 11th Edition Page 1674, Sabiston 20th Edition Page 936, Bailey 27th Edition Page 827

Ans: (A) Brachioradialis

Chapter 13

OBSTETRICS AND GYNECOLOGY

1. A post-operative cesarean section patient presents with 2 weeks of fever of 102 degree F despite antibiotics. On investigations she is diagnosed to have septic pelvic thrombophlebitis. What should be next step in management?

A. Hysterectomy

B. Stop antibiotics and perform surgical embolization

C. Continue antibiotics and perform surgical embolization

D. Continue antibiotics and start heparin

Key:

Clinical description is a case of Postpartum septic thrombophlebitis. Management would include Continue antibiotics and start heparin if already patient is on Antibiotics

Postpartum Thrombophlebitis

- Originates in thrombosed veins at the placental site by organisms such as anaerobic **Streptococci or Bacteroidesfragilis.**
- ***When localised in pelvis, it is termed as Septic pelvic thrombophlebitis (SPT).***

Pathogenesis

- Injury to the **intima** of the **pelvic vein** caused by spreading uterine infection, bacteremia, and endotoxins, which can occur secondary to the trauma of delivery or cesarean section.
- ***Suspicion of SPT*** *should arise when* ***fever continues for more than a week in spite of antibiotic therapy.***

Clinical Features

- Patients often complain of flank and lower abdominal pain.
- Pain may be of variable intensity and may radiate to groin/upper abdomen.
- ***Paralytic ileus.***
- On examination, patient usually doesn't appear toxic and tenderness may be present in lower abdomen.
- Occasionally, tender abdominal mass described as **rope/sausage-shape** may be identified–this is ***most diagnostic finding in an abdominal exam,*** but it is rare.

Diagnosis

- Blood count shows polymorphonuclear leucocytosis.
- Diagnosis may be made by Venous USG, CT or by MRI.
- ***In MRI, thrombosed vessel will appear bright, whereas normal blood flow looks dark.***

Treatment

- Surgical excision of thrombosed vein–Treatment of choice in earlier days.
- ***Current recommendation is to treat with heparin anticoagulation in conjunction with antibiotic coverage.***

Contd.

Contd.

- **"Triple antibiotic regimen"**→*Clindamycin, Ampicillin and Gentamicin is recommended.*
- However, if fever persists after 5 days of antibiotics, it is suggested to use alternative antibiotics with broad spectrum and ***anti-pseudomonal activity*** *like* ***Imipenem or ertapenem.***
- **Venous thrombectomy** may be needed for **massive illiofemoral vein thrombosis** or for **massive pulmonary embolus.**

Complications

Extra pelvic spread can occur as follows:

- Through right ovarian vein into IVC to lungs–**Pulmonary thromboembolism**
- Through left ovarian vein to left renal vein to left kidney
- Retrograde extension to iliofemoral veins to produce clinico-pathological entity termed ***'phlegmasia alba dolens' or white leg.***

Ref: Dutta Textbook of Obstetrics 9th Edition Page 440

Ans: (D) Continue antibiotics and start heparin

2. **Which of the following can present as a nongestational Trophoblastic neoplasm?**

A. Placental site trophoblastic tumour
B. Partial mole
C. Invasive mole
D. Choriocarcinoma

Key:

Choriocarcinoma can present as Nongestational trophoblastic tumor

NONGESTATIONAL OVARIAN CHORIOCARCINOMA

- Primary nongestational ovarian choriocarcinoma **is rare**.
- It is most often seen as a **component of mixed germ cell tumors of the ovary**
- Choriocarcinomas display **abundant hemorrhage and necrosis** on gross examination
- Microscopically, these neoplasms show a plexiform pattern composed of an admixture of syncytiotrophoblast and cytotrophoblast cells. Numerous mitoses are present.
- Choriocarcinoma spreads by **blood vessel invasion**
- These tumors **produce hCG** due to the presence of Syncytiotrophoblast cells
- Choriocarcinoma may also **stain for cytokeratins, epithelial membrane antigen and carcinoembryonic antigen.**

Non Gestational Choriocarcinoma must be distinguished from gestational choriocarcinoma because former has worse prognosis and requires more aggressive therapy.

- **Identification of paternal genetic material indicates that tumor is of gestational origin.**

GESTATIONAL TROPHOBLASTIC DISEASES

- **"Gestational trophoblastic disease (GTD)"** covers heterogeneous group of clinical conditions characterized by disordered proliferation of trophoblastic epithelium.
- **WHO classification**–GTD is differentiated into **villous** and **non-villous GTD,** according to the presence or absence of **chorionic villi.**
- Villous and non-villous GTD include both benign and malignant disease, as well as lesions which progress from benign to malignant, for example, persistent postmolar trophoblastic gestational disease.
- **Nongestational trophoblastic disease (NGTD)** includes **choriocarcinoma of the ovary** as a rare variant of mixed or pure germ cell tumors.

WHO Classification of gestational trophoblastic disease (GTD)	
• **Molar pregnancy** o Partial hydatidiform mole (PHM) o Complete hydatidiform mole (CHM) o Invasive mole (IM)	Villous GTD
• **Benign lesions** o Exaggerated placental site (EPS) o Placental site nodule (PSN) • **Gestational trophoblastic neoplasia (GTN)** o Choriocarcinoma (CCA) o Placental site trophoblastic tumor (PSTT) o Epitheloid trophoblastic tumor (ETT)	Non - villous GTD

- ***Choriocarcinoma***–Mostly develops after molar gestation; Gestational trophoblastic neoplasia that develops after a normal pregnancy is often a choriocarcinoma
- ***Invasive mole***–Exclusively develops after molar gestation
- ***PSTT (Placental site trophoblastic tumor)***–Mostly develops following term gestation
- ***Epitheloid trophoblastic tumor***–Rare

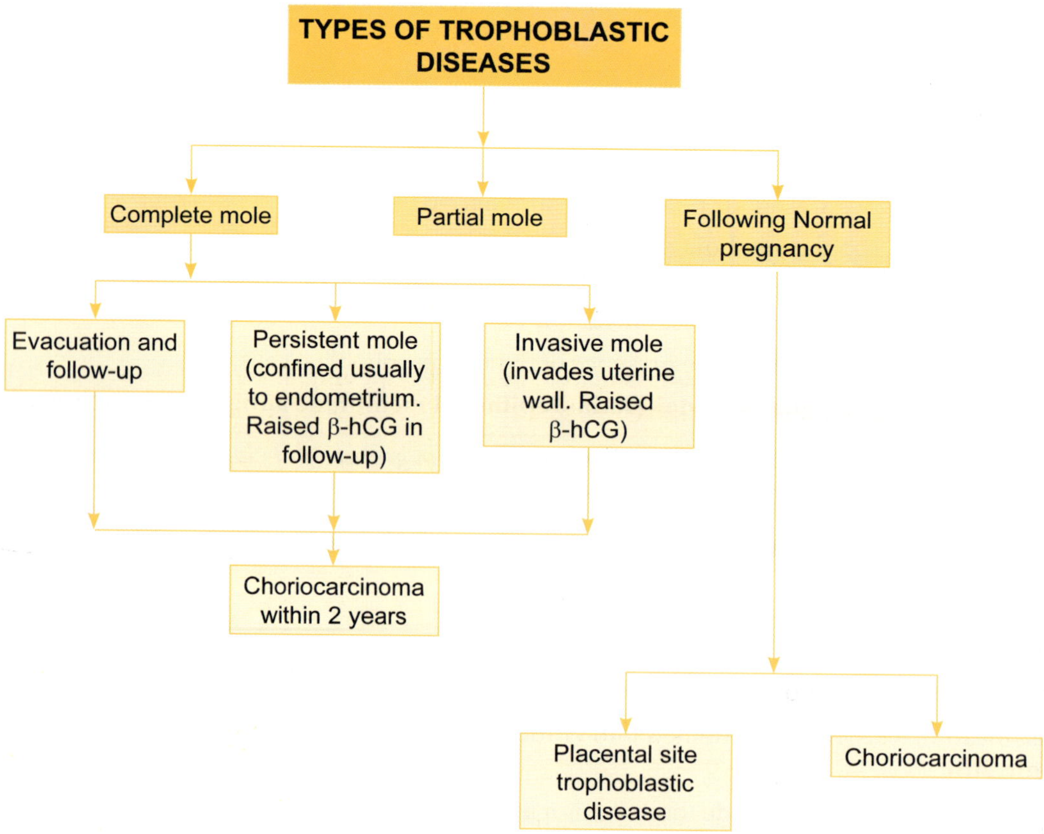

Ref: Dutta's Textbook of Obstetrics 9th Edition Page 190, William's Gynecology 3rd Edition Page 785

Ans: (D) Choriocarcinoma

A primipara presents at 41 weeks of gestation, sure of dates, confirmation of POG done by 1st trimester USG. Which is not used for induction of labor?

A. PgE2 gel
B. Intracervical Foley's
C. PgE1 tablet
D. PgF2α injection

Key:

Patient is of 41 weeks so there is need for termination of pregnancy by Cervical ripening and Induction of labour

Induction of Labor

- Refers to initiation of uterine contractions after the period of viability aiming for a vaginal delivery

Common indications for IOL include

- Post term pregnancy
- GDM
- Preeclampsia
- IUGR
- Rh isoimmunisation
- Premature rupture of membranes
- Major fetal malformations
- Intrauterine death

IOL in Post-term Pregnancy

- Post-term pregnancy is associated with increased perinatal mortality. Induction is usually started at 41 completed weeks of gestation, aiming for delivery before 42 weeks.
- **Success of IOL** depends on **degree of ripening of cervix.**
- **Bishop's score** is preinduction cervical assessment to assess the ripening of cervix.

Bishop's Score

Factor	Score 0	Score 1	Score 2	Score 3
Dilatation (cm)	0	1-2	3-4	>5
Effacement (%)	0-30	40-50	60-70	>80
Consistency	Firm	Medium	Soft	
Position	Posterior	Mid	Anterior	
Station	-3 or above	-2	-1 or 0	+1 or more

- *Bishop's score <6 indicates an Unfavourable for cervix for induction*
- *Bishop's score ≥6 indicates a Favourable cervix for induction*
- ***Modified Bishop's score**–Cervical length is included instead of cervical effacement in assessment of cervix for induction of labor.*

Contd.

Contd.

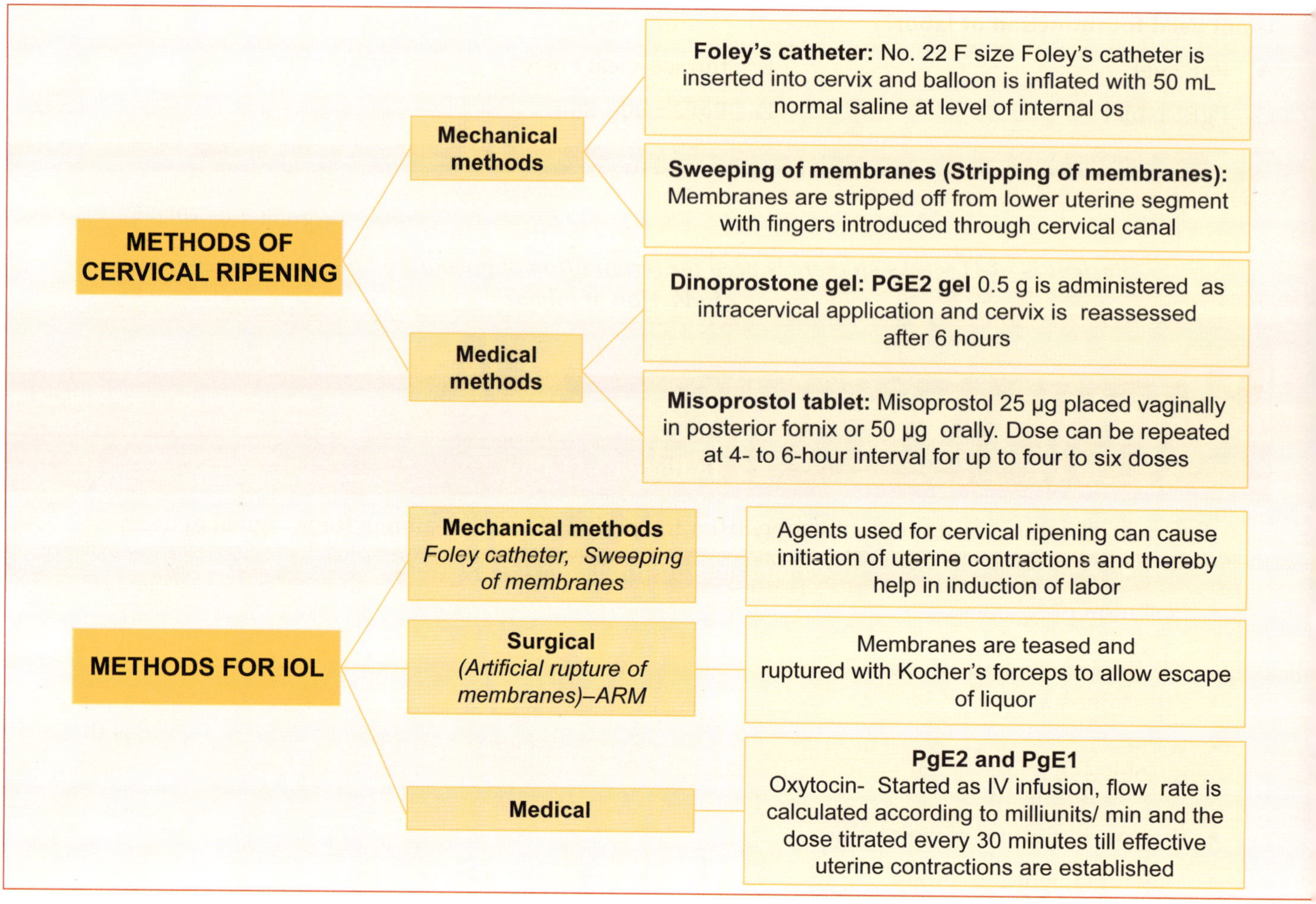

Choice of Uterotonics in Different Clinical Situations	
MTP	• ***Misoprostol*** *is the preferred drug*
Control of bleeding in abortion	• ***Misoprostol*** *is effective to hasten evacuation and to control bleeding* • ***Methergin*** *is also effective to control bleeding* • ***Oxytocin*** *can also be used to hasten evacuation and to control bleeding*
Induction of labor	• ***Cervix unfavorable–Prostaglandins (PGE2, PGE1)*** *are the preferred agents* • ***Cervix favorable****–Oxytocin and prostaglandins are equally good,* ***Oxytocin*** *is preferred*
Augmentation of labor	• ***Oxytocin*** *is the drug of choice*
Active management of 3rd stage of labor (Prevention of PPH)	• ***Oxytocin 10 units IV or IM is recommended***
Control of PPH	• ***Oxytocin*** *is drug of first choice* • ***Methergin*** *(IV or IM) can be given along with oxytocin* • *In severe bleeding,* ***Prostadin PGF2 alpha*** *injections are effective* • ***Misoprostol*** *is ideal in low resource setting*

Ref: Dutta Textbook of Obstetrics 9th Edition Page 522

Ans: (D) PgF2α injection

4. **Treatment of woman with recurrent pregnancy loss due to antiphospholipid antibody syndrome:**

A. Low dose Heparin only
B. Aspirin and Low dose Heparin
C. Aspirin only
D. Immunoglobulin

Key:

Aspirin along with Prophylactic anticoagulation with heparin throughout pregnancy and then 6 weeks post partum with either heparin or warfarin is recommended in APLA syndrome

Antiphospholipid Antibody Syndrome (APLA Syndrome)

- Autoimmune disorder characterized by **presence of antiphospholipid antibodies, recurrent vascular thrombosis, recurrent pregnancy loss and thrombocytopenia**

CLASSIFICATION
- **Primary** — ***Absence of other autoimmune diseases***
- **Secondary** — ***Associated with other autoimmune diseases like SLE***

Pathogenesis

- **Auto Antibodies are formed which are directed against phospholipids or plasma proteins** bound to phospholipids. Many of these proteins are anticoagulants in clotting cascade and hence there is disruption of physiological anticoagulation
- The basic pathological change is **thrombotic microangiopathy involving multiple organ system**
- Placental damage resulting from thrombosis is thought to be the reason for pregnancy loss in APLAS patients.

ANTI PHOSPHOLIPID ANTIBODIES
- **Anticardiolipin Antibody**
  - ***Detected by ELISA***
- **Lupus Anticoagulant antibody**
  - ***Detected by In vitro prolongation of coagulation studies***
    - Prolonged APTT, PT, Russel viper venom test, Platelet neutralization procedure and Kaolin clotting time

Diagnostic Criteria (Sapporo's Criteria) for APLAS

For diagnosis of APLA – one or more clinical AND one or more laboratory criteria must be present

Clinical Criteria

- One or more episodes of venous or arterial thrombosis
- Presence of pregnancy complications
  - >= 3 consecutive spontaneous pregnancy losses at < 10 weeks
  - >= 1 fetal death of morphologically normal fetus at > 10 weeks
  - >= 1 preterm births of morphologically normal newborn at < 34 weeks secondary to severe preeclampsia or placental insufficiency

Contd.

Contd.

Laboratory Criteria

- Positive plasma levels of ACA on >= 2 occasions 6 weeks apart
- Detection of LAC on >= 2 occasions 6 weeks apart

Obstetric complications in APLA Syndrome
• Recurrent 1st or 2nd trimester Pregnancy losses • Early onset preeclampsia • Uteroplacental insufficiency–IUGR • Preterm labor, Abruption, IUD

Indication for testing APLA Syndrome
• Recurrent abortions • Unexplained 2nd or 3rd trimester losses • Early onset severe preeclampsia • Unexplained IUGR • Venous or arterial thromboembolic events • Autoimmune or connective tissue diseases • False positive serological test for syphilis • Prolongation of coagulation studies

Treatment

- To improve maternal, fetal and neonatal outcome
- To reduce the risk of thromboembolism

General measures	Specific treatment
• Antenatal care in a tertiary care hospital • Patient explained about complications, treatment options and need for regular antenatal care • Frequent antenatal visits once in 2 weeks • Dating and anomalies scan are done • Obstetric scan done every month from 20 weeks • Fetal surveillance from 28 weeks onwards with DFMC, NST and Doppler	***Combined treatment with aspirin and heparin (UFH) or LMWH is recommended to reduce pregnancy loss and improve live birth rates in women with APLA*** • **Low dose aspirin** should be started at attempted conception or with a positive pregnancy test. *(Preconceptional aspirin has a possible beneficial effect on early stages of implantation).* • Prophylactic doses of **UFH** (5000-10000 units every 12 hours) or **LMW** (Enoxaparin 40 mg SC every 24 hours) should be started when viable intrauterine pregnancy is documented and continued until late in 3rd trimester. • Patient presents after conceiving, she should be immediately started on Low dose aspirin and heparin.

Ref: Dutta Textbook of Obstetrics 9th Edition Page 342, Williams Obstetrics 25th Edition Page 53

Ans: (B) Aspirin and Low dose Heparin

5. **Presenting diameter in well flexed fetal head in cephalic presentation is:**

A. Mentovertical
B. Suboccipitofrontal
C. Suboccipitobregmatic
D. Submentobregmatic

Key:

Presenting diameter in well flexed fetal head in cephalic presentation is Suboccipitobregmatic

Transverse Diameters of Fetal Skull

- **Biparietal diameter (9.5 cm)**–It extends between the two parietal eminences. This diameter is engaging transverse diameter most often.
- **Super subparietal diameter (8.5 cm)**–It extends from a point below one parietal eminence to point above other parietal eminence of the opposite side.
- **Bitemporal diameter (8 cm)**–Distance between antero inferior ends of coronal sutures.
- **Bimastoid diameter (7.5 cm)**–Distance between tips of mastoid process. This diameter is nearly incompressible.

Anteroposterior Diameters of Fetal Skull

Diameter	Extent	Length	Attitude of head	Presenting part
Suboccipitobregmatic	Extends from the nape of the neck to the center of bregma	**9.5 cm**	*Complete flexion*	Vertex
Suboccipitofrontal	Extends from the nape of the neck to center of sinciput	10 cm	*Incomplete flexion*	Vertex
Occipitofrontal	Extends from the occipital eminence to the root of nose (glabella)	11.5 cm	*Marked deflexion*	Vertex
Mentovertical	Extends from the chin to the highest point on sagittal suture	14 cm	*Partial extension*	Brow
Submentobregmatic	Extends from the junction of the floor of the mouth and neck to the center of bregma	**9.5 cm**	*Complete extension*	Face

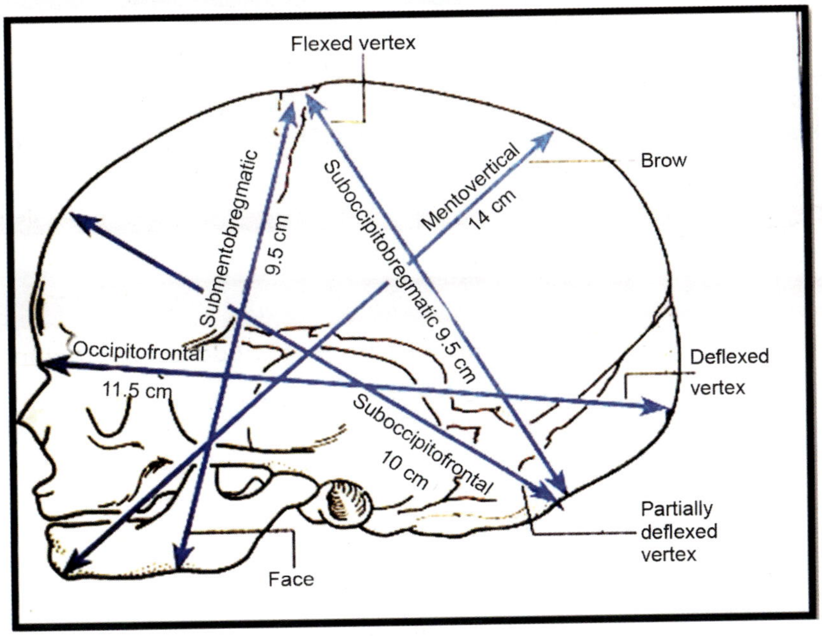

Anteroposterior Diameters of Fetal Skull

- Engaging AP diameters of fetal skull in **vertex and face presentations** are Suboccipitobregmatic and Submentobregmatic respectively which are 9.5 cm. Hence, a normal pelvis permits engagement of the fetal skull in vertex and face presentations.
- In brow presentation, Engaging AP diameter of fetal skull is mentovertical (14 cm). Hence, engagement does not occur and arrest of labor occurs.

Diameters of Obstetric Significance which are 9.5 cm

Diameters in Fetal Skull

- Bi parietal diameter
- Suboccipitobregmatic
- Submentobregmatic

Diameter in Maternal Pelvis

- **Sacrocotyloid diameter**–Distance from midpoint of sacral promontory to iliopubic eminence. Represents space occupied by Biparietal diameter of head while negotiating brim in a flat pelvis.

Ref: Dutta Textbook of Obstetrics 9th Edition Page 83

Ans: (C) Suboccipitobregmatic

6. A-45-year-old lady has heavy menstrual bleeding of 6 months. USG shows 2 cm intramural fibroid. She requires:

A. Hysterectomy
B. OCPs for 3 cycles
C. Progesterone therapy for 3 months
D. Endometrial sampling

Key:

Endometrial assessment should be done in any woman older than 45 years with AUB and those <45 years with history of unopposed estrogen exposure like Obesity/PCOD, Failed medical management and Persistent AUB

Indications for Endometrial Sampling in AUB

- Women with AUB at >45 years (perimenopausal AUB)—to exclude endometrial hyperplasia and carcinoma, as >90% of endometrial cancers are seen in this age group
- Women of reproductive age with persistent anovulatory AUB (>6 months), associated with risk factors such as obesity, PCOD, or tamoxifen therapy
- Ultrasound showing increased ET (>12 mm) in perimenopausal women
- Women not responding to medical therapy.

USG in given case shows small intramural fibroid which can be cause heavy menstrual bleeding. However, HMB due to associated endometrial pathology has to be ruled out, as woman belongs to perimenopausal age group.

General Investigations

- **Ultrasound** confirms diagnosis of fibroid and differentiates it from ovarian mass and adenomyosis
- Hemoglobin—to assess the severity of bleeding, and as a part of preoperative workup
- **Pap smear** in all cases
- **Fractional curettage [endocervical curettage (ECC) and endometrial curettage (EMC)]**—indicated in **patients with AUB in perimenopausal age group to rule out associated endometrial pathology**
- **Intravenous pyelography (IVP)** is recommended in **Large fibroids, cervical and broad ligament** fibroids to look for displacement of the ureter and for any signs of compression like hydroureter and hydronephrosis

Specific Investigations

If surgery is planned, other preoperative investigations required are following–**Special investigations used in fibroid evaluation:**

MRI Scan
- Superior to USG in diagnosis of fibroid, but very expensive (done only if diagnosis is doubtful)
- Can detect small fibroids
- Differentiates fibroids from adenomyosis
- Differentiates subserous fibroid from adnexal pathology
- Definitive diagnosis of adenomyosis and leiomyosarcoma
- Can clearly delineate the myometrium, junctional zone and endometrium

Hysteroscopy
- Can visualize and remove submucous fibroid and endometrial polyps (diagnostic and therapeutic)
- To differentiate submucous fibroid and endometrial polyps (which is difficult in USG)

Saline Infusion Sonography (SIS)
- Evaluation of endometrial cavity is enhanced by infusion of saline into endometrial cavity.
- Differentiates submucous fibroid from endometrial polyps
- Diagnosis of uterine synechiae
- Can assess tubal patency as evidence of spillage of saline into peritoneal cavity (in infertility cases)

Hysterosalpingography (HSG): In cases of infertility:
- Filling defects and distortion of endometrial cavity—noted in submucous fibroid and endometrial polyps
- To check for tubal patency

Treatment

Based on the following: Patient's age, Severity of symptoms, Desire for future fertility and Patient's preference

TREATMENT OPTIONS INCLUDE THE FOLLOWING:

Conservative/Expectant management: Asymptomatic fibroids

Medical management: Not curative, only a temporary therapy
- o Nonsteroidal anti-inflammatory drugs **(NSAIDs; mefenamic acid)**
- o Hemostatic agents **(tranexemic acid, ethamsylate)**
- o **Low-dose combined oral contraceptive (COC) pills**

Contd.

Contd.

- Progesterones **[oral medroxyprogesterone acetate (MPA)/norethisterone, depot medroxy progesterone acetate, levonorgestrel intrauterine device (LNG-IUD)]**
- GnRH agonists **(leuprolide, naferelin, goserelin)**
- GnRH antagonists **(cetrorelix, ganirelix)**
- Androgenic steroids **(danazol, gestrinone)**
- Antiprogestogens **(mifepristone)**
- **Newer drugs:** Selective estrogen receptor modulators **(raloxifene, ormeloxifene),** Selective progesterone receptor modulators **(ulipristal, asoprisnil)** and Aromatase inhibitors **(anastrozole)**

Surgical Management: Definitive Treatment

- **Hysterectomy:** Abdominal, vaginal, laparoscopic-assisted vaginal hysterectomy (LAVH), and laparoscopic hysterectomy
- **Myomectomy:** Abdominal, vaginal, hysteroscopic and laparoscopic myomectomy
- **Minimally invasive techniques:** Destruction of fibroid by various methods such as the following: Myolysis and Uterine artery embolization (UAE)
- **Noninvasive procedure:** Magnetic resonance guided focused ultrasound (MRFUS)

Ref: Lakshmi Seshadri Textbook of Gynecology 2nd Edition Page 117, Williams Gynecology 3rd Edition Page 184

Ans: (D) Endometrial sampling

7. **True regarding 'Acute fatty liver of pregnancy' is:**

A. Common in multiparous
B. Incidence is 1 in 1000 pregnancy
C. Incidence is more if fetus is female
D. Common in late trimester of pregnancy

Key:

Acute fatty liver of pregnancy almost always manifests late in pregnancy–typically presents between 30 and 38th week of gestation

AFLP (Acute Fatty Liver of Pregnancy)
Acute fatty metamorphosis/Acute yellow atrophy

- Typically occurs due to defect in intramitochondrial fatty acid oxidation during pregnancy.
- Incidence is approximately 1 in 10,000 pregnancies.
- **Most common cause of acute liver failure during pregnancy is acute fatty liver.**
- Deficiency of Fetal LCHAD (Long chain 3 hydroxy acyl coenzyme A dehydrogenase) is the major cause–Unmetabolized, long-chain fatty acids enter the maternal circulation.
- Accumulation of long-chain 3-hydroxyacyl metabolites produced by the fetus or placenta is toxic to the liver and ***results in fetal fatty oxidation defects*** and may be cause of maternal liver disease.

Risk Factors

- *Multigravid state*
- *Male sex*
- *Co existing liver disease–HELLP, Pre eclampsia*
- *Previous episode of AFLP*

Contd.

Contd.

Pathology

HOMOZYGOUS G1528C MUTATION (MOST COMMON

↓

Accumulation of fatty acid that have not undergone beta oxidation at required rate

↓

Inability to generate energy at rate required to sustain healthy pregnancy and labour

↓

Fetal energy deficiency

↓

Consumption of available glucose resulting in damaging hypoglycemia

Clinical Picture

- Typically present in 3rd trimester
- Anorexia, Nausea, Vomiting, Abdominal pain and headache–*Initial symptoms*
- Fatty liver is characterized by accumulation of microvesicular fat that "crowds out" normal hepatocytic function
- Multiorgan involvement–Acute pancreatitis, Transient Diabetes Insipidus and Upper GI Bleeding along with Acute kidney injury
- Most common clinical picture is Jaundice and Fever
- Most commonly associated abnormalities–Hypoglycemia and Raised serum Ammonia

Approximately only 20% of AFLP is associated with LCHAD deficiency

- Typically seen in mothers heterozygous for LCHAD deficiency with fetus homozygous for LCHAD deficiency.
- Maternal mortality rate= 20-75%
- Fetal mortality rate= 25-90%

Laboratory Tests

- Elevated Aminotransferases (5 to 10 times the upper limit of normal)
- Elevated Serum Bilirubin
- Elevated Prothrombin time
- Elevated Uric acid level, Elevated ammonia level, Elevated creatinine
- Elevated white blood cell count
- Low serum glucose
- Low fibrinogen

Diagnosis is mainly clinical

Spontaneous resolution usually follows delivery

- **Acute fatty liver can recur in subsequent pregnancies.** Women with a history of AFLP who are contemplating another pregnancy should be co-managed with a maternal-fetal medicine specialist.
- **Management**–Prompt delivery of the fetus, regardless of gestational age. Treatment is otherwise largely supportive with goals of maternal stabilization and recovery of liver dysfunction.

Ref: Williams Obstetrics 24th Edition Page 1086

Ans: (D) Common in late trimester of pregnancy

8. **Chromosome for partial mole:**

A. 46 XX
B. 46 XY
C. Trisomy 18
D. 69 XXY

Key:

Differentiating Features Between Partial and Complete Mole		
	Partial Mole	**Complete Mole**
Karyotype	69, XXX or 69, XXY	46, XX or 46, XY
Pathology		
Fetus	Often present	Absent
Amnion, fetal RBC	Usually present	Absent
Villous edema	Variable, focal	Diffuse
Trophoblastic proliferation	Focal	Diffuse
Clinical Presentation		
Diagnosis	Missed abortion	Molar gestation
Uterine size	Small for gestational age	Uterus larger than POG
Theca lutein cyst	Rare	25-30%
Medical complication	Rare	10-30%
Post molar GTN	2-7%	7-20%
Diagram	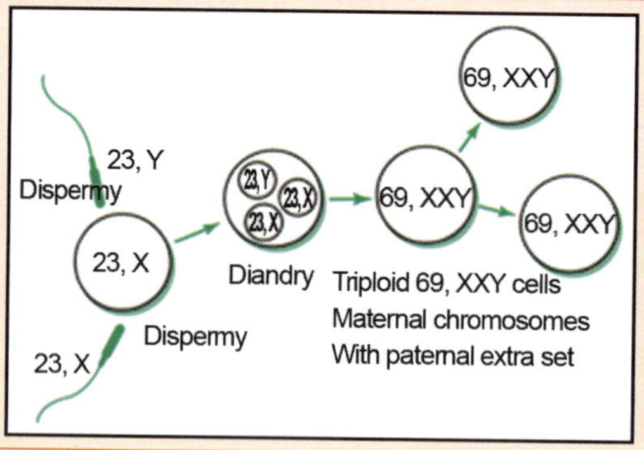	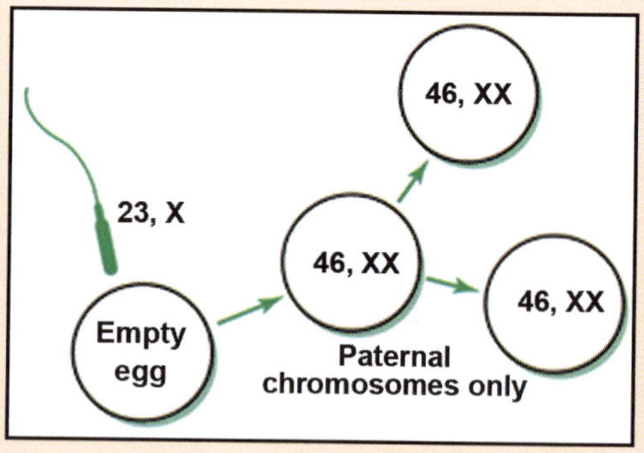

Ref: Dutta Textbook of Obstetrics 9th Edition Page 190

Ans: (D) 69 XXY

9. **Which of the following is not prevented by OCPs?**

A. Ovarian cyst
B. Thromboembolism
C. Iron deficiency anemia
D. Carcinoma Breast

Key:

Iron deficiency Anemia is not prevented by OC pill usage

Combined Oral Contraception Pills

- **Monophasic pills**–Contains the same amount of estrogen and progesterone
- **Phasic pills**–Contains varying amount of estrogen and progesterone over 2 weeks (biphasic pills) or 3 weeks (triphasic pills).

MECHANISM OF ACTION

- Inhibits Ovulation
- Thickens cervical mucus to prevent sperm penetration
- Makes endometrium non-receptive for Implantation

Brand name	Estrogen component	Progesterone component
Mala N (Govt. of India)	Ethinyl estradiol (30 μg)	Norethisterone (1.0 mg)
Mala D (Govt. of India)	Ethinyl estradiol (30 μg)	D-Norgestrel (0.5 mg)
Novelon	Ethinyl estradiol (30 μg)	Desogestrel (0.15 mg)
Femilon	Ethinyl estradiol (20 μg)	Desogestrel (0.15 mg)
Loette	Ethinyl estradiol (20 μg)	Levonorgestrel (0.1 mg)
Yasmin	Ethinyl estradiol (30 μg)	Drospirenone (3 mg)

COCs available free of cost in India are Mala N that contains 1 mg norethisterone and Mala D that contains 0.5 mg of D–Norgestrel

Advantages of OC Pills

Contraceptive benefits
- Very effective contraceptive method – Failure rate is 0.1 per 100 women years
- Usage is not related to sexual intercourse
- Reversibility rate is prompt
- It has additional non-contraceptive benefits

Non-contraceptive benefits
- Regulation of menstrual cycle
- Reduction of menorrhagia
- Reduction of dysmenorrhea
- Reduction of premenstrual tension syndrome

Protection against
- Pelvic inflammatory disease (thick cervical mucus)
- Ectopic pregnancy
- Endometriosis
- Functional ovarian cysts
- Benign breast diseases
- Hirsutism and acne
- Osteoporotic fractures
- Rheumatoid arthritis

Protection against malignancies
- Endometrial cancer
- Epithelial ovarian cancer
- Colorectal cancer

Contraindications

- History of valvular or Ischemic heart disease
- Uncontrolled hypertension
- Diabetes mellitus with vascular complications
- History of stroke
- Arterial or venous thrombosis
- Migraine with focal neurologic symptoms

Contd.

Contd.

- Breast cancer (Estrogen dependent neoplasms)
- Liver disease – adenoma, carcinoma
- Smoking at > 35 years
- Pregnancy
- Lactation
- Undiagnosed vaginal bleeding
- Major surgery or prolonged immobilization

Disadvantages

- COCs does not provide any protection against STDs or HIV infection
- Requires education and motivation for usage
- Requires initial check up and periodic supervision
- Inconvenience caused due to daily scheduling

Side Effects

Major side effects	Minor side effects
• Venous thromboembolism	• Irregular or breakthrough bleeding
• Myocardial infarction	• Breast tenderness
• Stroke	• Nausea
• Gallbladder disease	• Weight gain
• Endocervical cancer (High dose pills)	• Mood changes

Ref: Dutta Textbook of Gynecology 7th Edition Page 532,
Speroff Clinical Gynecologic Endocrinology and Infertility 8th Edition Page 1033

Ans: (B) Thromboembolism

10. A female has come to OG OPD with complaints of vaginal discharge. On examination, discharge was profuse, frothy with vaginal erythema. Vaginal pH is 5.9. Organism responsible:

A. Trichomoniasis
B. Gardenella vaginalis
C. Candidiasis
D. Neisseria gonorrheae

Key:

Vaginal discharge was profuse, frothy with erythema points Diagnosis of Trichomoniasis

Trichomonal Vaginitis

- **Most common cause for vaginitis in the reproductive age group.**
- **Causative agent**–Trichomonas vaginalis, a pear-shaped flagellated protozoa.
- Transmitted through sexual contact.

Clinical Features

- Profuse and offensive yellow green colored vaginal discharge
- Associated with itching and vaginal irritation and urinary symptoms like dysuria

Contd.

Contd.

On Examination

- Thin, greenish-yellow and frothy offensive discharge
- Vulval and vaginal edema and erythema
- Vaginal walls are red and inflamed with multiple punctate hemorrhagic spots giving appearance of **'strawberry vagina'**

Diagnosis

- pH is >4.5
- Identification of motile flagellated trichomonads by wet mount preparation

Treatment

- Metronidazole 400 mg BD orally for 1 week
- Metronidazole 2 g PO single dose
- Tinidazole 2 g PO single dose
- The partner should be treated simultaneously.

Distinguishing Features of Vaginitis			
	Bacterial vaginosis	Trichomoniasis	Candidiasis
Discharge	White, thin, homogeneous, Foul odour	Yellow, frothy, Foul odour	Thick, curdy, No odour
Other symptoms	-	Pruritus, dysuria	Pruritus, dysuria
Signs	No erythema	Strawberry vagina	Erythema ++
pH	>4.5	>4.5	<4.5
Diagnosis	Wet mount–Clue cells, (Whiff test–Amine odour with KOH)	Wet mount–Motile flagellated organisms	KOH mount–Pseudohyphae or spores

Ref: Dutta Textbook of Gynecology 7th Edition Page 160, Williams Gynecology 3rd Edition Page 61

Ans: (A) Trichomoniasis

11. Dose of Ulipristal used for Emergency contraception:

A. 30 micrograms
B. 300 micrograms
C. 30 milligrams
D. 300 milligrams

Key:

Various Regimens Used For Emergency Contraception		
Drug	Dosage	Time to be taken
Levonorgestrel	0.75 mg two doses, 12 hours apart or a single dose of 1.5 mg	Upto 72 hours following unprotected intercourse
Yuzpe regimen	100 μg of ethinyl estradiol + 500 μg Levonorgestrel in each dose given twice, 12 hours apart	Upto 72 hours following unprotected intercourse
Mifepristone	600 mg single dose	Upto 72 hours following unprotected intercourse

Contd.

Contd.

Ulipristal acetate	Single oral dosage of 30 mg	Upto 120 hours following unprotected intercourse
Copper IUCD	-	Upto 5 days following unprotected sexual intercourse

Ref: Dutta Textbook of Gynecology 7th Edition Page 492, William Gynecology 3rd Edition Page 131

Ans: (C) 30 milligrams

12. **Maximum dose of PGF2α used in Postpartum Hemorrhage (PPH):**

A. 200 micrograms
B. 200 milligrams
C. 2000 micrograms
D. 2000 milligrams

Key:

Carboprost (PgF2 alpha)

- **Indications**–Used for control of postpartum hemorrhage
- **Dosage**–250 microgram of PGF2 alpha is given as intramuscular injection and can be repeated at 15 minutes interval for a maximum of 8 doses (250 *8 = 2000 microgram)
- **Adverse effects:** Nausea, vomiting, diarrhea, Exaggeration of bronchial asthma

Postpartum Hemorrhage

- PPH is defined as cumulative loss >1000 ml accompanied by signs and symptoms of hypovolemia
- **Most common cause–Atonic PPH**
- **Drug of choice–Oxytocin (20 Units per litre if infusate @10-20 ml/min)**
- **Active management of third stage of labor (AMTSL) AMTSL** is a prophylactic measure for PPH prevention and has three components
  - Administration of uterotonics, preferably oxytocin (10 units IV/IM), immediately following the delivery of the baby
  - Delivery of the placenta by controlled cord traction (CCT)
  - Uterine massage

Uterotonics used in Medical management of PPH

- **Oxytocin IV infusion,** 20 units in 500 mL normal saline started at rate of 60 drops/min.
- **Injection Methergin** 0.2 mg IV or IM can be repeated up to two doses.
- **Injection carboprost** (PGF2 alpha 250 µg IM) can be repeated at intervals of >15 minutes, up to a maximum of eight doses. Intramyometrial injection of carboprost 250 µg may be given.
- **Misoprostol (PGE1)** 1000 µg can be given orally or placed per rectally.

If all the conservative measures fail to control PPH, then consider surgical intervention for controlling PPH.

Ref: Dutta Textbook of Obstetrics 9th Edition Page 410

Ans: (C) 2000 micrograms

13. FBS values for overt GDM:

A. 110 mg% B. 126 mg%

C. 140 mg% D. 200 mg%

Key:

Diagnostic Criteria for Overt DM
FBS >= 126 mg/dL or RBS >= 200 mg/dL or HbA1C >= 6.5

Whom to Screen?

Ideally GDM screening should be performed in all pregnant females but all those who have average/high risk for diabetes should definitely be screened.

ACOG recommends universal screening for diabetes in pregnancy.

Risk Stratification to Screen for Gestational Diabetes Mellitus in Pregnancy

Risk Category	Members Who Belong to the Risk Category	Screening for GDM
Low risk	All the following factors should be fulfilled: • Age <25 years • Normal prepregnancy body weight • No history of diabetes in first-degree relatives • No history of abnormal glucose metabolism • No history of poor obstetric outcome	No screening for GDM is required
Average risk	• Members of ethnic group belonging to Hispanic, African Americans, South East Asians, Native Americans	Screening for GDM is done at 24–28 weeks using two-step or one-step procedure. Indians belong to this risk group
High risk	• Age >30 years • Obesity • Family history of type 2 DM in first-degree relative • Previous history of GDM • Past history of bad obstetric outcome • Persistent glycosuria	Screening for GDM is done as soon as feasible and repeated at 24–28 weeks

Whom to Screen?

- Screening for GDM is usually done at **24–28 weeks of gestation** because placental hormone–mediated insulin resistance increases during the second trimester and glucose levels rise in women who cannot cope up with this insulin resistance.
- Screening in 1st trimester helps to identify cases of overt DM, diagnosed for 1st time during pregnancy.

Current Guidelines on Time of Screening of Pregnant Women for Gestational Diabetes Mellitus

Guidelines	Recommendation	Interpretation
IADPSG ADA	FBS or HbA1c or RBS is done for all women on the first prenatal visit	If results are not diagnostic of overt DM and FBS is ≥92 mg/dL, diagnosis of GDM is made If FBS is <92 mg/dL, 75 g OGTT is done at 24–28 weeks
DIPSI	Test is done at the first visit and if negative, repeat at 24–28 weeks and again at 32–34 weeks	

ADA, American Diabetic Association; DIPSI, Diabetes in Pregnancy Study Group in India; IADPSG, International Association of Diabetes in Pregnancy Study Group.

How to Screen?

Screening for Diabetes during Pregnancy: There is no consensus on single diagnostic method.

Two-Step Procedure for diagnosis of GDM: *Two step approach where initially screening is done followed by diagnostic test.*

- Includes screening with 50 g oral glucose challenge test (OGCT) followed by diagnostic 100 g OGTT for those meeting the threshold value in OGCT.

ACOG recommends 2 step approach

50 g Glucose Challenge Test (Screening Test)

Performed by administering 50 g of glucose orally, irrespective of previous meal and measuring venous plasma glucose 1 hour later.

Plasma Glucose	Interpretation
< 140 mg/dL	Further testing by GTT not required
≥ 140 mg/dL	Further testing required
≥ 200 mg/dL	Values > 200 mg/dL confirm diagnosis of diabetes – No further testing required

100 g Oral Glucose Tolerance Test

- Patients with abnormal screening test are followed by a 3 hours 100 g oral glucose tolerance test (GTT).
- The test should be performed with 100 gm of glucose load in the morning after an overnight fast of at least 8 hours but not more than 14 hours and after at least 3 days of unrestricted diet (> 150 g/d) and physical activity.
- Upper limit of normal for the 3 hours glucose tolerance test during pregnancy

Contd.

Contd.

Time	100 g Glucose (Carpenter coustan criteria)
Fasting	95 mg/dL
One hour	180 mg/dL
Two hours	155 mg/dL
Three hours	140 mg/dL

- **If two or more of these values are abnormal:** Gestational diabetes is confirmed.
- **If one value is abnormal:** Increased risk of complications like macrosomia and polyhydramnios.

One Step Approach

- **WHO and IADPSG recommend use of single step approach**–Both for screening and diagnosis of GDM.
- Patient is advised unrestricted diet for 72 hours, which is followed by fasting blood sample. Then 75 gm glucose given and 2 blood samples are taken—after 1 hour and 2 hours.

Time	75 gm Glucose
Fasting	92 mg/dL
1 hour	180 mg/dL
2 hours	153 mg/dL

In the single step approach, if one value is abnormal, GDM is diagnosed.

Extra Note

- ACOG recommends a 2 step approach for diagnosis of GDM
- ADA recommends either 1 step or 2 step procedure for diagnosis of GDM
- WHO and IADPSG recommends a single step procedure for diagnosis of GDM

Diabetes in Pregnancy Study Group in India (DIPSI) Criteria

- DIPSI recommends non-fasting 75 g OGTT with a second-hour cutoff of ≥140 mg/dL for GDM diagnosis
- **Procedure:**
  - Irrespective of the last meal, 75 g glucose load is given.
  - Second-hour blood glucose value is estimated.

DIPSI Recommendations on OGTT Cutoff Values	
Second-Hour Venous Plasma Glucose	**Interpretation**
>200 **(mg/dL)**	DM
140–200 **(mg/dL)**	GDM
120–140 **(mg/dL)**	Decreased gestational glucose tolerance (DGGT)–Risk of polyhydramnios

- DIPSI recommends OGTT at 1st antenatal visit and if negative, to be repeated at 24–28 weeks and again at 32–34 weeks.
  - Testing at 1st visit—identifies overt diabetic cases (prevalence of DM is high in India; second-hour value >200 mg/dL at the first antenatal visit is considered as pregestational DM)
  - Testing at 24–28 weeks (time period when glucose intolerance gets manifested)
  - Testing at 32–34 weeks (identifies cases with delayed onset GDM)

Ref: Dutta Textbook of Obstetrics 9th Edition Page 281

Ans: (B) 126 mg%

14. Best treatment for pruritis vulvae with atrophic vaginitis:

A. Antihistaminics
B. Topical steroids
C. Topical estrogen therapy
D. Tranquilizers

Key:

Best treatment for pruritis vulvae with atrophic vaginitis is Topical Estrogen therapy

Atrophic Vaginitis

- Inflammation of Vagina as a result of tissue thinning due to Estrogen deficiency following menopause or due to medications like GnRH analogues.
- **Symptoms:** Dyspareunia, Vaginal/ Vulval pruritis or Dryness, Burning micturition.
- **Diagnosis:** Based on symptoms
- **Treatment:**
  - **If symptoms are severe–*Topical estrogen therapy is effective*→**Relieves disruption in pH to restore normal flora of vagina.
  - **If urinary symptoms are present–**Systemic hormonal therapy can be used. Recommendation is to use lowest effective dose for the shortest duration to prevent adverse endometrial effects.
  - **Recent treatment modality include–**Selective estrogen receptor modulators, vaginal dehydro-epiandrosterone, and laser therapy. Other treatment measures include vaginal lubricants and moisturizers.

Ref: Dutta's Textbook of Gynecology 3rd Edition Page 554

Ans: (C) Topical estrogen therapy

15. A P2 L2 complaints of menorrhagia and dysmenorrhea for 6 months. Hysterectomy specimen is shown. What is the probable diagnosis?

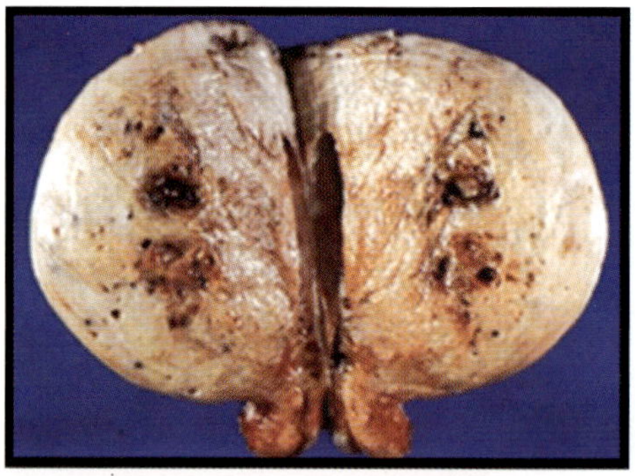

A. Fibroid
B. Adenomyosis
C. Hydrometra
D. Endometriosis

Key:

Given image is that of Adenomyosis–Note absence of capsule and presence of dark blood spots

Cut section shows thickening of the uterine wall with characteristic trabeculated appearances. Unlike fibroid, there is no capsule surrounding growth. There may be visible blood spots at places

Adenomyosis

- Condition where there is in growth of Endometrium, both glandular and stromal components, directly into the myometrium.
- Pelvic endometriosis co-exists in about 40%.

Contd.

Contd.

Etiology

- Repeated childbirths
- Vigorous/ repeated curettage
- Excess of estrogen effect

Pathology

- There is **hyperplasia of the myometrium** producing diffuse enlargement of the uterus, symmetrically but at times, more on the posterior wall.

Naked Eye Appearance

- **Diffuse symmetrical enlargement** of uterus; posterior wall is often more thickened than anterior one.
- The size usually does not increase more than 14 weeks pregnant uterus.
- Cut section shows thickening of the uterine wall with characteristic trabeculated appearances. **Unlike fibroid, there is no capsule surrounding the growth.** There may be visible blood spots at places.
- The given image is that of Adenomyosis–Note the absence of capsule and presence of dark blood spots.

Histological examination

- Characterized **by extension of endometrial glands and stroma beneath the endometrial—myometrial interface (EMI).** As the submucosa is absent, endometrial glands lie in direct contact with the underlying myometrium.

Clinical Features

- Patients are usually **parous with age usually above 40.**

Symptoms	Signs
Menorrhagia (70%)–Excessive bleeding is due to increased uterine cavity, associated endometrial hyperplasia and inadequate uterine contraction. **Dysmenorrhea (30%)**–Progressively increased colicky pain during period is due to retrograde pattern of uterine contractions. When depth of penetration is >80% of myometrium, pain is severe. **Dyspareunia**–Due to enlarged and tender uterus.	Uterine size does **not exceed 14 weeks** pregnant uterus. **Pelvic examination**—reveals **uniform enlargement** of uterus, and is tender on palpation **Ultrasound (TVS) and Color Doppler Characteristics** ***Subendometrial halo is characteristic of adenomyosis.*** Other features are: (i) heterogenous echogenecity, (ii) hypoechoic myometrium with multiple small cysts in the myometrium (honeycomb appearance), (iii) increased vascularity within the myometrium
'Swiss cheese' pattern of endometrium with increased vascularity in histopathology is suggestive of adenomyosis	

- **MRI**–More specific diagnosis. Low signal intensity JZ < 8 mm excludes the disease. Whereas **JZ thickness > 12 mm is suggestive of adenomyosis.** MRI shows a Junctional zone with low signal intensity on T2 weighted images at the innermost layer of myometrium. **Disturbance of normal junctional zone (JZ)** may predispose to secondary infiltration of endometrial glands and stroma to inner myometrial zone.

Treatment

- Treatment is **predominantly surgical.**
- There is little place of hormone therapy–Response of the ectopic endometrial tissue to ovarian hormones is minimal as the invasion is predominantly in the basal layer.
- Treatment with progestins or cyclic estrogen and progestin have got little benefit.
- **Levonorgestrel-releasing**–IUS is found to improve menorrhagia and dysmenorrhea.

Contd.

Contd.

Surgical Management

- **Hysterectomy** (parous and aged women)
- **Conservative surgery**–Adenomyomectomy (in young women with localized adenomyoma, localized excision can be tried)

Ref: Dutta's Textbook of Gynecology 3rd Edition Page 314, Shaw 16th Edition Page 420

Ans: (B) Adenomyosis

16. Which of the following hormone acts in this period?

A. Progesterone
B. LH
C. FSH
D. Estrogen

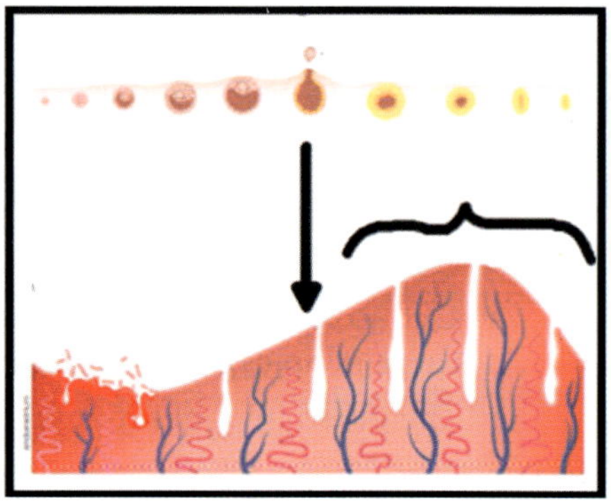

Key:

Given picture shows luteal phase and the predominant hormone during luteal phase is progesterone

Fluctuation of Different Hormonal Levels During Menstrual Cycle (Ovulatory)

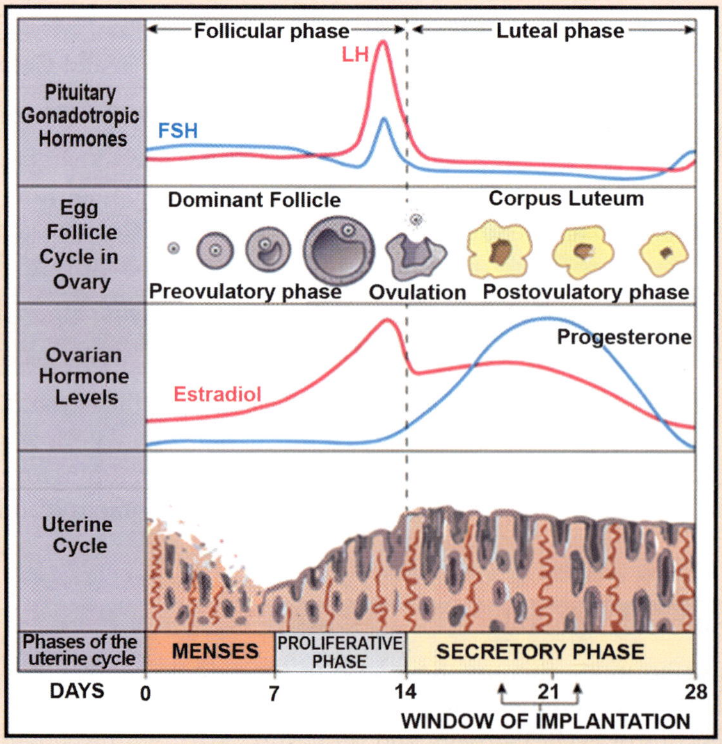

- Principal hormones secreted from ovaries are–Estrogens, Progesterone, Androgens and Inhibin

Contd.

Contd.

Mechanism of Steroid Hormone Production

- **Two cell, two gonadotropin concept of ovarian steroidogenesis**–Two cells **(theca cells and granulosa cells)** produce different hormones under the influence of **two gonadotropins (LH and FSH).**
- During **follicular phase,** under influence of LH, androgens (androstenedione and testosterone) are produced in theca cells. These androgens diffuse into granulosa cells where they are aromatized under influence of FSH to estrogens.
- **After ovulation,** progesterone is synthesized from the precursor-LDL in the luteinized granulosa cells under the influence of LH.
- **During luteal phase,** androstenedione produced by theca luteal cells diffuses into the granulosa luteal cells to be converted into estradiol by LH.

Note

- o During follicular phase, FSH enhances aromatase activity in the granulosa cells.
- o During the luteal phase, LH enhances the aromatase activity in luteinized granulosa cells.

Comparison of Hormones–Estrogen and Progesterone

	Estrogens	Progestogens
Composition	**C18 compounds** **E1–estrone; E2–estradiol; E3 – Estriol** **Estradiol is the most potent:** estradiol >estrone>estriol	Natural progesterones–C21 compounds Synthetic progesterones–C19 compounds
Sources	Predominant sites are granulosa cells of the follicles –E2 Small quantity is produced from the theca cells and ovarian stroma Corpus luteum, Placenta (with precursors from fetus)–**E3**	Corpus luteum Placenta (with maternal precursors)
Receptor	**Intranuclear receptor** *Estrogen receptors upregulate Progesterone receptors*	**Intracytoplasmic receptor** *Progesterone receptors downregulate estrogen receptors*
Metabolism	Bound to sex hormone binding globulin (SHBG) in 69% and albumin (30%) **Only 1% is free–biologically active form** Estrogens–Inactivated by conversion to estriol Estriol is conjugated in liver with glucuronic acid and excreted in bile and urine. Bile fractions are broken down by intestinal flora and enter the enterohepatic circulation.	Mainly bound to albumin (79%) and corticosteroid binding globulin Metabolized in liver and excreted as pregnanediol in urine. Pregnanediol metabolite has no progesterone activity.

Contd.

Contd.

Blood levels	**Daily production of Estradiol** • 50 μg during early follicular phase • 150–300 μgnear ovulation. • 300–600 pg/mL at ovulation After a sharp fall, it rises again to • 150–200 pg/mL in luteal phase ***Total estradiol production during cycle–10 mg***	**Daily production** • 2–3 mg in follicular phase • 20–30 mg in luteal phase. Daily excretion of pregnanediol in the urine • < 1 mg in follicular phase • 3–6 mg in luteal phase.

Physiological Action of Estrogen and Progesterone

Target organ	Estrogen	Progesterone
Uterus	- Increases vascularity and causes hyperplasia of the muscles. - Produces proliferative endometrial changes - **Produces receptors for progesterone.**	- Diminishes contractility of myometrium - Increases tone of the circular muscle fibers at isthmus - Produces secretory changes in endometrium ***NOTE*–Progesterone acts only in estrogen primed endometrium**
Cervix	- Cervical mucous becomes watery, profuse and stretchable (Spinbarkeitt effect) - Less protein and more electrolytes - Favors sperm penetration - Characteristic fern pattern on drying and microscopy examination	Cervical mucus become thick, scanty and viscid, losses stretchability (termed 'tack') More protein and reduced electrolytes - Prevents sperm penetration - Looses fern pattern
Vagina	- Induces thickening of epithelium - Predominance of superficial cells–deposition of glycogen which is converted into lactic acid by the Doderlein's bacilli. - **Vaginal flora is maintained by estrogen.**	- Predominance of intermediate cells
Fallopian tubes	Increases tubal motility	- Decreases tubal motility - Increases mucous secretion
Breasts	- Proliferation of the ductal component - Increase in vascularity and pigmentation of areola.	Causes proliferation of alveoli component
General	Responsible for feminine body configuration, change in voice and deposition of fat on breasts, thighs and hips. Increases coagulability of blood by increasing procoagulants, chiefly fibrinogen Causes mineralization of bones Closure of epiphysis Increases sodium and fluid retention	Thermogenic hormone, raises BBT by 0.5°C. Relaxes smooth muscles and ligaments during pregnancy
Endocrinal system	Estrogen exerts negative feedback on FSH High levels of estrogen (>200 pg/mL) exert	At low concentration→positive feedback on FSH and LH

Contd.

Contd.

	positive feedback on LH (mid cycle LH surge) Inhibits GnRH	At high concentration→negative feedback on LH - Inhibits GnRH
Lipid profile	Cardioprotective effect Increases HDL, TG and Decreases LDL	Decreases HDL, TG Increases LDL

Ovarian phases	Uterine (endometrial phase)	Events
Follicular phase (Days 1-14)	Menstrual phase (Days 1-5)	Withdrawal of the hormonal support of the endometrium at this time causes necrosis and menstruation. Low estrogens and progesterone
	Proliferative phase (Days 6-14)	This phase is dominated by the effects of estrogen, which include the replacement of the endometrial cells lost during menses
Ovulation (Day 14)		Characterized by the LH surge, which actually induces ovulation
Luteal phase (Days 15-28)	Secretory phase (Days 15-28)	Dominated by the elevated plasma levels of **progesterone** which, along with the secreted estrogen, prepares the uterus for implantation

Ref: Dutta's Textbook of Gynecology 3rd Edition Page 74

Ans: (A) Progesterone

17. Magnesium sulphate does not protect against:

A. Seizures in Severe eclampsia
B. Pre-eclampsia
C. Fetal neuroprotection
D. Fetal respiratory distress syndrome in premature babies

Key:

Magnesium sulphate does not protect against Fetal respiratory distress syndrome

Magnesium Sulphate
Mechanism of Action • Magnesium sulfate is a blocker of N-methyl-D aspartate (NMDA) receptors in the brain. • It suppresses motor end-plate sensitivity to acetylcholine and the release of acetylcholine from nerve endings. • It acts as a competitive inhibitor of calcium ion (it acts as a tocolytic by competing with Ca^{2+} ions for entry into myometrium).

Contd.

Contd.

Indications

- Anticonvulsant: In eclampsia
- Prophylaxis for prevention of convulsions: In severe preeclampsia and imminent eclampsia
- Tocolytic agent: In preterm labor
- Also has a neuroprotective effect on the fetus

Route of administration: Intramuscular/intravenous route

Dosage: One ampoule of $MgSO_4$ contains 1 g in 2 ml

For management and prevention of eclamptic convulsions—Pritchard regimen is usually followed.

Pritchard Regimen for Magnesium Sulfate Therapy	
Dosage	**Administration**
Loading dose	4 g of 20% solution IV over 5–10 minutes, followed by 10 g of 50% solution given as 5 g in each buttock, deep IM
Maintenance dose	5 g of 50% solution every 4th hourly, on alternate buttocks

- Therapeutic level of $MgSO_4$ is 4–7 mEq/L.
- Drug is excreted in urine.
- Excess dose causes loss of patellar reflexes, and respiratory depression.

Following parameters are monitored before administration of each dose

- Respiratory rate should be >14/min.
- Patellar reflex should be present.
- Urine output should be >100 mL/4 hours.

- **$MgSO_4$ for tocolysis**→4–6 g IV (20% solution) is given over 20–30 minutes, followed by infusion of 1–2 gm/hour, continued up to 12 hours following stoppage of contractions.

Adverse Effects

- Respiratory depression
- Muscle weakness
- Reduced fetal heart rate (FHR) variability
- Respiratory and/or neuromuscular depression in the newborn, if the mother has received magnesium sulfate IV therapy, for a prolonged period prior to delivery.

Antidote–Calcium gluconate (10 mL of 10% solution given as slow IV)
Contraindications: Myasthenia gravis, Maternal renal disease

Note

- If convulsions recur after loading dose, additional 2 gm of 20% solution IV over 3–5 minutes can be given.
- Dose is the same for prophylaxis and treatment of convulsions.
- Drug should be discontinued 24 hours after delivery or 24 hours after last convulsion, whichever occurs later.

Ref: Dutta Textbook of Obstetrics 9th Edition Page 233

Ans: (D) Fetal respiratory distress syndrome in premature babies

18. True regarding Vaginal GBS infection in pregnancy:

A. GBS culture needs immediate antibiotic therapy

B. GBS needs antibiotics 4 weeks before and 2 weeks after delivery

C. Positive GBS culture does not require treatment

D. Previous pregnancy with a positive GBS screening culture does not require therapy

Key:

Previous pregnancy with positive GBS screening culture does not require therapy

Group B Streptococcus

- Streptococcus agalactiae is a group B organism–colonize the gastrointestinal and genitourinary tract in 20 to 30 percent of pregnant women.
- Throughout pregnancy, group B Streptococcus (GBS) is isolated in transient, intermittent, or chronic fashion

Maternal and Perinatal Infection

- Spectrum of maternal and fetal GBS ranges from asymptomatic colonization to septicemia.
- Streptococcus agalactiae has been implicated in adverse pregnancy outcomes, including preterm labor, prematurely ruptured membranes, clinical and subclinical chorioamnionitis, and fetal infections.
- GBS can also cause maternal bacteriuria, pyelonephritis, osteomyelitis, postpartum mastitis, and puerperal infections.
- It remains leading infectious cause of morbidity and mortality among infants in the United States.
- Neonatal sepsis has received most attention due to its devastating consequences and available effective preventative measures.
- **Early-onset GBS disease**–Infection < 7 days after birth.
- **Late-onset GBS disease** caused by GBS is usually manifests as meningitis 1 week to 3 months after birth.
- Mortality rate is less for late-onset meningitis than for early-onset sepsis. The surviving infants of both early- and late-onset disease may exhibit devastating neurological sequelae.

Prophylaxis for Perinatal Infections:

2010 Centers for Disease Control and Prevention GBS Guidelines recommend a culture based approach designed to identify women who should be given intrapartum antimicrobial prophylaxis.

- Women are screened for GBS colonization at 35 to 37 weeks gestation, and intrapartum antimicrobials are given to women with rectovaginal GBS-positive cultures.
- Selective enrichment broth followed by subculture improves detection.
- Previous sibling with GBS invasive disease and identification of GBS bacteriuria in the current pregnancy are also considered indications for prophylaxis.

Intrapartum GBS prophylaxis indicated in the following conditions:

- Previous infant with invasive GBS disease
- GBS bacteriuria during current pregnancy
- Positive GBS screening culture during current pregnancy (unless a planned cesarean delivery, in absence of labor or amnionic membrane rupture, is performed)
- **Unknown GBS status (culture not done, incomplete, or results unknown) and any of the following:**
  - Delivery at < 37 weeks' gestation
  - Amnionic membrane rupture $\geq$ 18 hours
  - Intrapartum temperature $\geq$ 100.4°F ($\geq$ 38.0°C)
  - Intrapartum nucleic acid amplification test (NAAT) positive for GBS

Contd.

Contd.

Intrapartum GBS prophylaxis not indicated in the following conditions

- Previous pregnancy with a positive GBS screening culture (unless a culture was also positive during the current pregnancy)
- Planned cesarean delivery performed in the absence of labor or membrane rupture (regardless of maternal GBS culture status)
- Negative vaginal and rectal GBS screening culture in late gestation during the current pregnancy, regardless of intrapartum risk factors

Regimens for Intrapartum Antimicrobial Prophylaxis for Perinatal GBS Disease

- **Recommended**–Penicillin G, 5 million units IV initial dose, then 2.5-3 million units IV every 4 hours until delivery
- **Alternative**–Ampicillin, 2 g IV initial dose, then 1 g IV every 4 hours or 2 g every 6 hours until delivery

Penicillin Allergic

- **Patients not at high risk for anaphylaxis**–Cefazolin, 2 g IV initial dose, then 1 g IV every 8 hours until delivery
- **Patients at high risk for anaphylaxis and with GBS susceptible to clindamycin**–Clindamycin, 900 mg IV every 8 hours until delivery
- **Patients at high risk for anaphylaxis and with GBS resistant to clindamycin or susceptibility unknown**–Vancomycin, 1 g IV every 12 hours until delivery

Ref: William's Obstetrics 24th Edition Page 1249

Ans: (D) Previous pregnancy with a positive GBS screening culture does not require therapy

19. An infant born at 34 weeks of gestation. Picture is shown. Mother most probably has:

A. DM
B. PIH
C. Anemia
D. APH

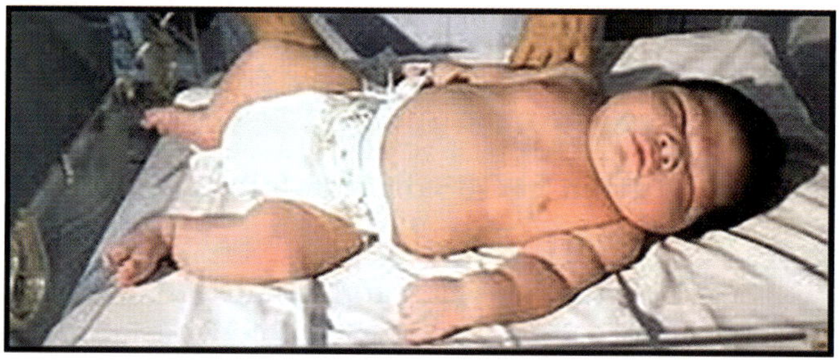

Key:

Given image is a macrosomic baby, born to a diabetic mother

Macrosomia in GDM (birth weight >4.5 kg) occurs due to the following reason:

Pederson's hypothesis: Maternal hyperglycemia→ fetal hyperglycemia → stimulates fetal pancreas to secrete insulin → fetal hyperinsulinemia → increased glycogen synthesis, lipogenesis, protein synthesis → deposition of fat in fetus → macrosomia

EFFECT OF DM ON PREGNANCY

Maternal Complications		
Antenatal	**Intrapartum**	**Postpartum**
Infections–Recurrent UTI,	Prolonged labor	Prolonged labor

Contd.

Contd.

pyelonephritis, vulvovaginal candidiasis Preeclampsia–25% incidence Polyhydramnios Preterm labor	Increase in instrumental delivery and LSCS Perineal trauma PPH	Puerperal sepsis
***NOTE* – Intrapartum complications are mainly due to macrosomia and shoulder dystocia**		

Fetal Complications	Neonatal Complications
Abortions (in overt DM) **Congenital malformations (in overt DM)** • Macrosomia • Prematurity • Sudden intrauterine deaths • Birth injuries during delivery	• Respiratory distress syndrome • Hypoglycemia • Hypothermia • Hypocalcemia • Hyperbilirubinemia • Polycythemia • Myocardial hypertrophy (overt DM) • Future risk of DM

Fetal Complications Specific to Pregestational or Overt DM

- Increased risk of **abortions and congenital anomalies** (in true GDM, hyperglycemia usually occurs in second trimester and hence late fetal complications like macrosomia and polyhydramnios occur in these women).
- Neonatal complications are similar in both true and pregestational DM.

Congenital Malformations

- These occur in overt DM when blood glucose levels are uncontrolled during organogenesis.
- **Incidence of Congenital Anomalies**–6–10% in DM (in normal population—3%).
- **Common congenital anomalies in fetuses of diabetic mothers are as follows:**
  - Cardiac anomalies (most common anomalies)—Transposition of great vessels, VSD, ASD, PDA, and coarctation of aorta
  - Neural tube defects—anencephaly and microcephaly
  - Renal and GIT anomalies
  - Most specific defect—caudal regression syndrome (very rare)

Note

Usually GDM is associated with fetal macrosomia. However, it may be associated with IUGR in certain conditions such as the following:

- Pregestational DM with vasculopathy such as nephropathy, and microangiopathy etc., (due to uteroplacental insufficiency)
- GDM associated with preeclampsia

Major Birth Defects in Infants of Diabetic Mothers (6-10%)				
CNS and Skeletal	**Cardiovascular**	**Renal**	**Gastrointestinal**	**Others**
• Neural tube defects • Anencephaly • Microcephaly • Caudal regression syndrome • Sacral agenesis	• VSD, ASD • Coarctation of aorta • Transposition of great vessels • Situs inversus • Fallot's tetralogy	• Renal agenesis • Hydronephrosis • Double ureter • Polycystic kidneys	• Duodenal atresia • Anorectal atresia • Omphalocele • Tracheoesophageal fistula	• Single umbilical artery
Good glycemic control with preconceptional counseling can reduce the incidence to 0.8-2%.				

Ref: Dutta Textbook of Obstetrics 9th Edition Page 281

Ans: (A) DM

20. True about HIV in pregnancy:

A. Chemoprophylaxis against Pneumocystis carinii pneumonia initiated when CD4 count is < 750 cells/cu. mm

B. Pregnancy increases viral load

C. Increased risk of opportunistic infections

D. Maternal to child transmission rate is 15-30%

Key:

Without antiretroviral therapy, rates of MTCT: ***15–30% without breastfeeding and 30–45% with prolonged breastfeeding***

With appropriate ART, ***rate of MTCT <2%***

Human Immunodeficiency Virus (HIV) and Pregnancy
• HIV is a **lentivirus (Subgroup of retrovirus)** that causes acquired immunodeficiency syndrome (AIDS). • In AIDS, there is progressive failure of immune system. • Life-threatening opportunistic infections and cancers flourish in this immunosuppressed state. • Without treatment, life expectancy after infection with HIV is estimated to be 9–11 years. • Infection with HIV occurs by the transfer of blood, semen, vaginal fluid, or breast milk. • India is home to the world's third largest population suffering from HIV/AIDS. • Women with **heterosexually acquired HIV infection represent most rapidly increasing group of HIV infected individuals** in the world, accounting for 1 in 4 new HIV diagnoses and deaths caused by AIDS.

Contd.

Contd.

Screening for HIV in Pregnant Women
• All pregnant women should be given **pretest counseling** regarding screening for HIV. • All pregnant women (except those who opt out) should undergo **HIV screening early in each pregnancy.** • **Repeat testing in the third trimester is recommended for those who are at high risk** of infection. • Women who present in labor without prior HIV testing should undergo rapid HIV testing. Results are obtained in 20 minutes.
Effect of Pregnancy on HIV Infection
• Disease **does not worsen during pregnancy and the rate of progression is not altered.**
Effect of Maternal HIV Infection on Pregnancy
An HIV-infected pregnancy is associated with fetal sequelae such as: • Spontaneous **abortion, low birth weight and stillbirth** • Increased risk of **preterm delivery** • Most important and worrisome sequelae is the vertical transmission of disease to the fetus and infant **(maternal to child transmission–MTCT).** • MTCT is responsible for 90% of HIV infection in children worldwide. • **Sequelae can be minimized by the appropriate use of antiretroviral therapy (ART).**
Route of Transmission From Mother to Child

• Intrauterine transmission 5–10%
• During delivery 10–20%
• Postdelivery transmission 5–20%
• **Without antiretroviral therapy, rates of MTCT**
  o 15–30% without breastfeeding
  o 30–45% with prolonged breastfeeding
• **With appropriate ART, rate of MTCT <2%**

Factors that Increase Risk of MTCT
• **Virus-related factors:** Maternal viral load, Low CD4 count • **Maternal disease-related factors:** Seroconversion during pregnancy, Advanced stage • **Obstetric factors:** Vaginal delivery, Prelabor rupture of membranes, Preterm labor, Chorioamnionitis, Ventouse delivery, Antepartum invasive procedures, Fetal scalp blood sampling and Use of fetal scalp electrode • **Breastfeeding**
Diagnosis–HIV antibody tests are used most commonly for screening and diagnosis.
Antibody tests are: • **Enzyme-linked immunosorbent assay (ELISA)**–Primary screening test. False positives can occur with ELISA. Hence, if the ELISA test is positive, Western blot should be performed for confirmation • **Western blot**–Western blot tests are more specific and are used as confirmatory tests. • **Rapid tests**–Used when results are required within a short period of time, like a woman in labor. Positive tests should be confirmed by Western blot tests. • **Nucleic acid tests**–Used when initial tests are inconclusive, especially for determination of HIV-1/HIV-2. They are expensive and not offered routinely.
Management of HIV in Pregnancy Hinges on Four Main Factors
• Universal testing of pregnant women for HIV infection • Use of ART to prevent vertical transmission • Perform cesarean section, when appropriate • Avoidance of breastfeeding, when feasible

Contd.

Contd.

Monitoring of HIV–HIV disease progression and response to antiretroviral treatment are monitored using two markers:

- **CD4 T-lymphocyte (CD4) cell count–**Defines overall immune function of an HIV infected patient. Progression to AIDS signified by a count of <200 cell/mm^3
- **HIV RNA (viral load)–**Marker of response to ART

Laboratory evaluation in the pregnant patient with HIV (in addition to routine investigations):

- CD4 –T lymphocyte count
- Viral load measurement
- Viral hepatitis markers [hepatitis B surface antigen (HBsAg) and hepatitis C virus (HCV) antibodies]
- Screening for gestational diabetes
- Screening for sexually transmitted infections (STIs)
- Screening for genital infections
- Testing for tuberculosis

Antiretroviral Therapy Regimen in Pregnant and Breastfeeding Women (WHO 2013)

- Recommended that **all pregnant HIV infected women receive a combination antiretroviral drug regimen,** regardless of CD4 T-lymphocyte count or plasma HIV RNA copy, to prevent perinatal transmission.
- ART should **be initiated by 14 weeks' gestation.**
- Women should be started on the following regimen as soon as the diagnosis of HIV infection is made and should continue the same regimen throughout pregnancy, labor, and breastfeeding and lifelong thereafter

  Once-daily combination of:
  - **Tenofovir (TDF) 300 mg**
  - **Lamivudine (3TC) 300 mg (or) Emtricitabine (FTC) 200 mg**
  - **Efavirenz (EFV) 600 mg**

Because of the increased risk of **pneumocystis pneumonia, chemoprophylaxis with trimethoprim–sulfamethoxazole (one double-strength tablet daily) is recommended** for all pregnant women with a **CD4 count of <250 cells/mm^3.**

Infants prophylaxis should begin at birth or when HIV exposure is recognized postpartum

- **Infants of mothers who are receiving ART and are breastfeeding–**Should receive 6 weeks of infant prophylaxis with daily nevirapine (NVP)
- **Infants receiving replacement feeding–**Should receive 4–6 weeks of prophylaxis with daily NVP or twice-daily zidovudine (AZT)

Mode of Delivery–Cesarean section is the preferred mode of delivery. Universal precaution should be followed (Estimated risk of infection after parenteral or mucous membrane exposure is 0.36%).

Breastfeeding–Avoidance of breastfeeding is a definite way to prevent HIV transmission via breast milk during the postnatal period

- Replacement feeding is recommended for infants born to HIV-infected mothers in developed countries.
- However, in developing countries, replacement feeding is associated with greater infant morbidity and mortality from diarrheal disease, pneumonia, and other infectious diseases. 2010 WHO guidelines recommend exclusive breastfeeding for 6 months in developing countries, in combination with maternal or infant antiretroviral prophylaxis.
- Feeding should be either exclusive breastfeeding or exclusive replacement feeding for the first 6 months.

Mixed feeding is not recommended for infants of HIV-positive mothers

Contraception: Barrier methods of contraception (condom or female condom) is effective in preventing transmission of the virus. **Disease could be prevented predominantly by health education and by practice of safer sex.**

Ref: Lakshmi Seshadri Textbook of Obstetrics Page 850

Ans: (D) Maternal to child transmission rate is 15-30%

21. In poor ovarian reserve, value of anti-mullerain hormone:

A. > 3 mg/ml
B. >10 mg/dL
C. 1– 3 mg/ml
D. < 1 mg/ml

Key:

AMH level in Mature women reflects Ovarian follicle reserve–3 ng/ml at 25 years and this is dropped to 1 ng/ml at 35-37 years
In case of Low Ovarian reserve, levels are <1 ng/ml

AMH

- **Anti Mullerian Hormone (AMH)** levels are **indicative of the size of the growing follicle pool** and considered as a **marker of ovarian aging**
- **AMH levels decline with age,** hence decline in AMH levels may be the **earliest marker of ovarian aging**
- Changes in serum AMH levels occur relatively early in the sequence of events associated with ovarian aging
- Changes in serum levels of FSH, Inhibin B and E2 occur relatively late in the reproductive aging process
- There is a **strong correlation of serum AMH levels with Antral follicular count (AFC)**
- AMH is **marker of ovarian responsiveness in women undergoing treatment for infertility. It helps to predict outcome of IVF procedures**

Tests to Determine Ovarian Reserve

Parameter	Indicator of reduced ovarian reserve
Serum FSH on day 3	>15 mIU/ml
Serum Estradiol on day 3	<80 pg/ml
Serum inhibin (produced by developing antral follicles)	<400 pg/ml
Serum anti-Mullerian hormone (normal value >1 ng/ml)	<1 ng/ml (Levels >3 ng/ml seen in polycystic ovarian disease)
Antral follicle count by transvaginal ultrasound	<10 follicles of 2–10 mm diameter
***Clomiphene citrate challenge test**—Clomiphene 100 mg from day 5 to 9; FSH measured on days 3 and 10*	Day 3 and Day 10 FSH >15 mIU/ml

Serum AMH levels and the predictive outcome of IVF procedures

AMH Level mg/ml	Interpretation	Expected Response to FSH	Anticipated Cancellation Rate with IVF	Anticipated Pregnancy Rate with IVF
> 3.0	High, often PCOS	Very High	Low	Normal
1.0-3.0	Normal	Good	Low	Normal
0.4-0.9	Low	Reduced	Increased	Reduced
< 0.4	Very Low	Very Poor	Very High	Very Low

Ref: Lakshmi Seshadri Essentials of Gynecology by 2nd Edition Page 306

Ans: (D) < 1 mg/ml

22. What type of placenta previa is shown?

A. Type 1

B. Type 2

C. Type 3

D. Type 4

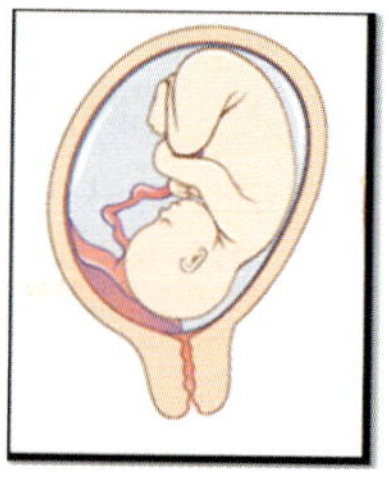

Key:

Picture shows Type 3 placenta previa–Placenta partly covering internal os

Placenta Previa

- When the placenta is implanted partially or completely over the lower uterine segment, it is termed placenta previa.
- **Types of Placenta Previa:** Classified according to proximity of placenta to internal os as follows:

Type	Description
Type I placenta previa (Low-lying)	Placenta is implanted in lower uterine segment, but doesn't reach up to cervix.
Type II placenta previa (Marginal)	Placenta reaches upto edge of cervix but doesn't cover internal os.
Type III placenta previa (Partial)	Placenta partly covers internal os.
Type IV placenta previa (Total/Central)	Placenta completely covers internal os as observed on TVS.

Risk Factors

- Multiparity, Multiple pregnancy, Previous cesarean section and Previous history of placenta previa

Clinical Features

- History of **sudden-onset, painless, causeless, recurrent fresh vaginal bleeding** is the hallmark of placenta previa.
- **Pallor is proportional** to the amount of visible blood loss.
- Signs of hemodynamic compromise (tachycardia, hypotension, features of shock) may be present in severe cases of placenta previa.
- **Uterine size is proportional** to the period of gestation.
- **Uterus is relaxed and nontender** on palpation
- Fetal **presenting part is usually high up** and cannot be pushed into pelvic inlet due to presence of placenta
- **Fetal malpresentations are common** (e.g., breech, transverse lie)
- **Fetal heart rate is usually normal** in cases of placenta previa. Rarely, fetal distress or fetal death may occur as a result of maternal shock.

Vaginal Examination

- **Vaginal examination is contraindicated** in cases of APH with suspected diagnosis of placenta previa, as it may cause further bleeding
- Local inspection and per speculum examination can be performed to rule out local causes of APH.

Management of Placenta Previa

- Management is **either active interference or expectant management** depending on the **maternal and fetal condition and POG.**

Expectant management– Termed Macaffee – Johnson regime	Active management
AIM: To continue pregnancy till term with aim of achieving fetal lung maturity without jeopardizing the maternal condition. **Candidates suitable for expectant management:** • No active bleeding present • Mother is Hemodynamically stable • POG <37 weeks • Fetal well being is assured • No fetal anomaly on USG	**AIM:** To terminate pregnancy immediately irrespective of gestational age. **Indications:** • If active bleeding is present • Hemodynamically unstable/shock • Gestational age >37 weeks and patient in labour • Fetal distress present/ FHS absent • USG shows fetal anomaly or dead fetus

Prerequisites for expectant management:
- Availability of blood for transfusion whenever required
- Facilities for emergency caesarean section

Expectant management–MacAfee and Johnson regime includes:
- Hospitalisation till active bleeding stops and then readmission at 34 weeks
- Anaemia corrected with blood transfusion and Blood is cross matched and kept ready as bleeding can recur
- Complete bed rest
- **Antenatal Steroids** given to hasten fetal lung maturity–Inj betamethasone (12 mg IM for 2 doses, 24 hours apart, if POG < 34 weeks)
- **Tocolytics** are given if uterine contractions are present at POG < 34 weeks to buy time for steroids to act. Tocolytics should not be used for more than 48 hours.
- **Anti D** is given in Rh-negative women

Expectant management should be **continued till 37 weeks**

Expectant management is abandoned and pregnancy is terminated in the following situations:
- Pregnancy reaches 37 weeks
- Severe hemorrhage at any time endangering the life of the mother
- Fetus is dead or malformed
- Onset of labor or rupture of membranes

In active management: Pregnancy is **immediately terminated.**

Mode of Delivery	
Major degree placenta previa—**types II (posterior), III and IV**	**CS** is done
Minor degree placenta previa—types I and II (anterior)	**Vaginal delivery** can be allowed

Steps to control postpartum hemorrhage in cases with placenta previa
- Uterotonic agents such as oxytocin, methergin, PG F2 alpha, and misoprostol are administered to control bleeding
- Application of B-Lynch sutures or multiple CHO sutures (multiple square sutures involving the anterior and posterior walls of uterus)
- Intrauterine compression packing
- Bilateral uterine artery ligation
- Internal iliac artery ligation

Contd.

Contd.

- Uterine artery embolization
- **Peripartum or Cesarean hysterectomy is the final option** to control bleeding, if all conservative measures fail.

Ref: Dutta's Textbook of Obstetrics 9th Edition Page 241

Ans: (C) Type 3

23. A 60 years old female with 3rd degree UVP along with cystocele and rectocele. Treatment of this condition is:

A. Hysterectomy
B. Manchester repair
C. Vaginal hysterectomy with Pelvic floor repair
D. Sling surgery

Key:

Vaginal Hysterectomy with Pelvic floor repair is suitable for women with uterovaginal prolapse aged > 40 years who have completed family

Treatment Options for Uterovaginal Prolapse

- Expectant management – Kegel's exercise
- Non surgical management – Pessary
- Surgical management

Expectant Management

Kegel's Exercise

- To strengthen Pelvic floor muscles
- Patient is taught to voluntarily contract her sphincters – 15 times, each of 10-15 sec duration, 6 times per day

Indications

- Minor degrees of UVP
- During 6 months following delivery

Non Surgical – Pessary Treatment

- A pessary is a device placed into the vagina to support the prolapsing vaginal walls.
- Pessary can be used to relieve symptoms of prolapse and of urinary stress incontinence.
- Pessary provides temporary treatment only–supports vagina but doesn't prevent progression of prolapse

Indications for Pessary

- During pregnancy
- Lactation
- Poor surgical candidates–uncontrolled HT, DM etc.,
- Patient refuses surgery
- For healing of decubitus ulcer

SURGICAL MANAGEMENT

- **Ward Mayo's Surgery**
  - **Vaginal hysterectomy with pelvic floor repair** *(VH with anterior colporrhaphy and posterior colpoperineorrhaphy)*
  - **Indications**
    Suitable for women aged >40 years who have completed family. Age limit can be relaxed to 35 years, if associated with problems like fibroid/adenomyosis
- **Manchester Operation**
  - **Indications**
    Suitable for women <40 years who have completed their family with intention of preserving menstrual function
    II or III degree uterine prolapse with cystocele / rectocele, with or without supravaginal elongation of cervix
- **Abdominal Sling Operations**
  - **Indications**
    Nulliparous prolapse
    If woman desires child bearing function
    Specially designed for young women with II or III degree prolapse, with no or minimal cystocele/rectocele and no supravaginal elongation of cervix

Sling Surgeries

Sling Surgery	Principle
Shirodkar's sling operation	- Mersilene tape (originally fascia lata was used) is fixed to the posterior aspect of **the isthmus** and to **anterior longitudinal ligament of the sacral promontory.** Sling is taken through psoas loop on left side due to presence of sigmoid colon on left.
Purandare's sling operation	- Mersilene tape is fixed anteriorly to the **isthmus of cervix** and brought between leaves of broad ligament to emerge at the lateral border of rectus abdominis on either side and **fixed to the rectus sheath** on either side.
Khanna's sling operation	- Mersilene tape fixed to **isthmus of cervix** posteriorly and fixed to **anterior superior iliac spine** on either sides.

Le Fort's Operation (Partial Colpocleisis)

Indications

- Very elderly women with prolapse who are unfit for surgery

Principal Steps

- Perform Pap smear and pelvic scan to R/o any pelvic pathology prior to the procedure.
- Le Fort's operation can be performed under local anesthesia.
- Rectangular flaps of anterior and posterior vaginal walls are excised and raw areas are opposed with catgut sutures with a small tunnel on either side to permit drainage.

Limitations

- Limits sexual function
- Inability to evaluate any bleeding from genital tract
- Enterocele formation

Contd.

Contd.

Contraindications
- Menstruating women
- Diseased cervix or uterus

Ref: Dutta Textbook of Gynecology 3rd Edition Page 201

Ans: (C) Vaginal hysterectomy with Pelvic floor repair

25. A major source of amniotic fluid in 3rd trimester is from:

A. Fetal urine
B. Fetal skin
C. Transudation across placenta
D. Fetal membranes

Key:

Major source of Amniotic fluid in 3rd trimester is from Fetal urine

Source of Amniotic Fluid (Secretion)

- ***Early pregnancy:*** Ultrafiltrate of maternal plasma across placenta
- ***Second trimester:*** Transudation across fetal skin
- ***From 20 weeks onwards:*** Fetal urine and fetal lungs–Main source
- *Overall Major source of Amniotic fluid*–Fetal Urine

Amniotic fluid is kept in balance by the following mechanisms (Absorption):
- Fetal swallowing
- Intramembranous flow across skin, cord and placental surface

Functions of Amniotic Fluid
- Acts as a Shock absorber—protects the fetus
- Maintains an even temperature
- Allows movement and growth of fetus—prevents adhesions
- Forms bag of membranes during labor that helps in dilatation of cervix

- **pH of Amniotic fluid**–7.1 to 7.3
- **Specific gravity**–1.008 to 1.010
- **Osmolality**–250 mOsm/L

Note: Amniotic fluid is not of much nutritive value.

Ref: Dutta's Textbook of Obstetrics 9th Edition Page 37, Mudaliar and Menon 12th Edition Page 28

Ans: (A) Fetal urine

26. Nuchal translucency assessment by ultrasound is done during:

A. 16-20 weeks
B. 14-16 weeks
C. 10-14 weeks
D. 7-10 weeks

Key:

Nuchal translucency assessment by ultrasound is done during 10-14 weeks
Maximum thickness of subcutaneous translucent area between skin and soft tissue overlying fetal spine at back of neck

Nuchal Translucency

- *Nuchal Translucency is a sonographic marker of Down syndrome/aneuploidy in 1st trimester*
- Increased nuchal translucency is not a fetal abnormality, but rather a marker or soft sign that confers increased risk of fetal abnormality.
- Component of 1st Trimester aneuploidy screening.
- It is the maximum thickness of the subcutaneous translucent area between the skin and soft tissue that overlies the fetal spine in sagittal plane.
- NT is measured in midsagittal plane, when Crown Rump Length is between 45-85 mm
- It is measured **between 11 and 14 weeks**
- Nuchal translucency **upto 3 mm = Normal**
- If **NT > 3 mm→Marker for Down syndrome**
- Best Approach for measuring NT – Transvaginal route

Causes of Increased Nuchal Translucency

- Down syndrome (Trisomy 21)
- Trisomy 18
- Trisomy 13
- Turner syndrome
- Klinefelter syndrome
- Triploidy
- Congenital heart disease

Prenatal Diagnosis: Biochemical and Biophysical Screening Test

	β-hCG + PAPP-A + NT	MSAFP	MSAFP, hCG, uE, (Triple Test)	MSAFP, uE, hCG, Inhibin A	Soft Tissue Marker (Nuchal Translucency, Nasal Bone)
Time (weeks)	11-14	15-20	15-18	15-20	11-14
Observation	β-hCG (↑); PAPP-A (↓)	MSAFP (↑)	MSAFP (↓); uE, ↓; hCG ↑	MSAFP(↓); uE, (↓); hCG (↑); Inhibin (↑)	Nuchal thickness (NT) > 3 mm, Nasal bone (NB) absent

Contd.

Contd.

Anomaly to detect	Down's syndrome	Open neural tube defects	Down's syndrome	Down's syndrome	Down's syndrome, Tumor's syndrome and other
Comment	A cut-off value 1 in 300 is screen positive	Cut-off level of 2.5 MOM can detect 90% of anenceph-aly, 80% open spina bifida	A cut-off value of 1 in 200 is screen positive	Detection rate is high	Detection rate of Down's syndrome is high (92%), when NT and NB are combined
Detection rate	85-92%	85%	73%	85-92%	85-92%
False-positve rate	5%	3-5%	5%	0.9%	3-5%

Ref: Dutta's Textbook of Obstetrics 9th Edition Page 650

Ans: (C) 10-14 weeks

Chapter 14

ORTHOPEDICS

1. **In painful arc syndrome pain occurs in which range of movement?**

A. Initial abduction
B. Full range of abduction
C. Mid range of abduction
D. Overhead abduction

Key:

In painful arc syndrome pain occurs in mid range of movement

Shoulder Impingement Syndrome

- Seen with repetitive overhead activities of shoulder
- This leads to mechanical impingement of rotator cuff and humeral head against lateral edge of acromion
- ***Supraspinatus***–Most susceptible to impingement and Rupture

Pathogenesis

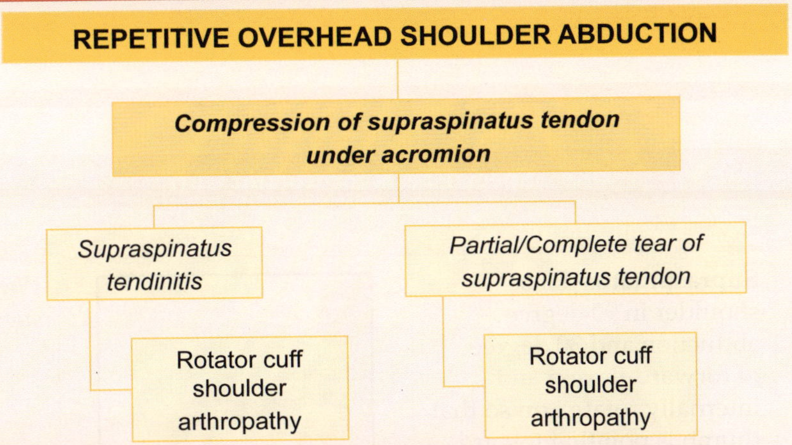

PAINFUL ARC SYNDROME (Supraspinatus tendinitis)

Swimmer's syndrome, Thrower's shoulder

- Pain occurs in middle of arc of abduction in range of 60 to 120°
- **This is called as Painful arc syndrome**
- Except that arc rest of the movements are painless
- Partial tear of supraspinatus tendon
- Most common muscle damaged in rotator cuff–Supraspinatus

Mechanism: Space between upper-end of humerus and acromion gets compromised, so that during mid-abduction tendon of rotator cuff gets nipped between greater tuberosity and acromion.

Contd.

Contd.

Causes

- **Chronic Supraspinatus tendinitis**–Most common cause
- Calcification of supraspinatus tendon
- Subacromial bursitis
- Fracture of the greater tuberosity
- Minor tears of the supraspinatus tendon

Treatment

- Anti Inflammatory drug and Ultrasound therapy to tender point
- Injection of hydrocortisone in subacromial space
- **Excision of anterior prominent part of acromion (rare)**

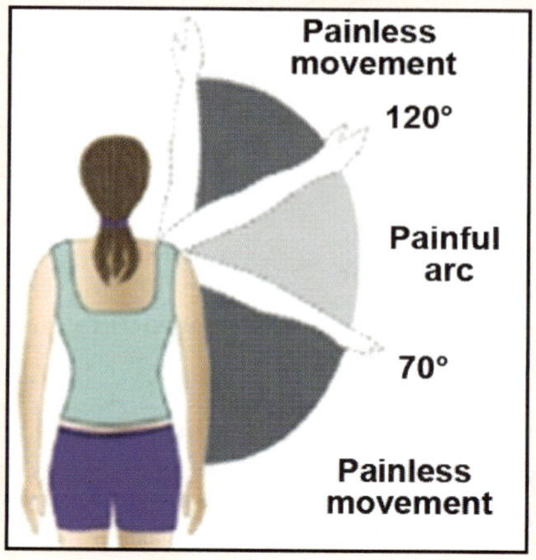

Complete Rupture/Tear of Supraspinatus tendon

- No pain
- ***Drop arm sign +ve***

Treatment

- **Small tears**–Repair by suturing
- **Large irrepairable tears**–Tendon transfer *(Particularly Younger patients)*
- **Reverse shoulder arthroplasty**–Metal ball is positioned to replace head of humerus *(Older patients)*

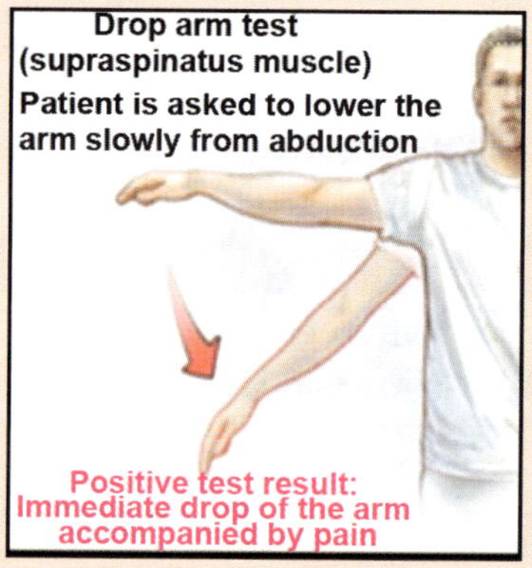

Special Tests for Rotator Cuff			
Test	**Examination**	**Picture**	**Inference (+ve test)**
Jobe's test/ Empty can test	**Supraspinatus**–Place shoulder in 90 degree abduction and 30 degree of forward flexion and internally rotate arm so that thumb is pointing toward floor	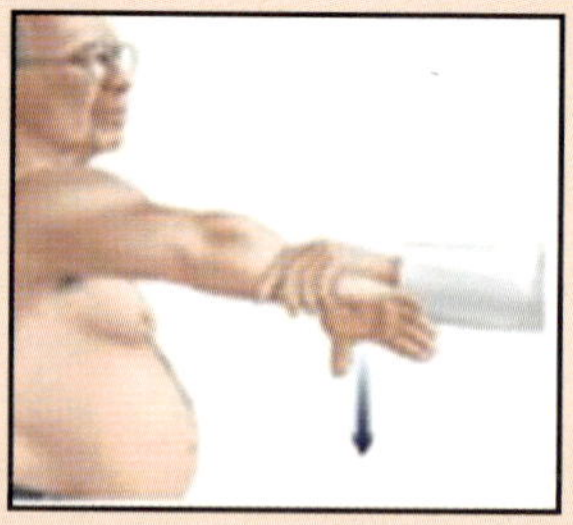	*Weakness with active resistance suggest supraspinatus tear*
Hawkin's Kennedy test	**Supraspinatus**–Patient arm is kept in throwing position and flexed forward 30 degrees. Examiner internally rotates humerus	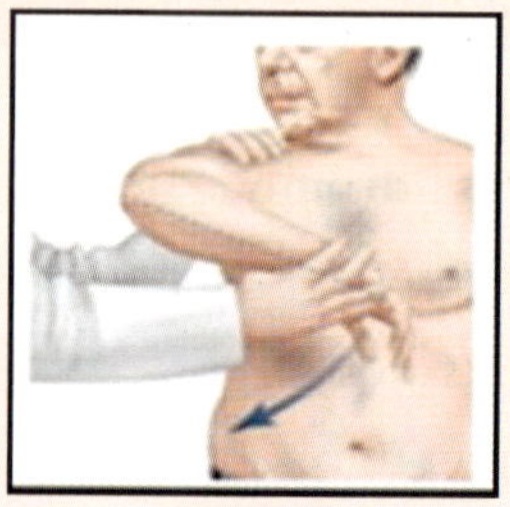	*Pain on testing infers test is +ve*

Contd.

Contd.

Drop arm test	**Supraspinatus**–Patient's arm is passively forward flex hand and bring to 90° abduction. Ask to hold hand in this position	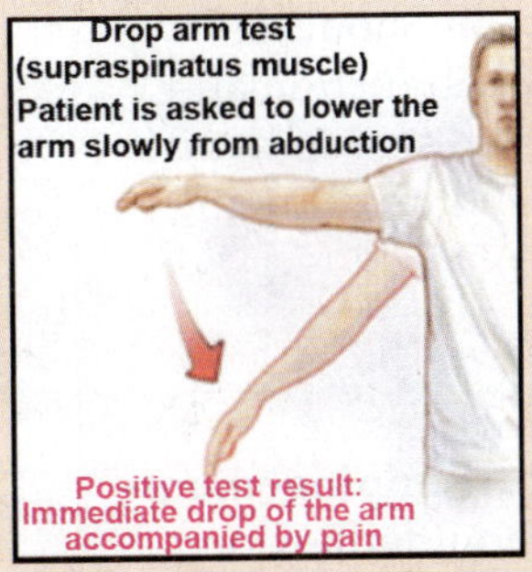	*Immediate drop of arm accompanied by pain*
Lift off test/ Gerber's test	**Subscapularis**–Internally rotate arm so dorsal surface of hand rests on lower back. Patient is instructed to actively lift hand away from back against examiner resistance	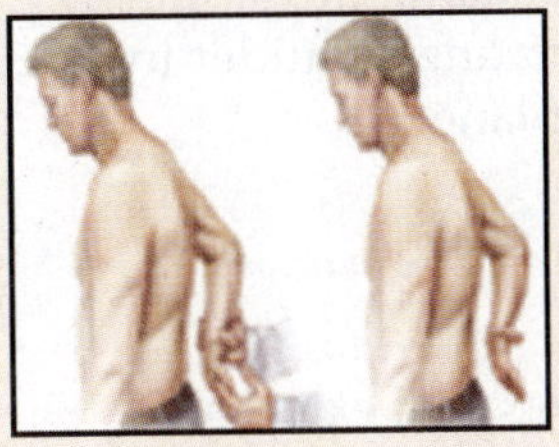	*Inability to actively lift hand away from back suggests Subscapularis tear*
Belly press test/ Napolean test	**Subscapularis**–Patient can't fully internal rotate shoulder. Patient is asked to push on their belly while keeping their elbow pushed forward	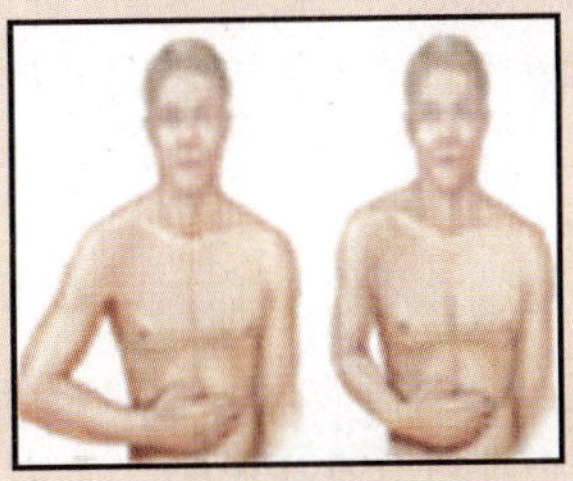	*If subscapularis is weak pressure on belly can be maintained by moving elbow back and flexing wrist*
Internal rotation lag test	**Subscapularis**–Arm is held in maximal internal rotation. Elbow is flexed to 90° and dorsum of hand is passively lifted away from lumbar region until almost full internal rotation is reached	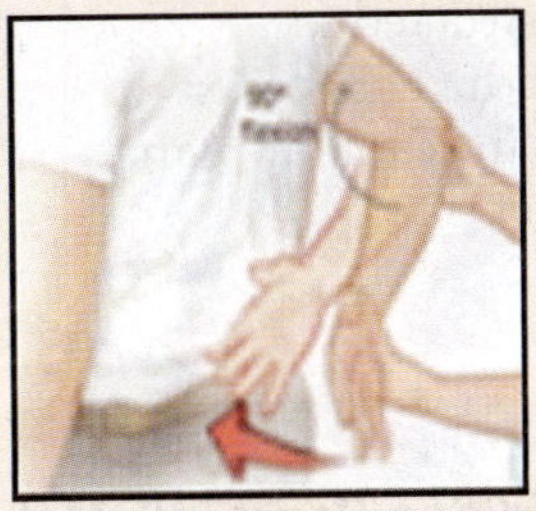	*Release wrist but support at elbow. Failure to maintain this position*
Bear hug test	**Subscapularis**–Patient hand is placed on opposite shoulder with elbow anterior to body. Examiner then attempts to maintain hand on shoulder	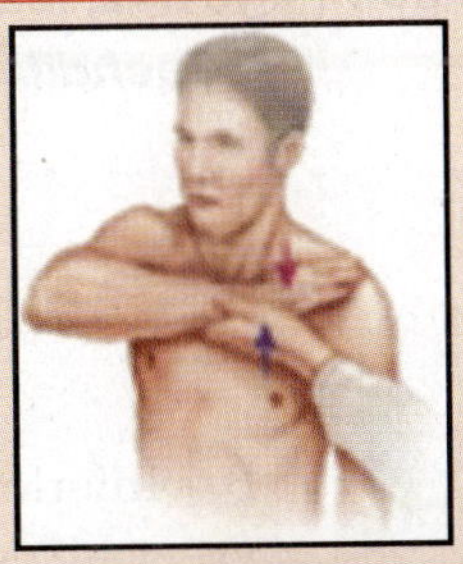	*Patient can't hold hand against shoulder as examiner applies external force–Indicates Subscapularis tear*
External rotation lag sign	**Infraspinatus**–Examiner holds arm in 20° forward elevation in scapular plane with elbow flexed 90° and arm in maximum external rotation	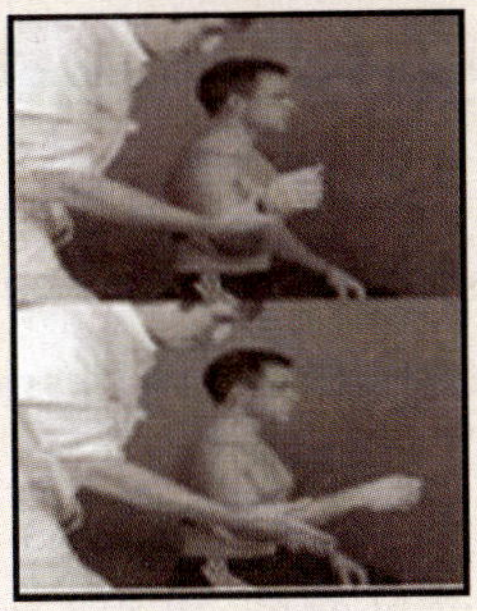	*Inability to maintain maximal external rotation–Posterior cuff integrity (Massive rotator cuff tear)*

Contd.

Contd.

Horn blowers test/ Patte's test	**Teres minor**–Shoulder is kept in 90° abduction and elbow flexed so that hand comes to mouth (blowing horn)	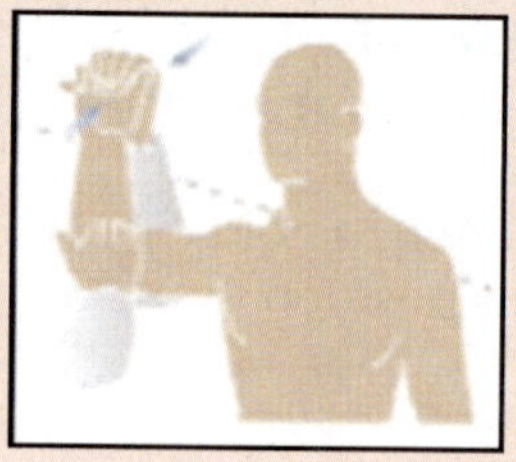	*Pain and Inability to maintain position–Indicates Teres minor Insufficiency (Massive rotator cuff tear)*
Neer Impingement test	**Rotator cuff impingement**–Passive shoulder flexion. Examiner stabilises scapula while elevating shoulder in scapular plane	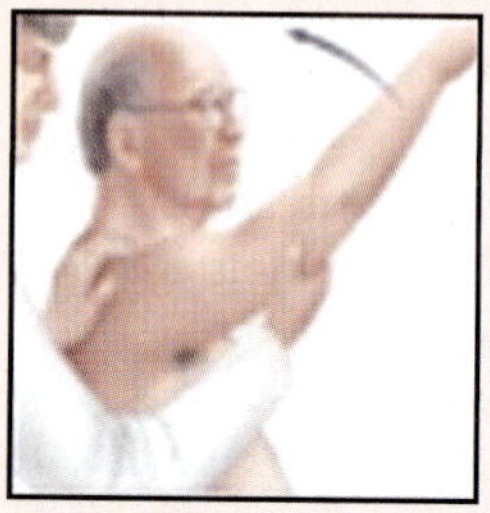	*Pain elicited between 130 and 170 degrees causes Impingement*
Internal Impingement sign	Arm in maximal external abduction at 90°	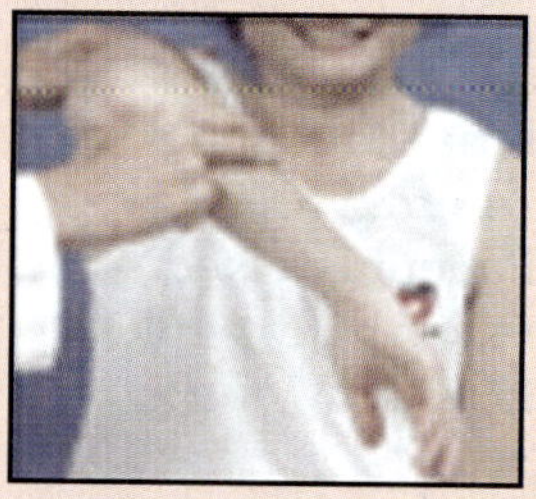	*Anterior pain indicates anterior instability and posterior pain indicates Internal Impingement*
Painful arc test	**Rotator cuff tendinopathy**–Patient instructed to actively abduct shoulder and move in scapular plane	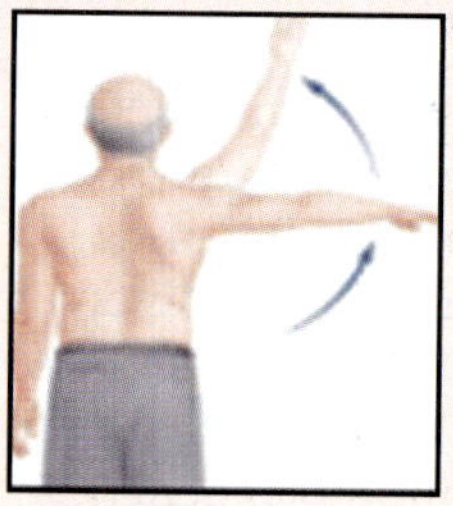	Pain with abduction 60-120 degrees suggest Supraspinatus tendinitis

Ref: Apley's 9th Edition Page 342, Maheswari 5th Edition 305, Rockwood 7th Edition Page 1563, Tachdjian 3rd Edition Page 2285, Campbell 11th Edition Page 3272, Watson Jones 6th Edition Page 951

Ans: (C) Mid range of abduction

2. **Foot drop results from injury to:**

A. Femoral nerve
B. Inferior Gluteal nerve
C. Common peroneal nerve
D. Tibial nerve

Key:

Foot drop is a result of injury to common peroneal nerve/Lateral popliteal nerve
Foot remains in plantar flexion due to weakness of dorsiflexors–Occurs in common peroneal nerve palsy

COMMON PERONEAL NERVE

- Supplies motor supply to muscles of anterior and lateral compartments of thigh
- Most commonly damaged nerve in lower limb–Common peroneal nerve

Clinical Features of Common Peroneal Nerve Injury

- **Foot drop**–Weakness of dorsiflexion and eversion of foot

  Patient walks with a ***'high-step gait'*** (while walking he has to lift the foot high in order to clear the ground).

  Causes of foot drop:

  Trauma, Diabetes, Motor neuron disease, Stroke, Polio, Tumors of brain and spinal cord, Charcot Marie tooth disease, Alcohol and Multiple sclerosis

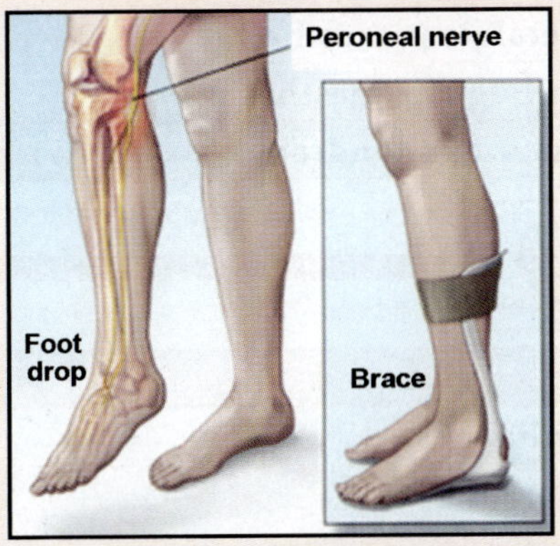

Inability to lift front part of foot off the ground

- Weakness of extensor hallucis longus
- Inversion and Plantar flexion are normal
- Anesthesia over lower lateral part of leg and dorsum of foot–*often little/no sensory loss*
- *All reflexes are intact–Ankle jerk is lost in sciatic nerve lesion*
- *Wasting of anterior tibial and Peroneal muscles*

Nerve Palsy	Deformity
Erbs palsy (C5,C6)	*Police man tips, Waiter's tip posture*
Klumpke's palsy (C8,T1)	*Claw hand*
Axillary nerve	*Deltoid paralysis*
Long thoracic nerve	*Winging of scapula*
Radial nerve (Crutch palsy, Saturday night palsy)	*Wrist drop*
Posterior interosseous nerve	*Finger drop*
Ulnar nerve	*Claw hand*
Median nerve	*Ape thumb deformity (Simian thumb), Pointing index*
Common peroneal nerve	*Foot drop*
Tibial nerve	*Claw toes*

Nerve Entrapment Syndromes

Carpal tunnel syndrome	*Median nerve*
Pronator syndrome	*Median nerve*
Kiloh Nevin syndrome	*Anterior Interosseous nerve*
Ulnar tunnel syndrome	*Ulnar nerve at wrist (Guyon's canal)*

Contd.

Contd.

Cubital tunnel syndrome	*Ulnar nerve at elbow*
Thoracic outlet syndrome	*C8 and T1*
Tarsal tunnel syndrome	*Tibial nerve*
Meralgia paraesthesia	*Lateral cutaneous nerve of thigh*
Chiralgia paraesthesia	*Superficial radial nerve*
Piriformis syndrome	*Sciatic nerve*

Nerve Injuries Associated With Trauma	
Radial nerve	*Humeral shaft fracture*
Ulnar nerve	*Medial humeral epicondyle fracture* *(Lateral humeral condyle non union–Tardy ulnar nerve palsy)*
Median nerve	*Dislocation of elbow*
Posterior interosseous nerve	*Monteggia fracture dislocation*
Anterior interosseous nerve	*Supracondylar fracture humerus*
Axillary nerve	*Shoulder dislocation, Surgical neck of humerus fracture*
Common peroneal nerve	*Fibular neck fracture*
Sciatic nerve	*Hip dislocation*

Ref: Apley's 9th Edition Page 282, Maheswari 5th Edition 68, Rockwood 6th Edition Page 212, Tachdjian 3rd Edition Page 1362, Campbell 11th Edition Page 3650, Ebnazer 2nd Edition Page 178

Ans: (C) Common peroneal nerve

3. Scissor gait is seen in which of the following condition?

A. Polio
B. Cerebral palsy
C. Hyperbilirubinemia
D. Hyponatremia

Key:

Scissoring gait is seen in Cerebral Palsy

- ***Scissoring gait**–Hypertonia and flexion in the legs, hips and pelvis leading to extreme adduction and even crossing.*
- *Caused by upper motor neuron (UMN) lesion like cerebral palsy.*
- *Among the options cerebral palsy is an UMN lesion.*

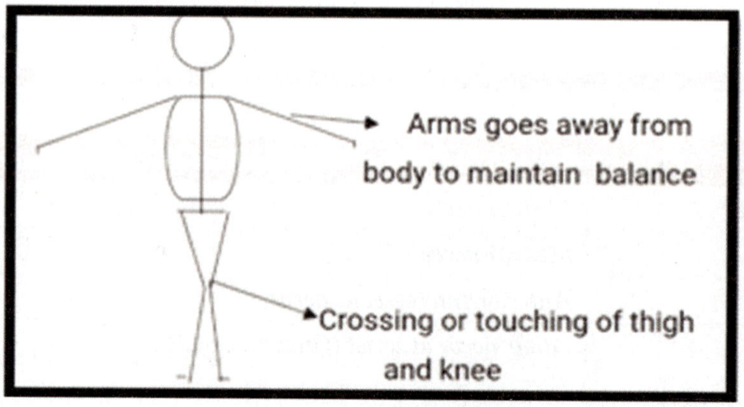

Gait Cycle

- Gait can be evaluated by observing a person walk in slow motion.
- Normal gait has a definite pattern. It is made up of a number of gait cycles.
- One gait cycle constitutes period from heel strike of a leg to its next heel strike.

- **Gait cycle can be divided into 2 phases:**
  - Stance phase
  - Swing phase

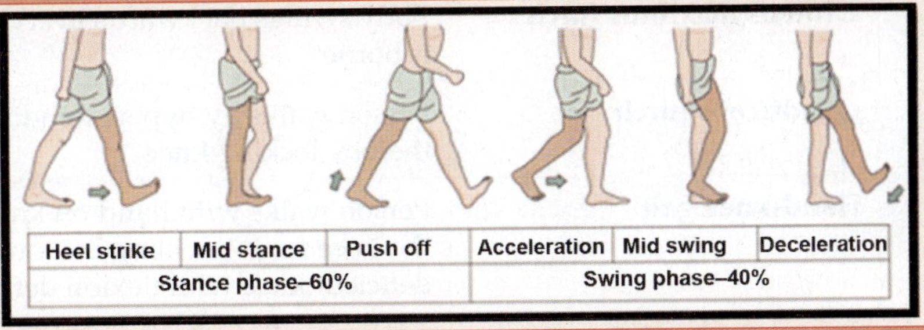

- **Stance phase**

- Part of gait cycle when foot is on the ground.
- Starts with heel strike and ends with toe off.
- ***Constitutes 60 percent*** of the gait cycle and consists of essentially three events:
  - ***Heel strike***–When heel strikes the ground.
  - ***Mid stance***–When whole foot is flat on the ground, and
  - ***Push off***–When body is propelled by taking push from foot; first heel goes off ground and finally toes.

- **Swing phase**

- Part of the gait cycle when the foot is off the ground.
- Starts with toe off and finishes when the foot is ready to strike the ground again.
- ***Constitutes 40 percent*** of gait cycle, and consists of following events:
  - ***Acceleration:*** Once the foot is off the ground, the leg moves forward with the help of hip flexors.
  - ***Mid swing:*** This is the mid part of the swinging leg.
  - ***Deceleration:*** Swinging leg is slowed down to get foot ready for heel strike.

- **Normal gait**

- In normal walking, each leg goes through stance phase and a swing phase alternately.
- Rhythmic repetition of such cycles provides grace to the gait.
- Normal gait is mechanically efficient and therefore, only minimal energy is consumed while walking.
- In case rhythm of gait is disturbed due to any reason, one lands up using extra energy for walking, and thus gets easily tired.

Abnromal Gait

Gait	*Pattern*	*Cause*
Antalgic/Painful gait	Time taken on affected leg is reduced. Body weight is shifted quickly to normal leg.	*Painful condition of the leg*
Stiff hip gait	Lifts pelvis, and swings it forward with leg in one piece	*TB hip, Rheumatoid hip, Ankylosing Spondylitis*

Contd.

Contd.

Stiff knee gait/ Circumduction gait	Leg is circumducted and brought forward in order to get clearance	*TB knee, Painful stiff knee*
Short limb gait	Becomes apparent only if the limb is < 2 inches. Body on affected side moves up and down every time weight is borne on affected leg	*Congenital short femur, Shortening secondary to fracture*
Trendelenburg/Gluteus medius gait	Body swings to affected side every time weight is borne on that side	*Dislocated hip, CDH*
Gluteus maximus lurch	Body swings backwards every time weight is borne	*Gluteus maximus paralysis*
Quadriceps lurch	Person walks by hyperextending and thereby locking knee	*Quadriceps paralysis*
Hand-knee gait	Person walks with hand on knee to prevent the knee from buckling in a quadriceps deficient knee with flexion deformity	*Polio*
High stepping/ Foot drop/Neuropathic/ Russian march gait	Due to drop of the foot, the leg is lifted more nerve in order to get clearance. First to touch the ground is forefoot and not heel	*Common peroneal palsy, Sciatic nerve palsy*
Scissor gait	**Legs are crossed in front of each other while walking due to *spasm of adductors of the hip***	***Cerebral Palsy***
Crouch gait	**Bilateral knee flexion contracture**	***Cerebral Palsy***
Waddling gait	Weakness of proximal muscles of pelvic girdle. Patient uses circumduction to compensate gluteal weakness	*Bilateral DDH*
In toeing/Pigeon toeing gait	Rotational variation of lower extremity where feet or toes point toward midline during gait	*Metatarsus adductus, Tibial internal rotation, Persistent femoral anteversion*
Festinent/Short shuffling gait	Patient is trying to catch up with centre of gravity which falls anteriorly	*Parkinsonism*
Charlie Chaplin gait	Caused faulty sitting or sleeping as in prolonged maintenance of spread eagle or frog leg position	*External tibial torsion and Alkaptonuria*
Choreiform/Hyperkinetic gait	Irregular, slow, spontaneous knee flexion and leg rising, wide based	*Sydenham chorea, Huntington disease*
Circumduction gait	Leg is stiff without flexion at knee and ankle and with each step rotated away from body. This forms a semicircle	*Hemiplegia*
Sailor gait	Child walks bent forward with feet wide apart. Takes irregular steps like a sailor on a rough or as if drunk	*Bilateral CDH*

Stumbling gait–*Bilateral CTEV*
Reeling gait–*Alcoholism, Cerebellar lesions*
Peg leg gait–*Congenital vertical talus*

Types of Abnormal Gait and Their Conditions	
Type of gait	**Causes**
Wide based gait	Normal 12 – 15 months of age Vitamin E deficiency Hartnup Disease
Waddling gait	Rickets Mucopolysaccharidosis IV Hip gridle weakness
Spastic gait	Contracture of Achilles tendon (Spastic cerebral palsy)
Hemiparetic/circumductive gait	Spastic Hemiplegic cerebral palsy
Reeling gait	Cerebral ataxia
Wide based steppage gait	Sensory ataxia
Trendelenburg gait	Duchenne muscular dystrophy
Antalgic gait	Trauma Pain (Legg Calve Perthes Disease) Infection

Ref: Apley's 9th Edition Page 449, Maheswari 5th Edition Page 347, Campbell 11th Edition Page 3650, Textbook of Orthopedics and Trauma Volume 3 2nd Edition Page 2706

Ans: (B) Cerebral palsy

4. Injury to which part of scaphoid bone is more likely to undergo Avascular necrosis?

A. Proximal 1/3rd
B. Middle 1/3rd
C. Distal 1/3rd
D. Scaphoid tubercle

Key:

Though injury to scaphoid most commonly occurs in waist region. Region most prone for AVN is proximal 1/3rd

Scaphoid Fracture

- Most common carpal bone fracture
- Occurs following a fall with wrist in dorsiflexion and radially deviated position
- *Most common site in Adults and Adolescents–Waist of scaphoid (70%)*
- *Most common site in children–Distal pole (Avulsion type)*
- Most commonly in males between 15 and 30 years
- Tenderness at anatomical snuff box

SCAPHOID FRACTURE

- **Proximal (20%)**
- **Middle/Waist (70%)**
- **Distal (10%)**

Contd.

Contd.

Vascularity of Scaphoid Bone

- Blood supply enters in reverse direction from distal to proximal direction
- Receives blood supply from dorsal and volar branches of radial artery ***(Both entering distally)***
- Volar/palmar branch enters scaphoid tubercle and supplies its distal end
- Dorsal branch enters through numerous small foramina along spiral groove and distal ridge–80% of blood supply
- Vascularity of proximal fragment is maintained by retrograde intraosseous blood flow from distal to proximal
- ***In waist fractures, vascularity may be compromised resulting in AVN of proximal fragment***

Investigations

- If fracture is not seen in standard AP/Lateral views then **Oblique view** may be useful
- Best radiological view–Oblique view
- Repeat X-ray at 2 weeks used for diagnosis of occult fractures–*Radiologically visible in 2 weeks*

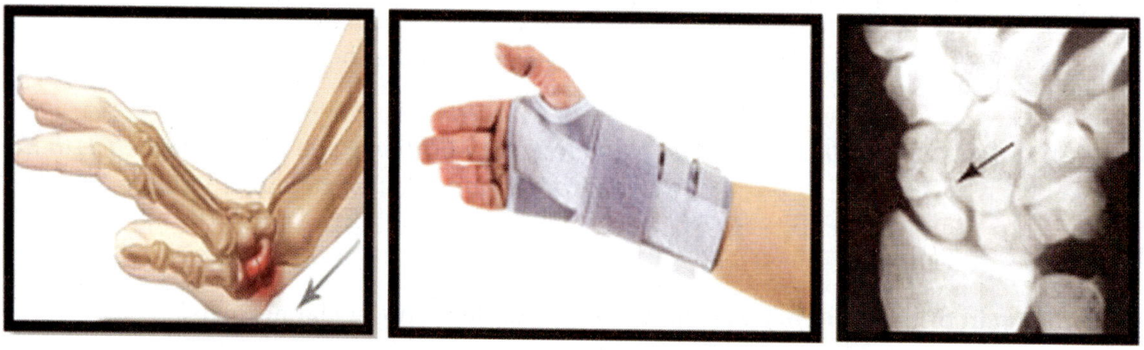

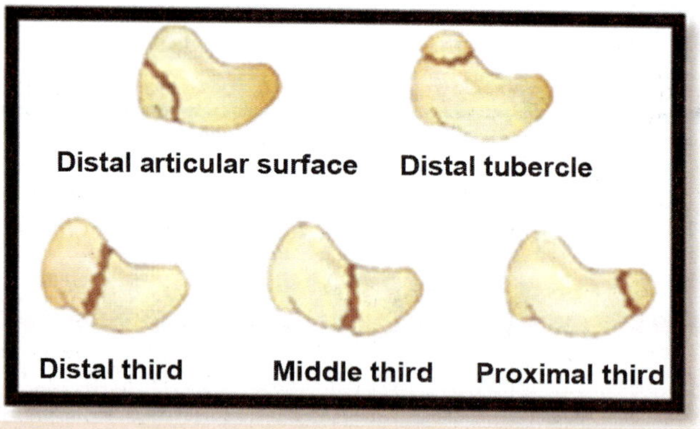

Treatment

- Undisplaced fracture–Immobilization in ***Scaphoid cast*** POP in glass holding position
- Displaced fracture–ORIF with Herbert screw
- If proximal pole is avascular and no significant radiocarpal arthritis is present, revascularization of scaphoid with vascularized bone graft from distal radius/preferably ***pronator quadrates graft***

COMPLICATIONS: Non union and AVN

Ref: Apley's 8th Edition Page 623, Maheswari 5th Edition Page 115, Rockwood 7th Edition Page 790, Tachdjian 4th Edition Page 2570, Campbell 11th Edition Page 4012, Watson Jones 6th Edition Page 718

Ans: (A) Proximal 1/3rd

5. Female complains of chronic low back ache with X-ray spine. Probable diagnosis is:

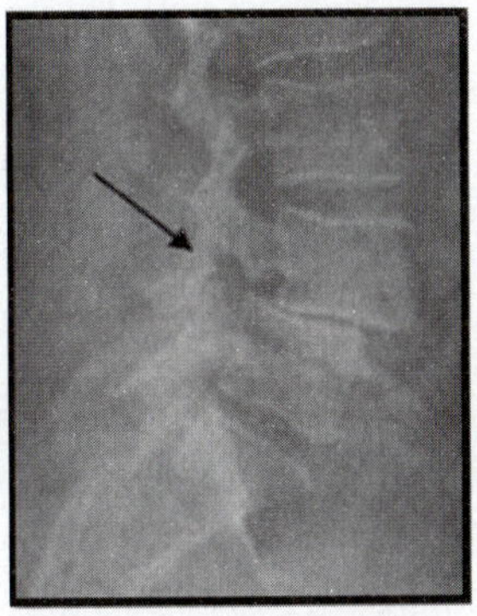

A. Osteoporosis

B. Potts spine

C. Spondylolisthesis

D. Paget's disease

Key:

X-ray Picture shows Anterior displacement of one vertebra over other can be seen on a lateral view of the spine seen in Spondylolisthesis

Spondylolisthesis

- Forward Displacement/Slip of one vertebrae over another vertebrae–Spondylolisthesis
- Most common location–L5-S1> L4-L5
- **X-ray lumbar spine:**
  - Lateral view–Forward slip of vertebrae best seen
  - Oblique view–Pars interarticularis gap is best see
    Scotty dog with broken neck appearance
- AP view–*Napolean hat sign*

Types of Spondylolisthesis		
Type 1	Dysplastic/ Congenital	Congenital abnormalities of upper sacral facets or inferior facets of L5 that allow slipping of L5 on S1 No pars interarticularis defect is present in this type
Type 2	Isthmic (Most common)	Defect in pars interarticularis that allows forward slipping of L5 on S1 **3 types:** Lytic–Stress fracture of pars interarticularis Healed fracture–Elongated but intact pars interarticularis Acute high energy fracture of pars interarticularis
Type 3	Degenerative	This lesion results from **intersegmental instability** of long duration with subsequent remodeling of articular processes at the level of involvement
Type 4	Traumatic	This type of lesion results from fractures in area of bony hook other than pars interarticularis like pedicle, lamina or facet
Type 5	Pathological	This type results from generalized or localized bone disease and structural weakness of bone
Type 6	Iatrogenic	Surgical excision of posterior elements

Contd.

Contd.

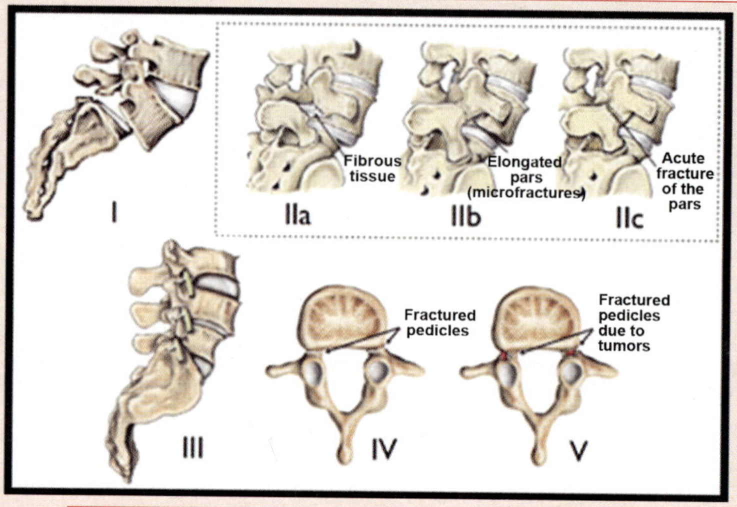

Type 1 and 2 are usually seen in Young children

- Children–Painless (Protruded abdomen and peculiar stance
- Adolescents and Adults–Intermittent back ache coming on exercise/strain
- **Phalen Dickson Sign:** Young patient regardless of extent of slippage there may be tight hamstrings and knee bent with hips flexed gait

Spondylolisthesis is staged according to percentage of vertebral body length that one vertebra subluxes over adjacent vertebra

- Stage I: 0 to 25%
- Stage II: 25 to 50%
- Stage III: 50 to 75%
- Stage IV: 75 to 100%

Treatment

- No treatment given–Asymptomatic and mild cases
- Physical therapy with lumbar stabilization exercises may be helpful (Brace)
- **Surgical:** Decompression of the compressed nerves if any, followed by fusion of the affected segments of the spine
- Use of internal fixation devices like pedicular screws and rods helped in early mobilisation of patient

EXTRA EDGE

- **Spondylolysis**–Defect in pars interarticularis
  X-ray lumbar spine–Oblique view–
  Scotty dog wearing a collar
- **Spondyloptosis**–Complete displacement of L5 in front of S1
- **Retrolisthesis**–Posterior displacement of 1 vertebrae over other

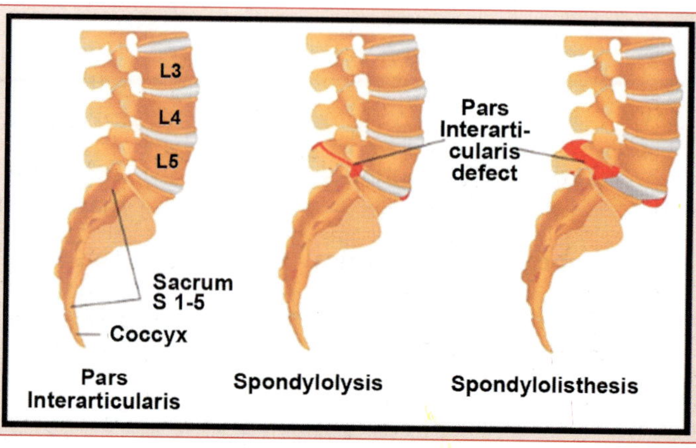

Condition	Features	Image
Osteoporosis	Decreased bone density Thinning of cortex of bone Biconcave vertebrae (Codfish/Fish mouth vertebrae) Compression fracture	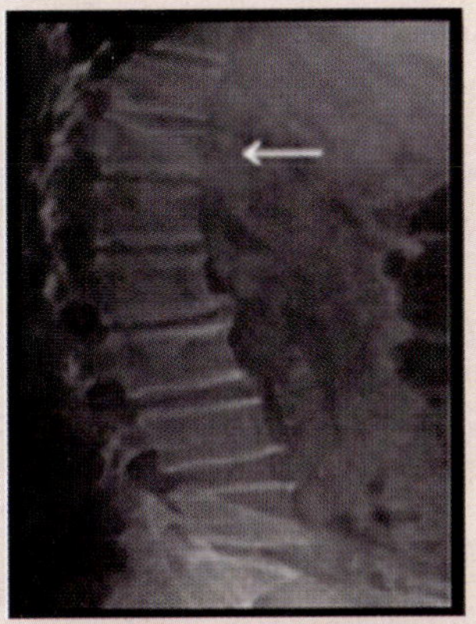
Potts spine	**Reduced disc space** Blurred paradiscal margins Destruction of bodies Loss of trabecular pattern Increased prevertebral soft tissue shadow Subluxation/Dislocation Decreased lordosis/Kyphosis	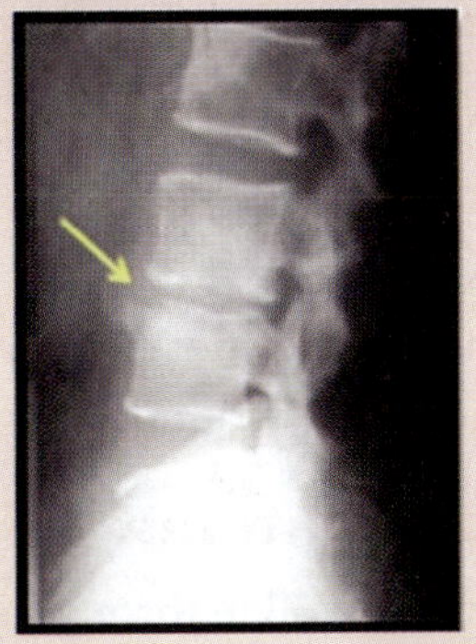
Spondylolisthesis	Forward slippage of vertebrae Scottish dog with a broken neck appearance–***Beheaded Scottish terring sign*** Pars interarticularis gap is present (Spondylolysis–Scottish dog wearing a collar–Scottish terring sign)	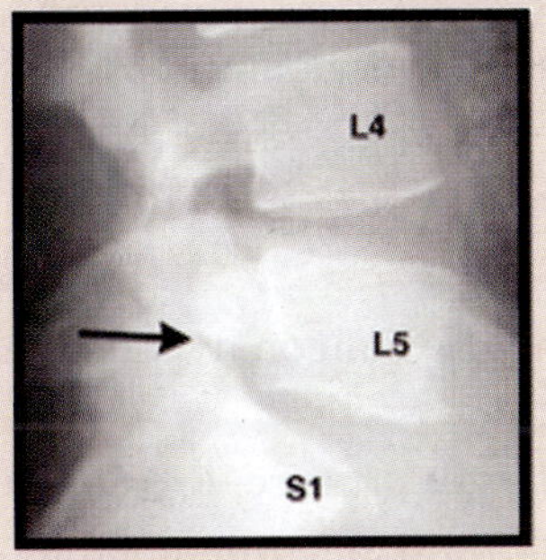
Paget's disease	Picture frame vertebrae Ivory vertebrae Osteoporosis circumscripta (Skull)	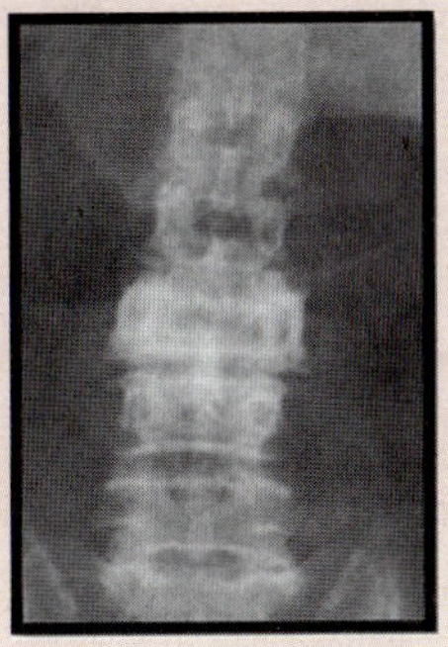

Ref: Apley's 9th Edition Page 449, Maheswari 5th Edition 347, Campbell 11th Edition Page 3650, Textbook of Orthopedics and Trauma Volume 3 2nd Edition Page 2706

Ans: (C) Spondylolisthesis

6. **True about Tenosynovitis of flexor tendon sheath is:**

A. Extension deformity at joint
B. Infection of little finger presents as localized swelling only
C. Associated with minimal pain and swelling
D. Treatment is antibiotics and splintage

Key:

Tenosynovitis of flexion tendon sheath results in placing finger in flexion, Intense pain on hyperextension, Manifests as uniform swelling of entire finger
Treatment is Antibiotics and Splintage

Tenosynovitis of Flexor Tendon Sheath

Etiology

- Pulp infection
- Puncture wounds in flexor crease
- Penetrating wounds are usually infected with staphylococcus aureus

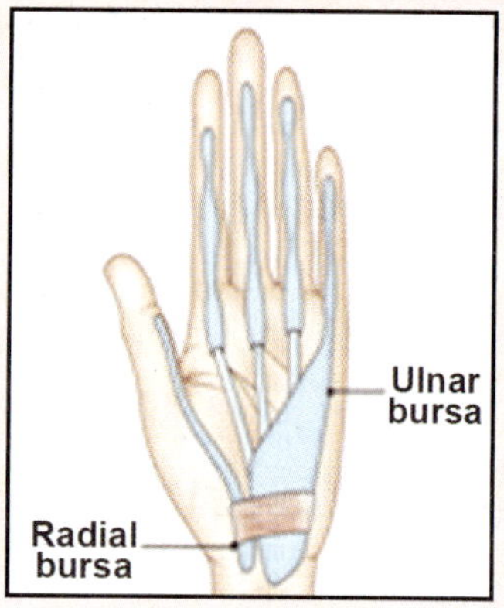

Clinical Features

- Finger–Swollen throughout its length and is acutely tender over flexor tendon sheath.
- It is held semi-flexed and active/passive extension at Interphalangeal joint is very painful.

Kanavel Signs

- Intense Pain on hyperextension of finger ***(Earliest and most important sign)***
- Flexion posture–***Rigid positioning of finger in flexion***
- ***Uniform swelling involving entire finger***
- Tenderness over flexor tendon sheath on percussion (Most significant sign)

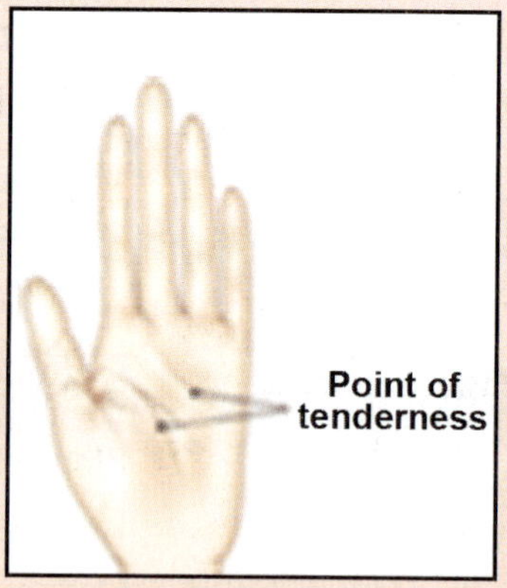

Kanavel sign

Treatment

- Early tenosynovitis for <48 hours can be treated with antibiotics and splinting.
- Prolonged infection causes flexor sheath pressure >30 mm Hg and Ischemia of tendon resulting in adhesion stiffness and functional impairment (Closed irrigation is better than open technique).
- Inflammation of the thin synovial lining of a tendon sheath is termed tenosynovitis.
- May arise from mechanical irritation or from bacterial infection.

Contd.

Contd.

TENOSYNOVITIS

Irritative

Commonly seen in tendons of hand
Results in pain and swelling
Treatment: Rest, analgesics and ultrasonic therapy
Need local hydrocortisone infiltration.

Infective

Infection of synovial lining of tendon by pyogenic/tubercular bacteria
Usually pyogenic origin.

Condition	Deformity	Picture
Trigger finger	Stenosing synovitis of flexor tendons Inability to extent flexed digit >45 years, Unknown etiology (DM, RA) Thickened A1 pulley of flexor tendon sheath Painful palpable nodules at MCP joint Ring finger–Most commonly involved	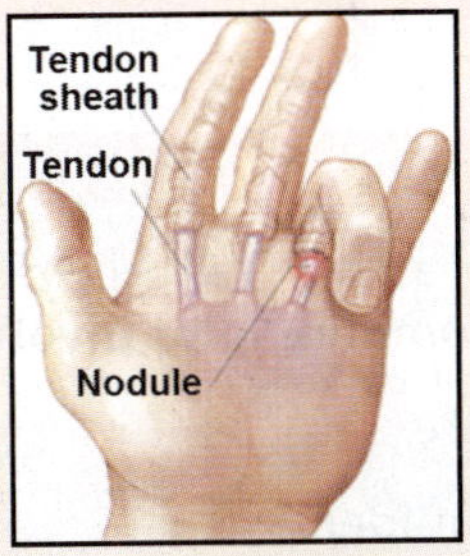
Mallet finger/ Baseball finger	Avulsion central slip of extensor tendon from distal phalanx Flexion deformity at DIP, Difficulty in extension of DIP	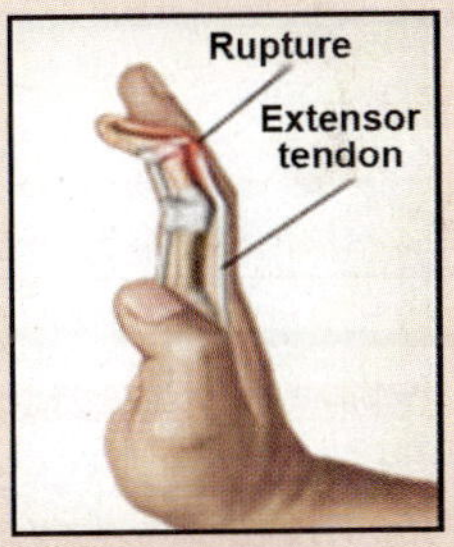
Gamekeeper's thumb/ Skier's thumb	Ulnar collateral ligament injury of thumb at MCP joint Forceful radial deviation of thumb ***Most common–Skier's and ball handling athletes***	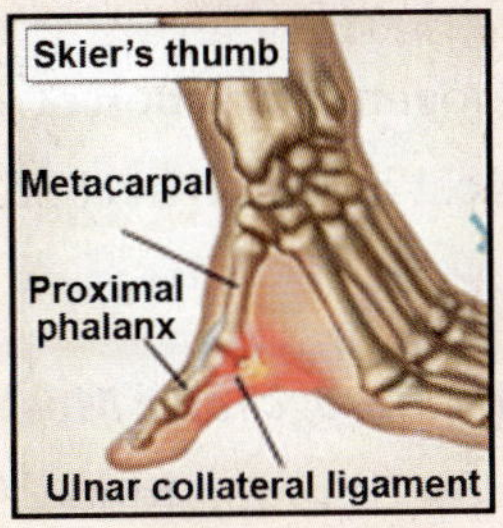
Jersey finger	Avulsion of flexor digitorum profundus tendon of fingers from distal phalanx	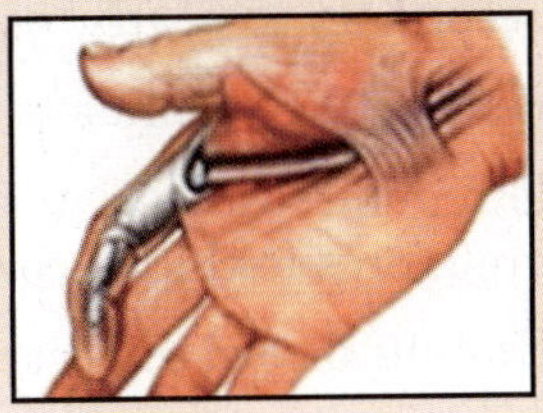

Contd.

Contd.

Bowler's thumb	Perineural fibrosis of ulnar digital nerve of thumb Repetitive compression while grapsing bowling ball Tingling and hyperaesthesia around pulp	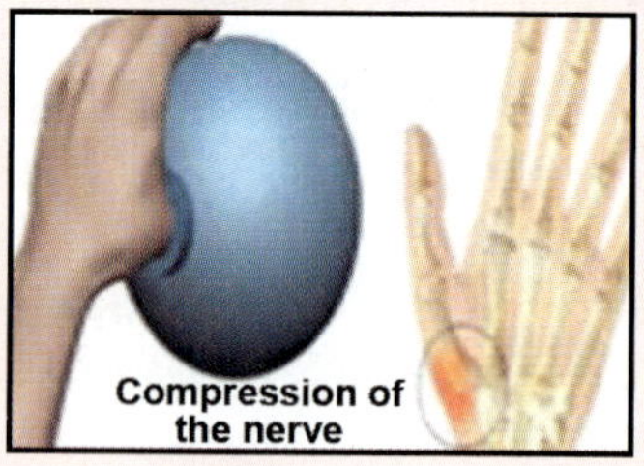
De Quervain's disease	Stenosing tenosynovitis of 1st extensor compartment of wrist Abductor pollicis longus and Extensor pollicis brevis–Involved **Finkelstein's test**–Flexion of thumb followed by ulnar deviation of wrist will produce pain	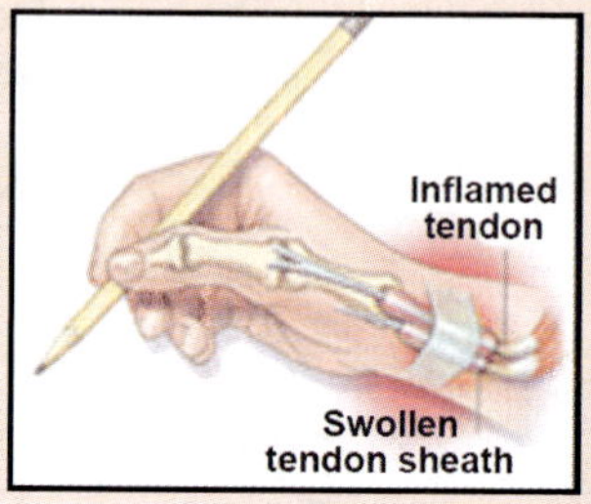

Ref: Apley's 9th Edition Page 798, Maheswari 5th Edition Page 304, Campbell 11th Edition Page 4351, Current Hand Surgery 13th Edition Chapter 44, CDTO 3rd Edition Page 546

Ans: (D) Treatment is antibiotics and splintage

7. **Most common joint involved in septic arthritis:**

A. Knee B. Hip
C. Shoulder D. Elbow

Key:

Most common joint involved in septic arthritis is Knee

Septic Arthritis/Pyogenic Arthritis/Suppurative Arthritis/Infective Arthritis

- Pyogenic infection of joint
- Most common in children <3 years old

Etiology

- ***Haematogenous: Most common route***
- Most common route of spread–Hematogenous
- Secondary to nearby osteomyelitis
- Penetrating wounds
- Iatrogenic–May occur following intraarticular steroid injections in different arthritis and during femoral artery punctures for blood collection
- Umbilical cord sepsis in infants can travel to joints

Contd.

Contd.

Pathogenesis

INFECTION
↓
Release of proteolytic enzymes
↓
Rapid destruction of joint
↓
SURGICAL EMERGENCY

Clinical Features

- Most commonly affected joints–Knee > Hip > Ankle > Elbow
- ***Most common joint involved in adults–Knee***
- ***Most common joint involved in children–Hip***
- Staphylococcus–Most common organism causing Septic arthritis in children
- Neisseria gonorrhea–Most common organism causing septic arthritis in adults and adolescents
- Most common organism causing Nongonococcal septic arthritis of adults of all ages–Staphylococcus
- Joint effusion–Warmth and Restricted joint movements in all directions–Pseudoparalysis

Joint	Position of ease
• Shoulder	Adduction, internal rotation
• Elbow	Flexion, mid pronation
• Wrist	Flexion
• Hip	Flexion, abduction, external rotation
• Knee	Flexion
• Ankle	Plantar-flexion

Diagnosis

- Mainly clinical
- **Synovial fluid aspirate–**Opaque and Non-viscous, WBC > 1,00,000 cells (Polymorphonuclear leukocytes >90%).

Treatment

- Open arthrotomy/Arthroscopic drainage of pus and Joint lavage

Complication

- Deformity and Stiffness
- Pathological dislocation
- Osteoarthritis
- Bony ankylosis

Ref: Apley's 9th Edition Page 44, Maheswari 5th Edition Page 178, Tichdjian's 4th Edition Page 2110, Mercer 10th Edition Page 225, Miller 6th Edition Page 101

Ans: (A) Knee

8. **Which of the following is not true about Osteogenesis Imperfecta?**

A. Blue sclera
B. Generalized Osteopenia
C. Fractures are very rare
D. Associated with Otosclerosis

Key:

Osteogenesis imperfecta is associated with generalized osteoporosis with weak bone which has liability to fracture
Most Important feature of Osteogenesis Imperfecta–Liability to fracture

Osteogenesis Imperfecta
(Brittle Bone Disease/Fragilitas Ossium/Lobstein Vrolik's Disease)

- Abnormal synthesis or deficiency of Type 1 Collagen
- Abnormalities of bone, skin, sclera and dentin

Clinical Features

Bone and Joint Features:

- Liability to fracture (Weak bone)–Most important feature
- *Multiple bilateral symmetrical fractures in newborn*
- Fractures may occur during intrauterine life and during parturition
- Tendency to fracture often reduces with age
- Fractures heal at normal rate
- Frequency of fractures decline sharply after adolescence or puberty
- New bone is pliable for long time due to defective osteoid formation→*Malunion and severe deformities*
- *Excessive laxity of joint ligaments produce Hypermobility*
- Patients with severe type don't survive beyond few years, but those with milder disease live their full life interrupted by frequent fractures.

Ocular Features

- **Blue sclera**–Uveal pigment shown through thin collagen layer
- **Saturn ring**–White sclera immediately surrounding cornea
- **Arcus juvenilis/Embryotoxon**–Opacity in periphery of cornea
- Hyperopia and retinal detachment may occur

Auditory Symptoms

- Deafness–Adolescence onset/Adult onset
- Conductive hearing loss–Otosclerosis

Dentigerous Imperfect/Crumbled Teeth

- Enamel is essentially normal
- Ectodermal origin
- Both deciduous and permanent teeth break easily
- Prone to caries, Yellowish brown/Bluish gray discoloration of teeth

Contd.

Contd.

Classification of Osteogenesis Imperfecta			
Type	**Inheritance**	**Sclera**	**Features**
Type 1	AD	Blue	***Most common type*** *Mildest type, Presents at preschool age, Hearing loss in 50%*
Type 2	AR	Blue	Lethal in perinatal period
Type 3	AR	Normal	Fractures at birth, Progressively short stature ***Most severe survivable form***
Type 4	AR	Normal	Moderate severity. Similar to Type 4
Type 5	***Hypertrophic callus after fracture. Ossification of interosseous membrane between radius–ulna and tibia–fibula***		
Type 6	***Moderate severity. Similar to Type 4***		
Type 7	***Associated with rhizomelia and coxa vara***		

Diagnostic Triad

- Generalized Osteoporosis (Osteopenia)
- Blue discolouration of sclera
- Dentinogenesis Imperfecta (Crumbling teeth)

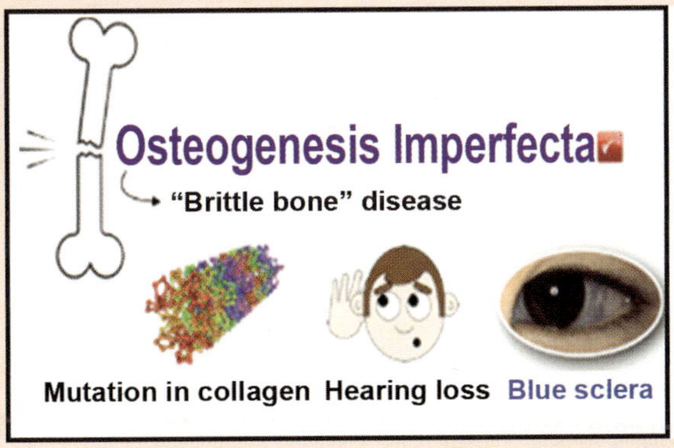

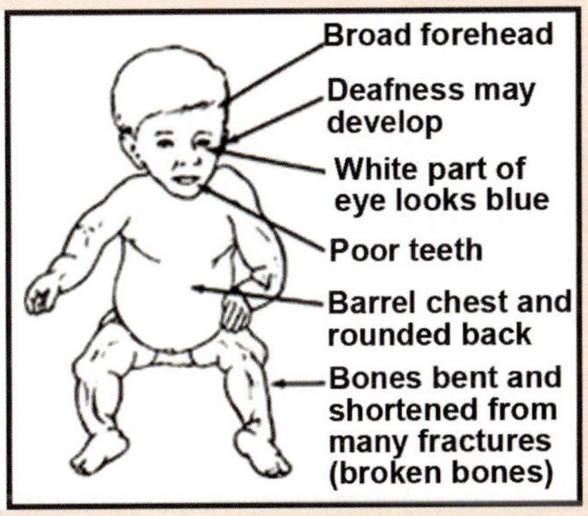

Diagnosis

- **Diagnosed by abnormal pro Alpha chain on Chorionic villous biopsy.**
- *Most striking abnormality is propensity to fracture following minor trauma*

X-Rays

- Generalized Osteopenia, Thinning of long bones
- ***Fractures in various stages of healing***
- Vertebral compression and spinal deformity
- **Wormian bones**–Areas of vicarious ossification in skull
- **Popcorn calcification and whorls of radiodensities**

Treatment

- Bisphosphonates, Multiple osteotomies, Telescopic nail fixation

Ref: Apley's 9th Edition Page 172, Maheswari 5th Edition Page 316, Tichdjian's 3rd Edition Page 1717, Mercer 9th Edition Page 242, Turek 6th Edition Page 325

Ans: (C) Fractures are very rare

9. **Incorrect about Giant cell tumor shown below is:**

A. Treatment of choice is Chemotherapy
B. Eccentric lesion
C. Occurs at Epiphysiometaphyseal junction
D. Clear demarcation of tumor

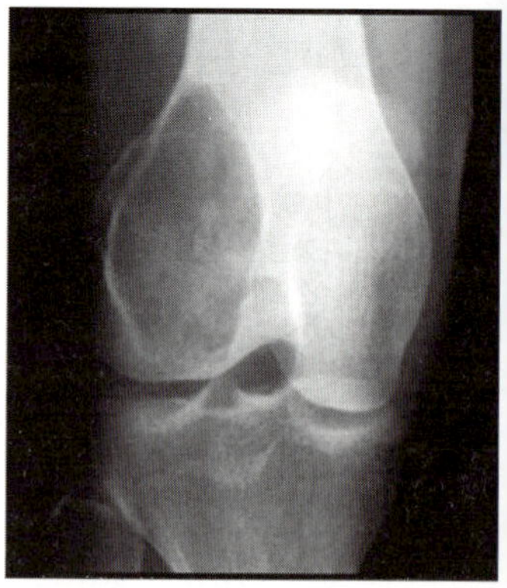

Key:

Treatment of choice for Giant cell tumor–Surgery (Not chemotherapy)

Giant Cell Tumor/Osteoclastoma

- Benign but locally aggressive, purely osteolytic lesion

Clinical Features

- Most common at site–*Distal femur > Proximal tibia > Distal radius*
- Most common age group–30 to 45 years
- More common in females
- Tumors are more aggressive at distal radius
- Presents with pain and slight swelling at end of long bones along with pathological fracture
- Occurs in epiphysis and extends into metaphysis

Histopathology

- Giant cells scattered on background of mononuclear stromal cells
- Mononuclear stromal cells express RANKL
- Overexpression of Osteoprotegerin ligand (OPGL)–suggests overactivity of osteoclasts
- Histological grading is unreliable predictor of tumor behaviour

Investigations

- X-ray–Radiolucent **Eccentrically** located lytic lesion **(Radiolucent)**
- Thinned cortex may expand ***(Ballooned/Soap bubble appearance)*** upto subchondral plate
- Tumor may break through cortex to extend upto soft tissues
- MRI and CT can determine extent
- Biopsy confirms diagnosis of tumor

Treatment

- ***Extended curettage is preferred*** (Curettage with adding adjuvants)
- Simple curettage–Associated with high rate of recurrence
- **Aggressive giant cell tumor of distal radius–**Primary resection and reconstruction with proximal fibular autograft is preferred.

Contd.

Contd.

TREATMENT OF GCT

- Curettage, Chemical cautery by PMMA and Bone grafting (Small unresectable lesions)
- Excision/ Complete resection (Lower end of ulna/Upper end of fibula)
- Excision and replacement by vascularized bone graft (Lower end of radius)
- Excision and arthrodesis or prosthetic replacement (Lower end of femur and upper end of tibia)
- Amputation (Malignant recurrent GCT extremity)
- Radiotherapy (Spine) Causes malignant transformation

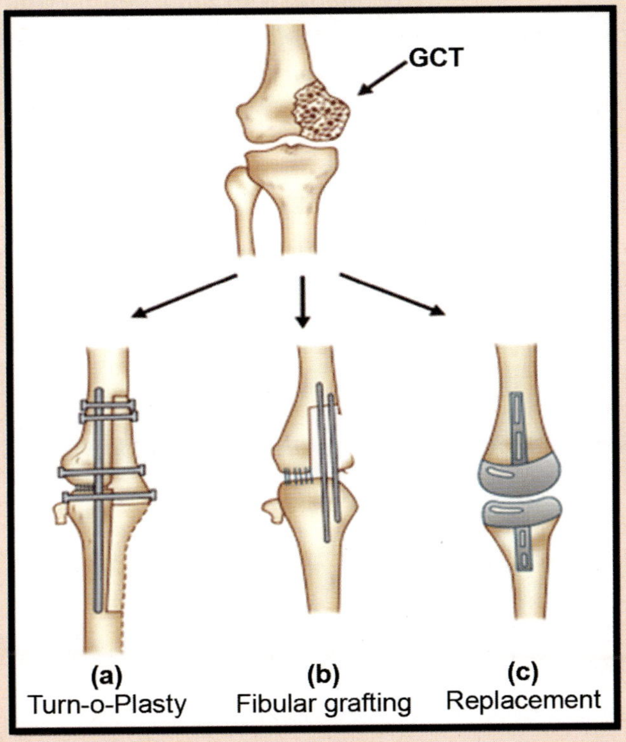

Arthrodesis by the Turn-o-Plasty Procedure

- In this technique, required length of the tibia is split into two halves.
- One half is turned upside down and fixed with the stump of the femur left after excising the tumour.
- A similar procedure can be used for a tibial lesion by taking half of the femur.

Site	Treatment of choice
Lower end of femur	Excision with Turn-o-Plasty
Upper end of tibia	Excision with Turn-o-Plasty
Lower end of radius	Excision with fibular grafting
Lower end of ulna	Excision
Upper end of fibula	Excision

Contd.

Contd.

Sites of Different Bone Tumors

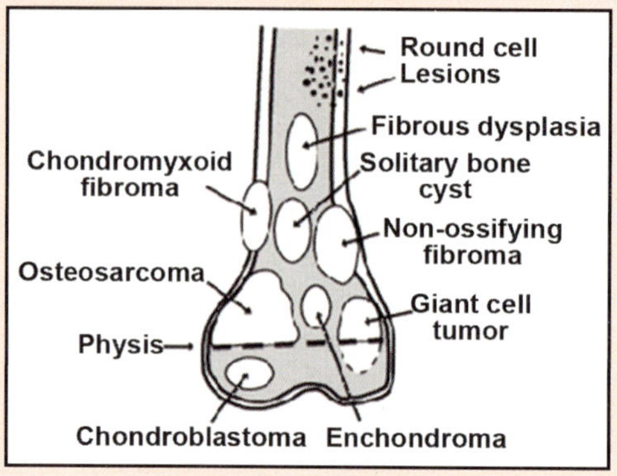

Ref: Maheswari 5th Edition Page 327, Apley's 9th Edition Page 202, Tichdjian's 4th Edition Page 2252, Mercer 10th Edition Page 889, Turek 6th Edition Page 305, Fechner-Tumors of Bones and Joints 3rd Edition Page 180, Campbell 11th Edition Page 887

Ans: (A) Treatment of choice is Chemotherapy

10. Which of the following attitude will be seen in patient with posterior dislocation of hip?

A. Flexion, Abduction, Internal rotation
B. Flexion, Adduction, Internal rotation
C. Flexion, Abduction, External rotation
D. Flexion, Adduction, External rotation

Key:

Attitude of patient with posterior dislocation of hip is Flexion, Adduction, Internal rotation

Posterior Dislocation of Hip

- Posterior dislocation of hip–Most common type (80%).
- Head of the femur is pushed out of acetabulum posteriorly.
- Etiology: Motor vehicle accidents.

Clinical Features

- Patient presents with history of severe trauma followed by pain, swelling and deformity (flexion, adduction and internal rotation) associated with shortening of the leg.

Able to feel head of the femur in the gluteal region

- **Dashboard injury**–Occupant of car is thrown forwards and his knee strikes against dashboard. Force is transmitted up femoral shaft, resulting in posterior dislocation of hip.

Radiological Features

- Femoral head is out of acetabulum.
- Thigh is internally rotated so that lesser trochanter is not seen.
- Shenton's line is broken.

Contd.

Contd.

Complications

- ***Most common–Osteoarthritis.***
- Avascular necrosis of femoral head.
- Sciatic nerve injury (10-20%)–Usually peroneal portion of nerve is affected.

Feature	Anterior	Posterior	Central
Incidence	10-15%	70%	Rare
Mechanism of injury	Deceleration dashboard/ Motor cycle injury with thigh abducted and externally rotated	Dashboard injury	Direct blow over trochancter due to fall in epilepsy
Deformity	Hip in flexion, abduction and external rotation	Hip in flexion, adduction and internal rotation	No shortening and limbs is in neutral position
Femoral head felt in	Groin	Gluteal region	Per rectal (PR)
Nerve injury	Femoral nerve	Sciatic nerve	–
Vascular sign of Narath	-ve	+ve	-ve
Hip movement	Decreased	Increased	Decreased

Common Dislocations in Body	
Spine	Anterior (C5-C6)
Hip	Posterior
Shoulder	Anterior
Elbow	Posterior
Wrist	Lunate

Only dislocation which results in lengthening of limbs-Anterior dislocation of hip

Injury	Deformity
Shoulder dislocation (Anterior)	Flattening of shoulder
Supracondylar fracture humerus	Cubitus Varus (Gunstock deformity)
Lateral condyle humerus fracture	Cubitus Valgus

Contd.

Contd.

Colles fracture	Dinner fork deformity (Velpeau)
Anterior dislocation of hip	Flexion, Abduction and External rotation (Mnemonic: **FABER***)
Posterior dislocation of hip	Flexion, Adduction and Internal rotation (Mnemonic: **FADIR***) ***Dashboard injury***
Trochanteric fracture	Coxa Vara
Condylar fractures of tibia (Bumper fracture)	Genu Valgum
Fracture neck of femur, Trochanteric fracture	External rotation of leg
Avulsion of insertion of extensor tendon	Mallet finger
Ulnar collateral ligament injury	Gamekeeper's thumb
Injury to long thoracic nerve	Winging of scapula
Fracture lateral condyle humerus	Trady ulnar nerve palsy

Ref: Maheswari 5th Edition Page 130, Apley's 8th Edition Page 681, Tichdjian's 3rd Edition Page 2273, Campbell 11th Edition Page 3285, Rockwood 7th Edition Page 1528, Watson Jones 6th Edition Page 902

Ans: (B) Flexion, Adduction, Internal rotation

Chapter 15

PEDIATRICS

1. A 7-year-old child presents with pain abdomen, nausea and rashes on buttock with normal platelet count. What is the most probable diagnosis?

A. Idiopathic Thrombocytopenic Purpura

B. Henoch-Schönlein Purpura

C. Hemolytic Uremic Syndrome

D. Hemorrhagic edema of infancy

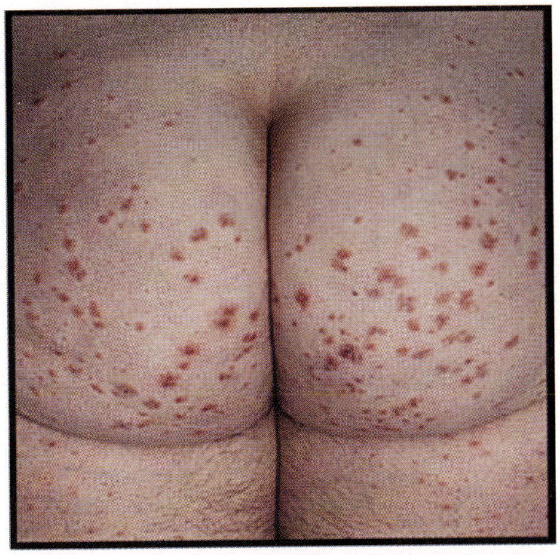

Key:

Typical symmetrical rash with abdominal complaints suggests Henoch-Schönlein Purpura

Normal platelet rules out–ITP and HUS

Age of 7-year rules out Hemorrhagic edema of infancy

HENOCH-SCHÖNLEIN PURPURA

- Most common vasculitis of childhood*
- Characterized by **Leukocytoclastic vasculitis** and **Immunoglobulin (Ig) A deposition** in the **small vessels** in the **skin, joints, gastrointestinal tract and kidney**
- Incidence – 14 to 20/100,000 children per year
- Males : female = 1.2-1.8 : 1
- 90% of HSP cases–ages of **3 and 10 years.**
- Follows **upper respiratory infection;** Common in the **winter and spring,** than in summer months

Pathogenesis

- Infectious triggers or genetically determined immune dysregulation→ Disease mediated by **IgA immune complexes***
- Infectious triggers – **Group A β-hemolytic streptococcus, Staphylococcus aureus, mycoplasma and adenovirus.**
- Skin biopsies – Vasculitis of the **dermal capillaries** and **postcapillary venules.**
- Renal histopathology – Endocapillary proliferative glomerulonephritis, with immunofluorescence (IgA deposition in walls of small vessels and deposition of C3, fibrin and IgM).
- Clusters in families – **HLA-B34 and HLA-DRB1*01** alleles linked to **HSP nephritis.**
- Increased risk–Familial Mediterranean fever, hereditary periodic fever syndromes, and complement deficiencies.

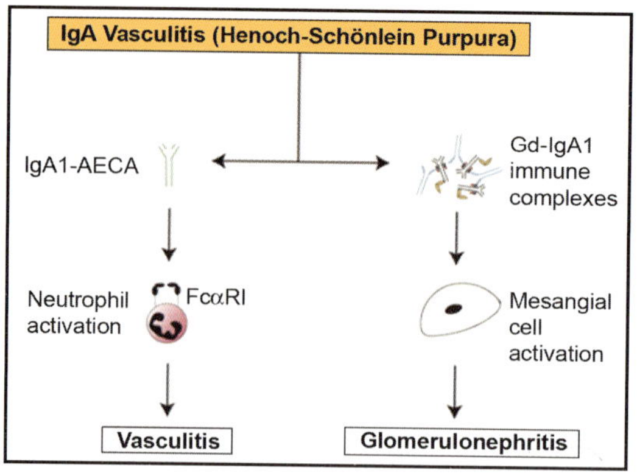

Clinical Features

- Hallmark of HSP is its **"Rash".**
- **Palpable purpura*** starting as pink macules or wheals and developing into **petechiae** or **raised purpura,** or **larger ecchymoses** (rarely bullae and ulcerations develop).
- **Symmetric** and occur in **gravity-dependent areas (lower extremities)** or on **pressure points.**
- Evolve in **groups** (3-10 days) after initial presentation.
- **Subcutaneous edema –** dorsa of hands and feet, periorbital area, lips, scrotum, or scalp.

Musculoskeletal (75%)
• **Arthritis** (self-limited and oligoarticular, with a predilection for the **lower extremities,** and does not lead to deformities and arthralgias), resolves within 2 weeks but recur.
Gastrointestinal Manifestations (80%)
• **Abdominal pain,** vomiting, diarrhea, paralytic ileus and melena; intussusception, mesenteric ischemia, intestinal perforation are uncommon. • Endoscopic evaluation–to identify purpura of the intestinal tract.
Renal Involvement (50%)
• Microscopic hematuria, proteinuria, hypertension, frank **nephritis,** nephrotic syndrome, and acute or chronic renal failure. • Rarely progression to end-stage renal disease (1-2%).
Neurologic Manifestations
• Caused by hypertension or central nervous system (CNS) vasculitis. • Intracerebral hemorrhage, seizures, headaches and behavior changes.
Miscellaneous
• Orchitis, carditis, Ureteritis, inflammatory eye disease, testicular torsion and pulmonary hemorrhage.

Laboratory Diagnosis

- Common nonspecific findings–Leukocytosis, mild anemia, and elevations of ESR and CRP.
- Platelet count is **normal or increased* (Thrombocytosis** and not thrombocytopenia).
- Occult blood in stool.
- **Serum albumin levels–Low*** due to renal or intestinal protein loss.
- **Serum IgA** values–elevated.
- Renal involvement–blood pressure, urinalysis, and serum creatinine.
- Ultrasound–bowel wall edema, associated **intussusception*.**

- **Barium enema–**diagnose and treat intussusception.
- Biopsies of skin and kidney–Characteristically show **IgA deposition** in affected tissues.

Treatment

- Mild and self-limited HSP – **Supportive** (adequate hydration, nutrition and analgesia).
- Significant gastrointestinal involvement or other life-threatening manifestations–Steroids*
  - Prednisone (1 mg/kg/day for 1-2 weeks, followed by taper).
  - Reduces abdominal and joint pain but does not alter overall prognosis nor prevent renal disease.
  - Rapid tapering of corticosteroids may lead to a flare of HSP symptoms.
- **Intravenous immune globulin*** and **plasma exchange*** – Severe disease.
- Chronic HSP renal disease – **Azathioprine, Cyclophosphamide, Cyclosporine** and **Mycophenolate mofetil.**
- End-stage renal disease develops in up to 8% of children with HSP nephritis.

Complications

(Can develop up to 6 months after diagnosis)

- Intestinal perforation
- Chronic Renal disease

Prognosis

- Excellent (Experience an acute, self-limited course lasting on average 4 weeks).
- 15-60% of children - experience 1/more recurrences, typically within 4-6 months of diagnosis
- 8% of those with HSP nephritis go on to have end-stage renal disease

Acute Hemorrhagic Edema (AHE)

- **Cutaneous leukocytoclastic vasculitis** (< 2 years of age, appears well except for the rash)
- Manifests as fever; tender edema–face, scrotum, hands and feet and ecchymosis (larger than purpura of HSP) on face and extremities
- Trunk is spared and petechiae–in mucous membranes
- Platelet count and urinalysis–normal.

Papular-purpuric Gloves-and-socks Syndrome

- Caused by **parvovirus B19***
- **Adolescents** are more often affected than young children
- Manifests with **symmetric edema** and **erythema** over the **hands and feet.**
- Well-demarcated lesions end at the ankle and wrist and evolve into purpuric papules.
- Infectious at the time of appearance of the rash.
- Fever, oral lesions, and leukopenia are inconsistent findings.
- Complications–**mononeuritis multiplex.**

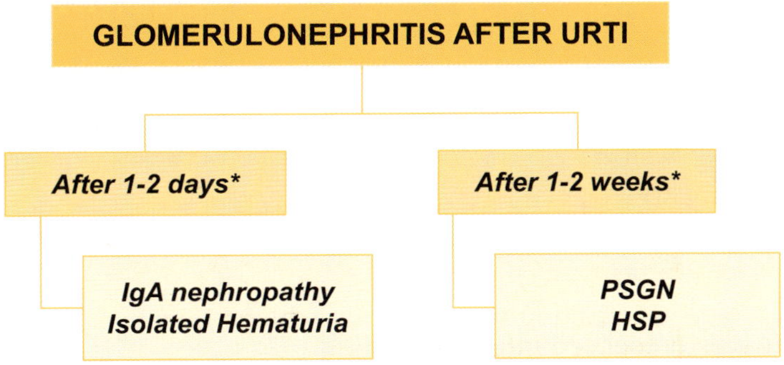

Disease Associated with Antibodies to Neutrophilic Cytoplasmic Antigens		
ANCA type	Antigen	Disease associated
c ANCA	Proteinase 3 (PR3)	*Wegener granulomatosis, Churg-Strauss*
p ANCA	Myeloperoxidase (MPO)	*Microscopic polyarteritis, Ulcerative colitis, Sclerosing cholangitis, Crohn's disease*
ANCA	Bactericidal/permeability-increasing protein (BPI)	*Cystic fibrosis*
p ANCA	Actin	*Autoimmune hepatitis type 1*

Ref: Nelson 20th Edition Page 1217, Ghai 8th Edition Page 480

Ans: (B) Henoch-Schönlein Purpura

2. **Boot shaped heart in Tetralogy of Fallot is due to enlargement of:**

A. Left Ventricular Hypertrophy
B. Right Ventricular Hypertrophy
C. Left atrium enlargement
D. Interventricular septal thickening

Key:

Boot shaped heart (Coeur en sabot): Appearance of upturned cardiac apex seen in conventional frontal chest radiograph due to RVH
Left Ventricular and Left atrial enlargements are NOT seen in Tetralogy of Fallot *In TOF there is ventricular septal defect, not thickening*

TETRALOGY OF FALLOT

COMPONENTS OF TOF

- VSD
- Aortic overriding of ventricular septum
- RVOT/PS
- RVH

Associated Features
• Anomalous origin of left anterior descending coronary artery from right coronary artery • *Right aortic arch–20%** • ASD • CATCH 22 • Associated with PDA • Persistence of left superior vena cava • Congenital absence of pulmonary valve

HEMODYNAMICS

- Hypoxemia and cyanosis depends on amount of pulmonary blood flow that is in turn controlled by degree of right ventricular outflow obstruction.

- Either increase in pulmonary vascular resistance/decrease in systemic vascular resistance will increase right to left shunt and hence the cyanosis.
- ***Severe obstruction*** – Systemic venous blood entering the RV will exit more easily through VSD into LV (right to left shunt), thereby causing systemic desaturation and cyanosis. *Associated with ductus dependent pulmonary circulation.*
- **PINK TOF (Mild obstruction):** Flow across VSD (left-to-right) and Pulmonary valve are normal.
- Mere presence of VSD and PS is not TOF. VSD in TOF should be as large as an aortic valve annulus to equalize pressure between RV and LV.

Pentology of Fallot–*TOF+ASD*
Triology of Fallot–*ASD+RVH+PS*
Tetralogy of Fallot–*ASD+RVH+PS+Aortic overriding*

Clinical Presentation

- **Mild (RVOT) obstruction–**Isolated murmur **(Pink tetralogy)-** Behaves similar to an isolated moderate VSD, since regurgitant VSD murmur masks ejection murmur of PS.
- **Severe obstruction (PS) presents with cyanosis–**Prominent left lower parasternal heave, S2 – loud and single (due to anterior position of aorta and soft closure of pulmonary valve respectively).
- ***Harsh ejection systolic murmur*** best heard in the left mid-parasternal area (due to sub-RV outflow tract obstruction and not due to VSD which is large and unrestrictive in TOF).
- *Intensity of the murmur is inversely proportional to the degree of obstruction, disappears during hyper cyanotic spell* (since most blood in the RV shunts through the VSD instead of going through the RV outflow tract).
- *Pan digital clubbing.*

Investigations

- **ECG:** Right ventricular hypertrophy and right axis deviation.
- **Chest X-ray** shows boot shaped heart (upturned cardiac apex due to RVH and concave pulmonary arterial segment); the toe of the boot forms an acute angle with the diaphragm (RVH).

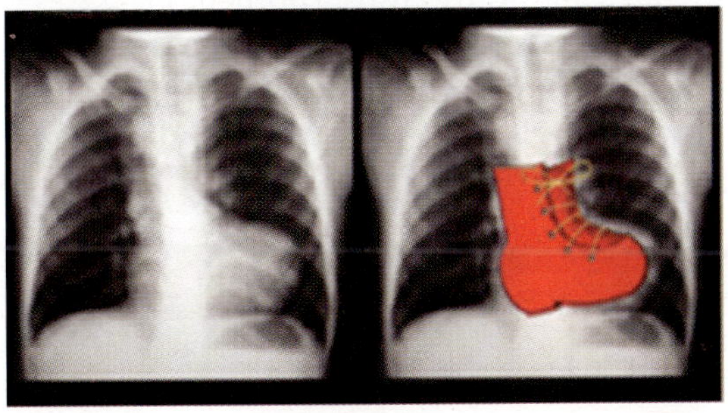

- Narrow upper part of the boot formed by the small or absent main pulmonary artery partly caused by a narrow infundibulum and hypoplastic main pulmonary artery.
- Lung fields may be oligemic/normal (due to PS or right to left shunt) or with right sided aortic arch.
- **ECHO** confirms the diagnosis, Coronary angiogram delineates the origin of the left anterior descending coronary.

Treatment	Effect	Mechanism of action
Knee chest position	Kinks vein of lower limb at hip. Kinks arteries of the lower limb at hip. Calms baby	Decreases systemic venous return to right heart and thus decrease amount of right to left shunt. Reduces arterial blood flow to legs and hence venous return from them. Increases systemic vascular resistance and hence right to left shunt. Decreases the anxiety/adrenergic surge

Contd.

Contd.

Administration of oxygen	Increases arterial oxygen saturation	Decreases hyperpnea
Morphine sulphate	Suppresses respiratory center	Decreases hyperpnea **(0.2 mg/kg) S.C.**
Ketamine	–	Increase systemic vascular resistance and sedates child
Propranolol use in acute situation	–	Slows heart rate and relieves infundibular spasm. Decreases vasodilating effect of beta adrenergic stimulants. In chronic use, propranolol Stabilizes vascular reactivity and thus paroxysmal fall in systemic vascular resistance which initiates spell
Vasoconstrictors like phenylephrine	–	Increase the systemic vascular resistance
Soda bicarbonate correction	To correct acidosis	Reduces respiratory centre stimulation by acidosis **1 meq/kg administered IV**

- **Oral propranolol therapy –** 0.5 to 1.5 mg/kg every 6 hourly
- **Iron replacement**

Surgical Correction

- Patch closure of the VSD and RV muscle bundle resection with or without a trans pulmonary valve annulus patch or pulmonary valvotomy at 6–12 months of life.
- **Blalock-Taussig shunt:** Palliative procedure when branch pulmonary arteries are hypoplastic regardless of associated anomalies followed by complete intracardiac repair. *Common complications are pulmonary insufficiency, ventricular arrhythmias and severe QRS duration prolongation on ECG*
- **Pott's shunt:** *Descending aorta to Pulmonary artery*
- **Waterson's shunt:** *Ascending aorta to Right pulmonary artery*
- **Brock's procedure:** Transventricular valvotomy/Infundibulectomy
- **Rastelli operation**

Complications

- **A**–Anemia, Arthritis
- **B**–Bleeding disorder
- **C**–Cyanotic spells
  CNS Complications: < 2 years–Cerebral thrombosis, > 2 years–Brain Abscess
- **D**–DIC
- **E**–Endocarditis
- **F**–Failure to thrive
- **G**–Gout
- **H**–Hemoptysis
- **I**–Infection, Iron deficiency anemia

Polycythemia *as result of increased erythropoietin stimulation due to low arterial oxygen saturation. Though they have polycythemia, smear shows microcytic RBCs due to relative iron deficiency*

Ref: Arun Babu Pediatrics for Medical Graduates 1st Edition Page 208, Nelson 20th Edition Page 2212, Ghai 8th Edition Page 422

Ans: (B) Right Ventricular Hypertrophy

3. **Diagnostic criteria for 'Severe Acute Malnutrition' as per WHO:**

A. Weight for Height < -3 SD

B. Weight for age < -3 SD

C. Height for age < -3 SD

D. Weight for Height < -2 SD

Key:

Diagnosis of Severe Acute Malnutrition (SAM)
(Children between 6 months and 59 months of age) with

- Weight/height or Weight/length < -3 Z score, using the WHO Growth Charts; **OR**
- Presence of visible severe wasting; **OR**
- Presence of bipedal edema of nutritional origin; **OR**
- Mid upper arm circumference (MUAC) < 115 mm.
- For infants below 6 months, Criteria 1 or 2 or 3 above should be used till data on MUAC below 6 months becomes available.

Parameter	Moderate malnutrition	Severe malnutrition
Weight for Height	Between 70-79% of expected or SD score between -2 and -3 **(WASTING)**	<70% of expected or SD score < -3 **(SEVERE WASTING)**
Height for Age	Between 85-89% of expected or SD score between -2 to -3 **(STUNTING)**	< 85% of expected or SD score <-3 **(SEVERE STUNTING)**

Management of Protein Energy Malnutrition	
Condition	**Treatment**
Hypoglycemia (<54 mg/dL)	**Asymptomatic:** 50 ml of 10% dextrose PO/NG **Symptomatic:** 5 ml/kg of 10% dextrose IV
Hypothermia (<35.5 C) **Severe hypothermia (<32 C)**	Warm clothes, KMC, warmer care, frequent feeds, antibiotics Oxygen, IV fluids (prewarmed), warmer care, antibiotics, temperature monitoring
Dehydration	**Some dehydration:** ORS 5 ml/kg every 30 min for 2 hours, then 5-10 ml/kg/hr for 5-10 hours **Severe dehydration/shock:** RL with 5% D or ½ DNS @ 15 ml/kg over 1 hour, repeat after 1 hour consider septic shock if no improvement. ORS once stable
Electrolyte Imbalance	Potassium and magnesium supplements for 2 weeks
Infection	Ampicilin/gentamicin Cloxacillin for suspected staphylococcal infection Cefotaxime (meningitis) Third generation cephalosporins (septic shock) Ciprofloxacin (dysentery)

Contd.

Contd.

Micronutrient Deficiency	Vitamin A, D supplements, Vitamin B (twice RDA) Folic acid (5 mg on D1 then 1mg/day), zinc (2 mg/kg/day) and copper (0.3 mg/kg/day) Iron in rehabilitation phase
Start Cautious Feeding	F75 diet (75 kcal+ 0.9 g protein/100 ml) ***(Rich in carbohydrate, Low in protein/ fat)***
Catch Up Growth	F100 diet (100 kcal+2.9 g protein/100 ml) (rich in protein/fat)
Sensory Stimulation	Emotional support
Discharge and Follow Up	Sensitize caretaker, immunization complete, feeding and follow-up advised

EXTRA EDGE

- **Gomez classification:** Weight for Age
- **IAP Classification:** Weight for Age
- **Waterlow classification:** Height for Age and Weight for Height
- **Monkey facies and Baggy paints appearance:** Marasmus
- *Triad of Kwashiorkor*–Edema, Growth retardation and Psychomotor changes
- **Best indicator for acute malnutrition:** Decrease in weight for height
- **Best indicator for chronic malnutrition:** Decrease in height for age

Ref: Arun Babu Pediatrics for Medical Graduates 1st Edition Page 46, Ghai Essential of Pediatrics 8th Edition Page 98, Nelson 20th Edition Page 296

Ans: (A) Weight for Height < -3 SD

4. **Triad of congenital rubella syndrome:**
   A. Chorioretinitis, hydrocephalus, intra cerebral calcification
   B. Chorioretinitis, hydrocephalus, Heart disease
   C. Cataract, Sensory Neural Hearing Loss, Heart defects
   D. Chorioretinitis, Heart disease, intra cerebral calcification

Key:

*Congenital Toxoplasmosis Triad→Chorioretinitis, Hydrocephalus and Cerebral calcifications**

- No structural heart disease was mentioned as CVS feature of congenital toxoplasmosis except for myocarditis.

Triads	
Congenital toxoplasmosis	**Congenital rubella syndrome**
• Chorioretinitis • Hydrocephalus • Cerebral calcifications	• Cataract • Sensorineural hearing loss • Heart defects

TOXOPLASMOSIS

- Caused by Toxoplasma gondii
- Obligate intracellular protozoan
- **Mode of infection:** Acquired perorally, Transplacentally, Vaginal delivery or parenterally
- **Congenital:** Risk of fetal transmission increases with each trimester (15%, 25% and 60% in 1st, 2nd and 3rd Trimester)
- **Severity of infection is greatest in Early pregnancy**
- **Clinical Manifestations**
    - **Acquired:** Generally asymptomatic in immunocompetent children
    - **Congenital:** Clinical features range from Hydrops fetalis to SGA, Prematurity, Peripheral retinal scars, Persistent jaundice, Mild thrombocytopenia
    - **Systemic signs:** Lymphadenectomy, Hepatosplenomegaly, Pneumonitis, Nephrotic syndrome, Myocarditis
    - **Skin:** Rashes, Petichae, Ecchymosis (Secondary to thrombocytopenia)
    - **CNS:** Hydrocephalus, Spinal/Bulbar involvement, Microcephaly, Hearing loss
    - **Endocrine:** Hypothalamic/Pituitary involvement
    - **Eyes:** Chorioretinitis, Retinal detachment, Glaucoma
- **Diagnosis:** Blood/Body fluid culture, Lymph node histology, Cysts in placenta/fetal/newborn tissues, CSF/Amniotic fluid PCR, Serological tests
- **Treatment:** Pyrimethamine+Sulphadiazine and Leukovirin
- **Refer Q. No. 5 for further explanation**

Ref: Nelson 20th Edition Page 1550, Ghai 8th Edition Page 230, CPDT 22nd Edition Page 1345

Ans: (C) Cataract, Sensory Neural Hearing Loss, Heart defects

5. **In congenital rubella syndrome, classic cardiac lesion is seen:**

A. Pulmonary artery stenosis B. VSD

C. ASD D. Aortic stenosis

Key:

Cardiac disease seen in CRS in decreasing order of frequency: Patent Ductus Arteriosus (PDA), Right PS, Left PS, Valvular pulmonic stenosis, VSD and ASD
Next to Patent Ductus Arteriosus, Pulmonary Artery Stenosis was commonly associated cardiac defect in Congenital rubella syndrome

Rubella

- ss RNA virus (the toga virus family).
- **Incubation period:** 14-21 days
- **Period of communicability:** 5 days before to 6 days after appearance of rash
- **Forchheimer spots:** Tiny rose colored lesions on soft palate

CONGENITAL RUBELLA SYNDROME

- Frequency of congenital infection and risk of congenital defects after maternal rubella with a rash is related to gestational age at the time of infection.

Triads	
Congenital toxoplasmosis	**Congenital rubella syndrome**
• Chorioretinitis • Hydrocephalus • Cerebral calcifications	• Cataract • Sensorineural hearing loss • Heart defects

Maternal infection (Gestation)	Rate of fetal infection	Occurrence of fetal anomalies
First 12 weeks of gestation	81%	100% of infected fetuses had cardiac defects and deafness
13 to 16 weeks	54%	Deafness was found in one-third of fetuses
31 to 36 weeks	60%	No abnormalities were found when fetal infection occurred beyond 20th week of gestation
Beyond 36 weeks	100%	

Clinical Features

- Cataracts (can be both unilateral or bilateral), Sensorineural hearing loss ***(Single most common finding in CRS infants)*** and Congenital heart disease (PDA and PS), forms classical triad of CRS.
- **Common early features**–IUGR, ***Retinopathy (Salt and Pepper)***, Microphthalmia, Hypotonia, Meningoencephalitis, Electroencephalographic abnormalities, Dermatoglyphic abnor-malities, hepatosplenomegaly, thrombocytopenic purpura, ***Radiographic bone lucencies*** and DM.
- **Rare complications**–Myocarditis, glaucoma, microcephaly, chronic progressive panence-phalitis, hepatitis, anemia, hypogammaglobulinemia, thymic hypoplasia, thyroid abnor-malities, cryptorchidism and polycystic kidney disease.
- **Blueberry muffin syndrome**–Infant born with multiple blue/purple marks or skin nodules→ Associated with Rubella, Toxoplasmosis, CMV and HSV.

- **Most cases of postnatally acquired rubella are asymptomatic**
- ***Posterior cervical and Occipital lymph nodes with low grade fever appears 14 days after initial infection and often prior to onset of rash.***

Antenatal Diagnosis

- Determination of specific IgM in fetal blood obtained by PUBS.
- Direct detection of rubella antigen and RNA in a chorionic villus biopsy specimen

Postnatal Diagnosis

Diagnosis of congenital infection is made by one of the following:

- Isolation of rubella virus (oropharynx, urine).
- Detection of rubella-specific IgM in cord or neonatal blood.
- Persistent rubella-specific titers over time (i.e., no decline in titer as expected for transplacentally derived maternal IgG).
- If, in addition, there are congenital defects, diagnosis of CRS is made.

Treatment

- No specific therapy for either maternal or congenital rubella infection.
- ***Maternal disease is almost always mild and self-limiting.***
- Primary maternal infection occurs during the first 5 months of pregnancy–termination options should be discussed with the mother.
- Infection is known to occur beyond 20th week of gestation, its unlikely to develop anomalies.
- Individuals with postnatal infection typically shed virus for 1 week before and 1 week after onset of rash.
- Infants with congenital infection may shed virus for many months, and contact should be avoided during the first year.
- Conception also should be avoided for 3 months following immunization.
- Immunization during pregnancy is not recommended because of theoretical risk to fetus.
- Inadvertent immunizations during pregnancy have occurred–Reassurance of little risk to the fetus can be given.

Maternal Infection

- **Symptoms:** Begin 2 to 3 weeks after exposure and include malaise, low-grade fever, headache, mild coryza, posterior cervical lymphadenopathy, arthralgias and conjunctivitis.
- Occurring 1 to 5 days before the onset of rash (salmon-pink macular or maculopapular exanthem that begins on the face and behind the ears and spreads downward over 1 to 2 days and disappears in 5 to 7 days from onset).
- **Confirmation**–Demonstrating four-fold or higher rise in serum IgG titers when measured at the time of symptoms and approximately 2 weeks later.
- If a woman exposed to rubella is known to be seropositive, she is immune, and the fetus is considered not to be at risk for infection.
- If the exposed woman is known to be seronegative, a serum sample should be obtained 3 to 4 weeks after exposure for determination of titer.
- Negative titer indicates that no infection has occurred, whereas positive titer indicates infection.

- *Most common manifestation of CRS–SNHL*
- *Most common CVS manifestation of CRS–PDA*
- *Most common eye manifestation–Salt and Pepper retinopathy*
- *Most serious eye manifestation–Cataract*
- *Most serious complication of post natal rubella–Encephalitis*

	Toxoplasmosis	CMV	HSV	Rubella
Hydrocephalus	++	+	+	Rare
Microcephaly	++	++	+	+
Intracranial calcification	++	++	+	+/–

Ref: Nelson 20th Edition Page 1550, Manual of Neonatal Care Cloherty 7th Edition Page 619, Ghai 8th Edition Page 218

Ans: (A) Pulmonary artery stenosis

6. **A 10 days old newborn has poor feeding, abdominal distension with blood in stools without diarrhea. X-ray is shown. Which of the following lab findings are compatible with this condition?**

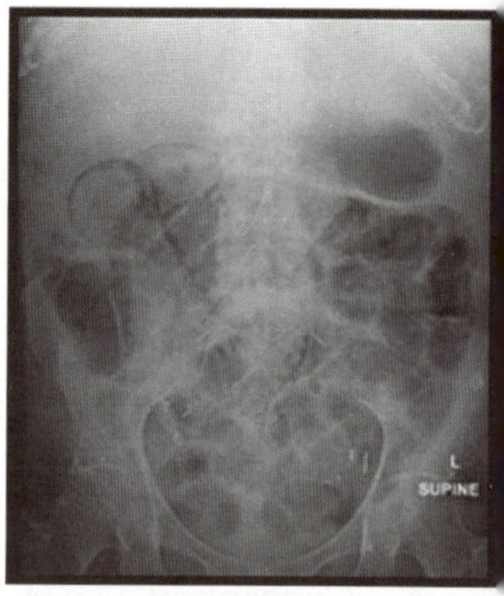

A. Hyponatremia + Metabolic acidosis + Thrombocytopenia
B. Hyponatremia + Metabolic alkalosis + Thrombocytopenia
C. Hyponatremia + Metabolic acidosis + Thrombocytosis
D. Hypokalemia + Metabolic acidosis + Thrombocytopenia

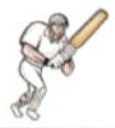

Key:

Neonate presenting in day 10 of life with abdominal distension and blood in stools could be due to milk protein allergy, Hirschsprung's disease with enterocolits, intussusception, Meckel's diverticulum and NEC. ***History of poor feeding, absence of diarrhea and plain X-ray abdomen with features of pneumatosis intestinalis suggests NEC***
(Curvilinear lucencies surrounding several loops of dilated small bowel in right side of abdomen)
Triad of NEC: Thrombocytopenia, Persistent metabolic acidosis, Severe refractory hyponatremia

NECROTISING ENTEROCOLITIS

- ***Most common life threatening emergency of GIT in newborn period***

Risk Factors

- ***Prematurity is single greatest risk*** factor (Decreasing gestational age is associated with an increased risk of NEC)
- 10% of infants with NEC are full term
- **Enteral feeding**–Next greatest risk factor and exposure to bovine milk-based products may increase NEC risk.
- **Use of H_2 blockers**–Higher risk of NEC in extremely low birth weight (ELBW) infants.
- **Mean gestational age**–30 to 32 weeks (weight appropriate for gestational age) and mean age at onset of 12 days.
- **Other risk factors**–Maternal disorders (e.g., toxemia), Infant's course (Asphyxia, PDA), and Type of management (Umbilical artery catheterization), congenital heart disease, polycythemia, sepsis and hypotension.
- Complex interactions between immaturity, mucosal injury (Ischemia, Luminal substrate, and infection) and Poor host work response to injury.
- Hypoxic/Hemodynamic insult, resulting in splanchnic vasoconstriction and reduced mesenteric flow, inducing bowel mucosal hypoxia, and rendering intestine susceptible to injury
- Osmolality of formula, lack of immunoprotective factors in formula and timing, volume and rate of feeding.
- Platelet activating factor (PAF), endotoxin lipopolysaccharide (LPS), tumor necrosis factor a (1NF-α), interleukins and nitric oxide–have a role in pathophysiology of NEC.

Diagnosis

- High index of suspicion and careful clinical observation for signs in infants at risk.
- "Walsh and Kleigman modification of Bell staging criteria" for diagnosis NEC.

Clinical Features

Systemic signs	Abdominal signs
Respiratory distress, apnea and/ or bradycardia, lethargy, temperature instability, irritability, poor feeding, hypotension (shock), acidosis, oliguria, or bleeding diathesis.	Abdominal distension or tenderness, Gastric aspirates (feeding residuals), vomiting (of bile, blood, or both), ileus (decreased/absent bowel sounds), bloody stools, abdominal wall erythema or induration, persistent localized abdominal mass, or ascites.

Laboratory Features

Radiology studies	Blood and serum studies
• Abdominal X-ray (AP and cross-table lateral or left lateral decubitus) • Abnormal gas pattern consistent with ileus. • Bowel wall edema • Fixed position loop on serial studies • ***Appearance of a mass, pneumatosis intestinalis (Radiologic hallmark used to confirm the diagnosis)*** • Portal or Hepatic venous air • Pneumobilia/Pneumoperitoneum taking appearance of gas under diaphragm.	**Triad of NEC** **Thrombocytopenia, Persistent metabolic acidosis, Severe refractory hyponatremia** • Serial measurements of C-reactive protein (CRP)– Assessment of response to therapy of severe NEC. • Blood cultures–Bacteremia with pathogenic organism. • Analysis of stool for blood–grossly bloody stools , occult hematochezia.

Treatment: Initial attention to respiratory, cardiovascular and hematological resuscitation.

Bell staging criteria	Clinical features	Radiological features	Treatment and monitoring	Antibiotics and Surgical treatment
Stage I (Suspect)	+	Non diagnostic	- NPO + IV fluids, Nasogastric drainage - CBC, electrolytes and abdominal radiograph q8h, Blood culture, Stool for occult blood	Ampicillin and Gentamicin for 48 hours
Stage II (Definite)	+	Pneumatosis intestinalis	- NPO + Parenteral nutrition, Nasogastric drainage - CBC, electrolytes and abdominal radiograph q8h, Blood culture, Stool for occult blood	Ampicillin, Gentamicin and Clindamycin for 14 days + Surgical consultation
Stage III (Advanced)	+ **Critically ill**	Pneumatosis intestinalis/ Pneumoperitoneum	***(Same as stage II)***	Same as Stage II+ Resection with enterostomy/primary anastomosis

Stage	I	IIa	IIb	IIIa	IIIb
Radiological feature	Normal/ Mild intestinal dilatation	Pneumatosis intestinalis	Portal vein gas	Peritonitis/ Ascites	Pneumo-peritoneum

- Antenatal steroids have been shown to improve the maturity of the GI tract.
- Breast milk has been shown to have protective factors.

Ref: Manual of Neonatal Care Cloherty 7th Edition Page 619, Nelson 20th Edition Page 870, Ghai 8th Edition Page 165

Ans: (A) Hyponatremia + Metabolic Acidosis + Thrombocytopenia

7. **According to NRP, targeted preductal SpO_2 of newborn at 3 minutes of life:**

A. 70 – 75% B. 75 – 80%
C. 80 – 85% D. 85 – 90%

Key:

Neonatal Resuscitation Programrecommends upper and lower limits of **preductal saturations (SpO_2)** *extrapolated from studies in infants resuscitated in room air. These preductal SpO_2 limits are used to monitor and guide oxygen therapy during neonatal resuscitation*

- SPO_2 monitoring and Optimal Oxygen Delivery (when pulse oximeter is available)
- Clinical assessment of skin color (for oxygenation) is not reliable, and may vary with the skin pigmentation.
- Normal transition to extra uterine life–take several minutes after birth to increase their blood oxygen saturation from approximately 60% (normal in intrauterine state) to more than 90%, which is the normal for a healthy newborn.
- These values may be lower in babies born by cesarean section compared to vaginally born babies.
- If central cyanosis persists–attach a pulse oximetry probe to determine if the baby's oxygenation is in the abnormal range.
- Acceptable preductal (right wrist) target SpO_2 for normal baby during the first 10 minutes transition.

Duration of life (min)	Acceptable preductal target SpO_2
1 Minute	60 – 65 %
2 Minutes	65 – 70 %
3 Minutes	70 – 75 %
4 Minutes	75 – 80 %
5 Minutes	80 – 85 %
10 Minutes	– 90 %

- Provide supplemental oxygen–if the levels are below the saturation targets established for a normal baby during transition and are not increasing.
- Free flow oxygen can be given to a spontaneously breathing baby by using one of the following delivering methods:
  - Oxygen Mask
  - Flow Inflating bag and Mask

- o Oxygen tubing held close to the baby's nose and mouth with cupped hand
- o T piece Resuscitator

- Free flow oxygen cannot be given reliably by a mask attached to the self-inflating bag.
- Avoid flow rates that are > 5 liters per minute (cause convective heat losses).

Ref: Neonatal Resuscitation India 1st Edition Page 23

Ans: (A) 70–75%

8. A baby has APGAR score of 3 at 1 minute of life. Which of the following is true?

A. Mildly depressed
B. Moderately depressed
C. Severely depressed
D. Normal baby

Key:

World Health Organization
Defined birth asphyxia as "failure to initiate and sustain breathing at birth" and based on Apgar score as an Apgar score of < 7 at 1 minute of life.
National Neonatal Perinatal Database (NNPD)
• **Moderate asphyxia**–Slow gasping breathing or an Apgar score of 4-6. • **Severe asphyxia**–No breathing or an Apgar score of 0-3 at one minute of life.

Birth Asphyxia
Clinically birth asphyxia defined as presence of any one of the following
• *Gasping or ineffective breathing or lack of breathing at 1 minute of life* • *Need for positive pressure ventilation for >1 minute* • *Apgar score < 3 at 5 minutes or longer*

Apgar Scoring System

Sign	0	1	2
Appearance (color)	Blue/Pale	Pink body, Blue extremities	All pink
Pulse (heart) rate	Absent	<100 per minute	>100 per minute
Grimace (Reflex irritability)	No response	Grimace	Cough / sneeze
Attitude (tone)	Limp	Some flexion of extremities	Active motion
Respiratory effort	Absent	Slow (irregular)	Good crying

- Apgar score is **NOT** used to guide resuscitation
- Total score: 10
- No depression: 7-10
- Apgar Score 0-3 for 75 min is seen in severe birth asphyxia

- *1 min Apgar score*→Indicates Intrapartum depression
- *5 min Apgar score*→Reflects adequacy of resuscitative effort

- Apgar Score > 7 is normal
- If Apgar score is < 7, Extended Apgar Score should be obtained for every 5 min upto 20 minutes.

Expanded Apgar score is proven to be useful in setting of delayed cord clamping, in which time of birth (complete delivery of the infant), time of cord clamping and time of initiation of resuscitation can all be recorded.

- Apgar 4 to 6→ Baby needs some resuscitation measures
- American Academy of Pediatrics defines perinatal asphyxia as APGAR Score < 3 for > 5 min

Neonatal Resuscitation Algorithm–2015 Update

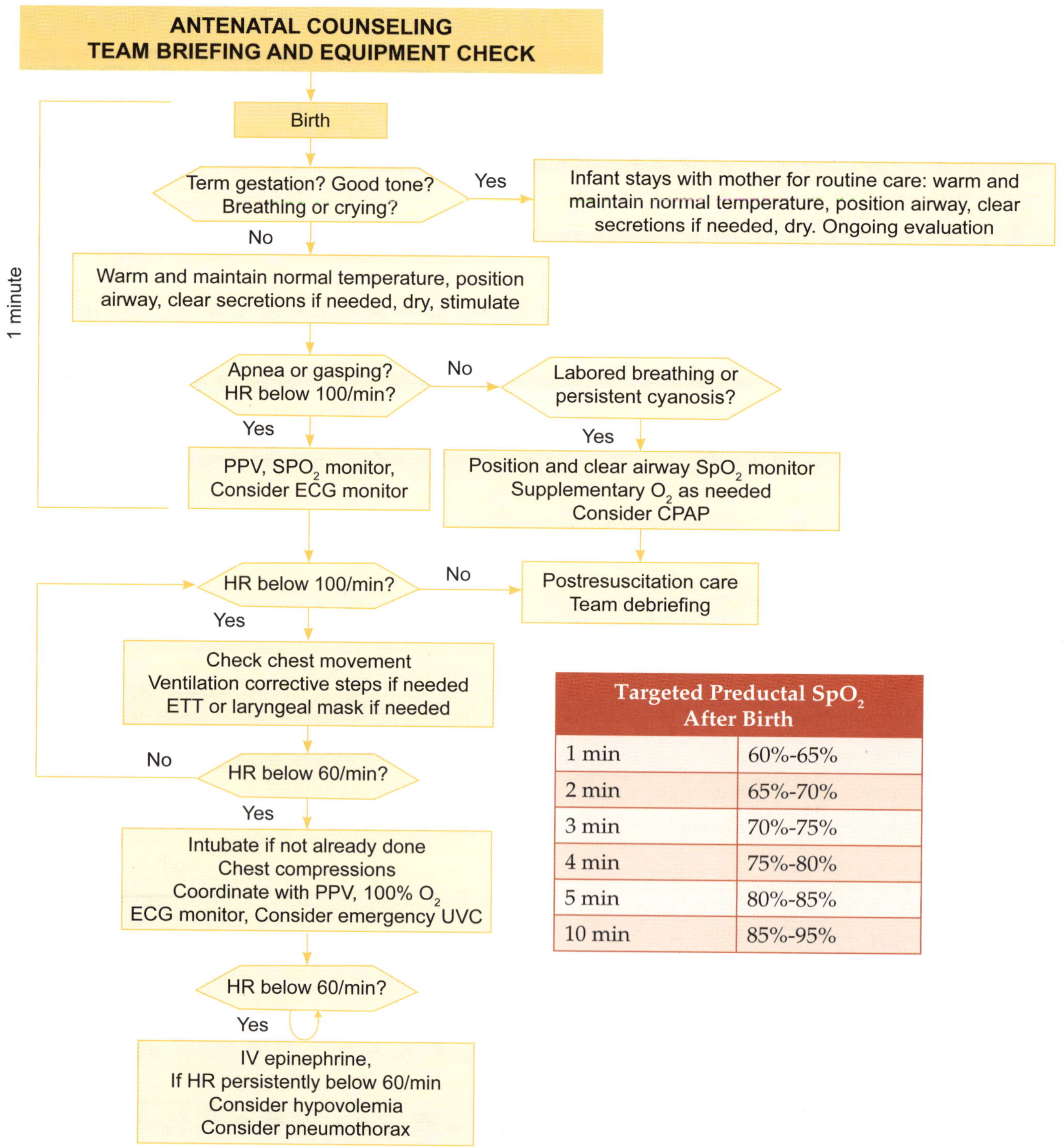

Targeted Preductal SpO_2 After Birth	
1 min	60%-65%
2 min	65%-70%
3 min	70%-75%
4 min	75%-80%
5 min	80%-85%
10 min	85%-95%

Major Recommendations (2015 American Heart Association)
• Delayed cord clamping > 30 seconds • Temperature of non-asphyxiated infants should be asphyxiated infants maintained between 36.5 and 37.5°C • In infants < 32 weeks • Radiant warmer with plastic wrap with cap • Warmed humidified resuscitation gases • Warming unintentionally hypothermic newborn • Either rapid – > 0.5 deg C per hour or • Slow – < 0.5 deg C per hour • Skin to Skin contact (Kangaroo Mother Care) • Routine intubation for tracheal suctioning for non-vigorous baby is not suggested • Use of 3 Lead ECG for measurement of newborn heart rate • In < 35 weeks baby – resuscitate with low oxygen (21% to 30%) and triturate according to preductal saturation • In spontaneously breathing preterm infant – CPAP is preferred than routine intubation • Induce Therapeutic Hypothermia

Ref: Post-Resuscitation Management of An Asphyxiated Neonate: NNF Teaching Aids: Newborn Care, Updated Neonatal Resuscitation Guidelines 2015 – Major Changes, Indian Pediatrics Volume 53 May 2016 Page 403-407, Ghai 9th Edition Page 127

Ans: (C) Severely depressed

9. **In PDA, preductal SpO_2 is measured with probe at:**

A. Right upper limb
B. Left upper limb
C. Right lower limb
D. Left lower limb

Key:

In PDA, preductal SpO_2 is measured with probe at Right Upper limb
Ductus arteriosus connects to the aorta distal to left subclavian artery, hence portion of body supplied (by aorta) proximal to ductus attachment is preductal and distal to ductal attachment is postductal
Since ductus connects distal to right subclavian artery–preductal flow from aorta enters right upper limb through right subclavian artery (branch of brachiocephlic trunk)

STRUCTURE OF DUCTUS ARTERIOSUS

- Ductus arteriosus (Ductus of Biotalli) – derived from 6th aortic arch.
- Connects the pulmonary artery (junction of main pulmonary artery and origin of left pulmonary artery) to proximal descending aorta just after origin of left subclavian artery.
- Passes from anterior aspect of the pulmonary artery to posterior aspect of aorta.
- Ductus has conical shape with large aortic end tapering into small pulmonary connection.

Since ductus connects distal to right subclavian artery–preductal flow from aorta enters right upper limb through right subclavian artery (branch of brachiocephalic trunk).

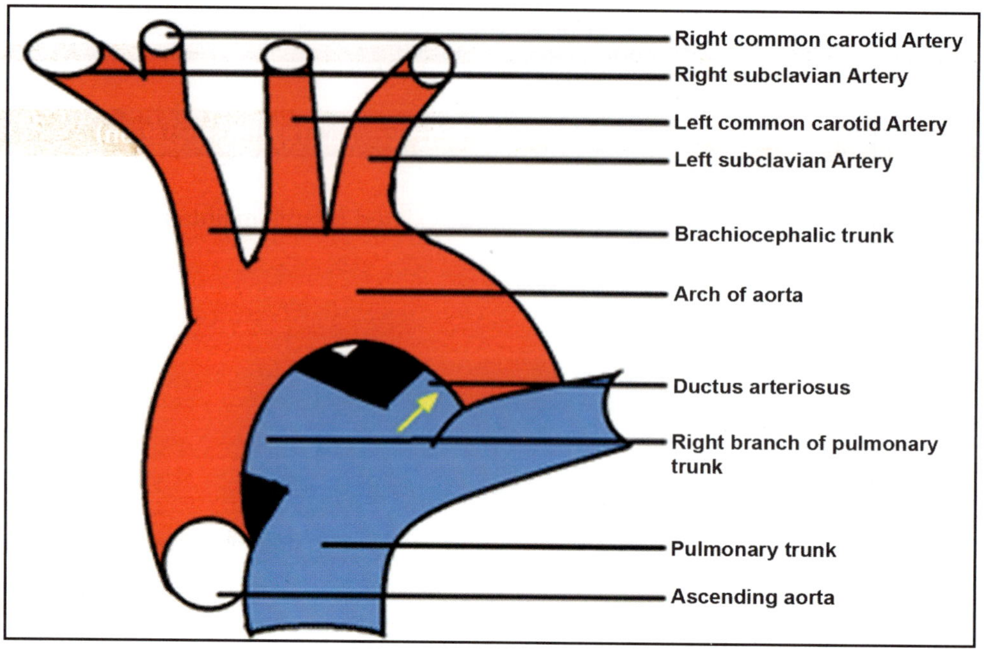

- **Hence the preductal oxygen saturation is measured in the right upper limb.**
- Post ductal flow of the aorta distal to left subcalvian artery contains blood from both aorta and pulmonary trunk, hence the post ductal oxygen saturation is seen in any of the lower limb.

PATENT DUCTUS ARTERIOSUS

- In PDA with reversal of shunt, the deoxygenated blood from right ventricle enters aorta through PDA and produce differential cyanosis.
- ***Prostaglandin E1 maintains ductus patency after birth***
- ***In fetal stage ductal patency is maintained by PgE2***
- ***Clinical findings:*** S1 loud, S2 narrow split, Aortic ejection click, Continuous machinery murmur, S3+
- ***ECG:*** Deep Q waves with tall T waves
- **Diagnosis of PDA is confirmed by ECHO**
- **Preterm**–Can close spontaneously or with medication *(Indomethacin)*
- **Term**–Never closes spontaneously/with medication *(Only surgery effective)*
- Drugs used to closure–Indomethacin and Ibuprofen
- Child with PDA–Ideal time for surgery is as and when diagnosed (Preferably <1 year)
- Recurrent laryngeal nerve–just anterior and caudal to ductus and loops posteriorly around the ductus to ascend behind the aorta–***Most commonly injured anatomic structure in ductal ligation.***
    - **Surgery for PDA**–*Double ligation of smaller ductus, Division and suture for Large PDA*
    - **Coil occlusion**–*Smaller PDA (< 4 mm)*
    - **Device closure using Amplatzer**–*Large PDA and Smaller infants*
- **Treatment to keep duct open–PgE1 infusion**
- Most common side effect of PgE1 infusion–Fever
- Most common complication of PDA–Congestive heart failure

Physiological closure of ductus→ 15-20 hours of birth
Anatomical closure of ductus→ 10-21 days

Ref: Perloff's Clinical Recognition of Congenital Heart Disease 6th Edition Page 368, Nelson 20th Edition Page 2197, Ghai 8th Edition Page 417

Ans : (A) Right upper limb

10. Which of the following is a stimulus for closure of ductus arteriosus after birth?

A. Loss of PGE2 from placenta
B. Decrease in O_2 tension in newborn blood
C. Increase in PGI2
D. Increase in PGF2α

Key:

Loss of PGE2 from placenta is a stimulus for closure of ductus arteriosus after birth

- Increase in oxygen and decrease in prostaglandin closes ductus arteriosus in general.

Closure of Ductus Arteriosus

- Functional closure begins within 10 to 15 hours after birth and completes by 2nd week of life.
- By constriction of medial smooth muscle in ductus.
- Anatomical closure to ligamentum arteriosum takes 3 weeks of life.
- By permanent change in the endothelium and sub intimal layers of ductus.

Physiological closure of ductus→ 15-20 hours of birth
Anatomical closure of ductus→ 10-21 days

FACTORS INFLUENCING CLOSURE OF DUCTUS

Oxygen and Ductus Arteriosus

- Strongest stimulation for closure–Post natal increase in oxygen saturation in the ductus (from 25 to 500 mm of Hg due to lung expansion).
- Responsiveness to oxygen induced closure is better in term than in preterm.

Prostaglandin E2 and Closure

- Decrease in PgE2 after birth result in ductal closure.
- Removal of placental source of PgE2
- Increased blood flow to lung–Effective removal of PgE2 in the lung
- Constriction effect of prostaglandin synthesis inhibitor (indomethacin, ibuprofen) and dilator effect of PgE2 and PgI2 were greater in preterm than in term infant.

Fetal Circulation

- In fetal circulation, the right and left ventricles exist in a parallel circuit, whereas in children and adults, it is in series.
- Ductus venosus, foramen ovale and ductus arteriosus are the important structures needed for maintaining this parallel circulation.
- Placenta provides gas and metabolites for exchange while the lungs do not provide gas exchange, and vessels in the pulmonary circulation are constricted.

Fetal Circulatory Flow

- Oxygenated blood from the placenta flows to the fetus through the umbilical vein (UV). Approximately 50% of UV blood enters the hepatic circulation while the rest bypasses liver and joins the inferior vena cava via ductus venosus.

Contd.

Contd.

- This combined lower body plus umbilical venous blood flow enters right atrium and is preferentially directed across the foramen ovale to the left atrium. The blood then flows into the left ventricle and is pumped into the ascending aorta.
- From fetal SVC blood enters right atrium and preferentially traverses tricuspid valve, rather than foramen ovale, and flows primarily to right ventricle.
- From right ventricle, the blood is ejected into the pulmonary artery.
- Since pulmonary arterial circulation is vasoconstricted, only about 10% of right ventricular outflow enters the lungs. Major portion of this blood bypasses the lungs and flows through the ductus arteriosus into the descending aorta to perfuse the lower part of fetal body, after which it returns to the placenta via the two umbilical arteries.

Circulatory Adjustments at Birth

- Removal of placenta
- Increase in systemic vascular resistance and closure of ductus venosus
- Lung expansion results in:
  - Decrease in pulmonary vascular resistance (PVR)
  - Functional closure of foramen ovale
  - Closure of Patent ductus arteriosus
- As a result of increase in SVR and decrease in PVR, there is reversal of shunt in ductus arteriosus from aorta to pulmonary artery, which was from pulmonary artery to aorta in fetal circulation.
- Perinatal changes influencing left to right shunt.

Before Birth

- Gas exchange in the fetus is primarily a placental function
- Minimal pulmonary blood flow (PBF), higher pulmonary vascular resistance (PVR) and low systemic vascular resistance (resistance in placental circuit is low) are characteristic.

After Birth

- Increase in arterial PaO_2 decreases the PVR through arteriolar dilation but pulmonary artery pressure (PAP) remains elevated.
- Pulmonary smooth muscle regression and a postnatal increase in cross-sectional area of the pulmonary vascular bed allows progressive reduction in PVR over the initial 8–12 weeks and then till 4–5 years of age.
- Elimination of the low resistance placental circuit increases systemic vascular resistance (SVR) thereby promoting left–to–right shunting.
- Timing of changes in vascular resistances in the perinatal period dictates the onset of clinical symptoms. Hemodynamically significant left-to-right shunting starts at approximately 8–12 weeks.
- Size of defect is the primary determinant of the magnitude of shunting, larger defects allowing larger shunts leading on to earlier heart failure.

Parameters	
Oxygen Saturation of IVC	70%
Oxygen Saturation of SVC	40%
Partial pressure of Oxygen in Umbilical Vein	32 mm Hg (Highest)
Partial pressure of Oxygen in Umbilical Artery	24 mm Hg
Partial pressure of Oxygen Aorta	28 mm Hg
Partial pressure of Oxygen Pulmonary Artery	19 mm Hg

Ref: Pediatric Cardiology for Practitioners 5th Edition Page 123, Perloff's Clinical Recognition of Congenital Heart Disease 6th Edition Page 368, Nelson 20th Edition Page 2197, Ghai 8th Edition Page 417

Ans: (A) Loss of PGE2 from placenta

11. True regarding Congenital varicella syndrome:

A. Can lead to prematurity

B. Virus is shed even after 6 months of birth

C. Defects are more when it occurs in last trimester

D. Causes cataract, cardiac defects and Mental Retardation

Key:

- *CVS can lead to* ***prematurity*** *or* ***IUGR***
- *Virus* ***NOT*** *shed after birth*
- *Risk of defect is greater during* ***first 20 weeks*** *of gestation*
- *Cardiac defect has* ***NOT*** *been document in the CVS defects.*

CONGENITAL VARICELLA SYNDROME / FETAL VARICELLA SYNDROME

- When mother has her first exposure to VZV during first half of pregnancy.
- Incidence–varicella during pregnancy is 1–5 cases per 10,000 pregnancies.
- **Overall risk of the congenital varicella syndrome**
  - 0.4% in the first 12 weeks of pregnancy
  - 2% from 13 to 20 weeks' gestation.
- Incidence of embryopathy after maternal varicella infection in the first 20 weeks is **~1%.**
- When the rash develops in the newborn **within 10 days,** it is presumed to result from in utero transmission.
- *Greatest risk for severe disease is seen when maternal varicella occurs* ***5 days before/2 days after delivery*.***

Risk Factors

- Pregnant woman with no history of varicella infection or vaccination.
- Exposed to VZV between the 8th and 20th weeks of gestation.

Clinical Features	Diagnosis
• **Skin lesions** (70%)–**Cicatricial** scars and skin loss. • **Central nervous system defects (60%).** Microcephaly, seizures, encephalitis, cortical atrophy and spinal cord atrophy, mental retardation and cerebral calcifications. • **Ocular abnormalities (60%)–**Microphthalmia, chorioretinitis, cataracts, optic atrophy, nystagmus, and Horner syndrome (ptosis, miosis and enophthalmos). • **Limb hypoplasia** and other skeletal defect (50%) • **Prematurity and IUGR** (35%).	• Appearance of maternal varicella during pregnancy. • Presence of congenital skin lesions in dermatomal distribution and/or neurologic defects, eye disease, or limb hypoplasia. • ***Proof of intrauterine VZV infection by*** o Detection of viral DNA in infant by polymerase chain reaction o Presence of VZV-specific IgM, persistence of VZV IgG beyond 7 months of age, ***or*** o Appearance of zoster during early infancy.

Management

- Damage caused by fetal VZV infection does not progress in postnatal period, which is an indication that there is no further viral replication or shedding.

Mother	Infant
• Exposed to VZV infection (1st/2nd trimester) • Treat mother with varicella-zoster immune globulin (VZIG) if her past history of varicella infection or vaccination is –ve/uncertain. • VZIG should be given within **72–96 hours** and appears to protect both mother and fetus. • If VZIG is not available, **intravenous immunoglobulin (IVIG)** can be used. • If chickenpox is diagnosed during pregnancy, antiviral therapy with **acyclovir** (safe during pregnancy) is considered.	• Supportive care of infant is required because there is usually profound neurologic impairment. • **Acyclovir** therapy may be helpful to stop the progression of eye disease or to treat recurrent zoster (shingles), which is common in first 2 years of life. • 30% of these infants die in first months of life–**intractable gastroesophageal reflux, severe recurrent aspiration pneumonia and respiratory failure.** • ***Survivors usually suffer profound mental retardation and major neurologic disabilities.***

Ref: Manual of Neonatal Care Cloherty 7th Edition Page 615, Neonatology Gomella 7th Edition Page 935, Nelson 20th Edition Page 1582, Ghai 8th Edition Page 215

Ans: (A) Can lead to prematurity

12. Bidextrous grasp develops at:

A. 3 months B. 6 months

C. 8 months D. 10 months

Key:

Fine Motor /Visual Motor	
Birth	• Visually fixes on an object
2 months	• Follows past midline
3 months	• Hands open • **Hand regard** • Holds an object
4 months	• Reaches with both arms together • Hands to midline • **Bidextrous grasp (4-5 months)**
6 months	• **Unilateral reach** • **Transfers object**
7 months	• **Unidextrous/Palmar** grasp
9 months	• **Immature pincer grasp** • Holds bottle • Throws object (overhead)
12 months	• **Mature pincer grasp** • Crayon marks

Contd.

Contd.

15 months	• **Scribbles** and builds towers of 2 blocks in imitation
18 months	• Scribbles spontaneously • Builds tower of **3 blocks** • Feeds self with **spoon** • Turns **2-3 pages** at a time
2 years	• Imitates stroke (up or down) with pencil • Builds tower of 7 blocks • Removes clothing • Turns **1 page** at a time
3 years	• Copies a **circle** • Undresses completely • Dresses partially • **Unbuttons** • **Handedness** • **Tower of 9 blocks**
4 years	• Copies a **square/Cross** • **Buttons** clothing • Dresses completely
5 years	• Copies **triangle** • Ties shoes • Spreads jam with knife

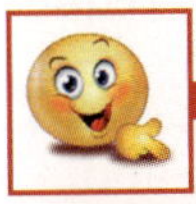

Development Milestones				
Age	**Gross Motor**	**Visual Motor**	**Language**	**Social Adaptive**
Birth	• Head flat in prone	• Visually fixes on an object	• Alerts to sound	• Regards face
2 months	• Raises head in prone • Begins to lift chest	• Follows past midline	• Smiles on touch and voice • Vocalizes	• **Recognizes mother***
3 months	• In Ventral suspension, head above the plane of body • **Neck holding***	• Hands open • **Hand regard*** • Holds an object	• **Cooing***	• **Social Smile***
4 months	• **Holds head steadily*** • Supports on forearms in prone • **Rolls** from **prone to supine***	• Reaches with both arms together • Hands to midline • **Bidextrous grasp (4-5 months)**	• Laugh aloud	• Likes to look around
6 months	• Sits with support **(tripod)** • **Feet in mouth** in supine	• **Unilateral reach*** • **Transfers object***	• Babbles • **Monosyllables***	• Recognizes stranger • **Mirror play***

Contd.

Contd.

7 months	• **Rolls** from **supine to prone*** • **Pivoting in Prone*** • May **crawl*** • **Sitting without support***	• **Unidextrous/ Palmar** grasp*		• **Stranger anxiety***
9 months	• **Crawls well*** • Pulls to stand • Standing with support* • Starting to cruise*	• **Immature pincer grasp*** • Holds bottle • Throws object (not overhand)	• **Bisyllables** – "Mama", "dada", indiscriminately • Understands "no" • Understands gestures	• Plays gesture games • Explores environment (crawling and cruising) • Waves bye bye • Plays peek a boo (10 months) • **Object permanence***
12 months	• **Walking with support*** • May walk alone • **Creeps well*** • **Bear walking/ crawling***	• **Mature pincer grasp*** • Crayon marks	• 1-2 words other than "mama" and "dada" • Follows 1-step command with gesture	• Imitates actions • Comes when called • **Plays simple ball game*** • Kisses on request
15 months	• Creeps up stairs • **Walks backward***	• **Scribbles** and builds towers of 2 blocks in imitation	• 4-6 words • Follows 1-step command without gesture • **Jargon speech***	• Uses cup and spoon (variable until 18 months) • Indicates wet pants
18 months	• Runs • Throws objects overhand while standing • **Goes upstairs/ downstairs holding railing**	• Scribbles sponta-neously • Builds tower of **3 blocks** • Feeds self with **spoon** • Turns **2-3 pages** at a time	• 15-25 words • Knows 5 body parts	• Imitates parents in tasks **(Domestic mimicry)** • Plays in company of other children • **Dry by day***
2 years	• **Walks up, and down stairs one foot at a time*** • **Running** • **Kicks a ball**	• Imitates stroke (up or down) with pencil • Builds tower of 7 blocks • Removes clothing • Turns **1 page** at a time	• 50 words • 2-word sentences • Follows 2-step commands • Uses pronouns inappropriately	• Parallel play • Indicates need for food/drink*

Contd.

Contd.

3 years	• **Alternates feet going up the stairs*** • **Pedals tricycle***	• Copies a **circle** • Undresses completely • Dresses partially • **Unbuttons** • **Handedness***	• ≥250 words • 3-word sentences • Uses plurals and past tense • All pronouns	• Takes turns / Group play • Shares • Knows **full name, age and gender** • **Dry by night**
4 years	• **Alternates feet going downstairs*** • Hops and skips	• Copies a **square/ Cross** • **Buttons** clothing • Dresses completely	• Knows colors • Recites songs from memory • Tells small stories	• Plays cooperatively • Tells "tall tales" • Asks **Questions**
5 years	• **Skips alternating feet***	• Copies **triangle** • Ties shoes	• Prints first name • Asks what a word means	• Plays cooperative games
	• Jumps over lower obstacles	• Spreads jam with knife	• Answers all "wh-" questions • Tells a story • Plays pretend • Knows alphabet	• Abides by rules • Likes to help in household tasks

Ref: Arun Babu Pediatrics for Medical Graduates T 1st Edition Elsevier Page 14, Nelson 20th edition Page 65, Ghai 9th Edition Page 47

Ans: (B) 6 months

13. Therapeutic dose of vitamin A for treatment of vitamin A deficiency in 2 years old child:

A. 2 Lakh IU on 0, within 24 hours and after 1 week

B. 1 Lakh IU on 0, within 24 hours and after 1 week

C. 20,000 IU on 0, within 24 hours and after 2 weeks

D. 10,000 IU on 0, within 24 hours and after 2 weeks

Key:

*Therapeutic dose of Vitamin A for treatment of vitamin A deficiency in 2 years old child is **2 Lakh IU on 0, within 24 hours and after 1 week***

Age	<6 months	6-12 months	>1 year
Vitamin A dose	50,000 IU	1,00,000 IU	2,00,000 IU

Age	Immediately on diagnosis	Next day	2 weeks later
< 6 months	50,000 IU	50,000 IU	50,000 IU

Contd.

Contd.

6-12 months	100,000 IU	100,00 IU	100,00 IU
> 12 months	200,000 IU	200,000 IU	200,000 IU
Women of reproductive age	200,000 IU	200,000 IU	200,000 IU

Treatment Protocol

Treatment of vitamin A deficiency:

- Schedule – 3 doses (Day 0, 1 and 14)
  - 1st dose–Immediately upon diagnosis and
  - 2nd dose–Next day,
  - 3rd dose–Third dose is given after 1-4 weeks (to replenish liver reserves), usually at 14 days.
- **Vitamin A Dose:**
  - **Age >12 months: 2 lakh units** of oral Vitamin A **(110 mg retinylpalmitate or 66 mg retinyl acetate).**
  - **Age 6 – 11 months,** half the dose is given **(1 lakh units).**
  - **Age < 6 months:** Quarter dose is given **(50000 units).**
- Oral vitamin A concentrate is the preferred treatment as it is safe, cheap and highly effective.
- **Indications for Parenteral (IM) vitamin A:**
  - When children with severe stomatitis (seen in severe measles), cannot swallow.
  - In case of persistent vomiting or
  - Severe malabsorption (e.g., cystic fibrosis).
- **Oil miscible** preparations–never given parenterally (poorly absorbed from injection site).
- **Water miscible** preparations–given intramuscularly do not replenish liver stores. So, they should always be followed with oral vitamin A concentrates.

Keratomalacia

- Treat with intramuscular vitamin A–**5000 IU / kg** / day for 5 days followed by **2500 IU** / day till recovery.

Treatment During Pregnancy

- Vitamin A is a class X teratogen (Safe limit for oral vitamin A is **10000 IU /day**).
- If night blindness or **Bitot's spots, 10000 IU of vitamin A** is given daily for **at least 2 weeks.**
- If corneal lesions are present–the risk of blindness overweighs the risk of congenital defects and so is treated with the full therapeutic schedule.

High Risk Groups

- These children are given age appropriate dose of vitamin A for 2 successive days.
  - Measles in a child < 2 years of age.
  - In case of severe acute malnutrition (SAM).
- The complete treatment schedule is instituted.
- Additionally, repeat doses of vitamin A are given every 2-4 weeks till recovery.

Periodic Supplementation

- According to **Vitamin A prophylaxis program:**
  - Children between **9 months and 3 years** are given five age appropriate mega doses of oral vitamin A concentrate at 6 months interval.
  - The first two doses are integrated with **MR vaccination and DPT first booster.**

Contd.

Contd.

- According to **National Immunization schedule (NIS) (Most recent) – Vit A – 9 doses within 5 years***
  - Vitamin A **1st dose** started at **9 months** along with MR vaccine (**1 lac** units orally)
  - Vitamin A **2 lakh** unit orally every **6 months upto 5 years.**

Hypervitaminosis A

- Manifestations of vitamin A deficiency that are not reversible–Bitot's spots.
- **Features**–Bulging fontanel, headache, vomiting, seizures, **pseudotumour cerebri,** changes in mental activity, pruritus, anorexia, hyperostosis of long bones (tender swelling of tibia), alopecia, craniotabes, desquamation of palms and soles, seborrheic cutaneous lesions and fissures in the corners of the mouth.
- Excess ingestion of β carotenoids can cause carotenemia, which is not toxic but manifests as yellowish discoloration of skin and plasma.
- It does not cause scleral discoloration.
- It does not result in hypervitaminosis A as the enzyme responsible for the conversion of β – carotenoids to vitamin A (dioxygenase) is inducible i.e. when vitamin A stores are replete, enzyme activity is suppressed and no vitamin A is formed from β – carotenoids.

Ref: Indian Journal of Practical Pediatrics (Infant and Child Nutrition Edition) Page 32–34, Nelson 20th Edition Page 320, Ghai 8th Edition Page 112

Ans: (A) 2 Lakh IU on 0, within 24 hours and after 1 week

14. For a 6 months old child, fast breathing is considered when respiratory rate is above:

A. 30 B. 40
C. 50 D. 60

Key:

Age-wise respiratory rate cutoff – to define fast breathing (IMNCI)	
Age of the child	**Respiratory cut off for fast breathing**
< 2 months	60 breaths per minute or more
2 months to 12 months	50 breaths per minute or more
12 months to 5 years	40 breaths per minute or more

Revised WHO classification and treatment of childhood pneumonia at health facilities (2014)

- **Change 1:** New classification is therefore simplified to include only 2 categories of pneumonia.
  - ***"Pneumonia" with fast breathing and/or chest indrawing,*** which requires home therapy with oral amoxicillin, and
  - ***"Severe pneumonia"***, pneumonia with ***any general danger sign,*** which requires referral and injectable therapy.
- **Change 2:** Oral amoxicillin replaces oral cotrimoxazole as 1st line treatment of pneumonia

S. No	Recommendations
1	Children with fast breathing pneumonia with no chest indrawing or general danger sign should be treated with oral amoxicillin: at least 40 mg/kg/dose twice daily (80 mg/kg/day) for 5 days (areas with low HIV prevalence, give amoxicillin for 3 days)

Contd.

Contd.

2	Children age 2–59 months with chest indrawing pneumonia should be treated with oral amoxicillin: at least 40 mg/kg/dose twice daily for 5 days.
3	Children aged 2–59 months with severe pneumonia should be treated with parenteral ampicillin (or penicillin) and gentamicin as a first-line treatment. Ampicillin: 50 mg/kg, or benzyl penicillin: 50000 units per kg IM/IV every 6 hours for at least 5 days Gentamicin: 7.5 mg/kg IM/IV once a day for at least 5 days Ceftriaxone should be used as a second-line treatment in children with severe pneumonia having failed on the first-line treatment.
4	Empiric cotrimoxazole treatment for suspected Pneumocystis jirovecii (previously neumocystis carinii) pneumonia (PCP) is recommended as an additional treatment for HIV-infected and -exposed infants aged from 2 months up to 1 year with chest indrawing or severe pneumonia.

- *Most common cause of Lobar pneumonia–Streptococcus pneumonia*
- *Most common cause of Primary Atypical pneumonia–Mycoplasma*
- *Most common cause of opportunistic infection in HIV–Pneumocystis carinii pneumonia*
- *Most common virus causing pneumonia–RSV and Rhinovirus*
- *Most common bacterial pathogen causing pneumonia in HIV Children–Streptococcus pneumonia*
- *Most common cause of pediatric pneumonia–RSV*
- *Most common bacterial cause of pediatric pneumonia–Streptococcus pneumonia*
- *Most consistent clinical manifestation of pneumonia–Tachypnea*

  - **Hehct's giant cell pneumonia**–Measles
  - **Interstitial plasma cell pneumonia**–Pneumocystis carinii
  - **Children with structural problems (Bronchiectasis, Cystic fibrosis)**–Pseudomonas aeuroginosa
  - **Focal lobar involvement**–Streptococcus pneumonia
  - **Diffuse infection with Interstitial pneumonia**–Group A streptococcus
  - **Confluent Bronchopneumonia (Often Unilateral)**–Staphylococcus aureus

Ref: Pediatrics for Medical Graduates 1st Edition, Arun Babu T, Page 346, Revised WHO Classification and Treatment of Childhood Pneumonia at Health Facilities "Quick Reference Guide", Nelson 20th Edition Page 2088, Ghai 8th Edition Page 380

Ans: (D) 60

15. A child has small ulcers and papules in oral mucosa. Similar lesions are found in hand and foot. Possible organism is:

A. Herpes zoster
B. Coxsackie A virus
C. Varicella
D. Ebstein Barr virus

Key:

*Hand, foot, mouth disease–Caused by Coxsackie virus A16**

Common Causes of Oral Ulceration in Children	
Condition	**Finding**
Aphthous (canker sore)	Painful and circumscribed lesions, Recurrences
Traumatic	Accidents, Chronic cheek biter, or After dental local anesthesia
Hand, foot, mouth disease	Painful; lesions on tongue, anterior oral cavity, hands, and feet
Herpangina	Painful; Lesions confined to soft palate and oropharynx
Herpetic gingivostomatitis	Vesicles on mucocutaneous borders; Painful, Febrile
Recurrent herpes labialis	Vesicles on lips; Painful
Chemical burns	Alkali, acid, aspirin; Painful

Human Enteroviruses

- Family – Picornaviridae, Genus – Enterovirus
- Small, single-stranded RNA viruses
- Enteroviruses, cause a variety of clinical syndromes with associated exanthems.
- **Subgroup:**
  - Poliovirus–3 Serotypes (1 – 3)
  - Coxsackie A virus–23 serotypes
  - Coxsackie B–6 serotypes
  - Echo virus–31 serotypes
  - Entero virus–4 serotypes (68 – 71) (72 reclassified as hepatitis A virus)

- Majority of enterovirus infections seen in practice are benign (hand-foot-and-mouth disease, herpangina, hemorrhagic conjunctivitis and pleurodynia).
- Some are severe or life-threatening (meningitis, encephalitis, myocarditis, neonatal sepsis and polio).

List of Enteroviral Exanthems	
Exanthem	**Causative Organism**
Hand-foot-mouth-and-disease	Coxsackievirus A or B, Enterovirus 71
Nail matrix arrest	Patients with preceding hand foot-and-mouth disease
Herpangina	Coxsackievirus A or B
Hemorrhagic conjunctivitis	Coxsackievirus A 24 and Enterovirus 70
Gianotti Crosti syndrome	Coxsackievirus A or B
Zoster-like eruption	Echovirus 6
EI-like eruption	Echovirus 12
Eruptive pseudoangiomatosis	Echovirus
Acute Generalized Exanthematous pustulosis	Coxsackievirus B4

Hand-Foot-and-Mouth Disease

- Caused by Coxsackie virus A16, sometimes (Enterovirus 71; Coxsackie A viruses 5, 6, 7, 9 and 10; Coxsackie B viruses 2 and 5; and some echoviruses).
- Mild illness, with or without low-grade fever, oropharynx is inflamed (scattered vesicles on tongue, buccal mucosa, posterior pharynx, palate, gingiva and/or lips).
- May ulcerate (leaving 4-8 mm shallow lesions with surrounding erythema).
- Maculopapular, vesicular, and/or pustular lesions–***hands and fingers (common),*** feet and buttocks and groin.
- ***Acral lesion***–Tender, 3-7 mm vesicles (dorsal surfaces), Vesicles resolve in about 1 week.
- ***Buttock lesions***–Don't usually progress to vesiculation.
- ***Enterovirus 71***–Frequently more severe than coxsackievirus A16 disease (Neurologic and cardiopulmonary involvement in young children).
- ***Coxsackievirus A16***–Complications such as Encephalitis, Acute flaccid paralysis, Myocarditis, Pericarditis and Shock.
- ***Onychomadesis (Nail shedding)***–Following Coxsackie virus A6.

Herpangina

- Enterovirus 71, although coxsackie A viruses are implicated most often.
- ***Sudden onset of fever (106°F), sore throat, dysphagia, and lesions in posterior pharynx.***
- Headache, backache, vomiting and abdominal pain were seen.
- Characteristic lesions present on anterior tonsillar pillars, soft palate, uvula, tonsils, posterior pharyngeal wall.
- Lesions are discrete 1-2 mm vesicles and ulcers that enlarge over 2-3 days to 3-4 mm and approximately 5 lesions are present, with a range of 1 to >15, surrounded by erythematous rings that vary in size up to 10 mm.
- Remainder of the pharynx appears normal or minimally erythematous.
- Fever generally lasts 1-4 days, and resolution of symptoms occurs in 3-7 days and most cases are mild, some are associated with meningitis or more severe illness.

Ref: Nelson 20th Edition Page 1564, Hurwitz Clinical Pediatric Dermatology 4th Edition Page 384, Ghai 8th Edition Page 223

Ans: (B) Coxsackie A virus

16. An infant presents with multiple injuries with various stages of healing. Diagnosis:

A. Battered baby syndrome B. Osteogenesis imperfecta
C. Shaken baby syndrome D. Rickets

Key:

Classical example of the battered baby syndrome presentation: Key points of diagnosis
• **Multiple injuries** o Can also be present in shaken baby syndrome, but always present in battered baby syndrome.

Contd.

Contd.

- o With various stage of healing – reveals that the insult or abuse have been there for long period and suggests battered baby syndrome.
- o And rules out osteogenesis imperfecta and rickets.
- *X-ray showing various stages of healing* (Can be present in all 4 options)

Osteogenesis imperfecta, scurvy, syphilis, and other diseases–mimic the radiographic findings of battered child syndrome usually are differentiated by

- Usually younger than the age of 2 years.
- Patient history of trauma is inadequate to explain the presenting injuries.
- Concurrent burns, bruises (different stages of healing).
- Retinal damage, subdural hemorrhages.
- Pulmonary infiltrates without fever representing lung contusion.

Specific Radiographic Findings

- Multiple fractures in various stages of healing.
- Other soft-tissue injuries may accompany the osseous injuries.
- Corner and bucket-handle metaphyseal fractures.

Shaken Baby Syndrome (Inflicted childhood neurotrauma)

- Form of Non Accidental Head Injury (NAHI)
- Victim is held by the torso or the extremities and violently shaken, causing abrupt uncontrolled head movements with a marked rotatory component
- Occurs secondary to violent, non-accidental, repetitive, unrestrained acceleration-deceleration head and neck movements, with or without blunt head
- Ocular manifestations are numerous
- Ecchymosis or laceration of the lids
- Hemorrhage in (retinal hemorrhage – most common ophthalmic finding) eye
- Cataract or dislocated lens
- Retinal detachment, or
- Fracture of the orbit
- **Other finding:** Acute encephalopathy and subdural hemorrhage

Osteogenesis Imperfecta (OI)/ (Brittle bone disease)

- Most common genetic cause of osteoporosis (Autosomal dominant disorder).
- Quantitative defects in type I collagen–heterotrimer, composed of two α1(I) chains and one α2(I) chain (primary component of the extracellular matrix of bone and skin).
- **Structural defects are 2 types:**
  - o 80%–point mutations, substitutions of helical glycine residues
  - o 20% are single exon splicing defects.
- One third of mutations in α1 chain are lethal while glycine substitutions in α2(I) are predominantly nonlethal.

Contd.

Contd.

- **Triad of Osteogenesis Imperfecta (OI)**

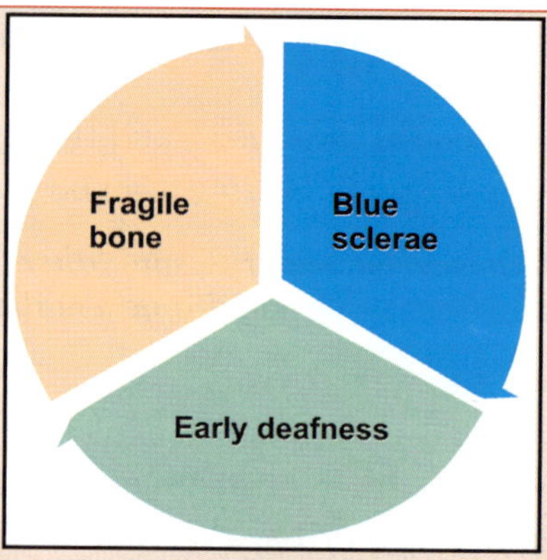

  - OI congenital–forms detectable at birth.
  - OI tarda–forms detectable later in childhood.
  - **Sillence classification** divides OI into 4 types based on clinical and radiographic criteria.

OI Type	Severity	Classical Features	Other Features
I	*Mild*	Blue sclerae, Recurrent fractures in childhood and Presenile hearing loss	Easy bruising, Joint laxity and Mild short stature
II	*Perinatal / Lethal*	Birthweight and length are small for gestational age, multiple intrauterine fractures of long bones, frog-leg position, dark blue to gray sclera	Respiratory insufficiency, Enlarged anterior and posterior fontanelles
III	*Progressive Deforming*	Most severe nonlethal form of OI, Fractures usually occur in utero, **"popcorn" appearance** at the metaphyses, sclera blue or white	Scoliosis and Vertebral compression, Extreme short stature
IV	*Moderately severe*	Moderate bowing even with infrequent fractures , recurrent fractures after ambulation, Fracture rates decrease after puberty, Sclera blue or white	Moderate short stature. Scleral hue may be blue or white
Other	*Type V (Hyperplastic Callus), Type VI (Mineralization Defect), Type VII (Autosomal Recessive).*		
	Both types I and IV are divided–absence (A) or presence (B) of dentinogenesis imperfecta		

Diagnosis

- Sequencing of cDNA using fibroblasts cultured from a skin punch biopsy.
- Severe OI can be detected prenatally by level II ultrasonography as early as 16 weeks of gestation.
- In the neonatal period, normal to elevated alkaline phosphatase levels present in OI distinguish it from hypophosphatasia.

Complications

- Recurrent pneumonias and declining pulmonary function occur in childhood, and corpulmonale is seen in adults.
- Other complications like basilar invagination, brainstem compression, hydrocephalus and syringohydromyelia.
- There is no cure for OI.
- GH improves bone histology in growth-responsive children (Usually I and IV).
- Short course of treatment of children with OI with bisphosphonates–beneficial for vertebrae (trabecular bone) than long bones (cortical bone) for 1–2 years results.

Ref: Nelson 20th Edition Page 3382, CPDT 19th Edition Page 401, Ghai 8th Edition Page 612

Ans: (A) Battered baby syndrome

17. Fatal liver condition in newborn baby:

A. Crigler-Najjar syndrome type 1
B. Crigler-Najjar syndrome type 2
C. Dubin Johnson syndrome type 1
D. Rotor syndrome

Key:

Crigler-Najjar syndrome type 1 is a severe form of unconjugated hyperbilirubinemia which requires liver transplantation to prevent kernicterus, while other options are compatible with life

INHERITED UNCONJUGATED HYPERBILIRUBINEMIA

- Congenital non-obstructive, Non-hemolytic, Unconjugated hyperbilirubinemia
- Bilirubin (metabolic end product of heme), before excretion into bile, it is first glucuroni-dated by the enzyme bilirubin-uridine diphosphoglucuronate glucuronosyl transferase (UDPGT).
- UDPGT (UGT1A1 is the primary UDPGT) activity is deficient or altered in 3 genetically distinct disorders
- **Crigler-Najjar [CN] syndromes type I –** complete absence (UGT1A1)
- **Crigler-Najjar [CN] syndromes type II –** decreased UGT1A1 activity
- **Gilbert syndrome** (30% decrease in UGT1A1 activity)
- Occurs after puberty; it is not associated with chronic liver disease and no treatment is required.
- **Mutations in UGT1A1 gene –** Cancer risk and predisposition to Drug toxicity (cancer chemotherapy).

Description	Crigler-Najjar syndrome Type I (Glucuronyltransferase deficiency)	Crigler-Najjar syndrome Type II (Partial glucuronyl-transferase deficiency)
Pathogenesis	**Autosomal recessive trait** (mutations that cause a premature stop codon abolish UGT1A1 activity). **Parents of affected children –** partial defects in conjugation *(Measurement of glucuronide formation but their serum unconjugated bilirubin concentrations are normal).*	**Autosomal recessive disease** (homozygous missense mutations in UGT1A1, partial enzymatic activity). **Marked decline in serum bilirubin level–**After treatment with phenobarbital (inducible phenobarbital response element on UGT1A1 promoter).
Clinical features	Persistence of Unconjugated hyperbilirubinemia >20 mg/dL after 1st week of life in absence of hemolysis Severe unconjugated hyperbilirubinemia (homozygous affected infants in 1st 3 days of life) Serum unconjugated bilirubin concentrations of 25-35 mg/dL are reached in 1st month ***Kernicterus, an almost universal complication (early neonatal period)*** ***Stools are pale yellow***	Unconjugated hyperbilirubinemia usually Occurs in the 1st 3 days of life **Elevated in 3rd week of life,** (range of 1.5-22 mg/dL) ***Kernicterus is unusual.*** ***Stool color is normal, infants are asymptomatic*** Liver enzymes and synthetic function tests are typically normal.
Diagnosis	Measuring hepatic glucuronyltransferase activity in liver specimen obtained by a closed biopsy.	Bilirubin concentration of in bile is nearly normal.

Contd.

Contd.

	Open biopsy should be avoided because surgery and anesthesia can precipitate kernicterus. DNA diagnosis is also available and may be preferable. Identification of heterozygous state in parents also strongly suggests the diagnosis	Respond readily to 5 mg/kg/24 hr of oral phenobarbital, with decrease in serum bilirubin concentration to 2-3 mg/dL in 7-10 days.
Treatment	**Requires repeated exchange transfusions and phototherapy** in immediate neonatal period (and also in early years of life). **Oral calcium phosphate** supplementation renders phototherapy **Phenobarbital therapy,** through CYP450 enzyme induction, should be considered to determine responsiveness and differentiation between types I and II (CN type I – no response to Phenobarbital). **Agents that bind photobilirubin products:** Cholestyramine/Agartreatment of intercurrent infections, febrile episodes, and other types of illness (prevent development of kernicterus) **Orthotopic liver transplantation** cures the disease / isolated hepatocyte transplantation **Other methods–**Plasmapheresis and Limitation of bilirubin production ***(Metalloporphyrin therapy).***	**Long-term reduction–**Achieved with continued administration of phenobarbital at 5 mg/kg/24 hr. **Orlistat–**Irreversible inhibitor of intestinal lipase, increases fecal fat excretion and decreases plasma unconjugated bilirubin concentrations (~10%) in patients with CN types I and II.

INHERITED CONJUGATED HYPERBILIRUBINEMIA

- Chronic mild conjugated hyperbilirubinemia–adolescence or early adulthood.
- Results of routine liver function tests are normal.
- Jaundice can be exacerbated–infection, pregnancy, oral contraceptives, alcohol consumption and surgery.
- There is usually no morbidity and life expectancy is normal.

Dubin-Johnson Syndrome	Rotor Syndrome
• Autosomal recessive defect with variable penetrance in hepatocyte secretion of bilirubin glucuronide. • Absent function of multiple drug-resistant protein 2 (MRP2), an adenosine triphosphate dependent canalicular transporter, is the responsible defect. • Bile acid excretion and serum bile acid levels are normal. • Total urinary coproporphyrin excretion is normal.	• Additional deficiency in organic anion uptake (Inactivating mutations in the linked genes SLCO1B1 and SLCO1B3. • Importantly, these mutations may confer significant drug toxicity risk. • Unlike Dubin-Johnson syndrome, total urinary coproporphyrin excretion is elevated, with a relative increase in the amount of the coproporphyrin I isomer. • Gallbladder is normal by roentgenography and liver cells contain no black pigment.
(Coproporphyrin I excretion increases and decrease in coproporphyrin III excretion).	

Contd.

Contd.

• Cholangiography fails to visualize the biliary tract and X-ray of the gallbladder is also abnormal. • Liver histology demonstrates normal architecture, but hepatocytes contain black pigment similar to melanin. • Liver function is normal. • Prognosis is excellent.	
Most commonly reported symptoms are abdominal pain and fatigue, jaundice, dark urine, and slight enlargement of liver.	
• Jaundice fluctuates in intensity and is aggravated by intercurrent disease.	

Ref: Nelson 20th Edition Page 1938, Ghai 8th Edition Page 320, Manual of Neonatal Care Cloherty 7th Edition Page 817

Ans: (A) Crigler-Najjar syndrome type 1

18. Condition mimicking Erythroblastosis foetalis:

A. EBV infection
B. Staphylococcus aureus
C. Cytomegalovirus infection
D. Fungal sepsis

Key:

Clinical features of Erythroblastosis foetalis like ***anemia, jaundice, hepatosplenomegaly*** *and* ***rash*** *mimics Congenital TORCH infections like CMV infection, syphilis and rubella*

CMV INFECTION

- Most common cause of congenital infection
- Double stranded DNA–Largest of the herpesviruses
- **Primary infection**–Seronegative, susceptible host.
- **Recurrent infection**–Reactivation of latent infection or reinfection of seropositive immune host (more severe than primary infection)
- *Risk for fetal infection is greatest with maternal primary CMV infection (30%) and much less likely with recurrent infection (<1%).*
- **Transmission**–Saliva, Breast milk, Cervical and Vaginal secretions, Urine, Semen, Stools, Blood and Tissue/Organ transplants.
- **Important perinatal sources of virus**–Genital tract secretions at delivery and Breast milk.
- **In CMV seropositive mothers**–Virus is detectable in Breast milk (96%) and Postnatal transmission in 38% of infants.
- Infected infants excrete virus for years in saliva and urine.
- Childcare centers contributing to rapid spread of CMV among children.
- 2nd peak occurs in adolescence as a result of sexual transmission.

Pathogenesis

- Depressed cellular immunity, uncontrolled viral replication, multiorgan involvement, and end-organ disease secondary to direct viral cytopathic effects.
- CMV infects placental cytotrophoblasts and can be transmitted to the fetus.
- Infected cells–large intranuclear and smaller intracytoplasmic inclusions (pathognomonic).

Clinical Manifestations

- **Infants and young children**–Primary infection causes pneumonitis, hepatomegaly, hepatitis and petechial rashes.
- **Older children, adolescents**–Mononucleosis-like syndrome characterized by fatigue, malaise, myalgia, headache, fever, hepatosplenomegaly, elevated liver enzymes, and atypical lymphocytosis, lasting 2–3 weeks.

Immunocompromised Persons

- Primary infection – pneumonitis (most common), hepatitis, chorioretinitis, gastrointestinal disease, or fever with leukopenia – severe and progressive.
- Risk is greatest in bone marrow transplant recipients and in patients with AIDS.

Congenital Infection

- Congenitally infected infants (5% have severe cytomegalic inclusion disease, 5% have mild involvement, and 90% are subclinical, chronic, CMV infection).
- Manifestation – intrauterine growth restriction, prematurity, hepatosplenomegaly and jaundice, blueberry muffin–like rash, thrombocytopenia and purpura, and microcephaly and intracranial calcifications.
- **Other neurologic problems**–Chorioretinitis, SNHL and mild increase in CSF protein.

Perinatal Infection

- Infections–maternal genital tract at delivery or in breast milk (despite the presence of maternally derived antibody).
- Present like pneumonitis and sepsis-like syndrome.
- Premature and ill full-term infants may have neurologic sequelae and psychomotor retardation.
- No increase in risk of hearing loss, chorioretinitis and microcephaly.

Diagnosis

- Active CMV infection is best confirmed by virus isolation from urine, saliva, bronchoalveolar washings, breast milk, cervical secretions, buffy coat, and tissues obtained by biopsy.
- Rapid quantitative detection of CMV antigens, and quantitative polymerase chain reaction (PCR) assays are also available.
- Primary infection is confirmed by seroconversion or the simultaneous detection of immunoglobulin M (IgM) and IgG antibodies with low functional avidity.
- 1st weeks after primary infection, the functional avidity of IgG class antibodies is very low and rises to a peak in 4–5 months.
- IgM antibodies can be demonstrated transiently in both symptomatic and asymptomatic infection at 4–16 weeks, which is during the acute phase of symptomatic disease.

Congenital Infection

- **Definitive diagnosis**–Virus isolation (Urine and saliva are the best specimens for culture) or PCR (performed at or shortly after birth).
- **IgG Antibody test**–Little diagnostic value (reflects maternal antibodies).
- **IgM test**–Lack sensitivity and specificity (unreliable for diagnosis of congenital CMV).

Fetal infection can be confirmed by viral isolation / PCR from amniotic fluid (Excellent sensitivity after 22nd weeks of gestation)

Treatment

- Not indicated for immunocompetent persons, but is recommended for immuno- compromised persons, and remains controversial for infants with symptomatic congenital infection.

- **Ganciclovir** combined with immune globulin (IVIG or hyperimmune CMV IVIG) to treat life-threatening CMV infections in immunocompromised hosts.
- CMV retinitis and gastrointestinal disease respond to therapy but recur on cessation.
- Toxicity with ganciclovir–neutropenia, thrombocytopenia, liver dysfunction, reduction in spermatogenesis, and gastrointestinal and renal abnormalities.
- **Foscarnet** is an alternative antiviral agent (limited information on its use in children).
- Prophylaxis with ganciclovir or acyclovir reduces the risk for morbidity in solid organ transplantation.
- **Oral valganciclovir,** the orally bioavailable prodrug of ganciclovir.
- Ganciclovir, cidofovir, and foscarnet are the systemic antiviral drugs that are currently licensed for treatment of human cytomegalovirus (CMV) infection.
- All 3 drugs in their active forms, target the viral DNA polymerase (pol) (CMV gene UL54)
- Resistance to ganciclovir–due to a mutation in the viral UL97 phosphotransferase gene.
- DNA polymerase mutant isolates are cross-resistant to ganciclovir, foscarnet and cidofovir.

Prevention

- Use of CMV free blood products, especially for premature newborns.
- Use of organs from CMV free donors for transplantation.
- Pregnant women who are CMV seropositive are at low risk for delivering a symptomatic newborn.
- Pregnant women who are CMV seronegative should be counseled regarding good handwashing and other hygienic measures and avoidance of contact with oral secretions of others.
- Pregnant women with primary CMV who receive CMV hyperimmune globulin may have a reduced risk for delivering a congenitally infected infant.
- Use of IVIG/CMV IVIG for prophylaxis of infection in solid organ and bone marrow transplant recipients reduces risk for symptomatic disease but does not prevent infection.

Ref: Nelson 20th Edition Page 1590, CPDT 22nd Edition Page 1265, Ghai 8th Edition Page 202

Ans: (C) Cytomegalovirus infection

Chapter 16

DERMATOLOGY

1. A-26-year-old man presents with alopecia as shown in picture. Which of the following finding is associated with this condition?

A. Pitting of nails

B. Pterygium of nails

C. Paronychia

D. Pigmentation of nails

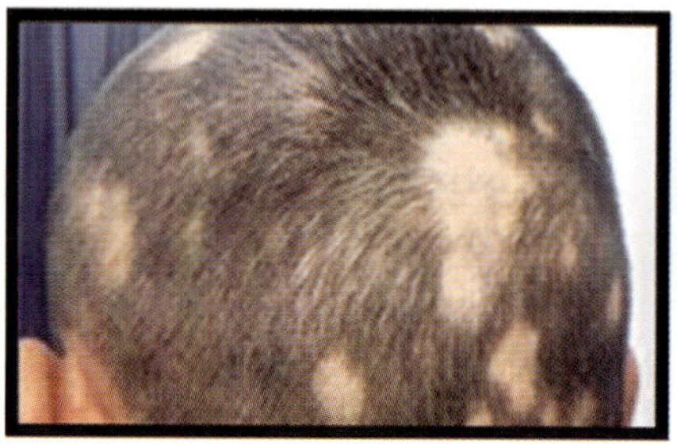

Key:

Picture shows non-scarring alopecia with exclamation mark sign in scalp region– Typically seen with Alopecia Areata. Nail finding in Alopecia areata is Pitting of nails

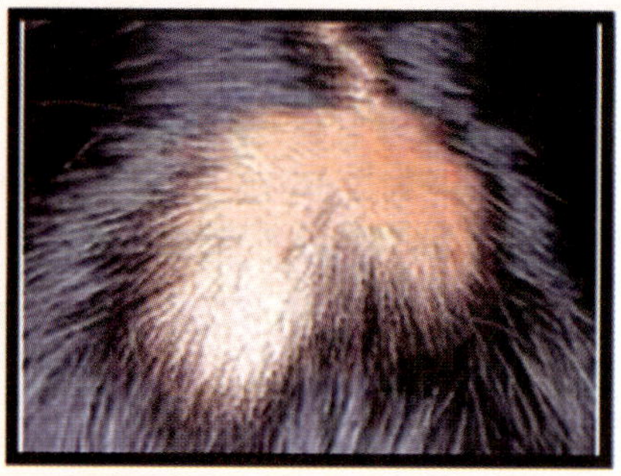

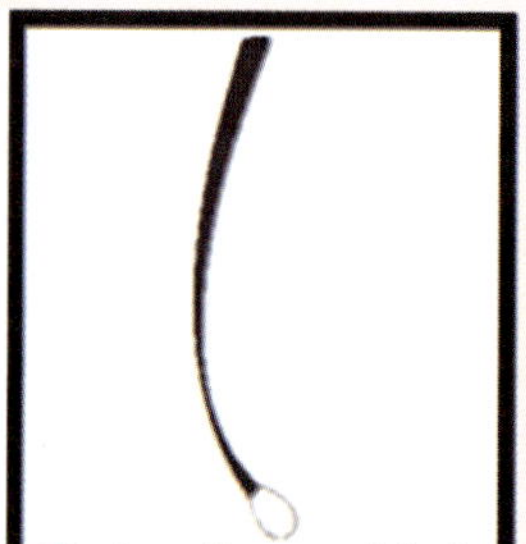

Exclamation mark hair

ALOPECIA

Scarring/Cicatricial
BCC, Cutaneous metastasis, Lichen planus, Folliculitis decalvans, Morphea,Sarcoidosis, HZV, ***Cutaneous lupus, DLE***

Non-scarring/Non-cicatricial
Androgenic alopecia, Alopecia areata, Tinea capitis, Traumatic alopecia, Telogen effluvium, Hypo/hyperthyroidism, Hypopituitarism, Iron, Zinc, Protein and Biotin Deficiency, Secondary syphilis, HIV, ***Lupus erythematosus***

Note: DLE (chronic lupus) causes scarring alopecia. Other cutaneous lupus (acute and subacute causes non scarring alopecia)

ALOPECIA AREATA

- **Alopecia areata** usually presents as smooth well circumscribed bald patch.
- Though not pathognomic ***exclamation mark hair*** is a characteristic finding seen in AA.
- ***Pathogenesis:*** T cell mediated autoimmune disease.
- ***Nail findings:*** Nail dystrophy, trachyonychia, fine pitting ("Hammered brass"), onychorrhexis.
- ***Types of AA:*** Patchy, reticulated, diffuse, ophiasis, sisaipho, totalis and universalis.

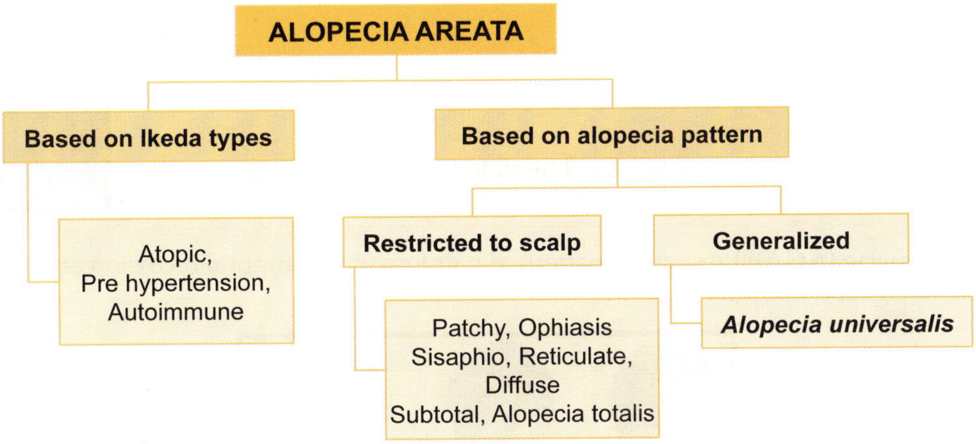

- *Ophiasis:* Alopecia along margin of scalp
- *Alopecia totalis:* Loss of hair on total scalp
- *Alopecia universalis:* Loss of hair on whole body

- *Pathology:* In histopathology the peribulbar lymphocytic infiltrate give it a **"swarm of bees"** appearance.

Clinical Features

- First site affected: Scalp
- Sharply defined alopecia with Sparing of grey/white hair
- *'Going white over-night' phenomenon*
- Exclamation mark hair
- Nails–'Hammered brass'→ Fine stippled pitting

- *Associated diseases:* SLE, myasthenia gravis, autoimmune thyroiditis, vitiligo and psoriasis.

Treatment

- **Few lesions:** Topical Minoxidil, Topical Corticosteroids, Topical Psoralen + UV-A, intra-lesional steriod
- **Extensive lesions:** Oral Corticosteroids, Oral Psoralen + UV-A

Diseases	Characteristic nail finding
Alopecia Areata	*Fine pitting* 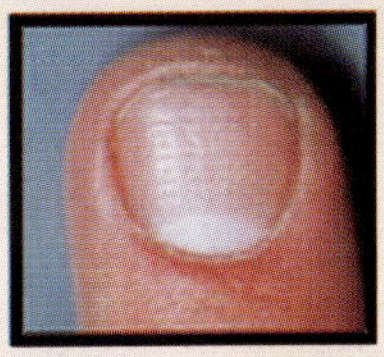
Psoriasis Vulgaris	*Coarse pitting* 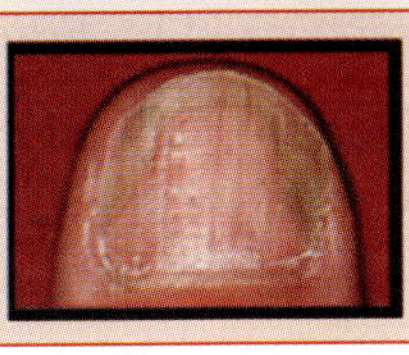

Contd.

Contd.

Lichen Planus	*Pterygium*	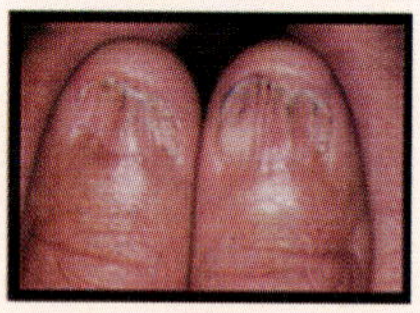

- **Androgenetic alopecia (AGA):** Presents as patterned hair loss with temporal recession and progressive hair loss in vertex sparing lateral and occipital region.

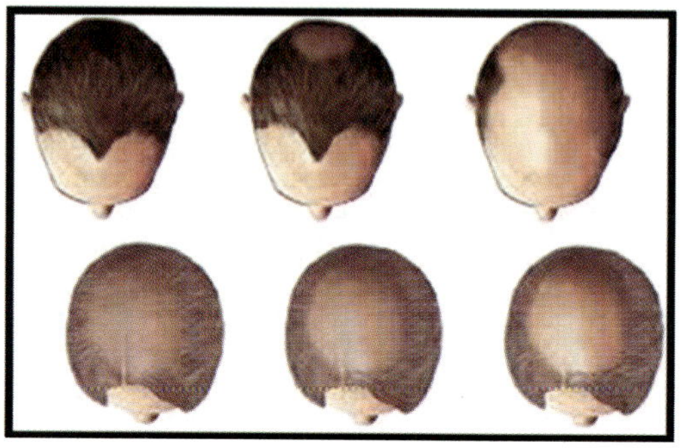

Grading for Patterned Hair Loss

- **Hamilton–Norwood:** Male pattern hair loss (AGA)
- **Ludwig scale and Olsen grading:** Female pattern hair loss

Ref: Rook's Textbook of Dermatology 9th Edition Page 89.28, Essentials in Dermatology 2nd Edition DM Thappa Page 191, IAVDL Textbook of Dermatology 4th Edition Page 902

Ans: (A) Pitting of nails

2. **A 2 months baby has papules, itching over face and trunk. Mother is a known case of bronchial asthma. Flexural involvement is also seen. Most probable Diagnosis is:**
   A. Atopic dermatitis
   B. Allergic contact dermatitis
   C. Seborrheic dermatitis
   D. Candidal intertrigo

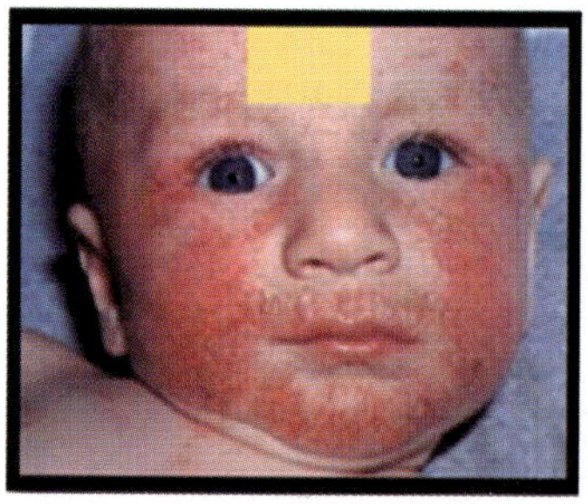

Key:

Pruritic rashes in flexural areas in a patient with known and family history of asthma/atopy suggests Atopic dermatitis
Associated with Itchy red swollen and cracked skin–Atopic eczema

ATOPIC DERMATITIS

- **Type 1 Hypersensitivity reaction**
- Characterized by Eczema, Family history of asthma or Allergic rhinitis
- Intensely pruritic lesions involving flexural areas
- Increased susceptibility to infection–Staphylococcus, Molluscum contagiosum and warts
- Age of onset is between 2 and 6 months in the majority of cases
- **Hanifin and Rajka critera** is used for the diagnosis

Hanifin and Rajka's criteria for diagnosis of atopic dermatitis	
Major features (must have 3 or more)	
1. Pruritus 2. Typical morphology and distribution: o Facial and extensor involvement in infants and children o Flexural lichenification in adults 3. Dermatitis, chronic or chronically relapsing 4. Personal or family history of atopy (asthma, allergic rhinitis or atopic dermatitis)	
Minor features and (must have 3 or more)	
Cataracts (anterior subcapsular) Cheilitis Conjunctivitis, recurrent Facial pallor/erythema Food intolerance Hand dermatitis: non-allergic, irritant Ichthyosis Elevated levels of IgE Immediate (type I) skin test reactivity Infections Itching, when sweating	Keratoconus Keratosis pilaris Nipple dermatitis Orbital darkening Palmar hyperlinearity Perifollicular accentuation Pityriasis alba White dermographism Wool intolerance Xerosis

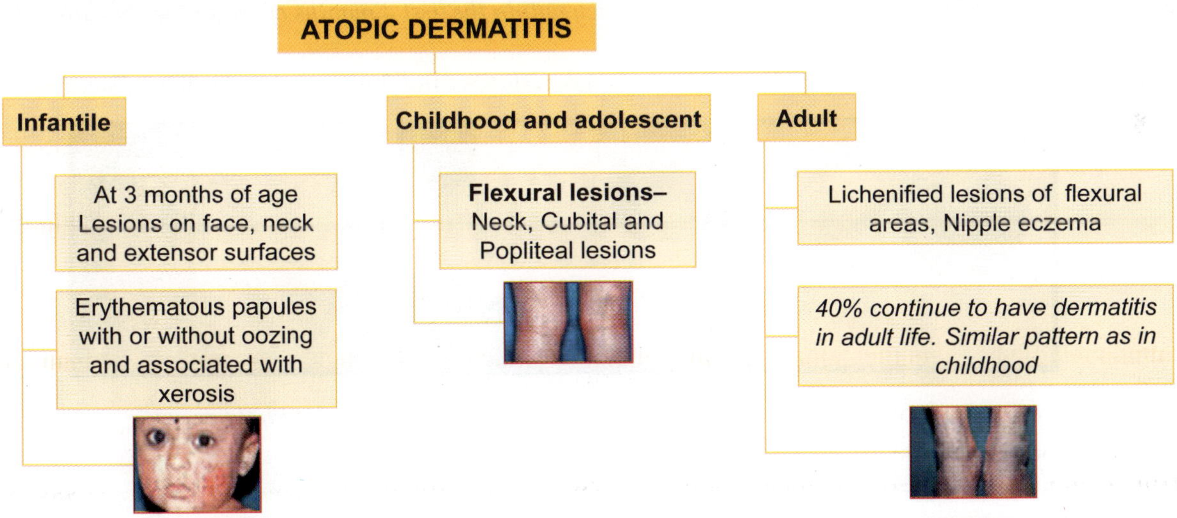

- **Filaggrin mutations are often present**
- Almost all cases usually have dry skin (Filaggrin maintains moisture–Here its mutated)
- IgE is elevated
- **Diagnosis**–Clinical features and History (HANIFIN and RAJKA CRITERIA)
- **Treatment**
  - **1st Line**–Moisturizers, Topical steroids (Soak and smear)
  - **2nd Line**–Topical calcineurin inhibitors (Tacrolimus/Pimecrolimus), Phototherapy
  - **3rd Line**–Steroids, Azathioprine, Mycophenolate mofetil, Cyclosporine and Methotrexate

CONTACT DERMATITIS

- **Irritant**
  - On exposure to irritant; More common than allergic
  - Common in eyelids and intertrigonous areas; Most common site–Hand
  - Wear and tear dermatitis; Napkin dermatitis; Household Eczema
- **Allergic**
  - On contact with allergen; Memory T cell mediated
  - Severe itching beyond area of contact; Nickel, Rubber and Dye

Contact Dermatitis	Candidal Intertrigo
On exposure to irritant/ allergen 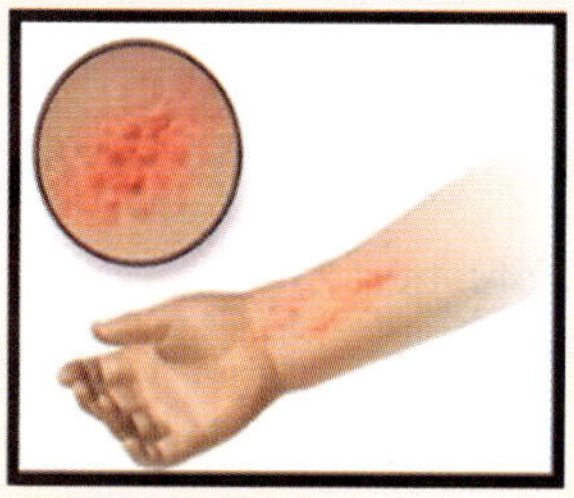	**Usually affects flexures** Presents as papules, pustules with satellite lesions and maceration. 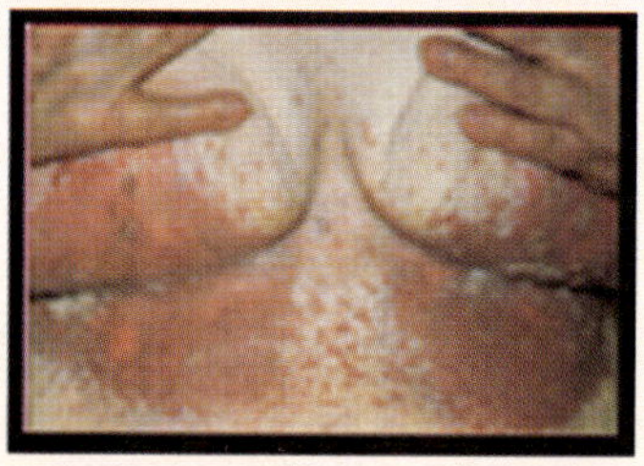

Seborrheic dermatitis ***(SD)*** *has two age peaks, one in infancy within the first 3 months of life and second around the second to third decade of life. Presents as erythema and scaling.*

Infantile SD: *Scalp (cradle cap), face including eyebrows, paranasal areas and flexures are commonly affected.*

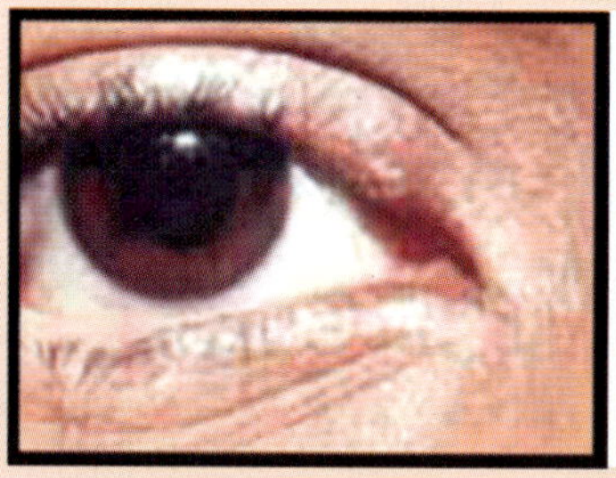

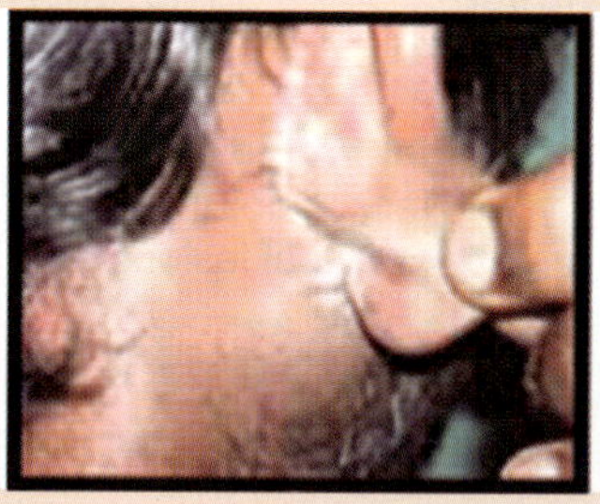

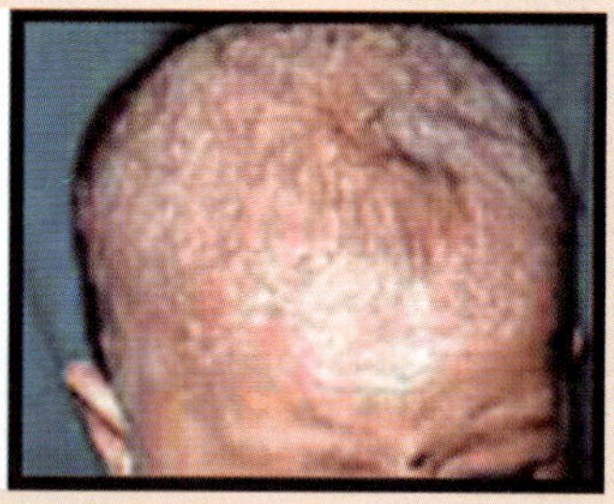

- Distributed over scalp, face, Retroauricular area, Sternum and Scapula→***Seborrheic areas***
- ***Etiology***–Seborrhea (oily skin)
- Colonization by Malassezia
- Initially presents as dandruff
- ***Frequent occurrence in Parkinson's disease, cerebrovascular accidents and HIV patients.***
- **Treatment:** Selenium Sulphide, Topical steroids, Topical antifungals, Oral Antifungals and Anti-dandruff shampoos

Seborrheic dermatitis in form of severe scaling of scalp in neonates is called cradle cap.

Ref: Rook's Textbook of Dermatology 9th Edition Page 41.19, Neena Khanna 4th Edition Page 181, Behl 10th Edition Page 403, IADVL Textbook of Dermatology 4th Edition Page 530

Ans: (A) Atopic dermatitis

3. **Causative organism for the condition depicted in the picture is:**

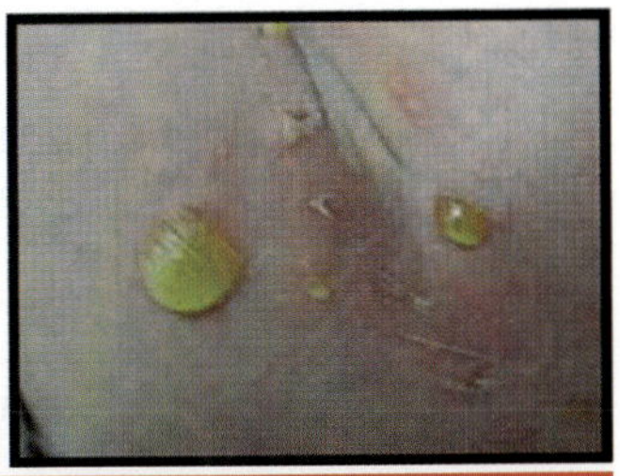

A. Candida
B. Streptococcus
C. Staphylococcus
D. Actinomycetes

Key:

Thin walled flaccid, superficial bullae with little erythema surrounding these forming varnish like yellow crusts later–Typical for Bullous Impetigo
Staphylococcus aureus is most common pathogen implicated in causing Bullous Impetigo

Types	Causative Organism	Features	Treatment
Bullous 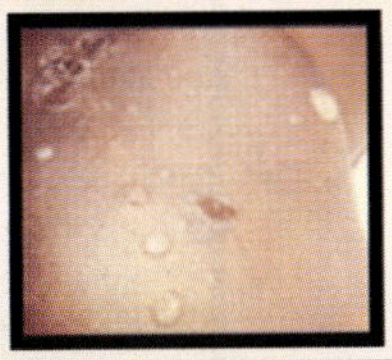	*Staphylococcus aureus** Gram +ve cocci in clusters	*Newborn and infants* *Blisters and erosions in flexures are typically seen*	**Localised** – Topical fusidic acid cream or mupirocin
Non Bullous 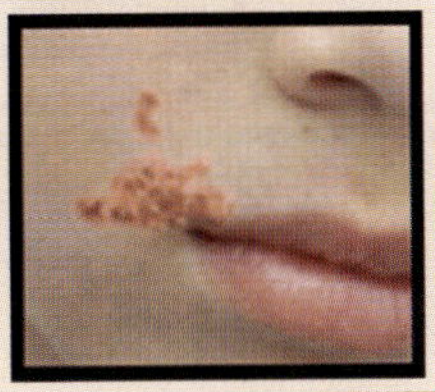	*Streptococcus pyogenes* (*More common in warm climatic regions*) Staphylococcus **Grams:** Gram +ve cocci in chains	*Preschool and young school aged* *Honey colored crusted lesions are typically seen over face*	**Extensive disease** – Oral cloxacillin, cephalexin, co-amoxiclav

Candidal Intertrigo

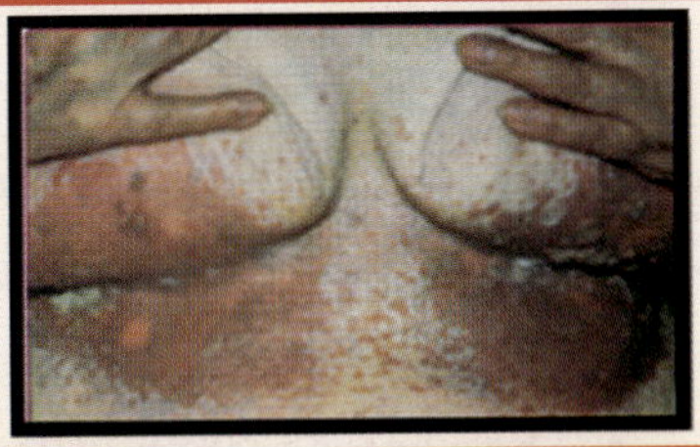

- **Etiology:** ***Candida albicans***
- **Clinical features:** Usually affects flexures and presents as papules, pustules with satellite lesions and maceration.
- **Investigations:** KOH smear from pustules shows budding yeast.

Actinomycosis

- Caused by Actinomyces Israeli
- Weekly gram +ve, **ANAEROBE,** non motile, non sporing, non capsulated bacteria with **long branching filaments** – Normal flora of oral cavity

ACTINOMYCOSIS

- **Cervicofacial–** ***Most common*** (LUMPY JAW)
- **Thoracic** *(Pleural and Pericardial)*
- **Abdominal** *(Caecum)*
- **PELVIC** *Associated with IUD*

Contd.

Contd.

- ***Culture: Spidery molar teeth*** colony in solid media ***and Fluffy ball*** at bottom of liquid medium.
- **Sulfur granules**–Pathognomonic (Granules consist of gram positive bacilli and surrounded by clubs–**sunray appearance**)

- **Drug of choice**–Penicillin

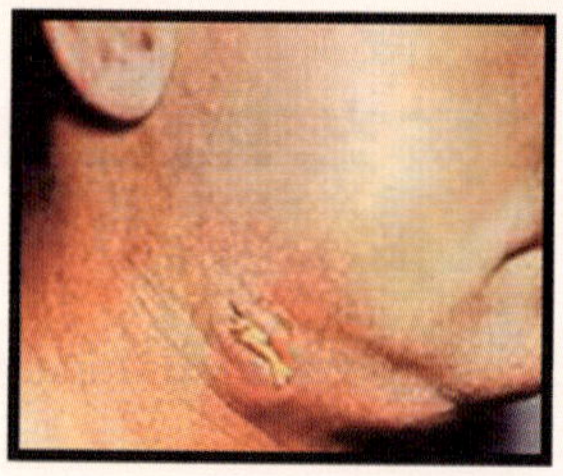

Ref: Essentials in Dermatology DM Thappa 2nd Edition Page 31, IADVL Textbook of Dermatology 4th Edition Page 226

Ans: (C) Staphylococcus

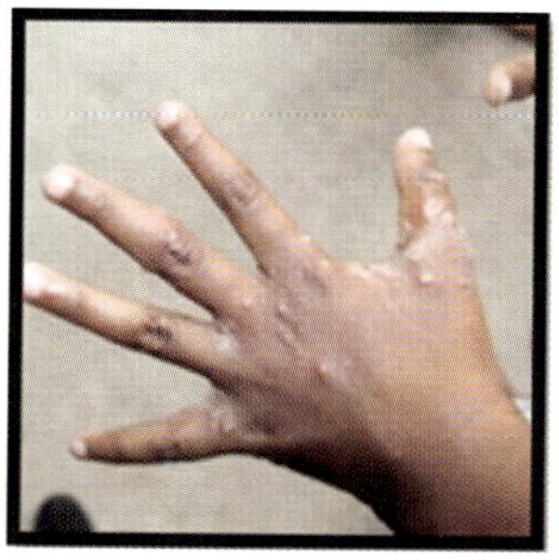

4. A boy has itching on hands webspaces. This condition is caused by:

A. Dermatitis herpetiformis
B. Scabies
C. Erythema multiforme
D. Psoriasis vulgaris

Key:

Picture shows papules in the finger web spaces–Pathognomonic of scabies
Occurs due to sarcoptes scabei mite

SCABIES

- Scabies usually presents as intensely pruritic excoriated papules and nodules with ***nocturnal exacerbation.***
- Common sites involved are interdigital spaces, wrists, elbows, the anterior axillary folds, umbilicus and genitalia ***("circle of Hebra").***
- ***Nocturnal itching at these sites***–Classical finding of Scabies.
- **Pathognomonic finding–*Intact "S" shaped or linear burrow harbouring mite.***
- Burrows are highlighted by India ink and also by dermoscopy which shows ***"jet in contrail" appearance.***
- **Sarcoptes scabiei mite:** *Sarcoptes scabei var hominis*

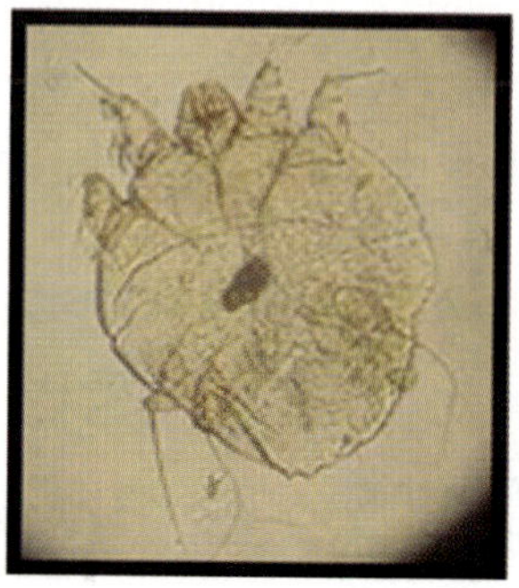

- **Treatment:** Topical–5% permethrin cream, Crotamiton, Benyl benzoate, Precipitated sulphur. Oral – Ivermectin 200 mcg/kg

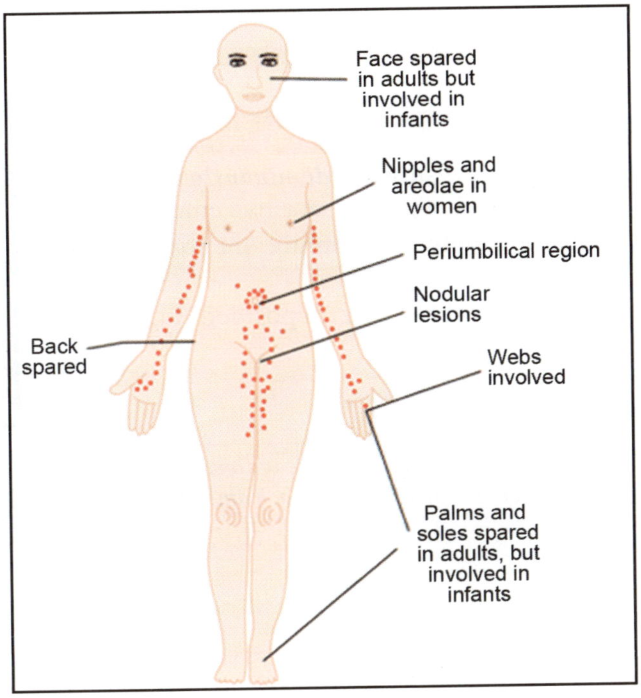

Other Types of Scabies

- **Animal scabies**–Presents as itchy papules at the site of contact (i.e., thighs, arms) of animals. ***No burrows seen***
- **Infantile scabies**–Palms and soles involved, pustules present
- Scabies incognito
- Norwegian or crusted scabies–Seen in immunocompromised

COMPLICATIONS

- Secondary bacterial infection
- Post streptococcal glomerulonephritis
- Eczematisation

High Yield Points About Scabies

- **Causative agent:** Sarcoptes scabiei
- **Type of disease:** Water washed
- **Incubation period:** 4 Weeks
- **Most common complaint:** Itching,
- **Pathogonomic lesion:** Burrow
- Burrow lies in ***stratum Corneum***
- Most common site–**Interdigital space**
- Most common site in infants–**Scalp and face**
- Drug of choice–***Permethrin followed by GBHC***
- Drug of choice in Pregnancy–***Permethrin cream***
- Drug given orally–***Ivermectin***

Note: GBHC is not used nowadays due to systemic toxicities (seizures)

Dermatitis Herpetiformis

- Presents as pruritic erythematous papulovesicles ***predominantly in extensor aspects*** of limbs, shoulders with underlying gluten sensitive enteropathy.
- ***Pathology:*** Sub epidermal blistering with neutrophilic microabscess in dermal papilla
- ***Investigations:*** Direct immunofluorescense: IgA deposition in dermal papillae

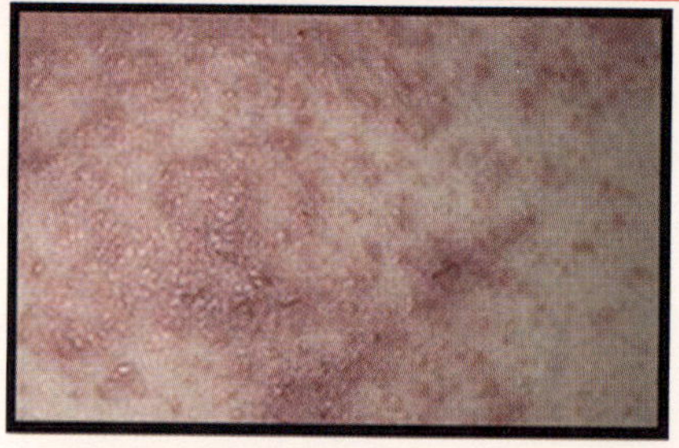

Psoriasis vulgaris: *Typical well-defined erythematous plaque with silvery-white scale mostly on extensor surfaces (elbows, knees), lower back and scalp.*

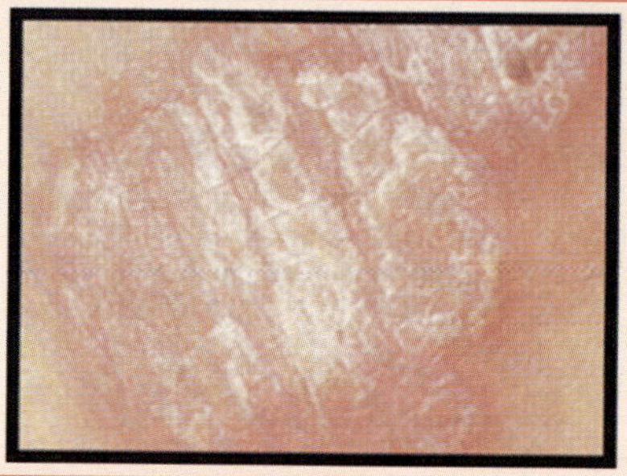

Erythema Multiforme

- Type III Hypersensitivity Immune complex mediated reaction
- Most common cause–***Herpes simplex virus***
- ***Drugs inducing EM***–Isoniazid, Antiepileptic drugs, penicillins, sulfonamides
- ***Types***–Major and minor
  - ***Major***–Skin lesions with mucous membrane involvement
  - ***Minor***–Skin lesions without mucous membrane involvement
  - ***Herpes associated EM***
  - ***Mucosal erythema multiforme***–(Fuchs syndrome, Ectodermosis pluriorificialis) Mucous membrane lesion without cutaneous involvement
- Severe mucosal involvement seen in erythema multiforme major
- ***Typical target Lesions symmetrically over acral areas***
- Centrifugal spread is seen
- ***Target lesion / Bull's eye / Iris Lesion has 3 zones***–Central bulla / dark dusky color, Edematous zone and Outermost erythematous zone

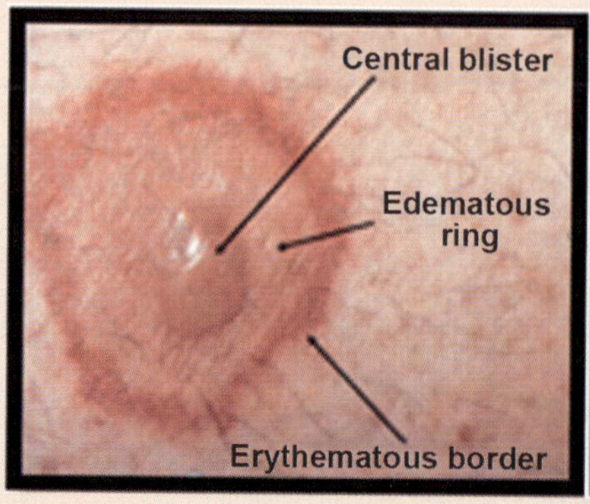

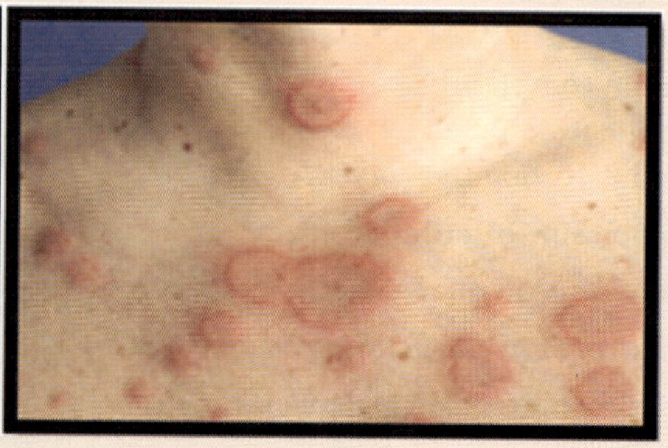

Contd.

Contd.

- Nikolsky negative
- Resolves in 2 weeks
- *Rowell's syndrome–Erythema multiforme with lupus erythematosus*

Treatment

- Symptomatic management
- Acyclovir if Herpes is suspected
- Topical steroids, antibiotics and Oral steroids in early stages

Ref: Essentials in Dermatology DM Thappa 2nd Edition Page 72, IADVL Textbook of Dermatology 4th Edition Page 424

Ans: (B) Scabies

5. **Identify this lesion:**
   A. Piebaldism
   B. Contact Leukoderma
   C. Vitiligo
   D. DLE

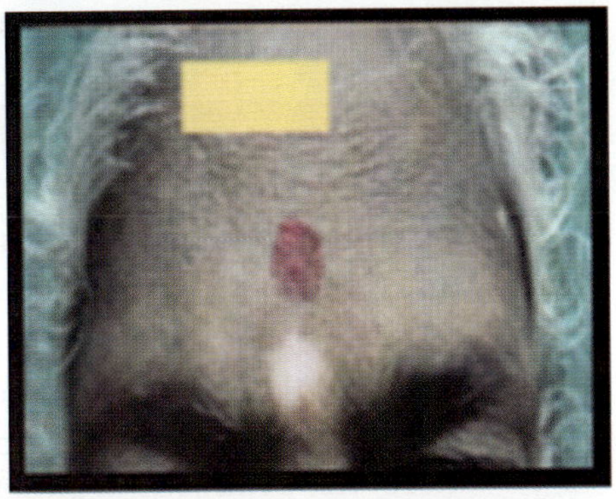

Key:

Hypopigmented skin lesion which occurs due to skin whitening induced by certain chemicals. These chemicals are responsible for depigmentation
In the above patient the usage of bindi has caused contact leukoderma

CONTACT LEUCODERMA

- Contact leucoderma is defined as acquired hypopigmented skin lesions produced by repeated exposure to specific chemicals.

Causative agents	Chemicals
Adhesive 'bindi'	**Para-tertiary butyl phenol**
Hair dye, black socks and shoes	Para-phenylene diamine
Rubber sandals	Monobenzyl ether of hydroquinone
Insecticides	Para-tertiary butyl phenol
Lipstick	Azo dyes

Treatment

Avoid contact with chemicals/cosmetics. Steroids are given in few cases.

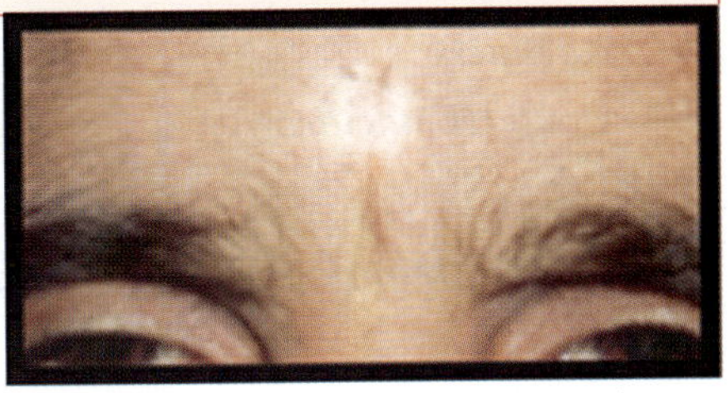

Piebaldism

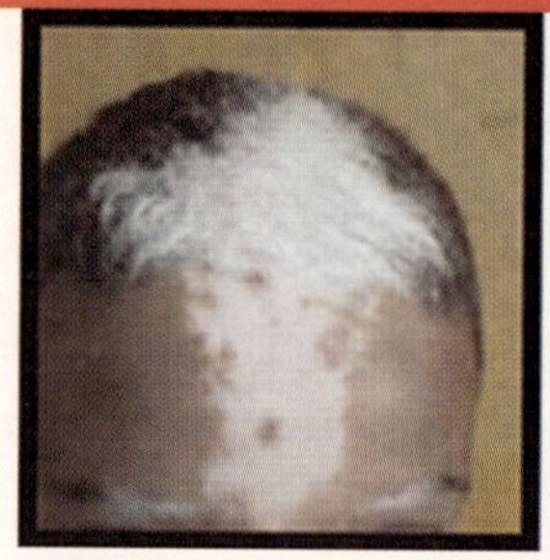

- Autosomal dominant leukoderma with ***white forelock*** and hence lesions are present from birth.
- Hyperpigmented macules within leucoderma is a typical finding
- Check for sensorineural deafness and heterochromia irides – ***Waardenburg syndrome***

Vitiligo

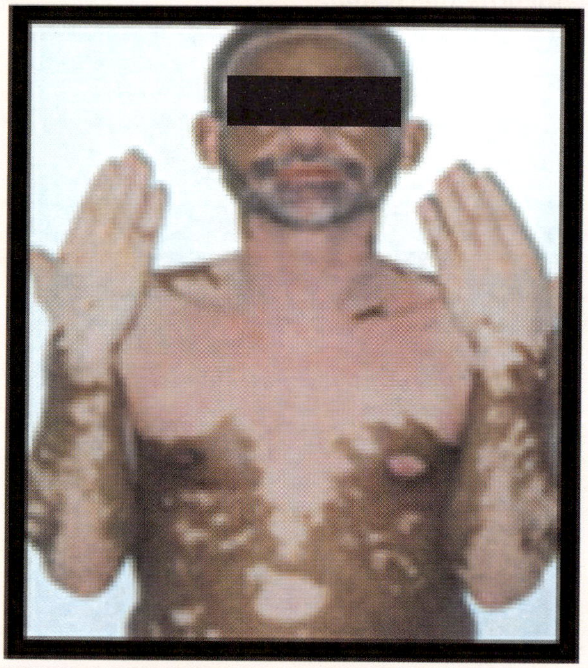

- Non pigmented patch
- **Location:** Anywhere on body
- Sharp scalloped hyperpigmented margins
- ***Koebner phenomenon***
- Leucotrichia (Loss of pigment in affected hair)
- ***Vitiligo vulgaris***–Multiple scattered lesions distributed in more/less symmetrical pattern;

  Most common presentation of Generalized vitiligo.
- ***Acrofacial vitiligo***–Affects distal end of fingers and facial orifices in circumferential pattern
- ***Mixed vitiligo***–Combination of acrofacial and vulgaris, or segmental and acrofacial types.
- ***Vitiligo universalis***–Complete / Nearly complete depigmentation of whole body

  Most severe form of Generalized vitiligo.
- ***Focal vitiligo***–Characterized by presence of one/few macule in one area but not distributed in a segmental pattern→ Considered Precursor form of Generalized vitiligo.
- ***Mucosal vitiligo***–Term reserved for depigmentation of mucous membrane alone.
- ***Segmental vitiligo***–Characterized by macules having U/L dermatomal distribution that don't cross midline.

	Chemical Leukoderma	Vitiligo
Trichome	–	+
Leukotrichia	–	+
Koebner	–	+
Confetti macules	+	–

Ref: IADVL Textbook of Dermatology 4th Edition Page 594, Ghosh, Mukhopadhyay Chemical Leucoderma: A Clinico-Aetiological Study BrJ Dermatol 2009 Jan; 160: 40-7

Ans: (B) Contact Leukoderma

6. **Identify this condition:**

A. Herpes simplex

B. Herpes zoster

C. Lichen planus

D. Irritant contact dermatitis

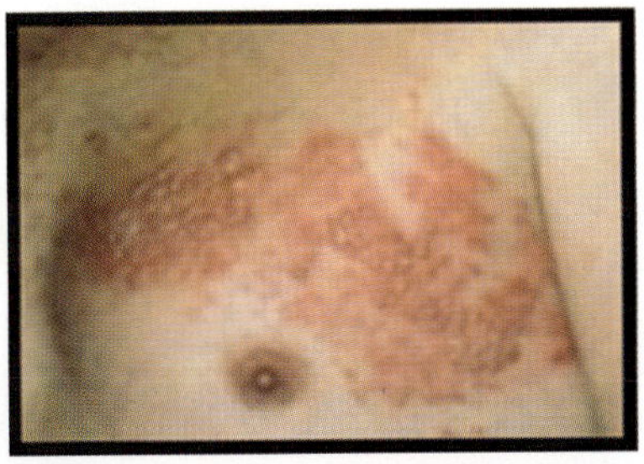

Key:

Picture shows vesicular eruptions predominantly involving thoracic region–Points towards diagnosis of Herpes zoster

Herpes Zoster

- **Causative agent:** Varicella zoster virus (HHV-3)
- Caused by reactivaton of latent virus from dorsal root ganglion.

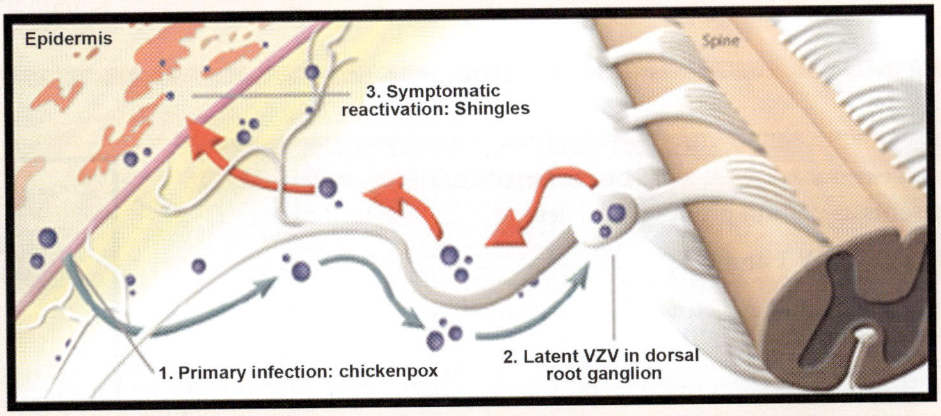

Clinical Features

- Presents as grouped painful vesicular eruption in dermatomal distribution. It can be unidermatomal, multidermatomal or disseminated.
- Decreasing order of frequency of dermatomal involvement is thoracic (53%), cervical (20%), ophthalmic (15%) and lumbosacral (11%).
- **Hutchinson's sign:** When patients develop ophthalmic herpes zoster, if tip of nose is involved then there is increased increased possibility for the patient developing ocular complications.
- **Ramsay Hunt syndrome:** Herpes zoster oticus with facial palsy.
- **Tzanck smear:** Multinucleated giant cells and intra-nuclear inclusion bodies.
  - **Treatment:** Oral acyclovir, Valacyclovir.
  - **Complications:** Motor weakness, post herpetic neuralgia, s

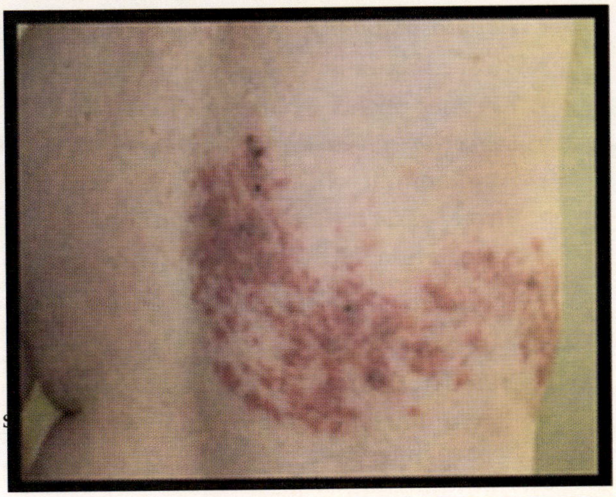

VARICELLA ZOSTER

- Produces vesicular eruption on skin and mucous membranes

VARICELLA ZOSTER VIRUS

Chicken pox/Varicella

Primary infection
Most common site involved–D3 to L2
Incubation Period–2 to 3 weeks
Period of infectivity–Infectious during initial stage–2 to 5 days of onset of rash until the vesicles are crusted
Rash–Usually starts in trunk, rapid evolution, appears in crops, centripetal distribution, bilateral and diffuse.
Localization in skin capillary endothelial cells
Secondary attack rates–70–90%
Acyclovir is drug of choice
Steroids contraindicated

ZOSTER

Sporadic, incapacitating disease of ***elderly/immunocompromised*** patients
Reactivation of latent virus
Most common site involved–T3 to L3
Site of latency–Trigeminal N (Ophthalmic branch)–***Zoster ophthalmicus***
Rash–Segmented and unilateral
Confined to segment of sensory nerve
Affects geniculate ganglion-Ramsay hunt syndrome
Tetrad: *Facial Nerve palsy, Vesicle on tympanic membrane, External auditory meatus and tongue*
Patient with Hodgkin's and NHL are at greatest risk for progressive Herpes zoster.
Famciclovir and valacyclovir are more effective than acyclovir

Herpes Simplex

- Usually presents as painful grouped vesicles.
- Causative agent: HHV 1 and 2.
- ***Herpes labialis:*** Following picture shows grouped vesicles around nose and mouth.

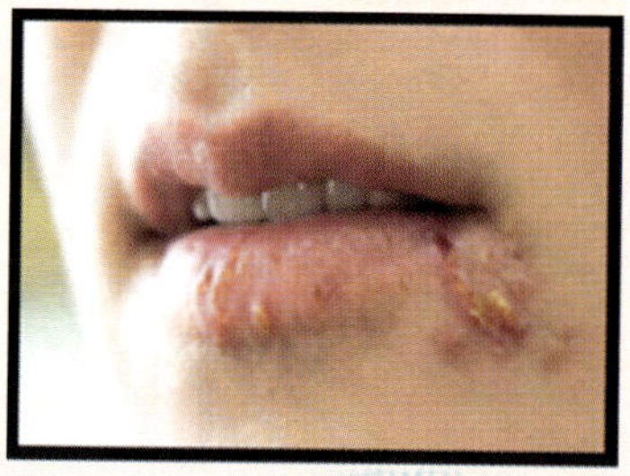

Lichen Planus

- Idiopathic Chronic inflammatory dermatosis involving skin, mucosa, nails and hair.
- ***Papulosquamous scaling disorder recognized by pruritic, polygonal, purple, plane topped papules and plaques.***
- Most commonly 30-60 years
- Koebner phenomenon is most characteristic
- ***Defective cell-mediated immunity***
- Autoimmune, chronic liver diseases, Hepatitis B and Hepatitis C
- ***Strong association with Hepatitis C virus***
- **Association:** HLA B8 in oral LP and HLA Bw-35 with cutaneous lichen planus in shins and oral mucosa
- ***Lacy reticular network in buccal mucosa/erosive stomatitis***
- ***Wickhams Striae is a network of whitish-gray lines along the papules seen due to hypergranulosis–characteristic of Lichen planus.***
- Pterygium, longitudinal ridging, onychoschizia or splitting of nail plate, pulp tenting of nail, onychodystrophy→ Nail changes

Contd.

Contd.

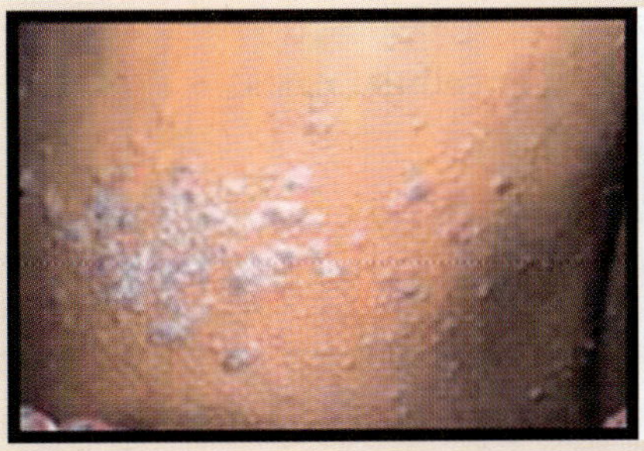

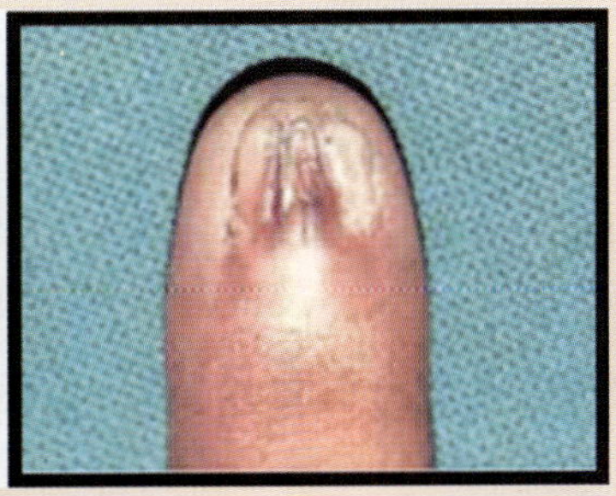

- Most important of the two is basal cell degeneration (Colloid bodies) and Lymphocytes at interface
- Can cause erosive stomatitis of mucosa
- Hypertrophic LP can increase risk of SCC
- Lichen planus pigmentosus: Slate gray macules over the photodistributed area

Treatment

- ***Commonly undergoes spontaneous remission***
- ***Topical steroids are mainstay of treatment***
- PUVA, Systemic steroids, Acitretin are systemic options available
- Oral Dapsone is used for oral Lichen Planus.

Ref: Essentials in Dermatology DM Thappa 2nd Edition Page 54 and Rook's Textbook of Dermatology 9th Edition Page 25.15, IADVL Textbook of Dermatology 4th Edition Page 594

Ans: (B) Herpes zoster

7. A female has small oral ulcers, skin rash on cheeks along with photosensitivity and relative sparing of Nasolabial fold. Likely diagnosis is:

A. SLE
B. DLE
C. Seborrheic dermatitis
D. Polymorphous light eruption

Key:

SLE often manifests as skin rash over forehead, chin, V area of neck and ears–Sparing of nasolabial folds
Most common manifestation is Malar rash–Photosensitive, Slightly raised erythema on face which worsens with flare of systemic disease

Systemic Lupus International Collaborating Clinics Classification Criteria for Systemic Lupus Erythematosus (SLE), 2012

Clinical Criteria

- Malar rash
- Discoid rash–depigmented plaque with adherent scaling *[cat tongue or tin tack or carpet tack sign]*
- Oral ulcers or nasal ulcers
- Non-scarring alopecia
- Synovitis

Contd.

Contd.

- Serositis: Pleurisy or pericarditis
- Renal disorder: Persistent proteinuria (>500 mg/day) or cellular casts
- Neurological disorder Seizures, psychosis
- Hemolytic anaemia
- Leukopenia (<4000/ mm^3 at least once) or lymphopenia (< $1000/mm^3$)
- Thrombocytopenia (<100 000/mm^3 at least once)

Immunological Criteria

- ANA above reference laboratory range
- Anti-dsDNA antibody above reference laboratory range
- Anti-Sm: Presence of antibody to Sm nuclear antigen
- Anti-phospholipid antibody positivity
- Low complement
- Direct Coombs' test in the absence of haemolytic anaemia

A patient is classified as SLE if four of clinical and immunological criteria, including atleast one clinical criteria.

Most Sensitive test for SLE	*Anti nuclear antibodies*
Most Specific test for SLE	*Anti Sm and Anti DNA antibody*
Best marker for Drug induced LE	*Anti histone antibodies*

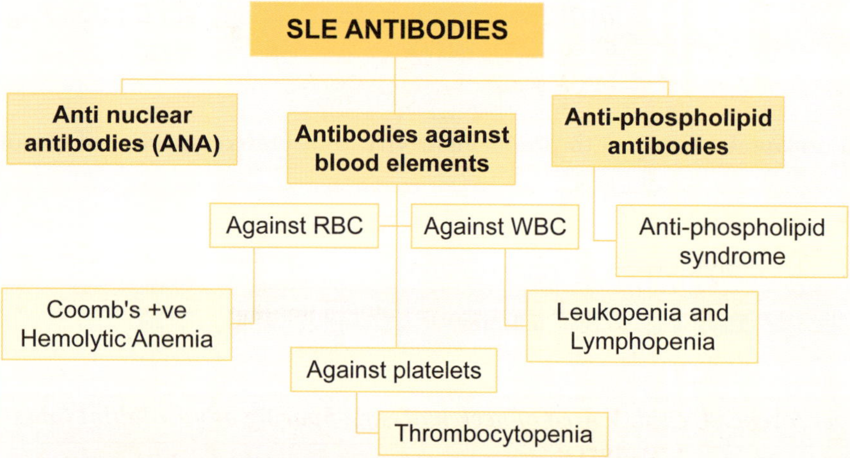

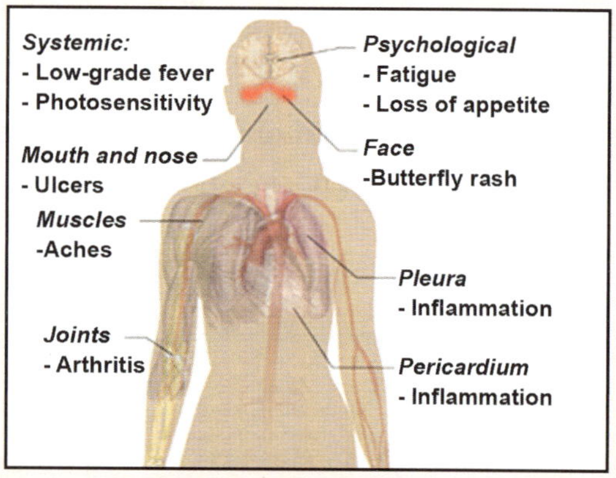

Frequently Asked Points

- ***Wire loop lesions–Most characteristic of Lupus Nephritis Class IV***
- ***Shrinking lung syndrome***–Pulmonary manifestation of SLE
- ***Most common pulmonary manifestation of SLE***–Pleuritis with/without pleural effusion
- ***Ocular manifestations***–Sicca syndrome, Non-specific conjunctivitis, Episcleritis, Retinal vasculitis and Optic neuritis
- ***Joints–Non-erosive arthritis***
- ***Most common cardiac manifestation of SLE–Pericarditis***

Polymorphic light eruption: Presents usually as itchy papules in sun exposed regions.

Ref: Rook's Textbook of Dermatology 9th Edition Page 51.15, IADVL Textbook of Dermatology 4th Edition Page 594, Harrison 20th Edition Page 2519

Ans: (A) SLE

8. **Diagnose the following condition (Patient came with axillary hyperpigmentation):**

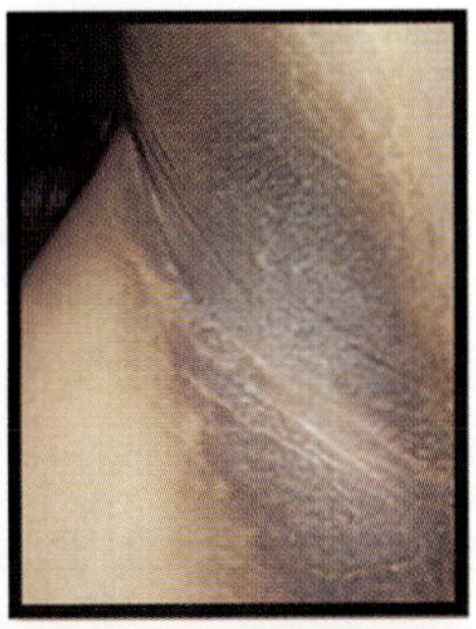

A. Erythrasma
B. Acanthosis nigricans
C. Trichomycosis axillaris
D. Tinea corporis

Key:

Picture shows hyperpigmentation with smooth symmetric velvety hyperpigmented plaque in axillary region– Indicates Acanthosis Nigricans

Acanthosis Nigricans

- Usually presents as ***smooth symmetric velvety hyperpigmented plaque*** in flexures (intertriginous areas) like neck, axilla, inframammary folds, cubital fossa and groin.

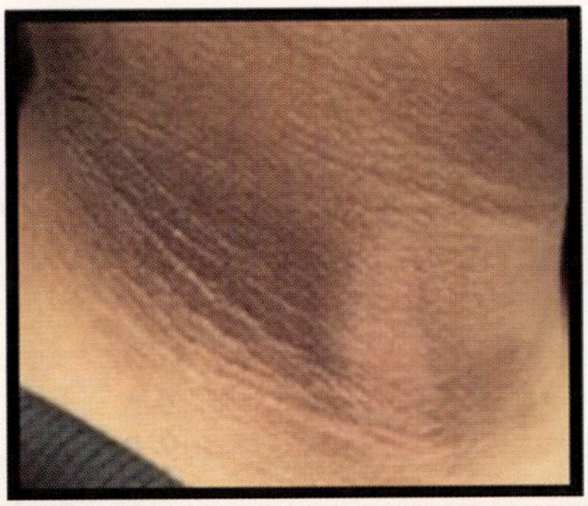

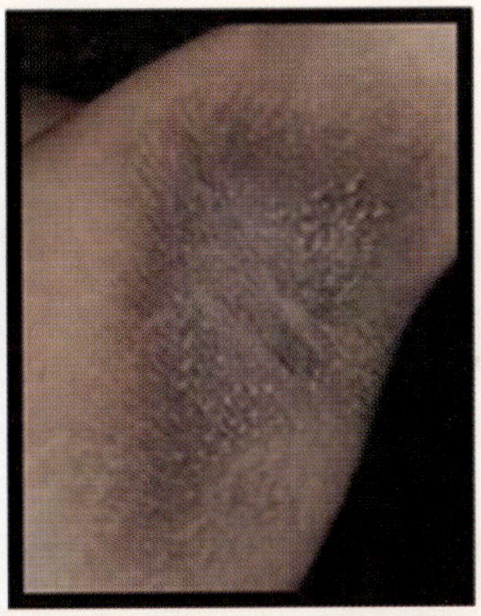

- Indication for hyperinsulinaemia and insulin resistance.

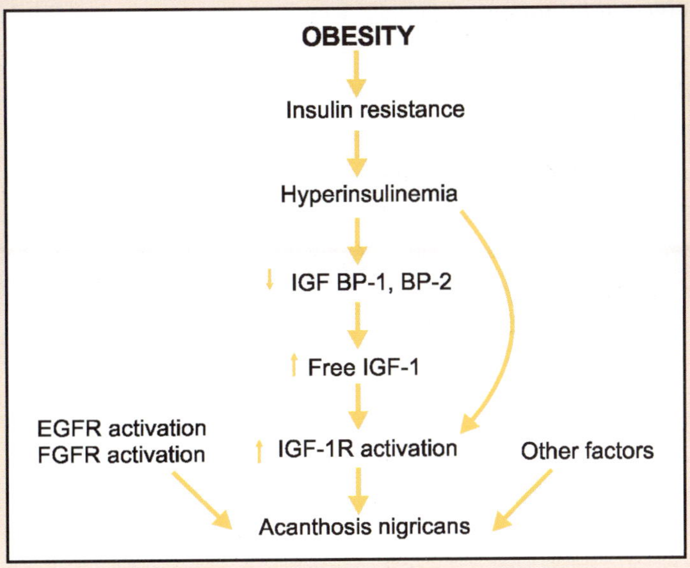

Contd.

Contd.

Etiology

1. ***Obesity (most common),*** diabetes
2. Familial
3. **HAIR AN syndrome**–Hyperandrogeneism, Insulin resistance, Acanthosis nigricans
4. Malignancy–*Gastric cancers* (most common)
5. Drug induced–Systemic steroids, oral contraceptives, nicotinc acid.

Curth Classification

- **Type 1**–Malignant AN
- **Type 2**–Benign AN/True AN (Present at birth/onset in childhood)
- **Type 3**–Pseudo AN (Associated with endocrinopathies)
- **Type 4**–Drug induced AN

Sinha and Schwartz Classification

- Obesity associated AN (Pseudo AN)
- Benign AN
- Syndromic AN
- Malignant AN
- Unilateral AN
- Acral AN
- Drug induced AN
- Mixed AN

Treatment

- Treatment of underlying condition
- Topical retinoids

Erythrasma

- Presents as symmetrical asymptomatic red brown scaly macules in flexures.
- Caused by ***Corynebacterium minutissimum***
- ***Gram stain:*** Gram positive bacilli
- *Woods lamp:* ***Coral red fluorescence***

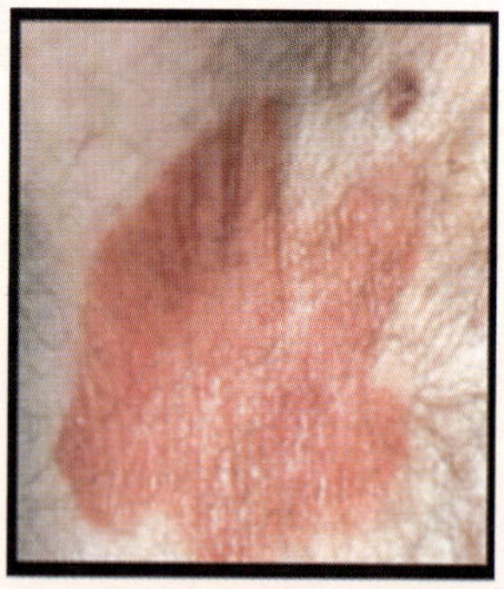

Trichomycosis Axillaris

- Presents as yellow concretions in axillary hair.
- Caused by *Corynebacterium tenuis*

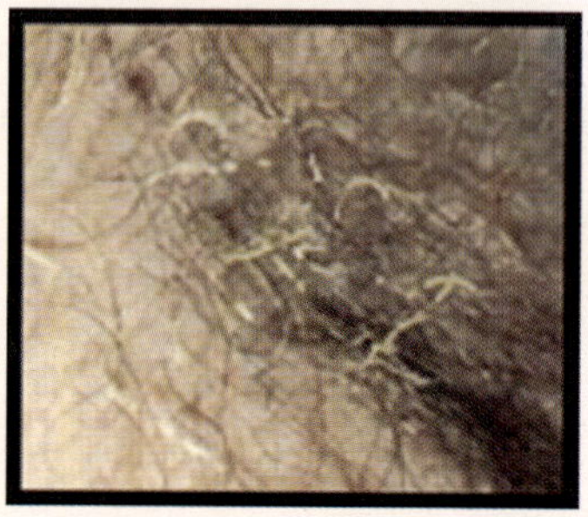

Contd.

Contd.

Tinea Corporis	
• Presents as well defined annular plaques with peripheral papulopustules and scaling • Caused by Dermatophytes ***(T. rubrum is most common organism)*** • **KOH smear**–Branched septate hyphae • **Treatment** o Oral Terbinafine or itraconazole is first line o Topical–Clotrimazole, terbinafine sertaconazole, luliconazole cream.	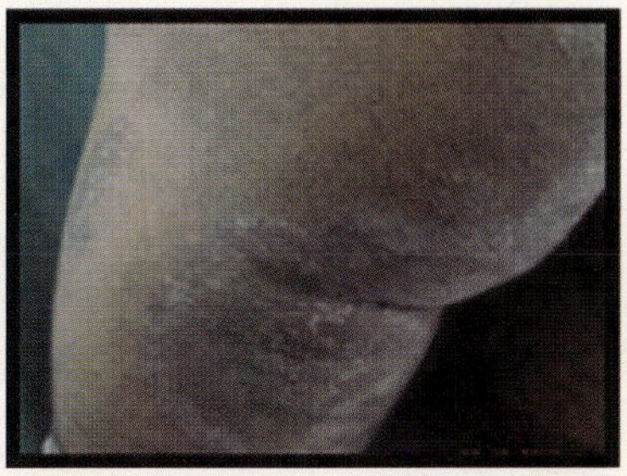

Cutaneous Markers of Malignancy	
Dermatomyositis	NPC, Ovarian, Breast, Lung, Stomach and Colon tumors Suspected if onset is after 6th or 7th decade
Necrolytic migratory erythema	Characterized clinically by erythematous, vesiculobullous areas with underlying erosion in perianal, perigenital and facial regions ***Considered a diagnostic marker for glucagonoma*** **NME without glucagonoma is known as pseudoglucagonoma**
Leser-trelat sign	Abrupt onset of seborrheic keratoses associated with an underlying cancer. ***Most commonly Gastric adenocarcinoma***
Sweet's syndrome	***Most often associated with AML,*** Involvement of eyes, muscle and internal organs. ***More severe form***
Erythroderma	Diffuse erythema and scaling in a generalized distribution. Usually is a manifestation of psoriasis, atopic dermatitis, or drug-induced allergic reactions Underlying malignant disorder such as Sezary syndrome or Mycosis fungoides (15%) or it can occur secondary to internal malignancies Suspected when there's no response to treatment
Erythema gyratum repens	Rare cutaneous marker Characterized by annular, erythematous plaques surrounded by areas of fine desquamation in ***distinctive and striking wood-grain pattern.*** Lesions expand rapidly in concentric rings after initial onset and usually pruritic ***Most commonly associated with Carcinoma lung***
Acquired ichthyosis	***Mainly lymphomas and leukemias***
Hypertrichosis lanuginosa acquisita	Abrupt appearance of Downy hair, commonly over face Most common–Lung and Colorectal carcinoma
Acanthosis nigricans	***Most common–Gastric Adenocarcinoma***
Tripe palms	***Most common–Lung Carcinoma***
Acanthosis nigricans and Triple palms	***Most common–Gastric Adenocarcinoma***
Migratory thrombophlebitis (Trosseau's syndrome)	Successive crops of tender nodules affecting blood vessels throughout the associated with Carcinoma pancreas (especially body and tail tumors)

OTHER MARKERS OF MALIGNANCY

- Paraneoplastic pemphigus associated with Hodgkins, CLL, thymoma and Castlemans disease.
- **Pyoderma gangrenosum:** Rarely a/w leukemia
- **Bazex syndrome:** Paraneoplastic acrokeratosis
- **Bowen's disease:** Intraepidemial carcinoma
- Acquired icthyosis
- **Multiple papillomata:** Cowden's disease (Multiple hamartoma syndrome)
- Erythema annulare centrifugum
- **Leser-Trélat:** Explosive onset of multiple seborrheic keratosis–ominous sign of internal malignancy as part of a paraneoplastic syndrome. Associated with gastrointestinal adenocarcinomas, Most common-stomach and colon. Also associated with paraneoplastic acanthosis nigricans (35% of patients).

Ref: Rook's Textbook of Dermatology 9th Edition Page 87.3, Essentials in Dermatology DM Thappa 2nd Edition Page 38, IADVL Textbook of Dermatology 4th Edition Page 1010

Ans: (B) Acanthosis nigricans

9. **All are true about skin except:**
   A. Dermis is derived from ectoderm
   B. Skin accounts for total of 15% of body weight
   C. Most of the cells in skin are keratinocytes derived from ectoderm
   D. Dermis is made up of type 1 and 3 collagen in 3 : 2 ratio

Key:

Dermis is derived from mesenchyme and neural crest cell

- Skin constitutes 16-20% weight of total body.
- **Skin has 3 Layers:** Epidermis, Dermis and Hypodermis (sub cutis).

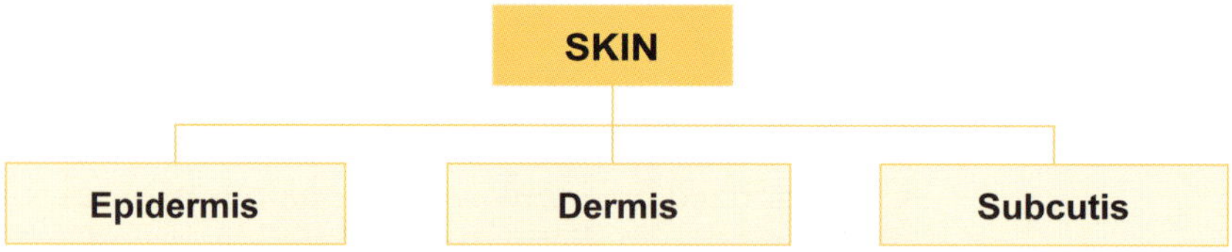

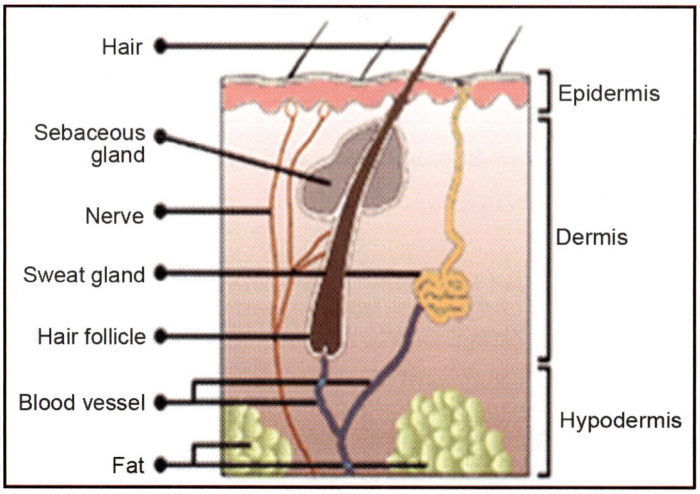

Epidermis

- Superficial stratified squamous layer
- 0.4 mm – 1.6 mm thick
- Keratinocytes – Predominant cell in epidermis
- Stratum corneum, lucidum (palms and soles), granulosum , spinosum, basale are the 5 layers seen in epidermis
- **Melanocytes, Langerhans cells, Merkel cells** are the immigrant resident cells intercalated among keratinocytes
- Embryological development–ectoderm

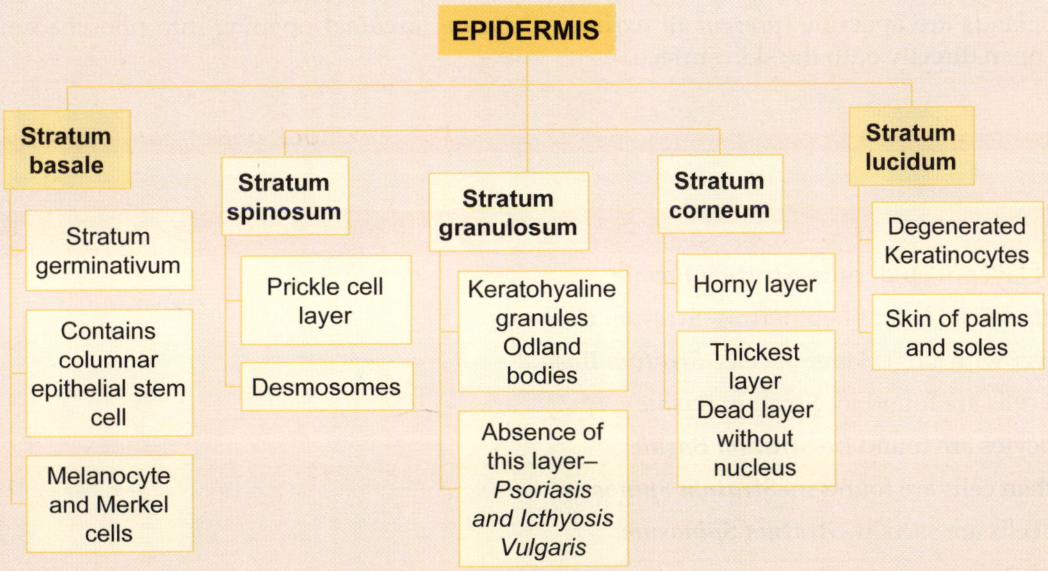

Component	Structure and Function
Stratum corneum	Semipermeable barrier with "bricks" (stacked cornified cells) and "mortar" (ceramides, cholesterol and fatty acids) like construction
Stratum granulosum	Contains keratohyalin granules that produce profilaggrin
Stratum spinosum	Contains desmosomes for intercellular adhesion
Langerhans cells	Dendritic cells, important in the modulation of the adaptive immune response
Merkel cells	Specialized cells with neuroendocrine function
Melanocytes	Dendritic cells that produce melanin for ultraviolet light protection
Basal cell layer	Contains the stem cells that divide and produce the rest of the keratinocytes in the epidermis
Basement membrane	Interface between the epidermis and dermis

Dermis

- Underlying layer consisting of connective tissue with dermal-epidermal junction basement membrane separating two.
- Contains connective tissue, **Fibres** (collagen, elastin and reticulin) + **Ground substance** (proteoglycans and GAGs)
- 1 mm (face)–4 mm (back) thick
- ***Collagen fibres: Type I (80%), Type III (10%)***
- Embryological development–***dermis from mesenchyme and neural crest cell.***

Contd.

Contd.

Subcutis

- Made up of adipocytes
- Embryological development – mesenchyme

Subcutaneous Fat (Panniculus)

- Consisting of fat lobules and fat septae (fibrous tissue).

Adnexa

- Appendages attached into skin are called as ***adnexae.***
- Pilosebaceous unit, nail and sweat glands are included in ***'appendages'.***
- Sweat glands are apocrine ***(present in axillae, perineum, areolae)*** opening into pilosebaceous unit or eccrine which open directly onto the skin surface.

High Yield

- Deepest layer of epidermis–***Stratum Basale***
- Most superficial layer of epidermis–***Stratum Corneum***
- Skin layer with single layer of cells–***Stratum Basale***
- Merkel cells are found in–***Stratum Basale***
- Melanocytes are found in–***Stratum Basale***
- Langerhan cells are found in–***Stratum Spinosum***
- Prickle cells are seen in–***Stratum Spinosum***
- Keratohyaline granules are found in–***Stratum Granulosum***
- Filagrin and Trichohyalin are found in–***Stratum Granulosum***
- Eleidin is found in–***Stratum Lucidum***

Ref: Essentials in Dermatology DM Thappa 2nd Edition Page 8,
IADVL Textbook of Dermatology 4th Edition Page 7,
Rook's Textbook of Dermatology 9th Edition Page 2

Ans: (A) Dermis is derived from ectoderm

Chapter 17

ANESTHESIA

1. **Injection of all of the following drugs is painful except:**

A. Propofol
B. Etomidate
C. Ketamine
D. Methohexitone

Key:

Ketamine doesn't result in pain on intravenous injection

Propofol

- Phenol based intravenous anaesthetic, Milky white powder
- Oil based preparation–contains soyabean, egg lecithin and glycerol
- Elimination half life–2 to 4 hours
- Regains consciousness–2 to 8 minutes
- No analgesia and No muscle relaxation
- Mechanism of action–GABA mediated
- ***Investigation of choice for Day care surgery***
- ***Agent of choice for Total intravenous anaesthesia***
- **Agent of choice for Induction in those susceptible to malignant hyperthermia**
- Used for control of status epilepticus
- ***Dose related surgical anaesthesia***
- Potential advantage of propofol for sedation of ICU–Antioxidant property
- **Systemic effects:** *Hypotension, Apnea, Cerebroprotective, Myoclonic, Bronchodilatation on COPD patients Anti emetic and Antipruritic*
- ***Arterial hypotension–Important side effect***
- Myoclonic movement may occur with propofol but short lived and not dangerous
- Propofol infusion syndrome–Occurs if given at rate of 4 mg/kg/hr or more for 48 hours/Longer

Etomidate

- Non barbiturate intravenous induction anaesthetic agent
- ***Depresses cortisol and aldosterone synthesis by inhibiting 11 beta hydroxylase***–Causes adrenocortical suppression
- ***Most cardiostable IV agent***
- ***Agent of choice for cardiac disease***
- Causes Vitamin C deficiency
- Doesn't depress arterial pressure
- ***Useful in sick and shock patients as induction agent***
- Neuroprotective
- Pain on injection and Thrombophlebitis
- Nausea and Vomiting on Recovery–Maximum incidence

Ketamine

- Phencyclidine derivative
- ***Produces Dissociative Anaesthesia***
  (State of profound analgesia, Light sleep, Increased muscle tone and Emergence delirium).
- Marked analgesia is prominent feature
- ***Primary site of action–Thalamo-neocortical projection***
- Inhibits thalamus and cortex but stimulates limbic system
- Exerts effect by inhibiting N methyl D aspartate receptors
- ***Intravenous agent of choice in burn patients–Ketamine***
- ***Anaesthetic agent of choice in shock–Ketamine***
- ***Anaesthetic agent of choice for asthmatics–Ketamine***
- Hallucination–Most common CNS side effect
- Strongest analgesic property
- Preferred in patients with R→L shunts, Congestive heart failure, Asthma and COPD
- Contraindicated in patients with raised ICT and Intracranial pathology

Methohexitone

- Ultra short acting Barbiturate
- 2-3 times more potent than thiopentone
- Less CVS depression
- Causes abnormal spike discharges in Epileptic patients–Induces seizures
- ***Agent of choice for Electroconvulsive therapy***

Pain on injection

Intra arterial injection
Thiopental

Intravenous injection

- **With thrombophlebitis**
  - Etomidate
- **Without thrombophlebitis**
  - Propofol
  - Methohexital
  - Thiopental

Features	Thiopentone	Propofol	Ketamine
Nausea and Vomiting	–	Antiemetic	+
Pain on intravenous injection	+	+ *(Max)*	–
Blood pressure	Decreased	Decreased *(Max)*	Increased
Cardiac output	Decreased	Decreased *(Max)*	Increased
Intracranial pressure	Decreased	Decreased	Increased
Intraocular pressure	Decreased	Decreased	Increased
Respiratory rate	Decreased	Decreased	Increased

☞ EXTRA EDGE (Intravenous Agents)

- *Most commonly used intravenous induction agent–**Thiopentone***
- *Agent of choice for cerebral protection–**Thiopentone***
- *Intravenous agent of choice for day care surgery–**Propofol***
- *Agent of choice for TIVA–**Propofol***
- *Agent of choice for induction of malignant hyperthermia susceptibility–**Propofol***
- *Agent of choice for ECT–**Methohexitone***
- *Most cardiostable intravenous agent–**Etomidate***
- *Intravenous agent causing maximum nausea and vomiting–**Etomidate***
- *Intravenous agent of choice for shock–**Ketamine***
- *Preferred agent for patients with full stomach–**Ketamine***
- *Intravenous agent of choice for asthmatics–**Ketamine***

Ref: Miller 7th Edition Page 567, Lee 13th Edition Page 129, Morgan 6th Edition Page 318, Yao 7th Edition Page 524, Aitkenhead 4th Edition Page 178, Ajay Yadav 4th Edition Page 148

Ans: (C) Ketamine

2. **Which intravenous anaesthetic agent doesn't cause cardiac depression?**

A. Etomidate
B. Ketamine
C. Propofol
D. Thiopentone

Key:

Etomidate doesn't cause cardiac depression–Most cardiostable IV agent

Etomidate

- Non barbiturate intravenous induction anaesthetic agent
- ***Depresses cortisol and aldosterone synthesis by inhibiting 11 beta hydroxylase***–Causes adrenocortical suppression
- ***Most cardiostable IV agent***
- ***Agent of choice for cardiac disease***–Cardiovascular stability after induction

Effects of etomidate induction dose

- Negligible increase in heart rate.
- Little decrease in blood pressure/cardiac output.
- Little effect on coronary perfusion pressure and reducing myocardial O_2 consumption

- Causes Vitamin C deficiency
- Doesn't depress arterial pressure–***Useful in sick and shock patients as induction agent***
- Neuroprotective
- Pain on injection and Thrombophlebitis
- Nausea and Vomiting on Recovery–Maximum incidence

Ref: Miller 7th Edition Page 567, Lee 13th Edition Page 129, Morgan 6th Edition Page 318, Yao 7th Edition Page 524, Aitkenhead 4th Edition Page 178, Ajay Yadav 4th Edition Page 148

Ans: (A) Etomidate

3. **Which of the following inhalational anaesthetic agent causes maximum respiratory irritation?**

A. Enflurane
B. Halothane
C. Sevoflurane
D. Desflurane

Key:

Desflurane when used for induction cause respiratory irritation due to their pungent smell leading to breath holding and coughing. Halothane and sevoflurane do not cause such effects

DESFLURANE

- Fluorinated congener of Isoflurane
- ***Colourless liquid***
- ***Pungent***–Induction is Unpleasant
- Highly volatile, Extremely low oil gas partition coefficient
- Very low solubility in blood and tissue, Vapour pressure is very high

- *Induction and Recovery is very fast–(MAC 0.42)*
- Minimal metabolism in humans
- Minimal cardiac depression like Isoflurane
- ***Safe anaesthetic agent for geriatric age group as its CVS effects are similar to Isoflurane but without coronary steel phenomenon***
- ***Commonly used as anaesthetic for Out patient departments***
- **Agent of choice–**Prolonged duration surgeries, Old age patients and Obese patients

Property	Isoflurane	Desflurane	Sevoflurane
Potency	Similar to halothane	Similar to isoflurane	Similar to desflurane
Analgesia	Strong	Strong	Strong
Induction	Rapid and smooth	Rapid and smooth	Rapid and smooth
Irritability	Non pungent	Pungent	Non pungent
Recovery	Rapid	Rapid	Rapid
Postop nausea	Not significant	Not significant	Not significant
Respiratory system	90% gets excreted through respiration	–	***Bronchodilator***
CVS	Doesn't sensitize heart to adrenaline, Hypotension	Transient sympathetic stimulation, tachycardia	–
Liver	Safer	Safer	Safer
Kidney	Non toxic	Non toxic	***Nephrotoxic*** *Biotransformed to fluoride ions*
CNS	Only mild vasodilatation, ***Preferred in CNS***	–	–
Muscle relaxation	–	–	–

☞ EXTRA EDGE (Inhalational Agents)

- *Maximum respiratory depression–**Enflurane***
- *Maximum bronchodilatation in non asthmatics–**Sevoflurane***
- *Agent of choice in children–**Sevoflurane***
- *Best maintenance of cardiac output–**Isoflurane***
- *Maximum Hypotension–**Isoflurane***
- *Agent of choice in cardiac patients–**Isoflurane***
- *Agent of choice for Maintenance in liver disease–**Isoflurane***
- *Agent of choice for Neurosurgery–**Isoflurane***
- *Maximum inhibition of ventilator response–**Halothane***
- *Agent of choice in Asthma–**Halothane***
- *Maximum bronchodilatation in asthmatics–**Halothane***
- *Inhibition of myocardial contractility–**Halothane***
- *Maximum sensitization of heart to adrenaline–**Halothane***

Contd.

Contd.

- *Maximum hepatocellular damage–**Halothane***
- *Maximum nephrotoxicity–**Methoxyflurane***
- *Agent causing megaloblastic and aplastic anemia–**Nitrous oxide***
- *Agent causing Subacute combined degeneration of Spinal cord–**Nitrous oxide***
- *Agent that causes maximum muscle relaxation–**Desflurane***
- *Agent of choice in kidney disease–**Desflurane***
- *Agent that causes maximum hyperglycemia–**Chloroform***
- *Agent contraindicated in renal disease–**Methoxyflurane***
- *Agent causing maximum analgesia–**Trielene***
- *Agent of choice for maintenance in dental procedures–**Enflurane***

Ref: Ajay Yadav 6th Edition Page 61, Miller 7th Edition Page 307, Lee 12th Edition Page 328, Morgan 5th Edition Page 169, Yao 7th Edition Page 524, Aitkenhead 4th Edition Page 153

Ans: (D) Desflurane

5. **Advantage of cisatracurium over atracurium is:**
   A. Short duration of action
   B. Rapid onset
   C. Less allergic
   D. Releases less histamine

Key:

Cisatracurium undergoes Hoffmann elimination predominantly, Laudosine production is 5 times lesser than atracurium and No histamine release–5 times more potent than atracurium

HISTAMINE RELEASE–ATRACURIUM

- Observed in 40% of patients
- Transient hypotension and tachycardia with facial and truncal flushing
- Atracurium with minimal CVS side effects has histamine release
- Prevented by injecting drug slowly over 75 sec, reducing dose or prior treatment with chlorpheniramine or cemitidine intravenously

Non Depolarising Agents

Ultra short	Short	Intermediate	Long
Rapacuronium GW 280430	Mivacurium	Vecuronium Atracurium Cis-atracurium Rocuronium	Pancuronium d-Tubocurare Gallamine Metocurine Doxacurium Pipecuronium

Contd.

Contd.

Rapacurium

- Not used any more–Severe Bronchospasm

Mivacurium

- Shorte acting non depolarizing muscle relaxant (10-20 min)
- Metabolized by esterases (Pseudocholinesterase)
- Quick onset and Short duration
- No reversal required
- ***Muscle relaxant of choice in day care surgeries***

Atracurium

- Undergoes Hoffmann elimination (45%)
- Inactivated in plasma by spontaneous non enzymatic degradation and by choline esterase
- **Major metabolite–Laudosine (CNS Stimulant)**–*Results in epileptiform fits*
- Acrylate–Another metabolite
- Duration of action is not altered in hepatic and renal failure
- ***Muscle relaxant of choice in renal and hepatic failure***
- Histamine release–Flushing of Skin
- ***Muscle relaxant of choice in Mysthenia gravis***
- Reversal–Neostigmine
- Avoid in asthma patients

Cisatracurium

- Undergoes Hoffmann elimination predominantly (77%)
- No ester hydrolysis
- Laudosine production is 5 times ***lesser than*** atracurium
- No histamine release
- 5 times more potent than atracurium

Rocuronium

- Earliest onset of action among non depolarizing agents
- ***Muscle relaxant of choice in precurarization***
- ***Non depolarizing muscle relaxant of choice for Intubation***

Vecuronium

- Most commonly used muscle relaxant for routine surgery
- ***Muscle relaxant of choice in cardiac patients***
- Most cardiostable
- Site of action–Myoneural junction
- Metabolized in liver and Excreted in bile–Contraindicated in liver diseases
- Causes polyneuropathy on long-term usage

Pancuronium

- Quarternary amino Steroidal compound–Devoid of Hormonal activity
- Causes vagal blockade and releases noradrenaline–Tachycardia and HTN
- ***Muscle relaxant of choice in shock and hypotension***
- Doesn't cross BBB

Contd.

Contd.

- 5 times more potent than d tubocurare
- Safe in patients susceptible to malignant hyperpyrexia
- Metabolized by kidney–Avoid in Renal failure

Doxacurium

- Longest acting
- More potent non depolarizing skeletal muscle relaxant
- Doesn't release histamine

Pipecuronium

- Long acting steroid analogue of pancuronium
- No vagolytic activity or ganglionic blockade

D-Tubocurarine

- Highest histamine release–Asthma and Anaphylaxis
- Maximum ganglionic blockade and Severe hypotension
- Doesn't cross placenta–***Muscle relaxant of choice in Obstetrics***

Advantages of Smooth Muscle Relaxants	
Atracurium	Hoffman elimination, Useful in renal and hepatic failure
Cisatracurium	Less prone to cause histamine release
Pancuronium	1st steroid derived neuromuscular blockade, Causes slight tachycardia
Vecuronium	No histamine release
Rocuronium	Rapid onset of onset
Mivacurium	Shortest acting

EXTRA EDGE

- Muscle relaxant of choice in liver disease–***Atracurium/Cisatracurium***
- Muscle relaxant of choice in Renal disease–***Atracurium/Cisatracurium***
- Muscle relaxant of choice in CABG–Vecuronium
- Muscle relaxant of choice in IHD–Vecuronium
- Muscle relaxant of choice in Cyanotic heart disease–Pancuronium
- Muscle relaxant of choice to reduce BP–Tubocurarine
- Muscle relaxant of choice to increase BP–Pancuronium
- Muscle relaxant of choice in Myasthenia gravis–Atracurium

Ref: Miller 7th Edition Page 862, Lee 13th Edition Page 186, Morgan 5th Edition Page 215, Stoelting 5th Edition Page 136, Aitkenhead 4th Edition Page 227, Ajay Yadav 4th Edition Page 98

Ans: (D) Releases less histamine

6. **Most commonly used objective method for knowing depth of anaesthesia:**

A. CVP
B. Capnography
C. Esophageal contractility
D. Bispectral Imaging

Key:

BIS (Bispectral imaging) offers more effective method of assessing depth of anaesthesia

Bispectral Index

- 1st scientifically validated and commercially available monitor to check depth of anaesthesia.
- Analyses EEG data and quantitates anaesthetic effects on brain–*Especially hypnotic effect*
- **Composite numerical index–**Represents dimensionless numerical value that has been correlated with patients current hypnotic state/depth of anaesthesia and provides assurance that anaesthesized patient is asleep
- Utilizes parameters (EEG signals, eye blinks) to calculate depth score.
- *Reduces chance of patient awareness during anaesthesia*
- **Method of BIS:**
  - Combines power spectral analysis of phase relationships with component sine waves
  - EEG feature–best correlated with clinical depth of sedation and anaesthesia fitted to model.
- *BIS identifies EEG patterns with in 30 sec period*
- First it excludes artifact episodes and then periods of burst suppression are monitored
- Individual operative awareness is monitored by *Bispectral imaging index*
- **Disadvantage–**High cost and chance of Inaccuracy

BIS	Awareness Level and Depth of Anaesthesia
100	Awake (Memory intact, Respond to verbal command)
85-65	Sedation
65-40	*General anaesthesia* (No awareness, Deep hypnosis, Memory function lost)
<40	Cortical suppression becomes discernible, Increasing burst suppression
0	Cortical silence (Isoelectric), Deeply anaesthesized

Variations of BIS

- Better response with Isoflurane and Propofol than Opiates
- BIS values decrease in patients receiving NM Blocker and while fully conscious
- Unchanged/even elevated during N_2O anaesthesia
- Elevated during IV Ketamine anaesthesia

Capnography

- *Capnography is based on Luft principle*
- Continues measurement of End tidal carbon dioxide ($EtCO_2$)

Contd.

Contd.

- Normal 32-42 mm Hg
- **Flat capnogram**–Disconnection of anesthetic tubing, accidental extubation, mechanical ventilation failure

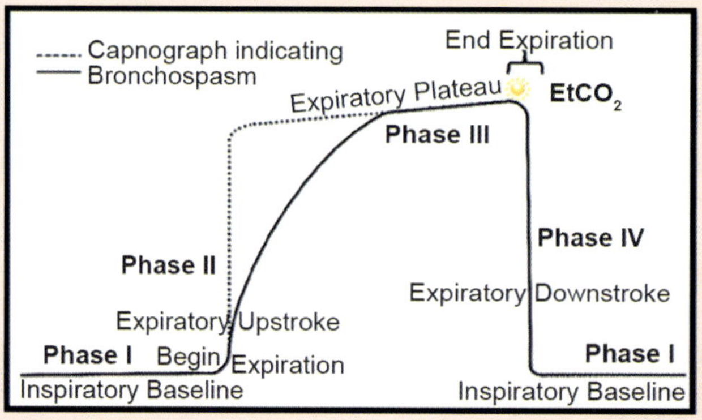

- **Phases of Capnogram:**
  - Phase 0–Inspiratory phase
  - Phase 1–Deadspace and little or no CO_2
  - Phase 2–Mixture of alveolar and dead space gas
  - Phase 3–Alveolar plateau with peak representing End Expiratory and End tidal CO_2

Uses of Capnography

- Confirming of correct intubations
- Intraoperative displacement of tube
- Diagnosis of malignant hyperthermia
- For detecting obstruction, disconnections
- Exhausted soda lime or defective valves
- Indicator of cardiac output

CVP

- Most common vein for CVP monitoring is ***Right Internal Jugular Vein***
- CVP monitoring–Most useful in guiding hemodynamic therapy

2D Transesophageal Echocardiography

- ***Most sensitive and practical technique to detect myocardial ischemia in perioperative period***–2D transesophageal echocardiography, regional wall motion abnormality can be detected

Must Know Points

- ***BIS offers more effective method of assessing depth of anaesthesia***
- End tidal CO_2 monitoring is commonly used in clinical practice to assess depth of anaesthesia–***Only possible when volatile anaesthetic agents are used.***

Ref: Miller 7th Edition Page 35, Lee 13th Edition Page 117, Morgan 5th Edition Page 132, Dorsch 5th Edition Page 807, Aitkenhead 5th Edition Page 201, Anaesthesia Science by Webster 1st Edition Page 434

Ans: (D) Bispectral Imaging

Chapter 18

RADIOLOGY AND RADIOTHERAPY

1. Identify the diagnosis from the chest X-ray of patient with low grade fever:

A. Interstitial lung disease
B. Bronchopneumonia
C. Miliary TB
D. Consolidation

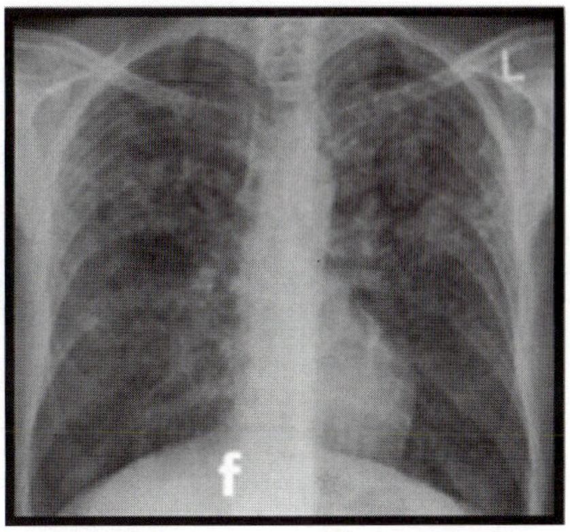

Key:

Picture shows multiple small discrete nodules scattered evenly through out both lungs on Chest X-ray–Points diagnosis to be Miliary TB
Don't reach beyond 5 mm size and associated with Low grade fever

MILIARY TUBERCULOSIS

- Uncommon pulmonary manifestation of tuberculosis.
- Represents haematogeneous dissemination of uncontrolled tuberculous infection and carries a relatively poor prognosis.
- Seen both in primary and post-primary tuberculosis.
- May be associated with tuberculous infection in numerous other tissues and organs.
- **Plain X-ray:** ***Miliary deposits appear as 1-3 mm diameter nodules, which are uniform in size and uniformly distributed.***
- **CT scan:** Similar findings to plain film but may more elaborately show extent and distribution.

Criteria for Diagnosis of Miliary TB

- Clinical presentation consistent with diagnosis of TB like pyrexia with evening rise of temperature, weight loss, anorexia, tachycardia and night sweats of >6 weeks duration responding to ATT.
- Classical miliary pattern on chest radiograph.
- Bilateral diffuse reticulonodular lung lesions on background of miliary shadows demonstrable either on plain radiograph or HRCT; and
- Microbiological or histopathological evidence of TB.

- **Differential Diagnosis:** *Metastasis, Fungal, Pneumoconiosis, Sarcoidosis and Eosinophilic granuloma*

Tuberculous Lesions

Primary TB

- ***Ghon's lesion***–Consolidation and enlarged lymph nodes (Commonly subpleural perifissural)
- ***Mimics community acquired pneumonia***
- ***Endobronchial spread****–Tree-in-bud appearance*
- Peripherally enhancing conglomerate lesions–Necrotic Lymph nodes on CT
- Nodal pressure can cause segmental collapse
- Lymphadenopathy is Hallmark with/without pneumonia
- ***Rasmussen Aneurysm***–Rare life threatening complication of cavitary TB caused by Granulomatous weakening of Pulmonary arterial wall.

Post Primary TB

- Previous infection/BCG vaccination hypersensitivity
- Apicoposterior of Upper and Superior segments of lower lobes–Most common site
- Poorly marginated nodular and linear opacities
- Greater inflammatory reaction and caseous necrosis

Secondary TB

- Involves apical segments of upper lower lobes
- Cavitations and Fibrosis

Miliary TB

- Pin-point mottling of millet seeds

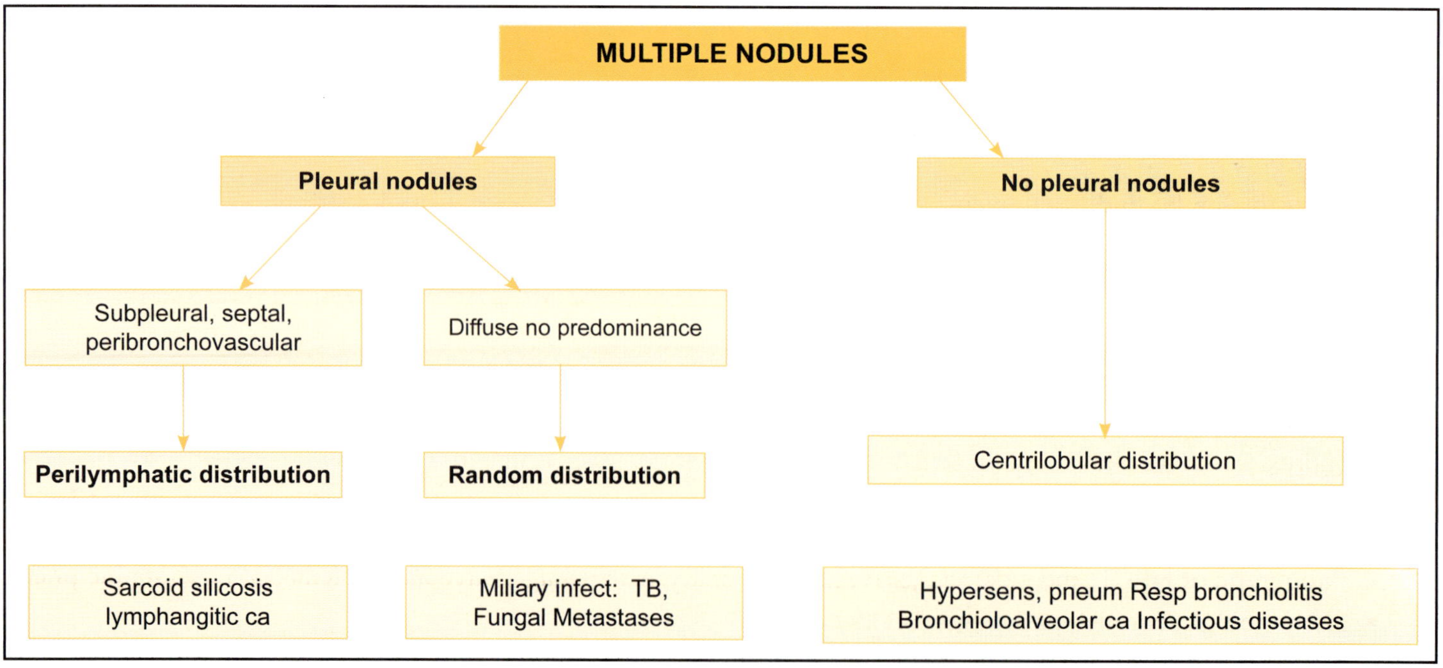

Pneumonia Right Upper Lobe	Consolidation Left Lower Lobe	Interstitial Lung Disease
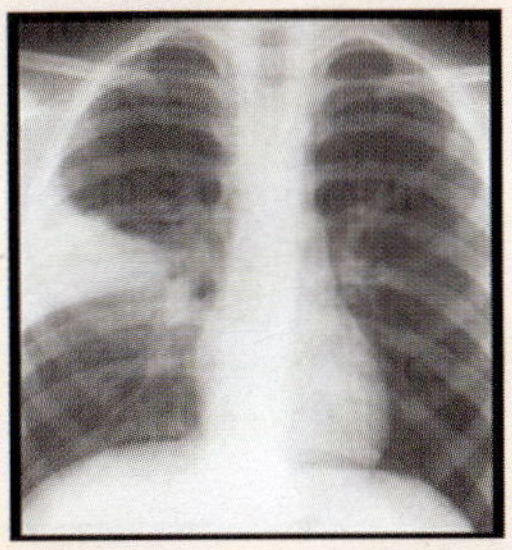	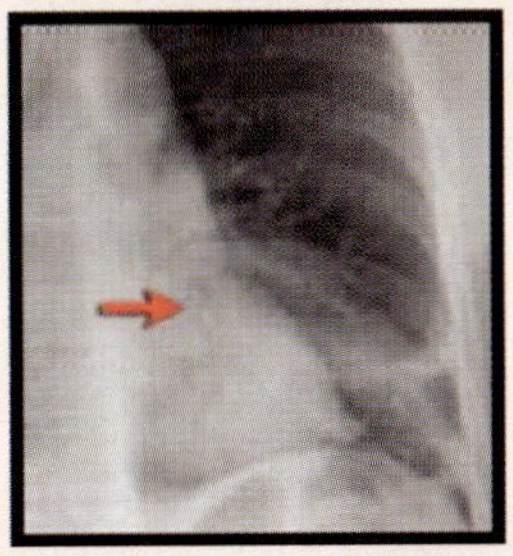	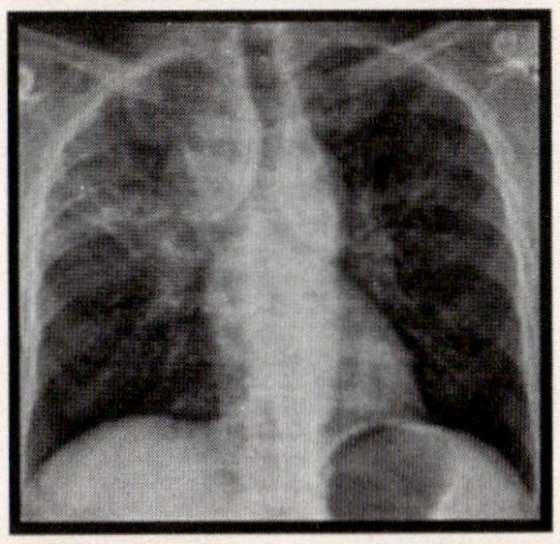
Atelectasis Left Lung	**COPD: Hyperinflated Lung Fields**	**Pulmonary Hamartoma**
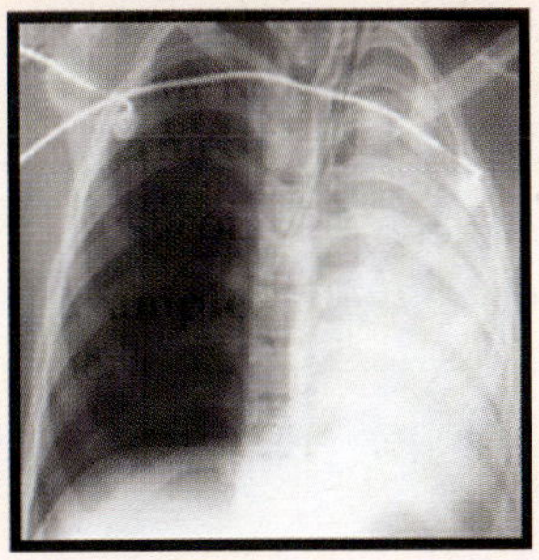	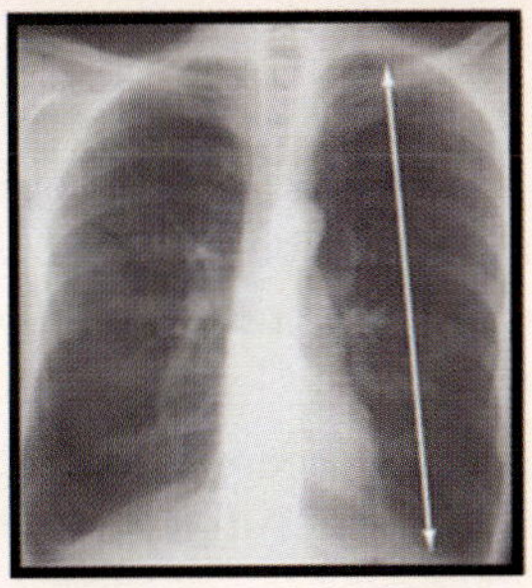	Pop-corn calcification and Irregular calcification 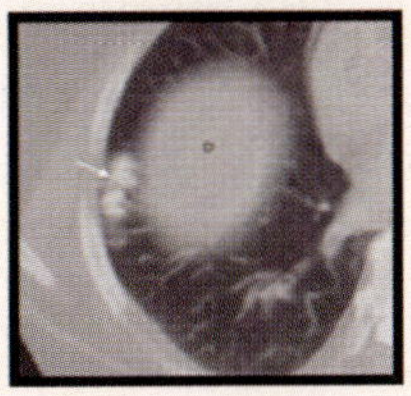

- *Isolated Anterior segment involvement excludes diagnosis of TB*
- **Ranke's complex:** ***Gohn focus + calcified nodes ipsilaterally + Draining lymphatics***
- **CECT–Investigation of choice for Consolidation and Collapse**
- **Pneumatocele–***Staphylococcal pneumonia*
- **Bulging fissure sign–***Klebsiella pneumonia (Right upper lobe)*
- **Pneumococcal pneumonia–***Opacity in Basal zone*
- **Mycoplasma pneumonia–***Fine reticulonodular shadows followed by consolidation*
- **Viral pneumonia–***Peribronchial shadowing, Fine reticulonodular shadows, Consolidation*

Interstitial Lung Disease	
Reticular pattern	Fibrosing alveolitis, Asbestosis, Sarcoidosis, Chronic allergic alveolitis, LCH and LAM
Nodular pattern	Silicosis, Coal worker pneumoconiosis, Sarcoidosis, TB
Reticulonodular pattern	LCH, Sarcoidosis, Lymphangitis carcinomatosa
Septal pattern	Interstitial pulmonary edema, Lymphangitis carcinomatosa
Ground glass pattern	Pneumocystis jerovecii, Pulmonary hemorrhage, Alveolar proteinosis, Eosinophilic pneumonia, Collagen vascular disease
Tree in bud	Endobronchial TB, Atypical TB

Version 2

A patient evaluated for PUO is having the following chest X-ray:

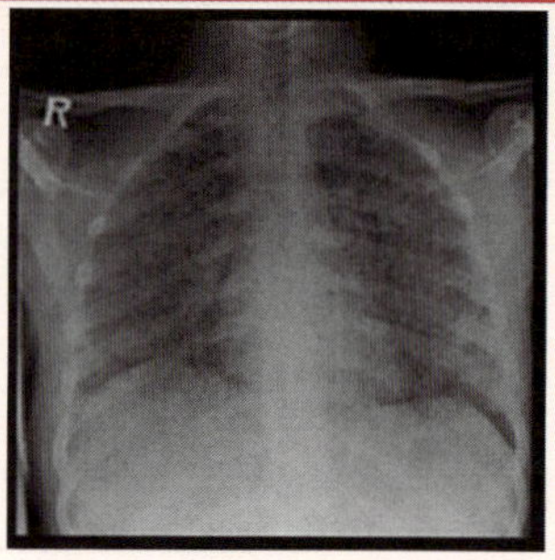

A. Malaria

B. Miliary TB

C. Sarcoidosis

D. Wegener's granulomatosis

MILIARY TUBERCULOSIS

- Form of tuberculosis that is characterized by a wide dissemination into the human body and by the tiny size of the lesions (1–5 mm).
- Miliary TB patients often have non-specific signs like cough and enlarged lymph nodes.
- Miliary tuberculosis can also present with enlarged liver (40% of cases), enlarged spleen (15%), inflammation of the pancreas (<5%), and multiple organ dysfunction with adrenal insufficiency ***(Adrenal glands do not produce enough steroid hormones to regulate organ function).***
- Sputum, pleural fluid, CSF, urine, bronchoscopic secretions, blood and tissue biopsy specimens have all been employed to confirm diagnosis of disseminated and miliary TB with varying results.
- Enzyme linked immunosorbent assay for detecting mycobacterial antigens, antibodies, and immunecomplexes in the blood and body fluids have been used for the diagnosis of disseminated and miliary TB.

Ans: (B) Miliary TB

Ref: Radiology Review Manual 7th Edition Page 472, David Sutton 7th Edition Page 190, Armstrong 5th Edition Page 78, Tuberculosis by Sharma 2nd Edition Page 511

Ans: (C) Miliary TB

2. **Water soluble radiopaque contrast most commonly contains:**

A. Barium B. Iodine

C. Bromium D. Calcium

Key:

Water soluble radiopaque contrast most commonly contains Iodine

Contrast Media for X-ray and CT

Positive contrast	Negative contrast
Contrast material is radiopaque High atomic number material White on film	Contrast material is not radiopaque Low atomic number material Black on film
Example: Barium sulphate	*Example:* Water, Air and CO_2

Condition	Dye
Myelography, Ventriculography, DSA	*Iopamidol, Iohexol, Myodil, Metrizamide*
Patency and Integrity of Recent anastomosis, Idiopathic Megacolon/Hirschsprung's disease	*Gastrograffin enema*
Esophageal atresia	*Dianosil*

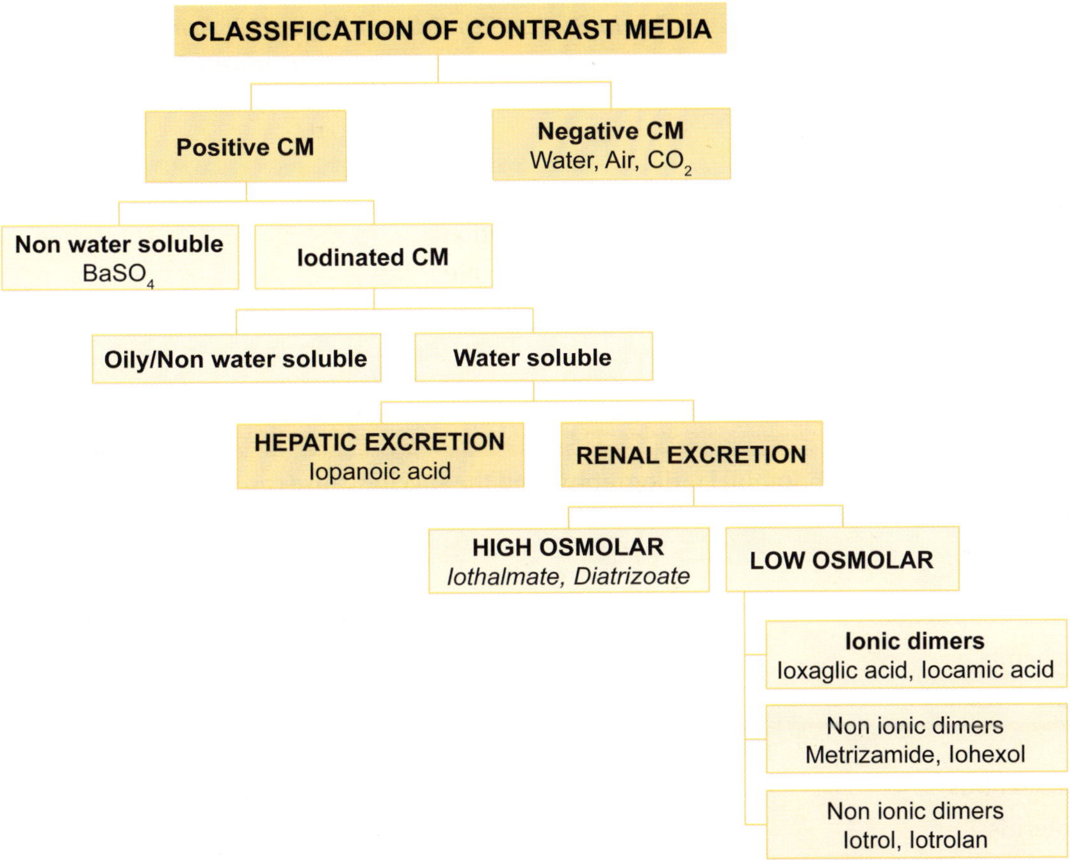

- **Myodil**–Contrast agent used for myelography is outdated now→ It results in Arachnoiditis
- **Metrizaide–Causes Flapping tremor**

Allergic reactions of iodine contrast media		
Severity	**Clinical features**	**Treatment**
Mild	Rash, Flushing, Feeling of warmth and Headache	Inj. Avil
Moderate	Severe urticaria, Fever, Perspiration, Rash and Hypotension	Inj. Avil, Inj. Hydrocortisone and IV Fluids
Severe	Bronchospasm, Convulsions, Hypotensive shock	IV Fluids, Inj. Adrenaline

Contraindications to iodinated contrast	
Absolute	**Relative**
CRF with Serum creatinine >2 mg% Previous history of allergic reaction Multiple myeloma (Acute renal shutdown)	Asthma Metformin therapy Severe cardiac therapy Sickle cell anemia Diabetic nephropathy

Ref: Radiology Review Manual 7th Edition Page 1147, David Sutton 7th Edition Page 418, Armstrong 5th Edition Page 430, Cannon Review of Radiology Page 627

Ans: (B) Iodine

3. **Gasless abdomen is seen in:**

A. Acute pancreatitis
B. Intussusception
C. Necrotising enterocolitis
D. Ulcerative colitis

Key:

Gasless Abdomen

- Refers to a paucity of gas on abdominal radiography, and the specific cause can usually be identified when patient's history is known.

Common Causes

- Small bowel obstruction
- Bowel ischemia
- Congenital atresia
- Ascites
- Acute Pancreatitis
- Gastroenteritis
- Large abdominal mass–due to displacement
- Post surgery following total colectomy, oesophagogastrectomy, gastrectomy, and low anterior resection
- Paucity of small bowel gas may be a normal finding in some adults

GASLESS ABDOMEN

- **Infants**
  - Esophageal atresia, Duodenal atresia
  - Volvulus, Annular pancreas
  - Hypertrophic pyloric stenosis,
  - Fluid filled bowel
  - Choledochal cyst, Excess vomiting,
  - Congenital diaphragmatic hernia
- **Adults**
  - High obstruction,
  - Acute pancreatitis,
  - Fluid filled bowel
  - Large abdominal mass
  - Ascites, Normal

Key Signs/Features in GIT

- *Antral beaking sign*–Congenital hypertrophic pyloric stenosis
- *Antral pad sign*–Pancreatic ductal adenocarcinoma
- *Bird beak/Rat tail*–Achalasia cardia
- *Bird of prey sign*–Sigmoid volvulus
- *Carman meniscus sign*–Carcinoma stomach
- *Chain of beads appearance*–Diffuse esophageal spasm
- *Coffee bean appearance*–Sigmoid volvulus
- *Concertina pattern/Herring bone pattern*–Jejunal obstruction
- *Cork screw esophagus*–Diffuse esophageal spasm
- *Creeping fat sign*–Crohn's disease
- *Crescentic shadow/Meniscus sign*–Gall stone
- *Copula sign*–Pneumoperitoneum
- *Football sign*–Pneumoperitoneum
- *Single bubble appearance*–Pyloric stenosis
- *Double bubble appearance*–Duodenal atresia, Midgut Volvulus, Duodenal stenosis, Annular pancreas, Preduodenal position of portal vein
- *Triple bubble appearance*–Jejunal atresia
- *Double duct sign on USG*–Pancreatic carcinoma
- *Frostberg inverted 3 sign*–Periampullary carcinoma
- *Lead pipe/Pipe stem colon*–Ulcerative colitis
- *Inverted umbrella sign*–Ileoceacal TB
- *Pincer sign*–Intussuception
- *Mercedes Benz sign*–Air in gall stones
- *Pseudopolyps*–Ulcerative colitis
- *Napkin ring/Purse string stenosis*–Ileocecal stenosis
- *Sentinel loop sign, Colon cut off sign, Renal halo sign*–Acute pancreatitis
- *Sterlin sign*–Ileoceacal TB
- *Saw tooth/Serrated appearance*–Diverticulosis
- *Scalloped edge of sigmoid colon*–Ulcerative colitis
- *String sign*–Congenital hypertropic pyloric stenosis
- *String of pearls/Chain of lakes/Hour glass appearance on ERCP*–Chronic pancreatitis
- *Wall Echo/Double Arc shadow sign*–Cholelithiasis with chronic cholecystitis
- *Widened Duodenal C loop*–Pancreatic head carcinoma

Ref: David Sutton 7th Edition Page 657, Radiology Review Manual 7th Edition Page 772, Armstrong 5th Edition Page 160, Chapman 5th Edition Page 128

Ans: (A) Acute pancreatitis

4. **IVP picture shows following picture:**

A. Ureterocele

B. VUR

C. TB urethra

D. Ureteic calculi

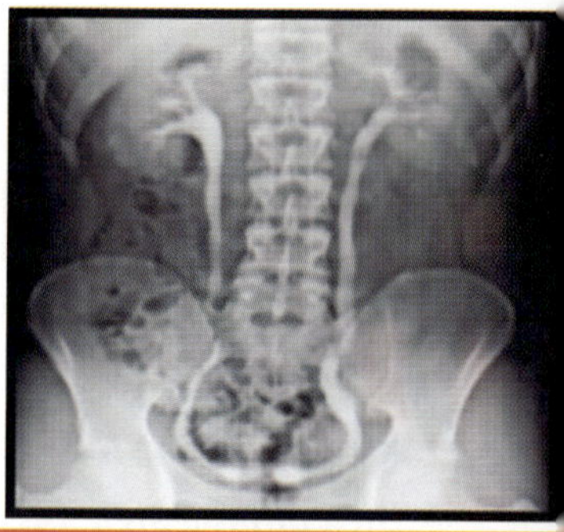

Key:

Picture shows Adder head/Cobra head appearance on IVP explains diagnosis of Ureterocele

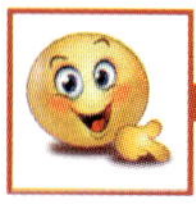

Ureterocele

Ultrasound

- Ureterocele appears as cystic structure projecting into bladder, often near normal location of the vesicoureteric junction (VUJ).
- Ectopic in majority of cases and therefore not at the expected location of the ureteric orifice. Associated ureter is usually noticeably dilated.

IVP

- Filling defect in bladder ***(Cobra head sign)*** which may be distended, collapsed/everted
- Radiolucent halo effect
- An everted ureterocele will appear like a bladder diverticulum

MCUG

- Round or oval lucency near trigone
- Effacement of the defect with increasing filling of the bladder

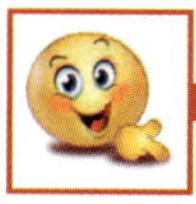

Types of Ureterocele

- **Single system ureteroceles** are those associated with single kidney, a single collecting system and solitary ureter.
- **Duplex system ureteroceles** are associated with kidneys that have a completely duplicated collecting system and two ureters.
- **Orthotopic ureterocele** is a ureterocele whose orifice is located in a normal anatomic position within the bladder. Commoner in adults.
- **Ectopic ureterocele** refers to those ureteroceles whose orifices are located in an ectopic position, such as bladder neck or urethra. They typically arise from upper pole moiety of a duplicated collecting system and are more common in the pediatric population

- Most sensitive imaging method of Renal TB–*IVP*
- Investigation of choice for renal TB in children–*IVP*
- Investigation of choice in Renal TB–*CT*
- Gold standard for diagnosis of Renal artery stenosis–***DSA/Conventional contrast renal arteriography.***

Key Signs/Features in Genitourinary System	
Swiss cheese nephrogram	Adult polycystic kidney
Putty kidney/Cement kidney	Renal TB
Saw tooth/Cork screw ureter	TB Urethritis
Thimble bladder	TB Cystitis
Soap bubble nephrogram	Hydronephrosis
Crescent sign, Rim sign	Hydronephrosis
Paint brush appearance	Medullary sponge kidney
Drooping lily/Drooping flower sign	Ectopic ureter
Flower vase ureter	Horse shoe kidney
Cobra head/Adder head deformity	Ureterocoele
Hand shaking sign	Horse shoe kidney
Sun burst Nephrogram	Polycystic kidney
Bilateral spider leg deformity	Polycystic kidney disease
Foetal head calcification bladder	Schistosomia
Fir tree/Pine tree/Christmas tree bladder	Neurogenic bladder
Lobster claw/Ball on ate of Renal pyramids	Renal papillary necrosis
Egg in cup appearance	Renal papillary necrosis
Tear drop bladder	Pelvic hematoma, Pelvic lipomatosis, Intraperitoneal bladder rupture
Goblet of urine glass/Surraco sign	Renal Hydatid
String of beads/Pile of plates appearance (Angiography)	Fibromuscular dysplasia
Chalice/Bregman sign	Transitional cell carcinoma
Kidney sweat sign	Renal failure

Ref: David Sutton 7th Edition Page 980, Lower Genitourinary Radiology by Jafri 1st Edition Page 528, Mandell Core Radiology 1st Edition Page 582, Radiology Review Manual 7th Edition Page 928

Ans: (A) Ureterocele

5. **A boy with chronic constipation and pain abdomen undergoes an imaging study. Picture is shown below. Identify the given study:**

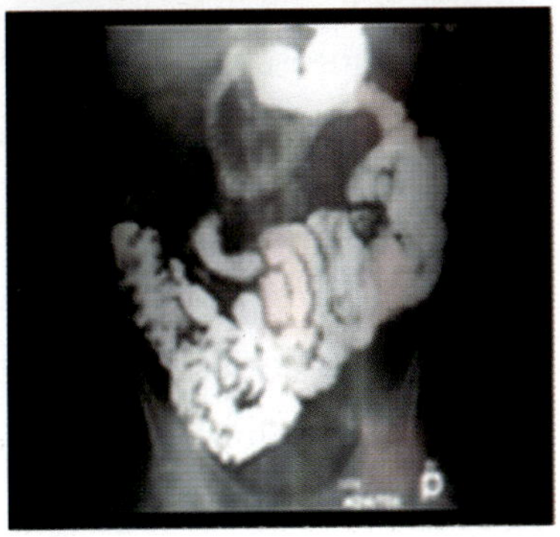

A. Enteroclysis
B. Barium meal follow through
C. Barium enema
D. Barium swallow

Key:

Enteroclysis–*Nasoduodenal tube will be visible distal to 2nd part of duodenum and there will be no contrast in stomach*
Barium Meal Follow Through–*Stomach, Duodenum, Small bowel loops upto Ileocecal junction and to some extent in Ascending colon are opacified*
Barium Enema–*Opacification of rectum, sigmoid colon and entire large bowel with Ileocecal junction*
Barium Swallow–*Opacification with contrast only from pharynx to lower esophageal sphincter rather than stomach and duodenum*

Barium swallow	Barium enema	Barium meal follow through
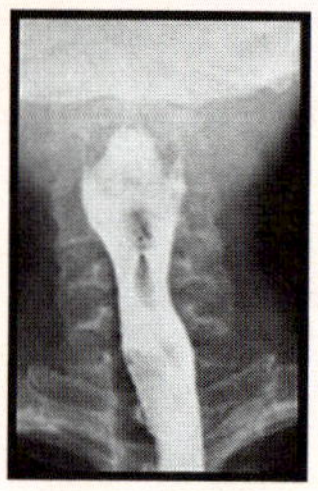	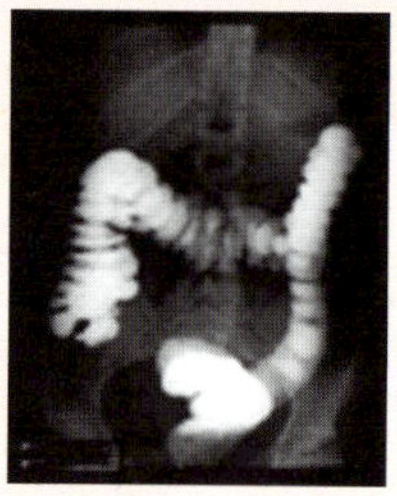	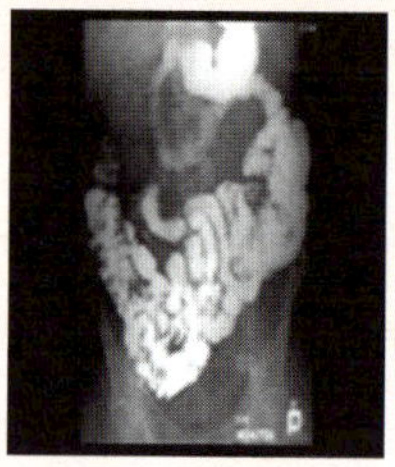

CONTRAST STUDIES

- **Barium studies**
  - Barium swallow, Barium meal, Barium enema, Barium meal follow through, Small bowel enema, Hypotonic duodenography
- **Non barium studies**
  - IVU, MCU, RCUG HSG (Hysterosalphingogram) Angiography, Dacrocystography, Myelography, Bronchography
- **Others**
  - CECT, Contrast enhanced MRI

Small Bowel Follow Through (SBFT)

- Fluoroscopic technique designed to obtain high resolution images of small bowel.
- Function of the small bowel can also be evaluated.

Indications

- Used for evaluation of small bowel abnormalities
  - Strictures, Obstruction, Diverticula, Masses
  - Extraluminal tethering, Abnormal motility

Contd.

Contd.

Limitations

- Intermittent passage of contrast through pylorus breaks up contrast column
- Less severe strictures and small masses may be difficult to see

Procedure

- Small bowel follow through is a single contrast study (oral contrast, either barium or water-soluble contrast). It is often performed after an upper GI fluoroscopic study, as contrast column moves from stomach and duodenum to small bowel.
- May also be performed by itself, without upper GI investigation of oesophagus, stomach and proximal duodenum, but this is less common.

SBFT is inferior to enteroclysis for evaluation of small bowel pathology, but enteroclysis has drawbacks that prevent it from being more widely used.

Enteroclysis

- Also called small bowel enema
- Barium X-ray examination used to display individual loops of small intestine by intubating jejunum and administering barium sulfate followed by methylcellulose or air
- ***Enteroclysis–GI technique designed to provide improved evaluation of small bowel.***

Indications

- Examination of mucosal detail of the small intestine
- Improved evaluation of small bowel tumours or inflammatory disease relative to small bowel follow through (SBFT)
- Conventional fluoroscopic technique is not widely used since it is somewhat invasive, time and labour intensive, and not particularly pleasant for the patient.
- Requires a degree of skill to perform and often information can be gathered through other techniques.
- ***In experienced hands, it is best radiographic technique for evaluation of small bowel mucosa.***
- Modifications of the traditional technique may involve CT/MRI.
- These should be differentiated from more routine CT and MR enterography.

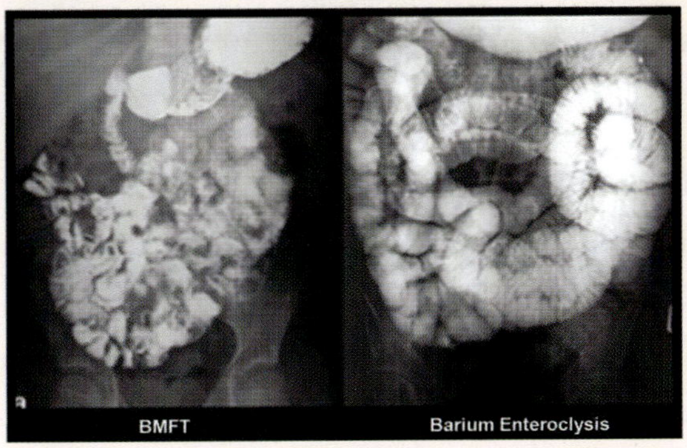

Contraindications of Barium Sulphate in GIT Studies
• Small bowel obstruction (Ionic contrast preferred)
• Intestinal perforation (Ionic contrast preferred)
• Tracheoesophageal fistula *(Non Ionic contrast preferred)–Risk of pulmonary edema with Ionic contrast*

Ref: David Sutton 7th Edition Page 552, Armstrong 5th Edition Page 160, Radiology Review Manual 7th Edition Page 772

Ans: (B) Barium meal follow through

6. Identify the marked structure in the given image:

A. Cerebellum

B. Cerebrum

C. Brainstem

D. Corpus Callosum

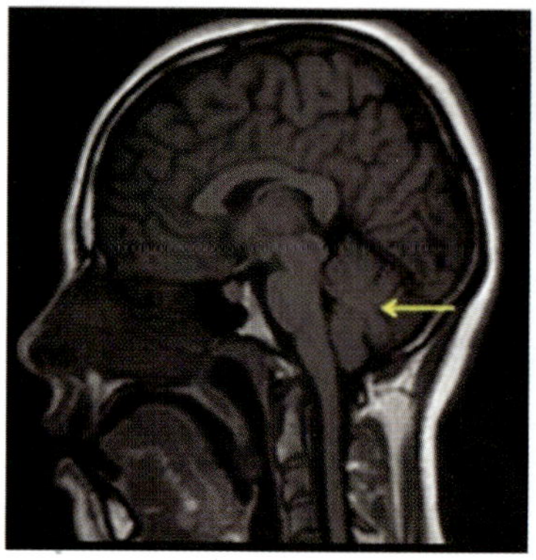

Key:

Picture depicts area which lies in hindbrain region–Cerebellum
Cerebellum is located inferior to occipital lobe of cerebrum lies in proximity to visual cortex of cerebrum and superior to pons and brainstem

Cerebrum–*Supratentorial structure consisting of 2 hemispheres*
Cerebellum–*Sits at base of brain in posterior cranial fossa below tentorium and behind brainstem*
Brainstem–*Most caudal part of brain, Adjoins and is structurally continuous with spinal cord*
Corpus callosum–*Midline supratentorial structure linking cerebral cortex of left and right cerebral hemispheres*

CEREBELLUM

- Part of hindbrain
- Lies inferior to occipital and temporal lobes
- Lies within posterior cranial fossa
- Separated from these lobes by tentorium cerebella (Tough layer of dura mater).
- Lies posterior to pons and medulla from which it is separated by 4th ventricle
- Consists of 2 cerebellar hemisphere united in midline by worm like vermis

FISSURES

- **Horizontal**
  - *Most conspicuous at junction between superior and inferior surfaces*
- **Posterolateral**
  - *Lies on inferior surface and separates flocculonodular lobe from rest of cerebellum*
- **Primary**
  - *Lies at junction of anterior 2/3rd and posterior 1/3rd*

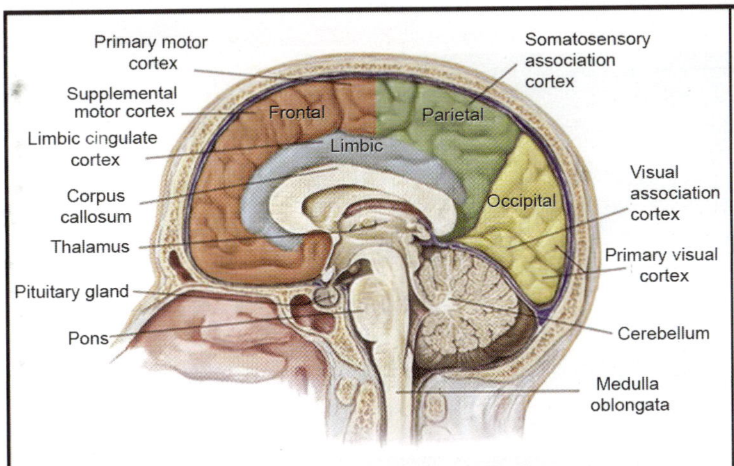

Medial aspect of the brain and brainstem

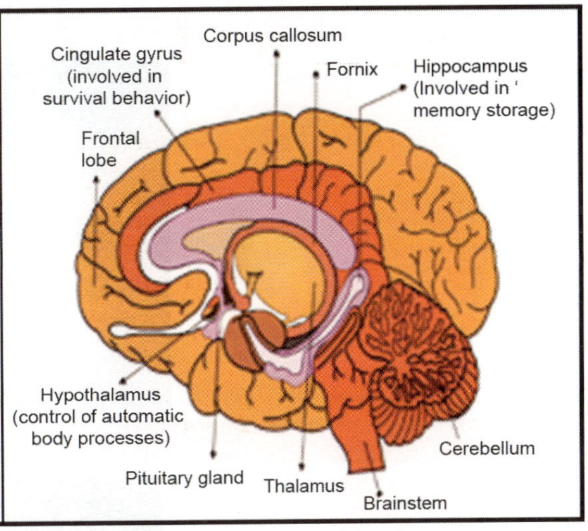

SUBDIVISIONS

- **Archicerebellum (Vestibular cerebellum)**
  - Consists of floculonodular lobe
  - Concerned with maintenance of equilibrium, tone and posterior trunk muscles
- **Paleocerebellum (Spinal)**
  - Consists of anterior lobe
  - Concerned with tone, posture and crude movements of limbs
- **Neocerebellum (Cerebral cerebellum)**
  - Most recent part and concerned with smooth performance of skilled motor activity

Lobes	Subdivisions of Vermis	Subdivisions of Cerebellar Hemisphere
Anterior lobe	**Lingula**–Central lobule and Culmen	Alae and Quadrangular lobe No lateral projection
Posterior lobe	**Declive**–Follum, Tuber, Pyramid and Uvula	**Lobulus simplex**–Superior and Inferior semilunar lobule, Biventral lobule and Tonsil
Flocculonodular lobe	Nodule	Flocculus

Version 2

Identify the structure marked in the image:

A. Cerebrum
B. Cerebellum
C. Brainstem
D. Corpus callosum

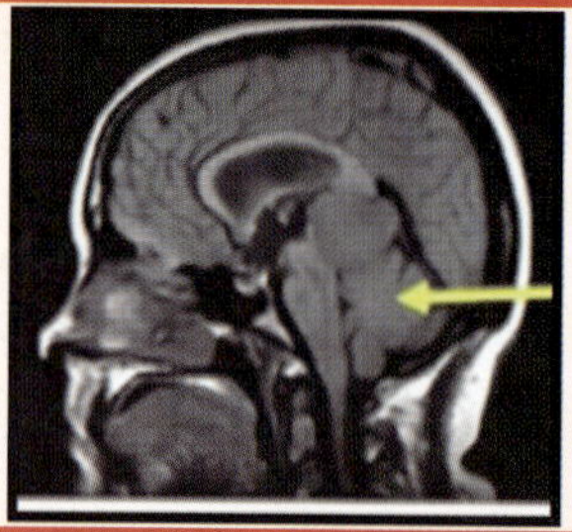

Normal Anatomy of Brain

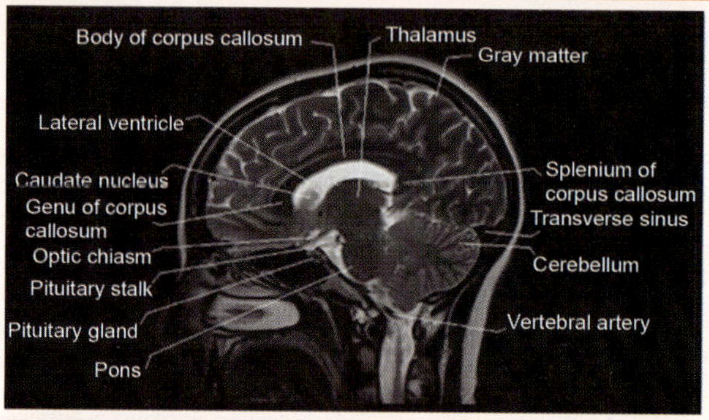

Sagittal view

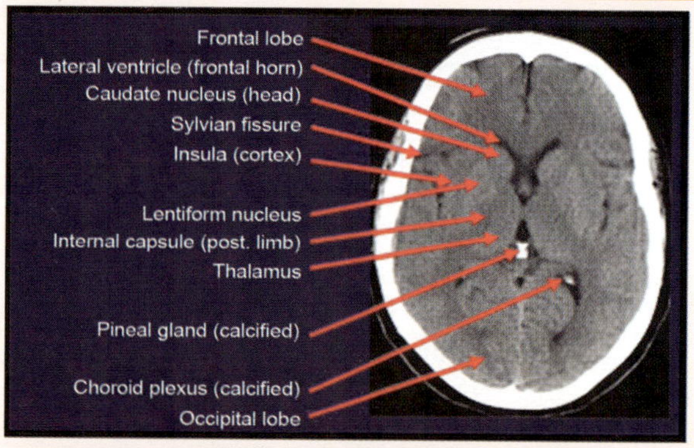

Axial view

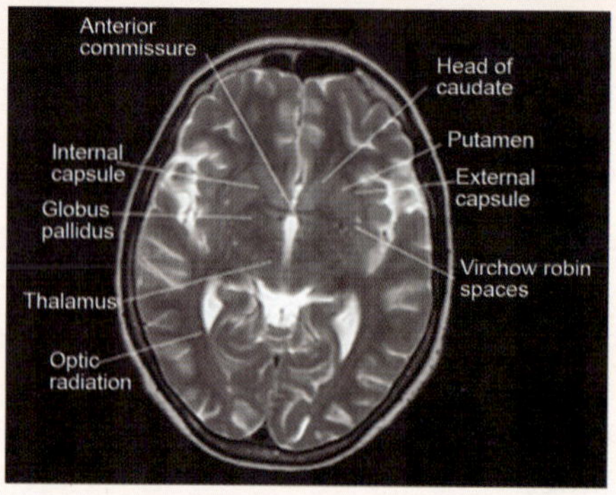

Ans: (B) Cerebellum

Ref: Radiopedia, Gray 41st Edition Page 331, Netter's Clinical Anatomy 2nd Edition Page 360, Mc Minn's Clinical Atlas of Human Anatomy 6th Edition Page 62

Ans: (A) Cerebellum

7. **CT scan image shows the following:**

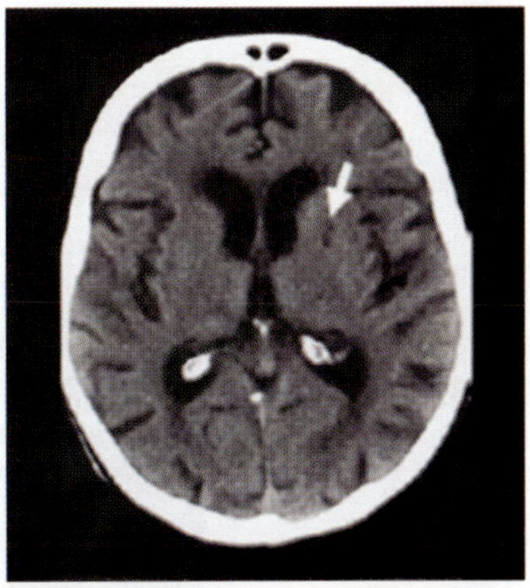

A. Left basal ganglia bleed
B. Lacunar infarct
C. Normal CT
D. Intraventricular bleed

Key:

Picture shows often rounded opacity with hazy outline suggests small infarcts
Small hypodense lesion in left gangliocapsular region isodense to CSF suggestive of chronic lacunar infarct

Other Options

- **Left basal ganglia bleed**–Lesion is not hyperdense to suggest bleed
- Lesion is not normal variant
- Lesion is far from ventricular system and no evidence of intraventricular extension to report as Intraventricular bleed.

Lacunar Infarcts

- Small (<15 mm) infarcts in the distal distribution of deep penetrating vessels ***(lenticulostriate, thalamoperforating and pontine perforating arteries, recurrent artery of Heubner).***
- Result from occlusion of one of the small penetrating end arteries at base of brain and are due to ***fibrinoid degeneration.***

Clinical Presentation

- ***Most lacunar infarcts are clinically silent,*** but repeated episodes are associated with vascular dementia.
- Symptomatic patients may present with lacunar stroke syndrome (LACS), one of five distinct syndromes.

Pathology

- Caused by occlusion small penetrating end-arteries and must be smaller than 15 mm. They are thought to result primarily from in situ microatheroma formation or lipohyalinosis 2.
- Pathologically, they are small holes of encephalomalacia and are traversed by a cob-web-like mesh of fibrous strands.

Contd.

Contd.

Radiographic Features	
CT	**MRI**
Acute lesions:	**Acute lesions:**
Appear as ill-defined **hypodensities.**	Following signal changes are seen: **T1:** Slightly hypointense **T2/FLAIR:** Hyperintense **DWI:** Restricted diffusion may demonstrate acute lesions not visible on other sequences **T1C+:** May enhance if acute (or early subacute)
Chronic lesions:	**Chronic lesions:**
Appear as **hypodense** foci (similar to CSF) 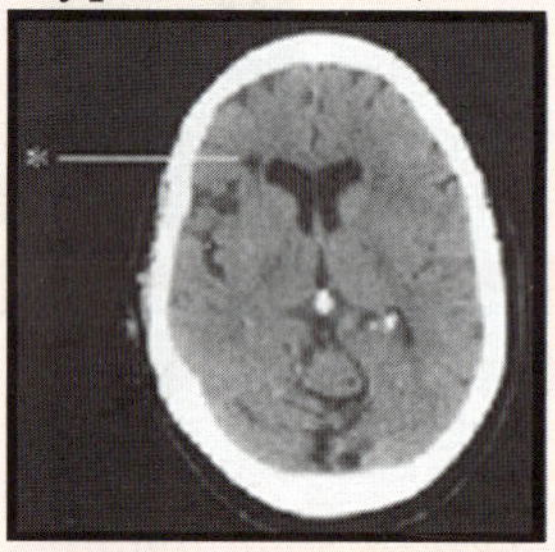	Isointense to CSF on all sequences but may demonstrate a peripheral T2/FLAIR hyperintense rim of marginal gliosis.

Differential Diagnosis

- Embolic stroke
- Enlarged Virchow-Robin spaces
- Neurocysticercosis
- Choroid fissure cysts
- Striatocapsular infarct

EXTRA EDGE

- Investigation of choice for suspected Intracranial bleed in Trauma–NCCT
- Investigation of choice for Acute Traumatic SAH–NCCT
- Investigation of choice for Acute Non traumatic SAH–Angiography
- Most common cause of SAH–Trauma
- Most common cause of Non traumatic SAH–Berry aneurysm rupture
- Investigation of choice for Chronic Intracranial bleed–MRI
- Investigation of choice for stroke in Unconscious patient–NCCT
- Investigation of choice for Non hemorrhagic infarct/stroke–MRI (Diffusion weighted)
- Investigation of choice for Hyperacute infarct–MRI (Best–DW1)

Ref: Radiology Review Manual 7th Edition Page 3131, David Sutton 6th Edition Page 215, Radiopedia Acute Ischemic Stroke by Lev 2nd Edition Page 43

Ans: (B) Lacunar infarct

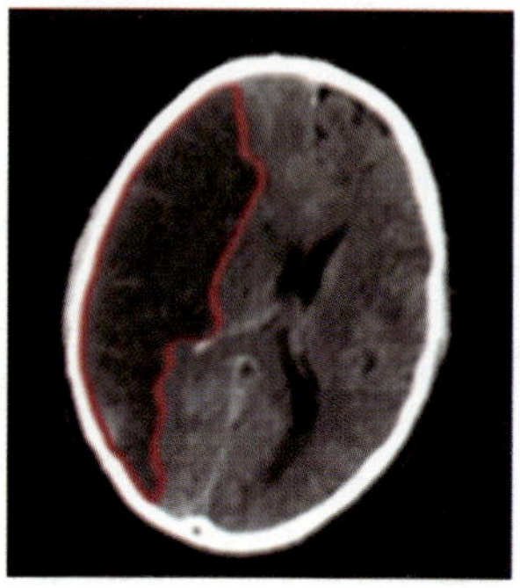

8. **A 40-year-old patient who is a known case of Diabetes, HTN and has left sided hemiplegia. His CT picture is shown. Most likey cause is:**

   A. Subarachnoid hemorrhage
   B. Intraparenchymal hemorrhage
   C. Acute infarct
   D. Intraventricular infarct

Key:

CT brain shows a large hypodense area at right cerebral region (fronto-parietal lobe, insular cortex and basal ganglia-capsular region). Patient with hypertension and diabetes presented with left sided hemiparesis. So diagnosis is acute infarct that appears as hypodense areas (Acute hemorrhage appear as hyperdense on CT scan). Therefore in our case CT brain shows acute infarct (hypodense area) in right cerebrum

CT BRAIN

- Non-contrast CT of brain remains mainstay of imaging in the setting of an acute stroke.

Goals of CT in the Acute Setting are:

- Exclude intracranial hemorrhage, which would preclude thrombolysis
- Look for any "early" features of ischemia
- Exclude other intracranial pathologies that may mimic stroke, such as tumor.

Immediate	Early Hyperacute
Earliest CT sign visible is hyperdense segment of vessel, representing direct visualization of intravascular thrombus / embolus and as such is visible immediately. It is most often observed in middle cerebral artery (see hyperdense middle cerebral artery sign and middle cerebral artery dot sign).	**Within first few hours, features include:** Loss of grey-white matter differentiation, and hypoattenuation of deep nuclei: Lentiform nucleus changes seen as early as 1 hour after occlusion, visible in 75% of patients at 3 hours. Cortical hypodensity with associated parenchymal swelling with resultant gyral effacement. Cortex which has poor collateral supply (e.g., insular ribbon) is more vulnerable.

CT Brain

• Earliest finding of middle cerebral artery occlusion–**Hyperdense middle cerebral artery sign**
• Seen immediately and represents direct visualisation of thromboembolism.
• Presence of calcification is important as it is a contraindication to angioplasty
• Early parenchymal signs include subtle blurring, decreased attenuation and swelling of the grey-white matter junction of affected regions.
• It should be noted that deep grey matter structures are affected before cortex due to lenticulostriate arteries being end arteries and cytotoxic oedema (intracellular fluid accumulation) occurring earlier
• **Lentiform nucleus; caudate nucleus**
  ○ As early as 1 hour after occlusion
  ○ Visible in 75% of patients at 3 hours

Contd.

Contd.

- **Insular ribbon**
  - Although cortical it is the furthest cortex from collateral circulation and is therefore also affected early
  - Insular ribbon sign describes loss of normal grey-white differentiation
- **Surface cortex (including peri-rolandic cortex)**
  - Collateral flow retards the development of CT signs with only 20% of cases demonstrating changes at 3 hours
- With time, hypo-attenuation and swelling become more marked, and in patients with majority of MCA territory affected the mass effect is often dramatic and life threatening, sometimes requiring decompressive craniectomy.
- As time passes infarct undergoes gradual reduction in swelling and mass effect

Signs of Hyperacute Infarct on NCCT	Signs of Acute Infarct on NCCT
• Hyperdense MCA sign • Cortical ribbon/Insular ribbon sign • Ill marginated lentiform nuclei • Sulcal effacement due to edema	• Wedge shaped cortical based hypodense area involving grey and white matter • Fogging effect in subacute stage of infarct

CT Findings of Stroke

Early CT Findings (<24 Hours)

1. **Hyperdense middle cerebral artery (MCA) or ACA sign:**
   - Due to clot in the MCA or ACA, the MCA or ACA will appear hyperdense.
   - Rare finding and Highly specific for an MCA/ACA stroke.
2. **Loss of gray/white differentiation: Early on, this is first seen in insular cortex.**
3. **Mass effect: Mild obliteration of sulci, adjacent ventricles, and subarachnoid space**

Late CT Findings (24 Hours to 21 Days)

- Hypoattenuations seen in MCA territory

Ref: Radiology Review Manual 7th Edition Page 3131,
David Sutton 6th Edition Page 215,
Radiopedia Acute Ischemic Stroke by Lev 2nd Edition Page 43

Ans: (C) Acute infarct

Chapter 19

PSYCHIATRY

1. **Extreme fear of darkness is known as:**

A. Xenophobia
B. Claustrophobia
C. Nyctophobia
D. Mysophobia

Key:

Extreme fear of darkness is known as Nyctophobia (Nycto-Night, Phobia-Fear)

PHOBIA

- Term ***phobia*** refers to an excessive fear of a specific object, circumstance, or situation.

THEORIES OF PHOBIA

- **Displacement** (Psychodynamic theory) *Anxiety is transferred from dangerous to neutral object*
- **Conditioned reflex** (Behavioural theory)
- **Hormone released by Amygdala** (Neurobiological theory)

Characteristic Features of Phobia

1. Presence of the fear of an object, situation or activity.
2. The fear is out of proportion to the dangerousness perceived.
3. Patient recognizes the fear as irrational and unjustified (Insight is present).
4. Patient is unable to control the fear and is very distressed by it.
5. This leads to persistent avoidance of the particular object, situation or activity.
6. Gradually, the phobia and the phobic object become a preoccupation with the patient, resulting in marked distress and restriction of the freedom of mobility (afraid to encounter the phobic object; *phobic avoidance*).

- ***Specific phobia is a strong, persisting and Irrational fear of an object or situation.***
- Diagnosis of specific phobia requires the development of intense anxiety, even to point of panic, when exposed to the feared object.
- ***Specific phobia is most common mental disorder among women and Second most common among men, second only to substance-related disorders.***
- Development of specific phobia may result from the pairing of a specific object or situation with the emotions of fear and panic.

DSM-5 Includes Distinctive Types of Specific Phobia
• Animal type • Natural environment type (Storms) • Blood-injection-injury type (Needles) – most familial • Situational type (Cars, Elevators, Planes) • Other type (For specific phobias that don't fit into previous four types).

Common Phobias	
Accidents	Dystychiphobia
Animals	Zoophobia
Ants	Myrmecophobia
Automobiles	Amaxophobia, motorphobia
Bees	Apiphobia, melissophobia
Birds	Ornithophobia
Blood	Haemophobia
Bridges	Gephyrophobia
Cats	Felinophobia
Choking/being smothered	Anginaphobia, pnigophobia, pnigerophobia
Contamination, dirt, or infection	Molysomophobia, mysophobia
Creepy, crawly things	Herpetophobia
Crossing streets	Agyrophobia
Darkness	Nyctophobia, scotophobia
Dentists	Dentophobia, odontophobia
Depth	Bathophobia
Doctors	Latrophobia
Dogs or rabies	Cynophobia
Everything	Panophobia, panphobia, pamphobia
Feathers	Pteronophobia
Flying	Aviophobia
Forests, at night	Nyctohylophobia
Frogs	Batrachophobia
Hair, fur, or animal skins	Chaetophobia, trichophobia, doraphobia
Horses	Equinophobia, hippophobia
Hospitals	Nosocomephobia
Injections	Trypanophobia
Jumping	Catapedaphobia
Lightning and thunder	Brontophobia, karaunophobia
Moths	Mottephobia
Needles	Aichmophobia, belonephobia
Open high places	Aeroacrophobia
Operations-surgical	Tomophobia
Places: enclosed	Claustrophobia
Railways/trains	Siderodromophobia
Rain	Ombrophobia, pluviophobia
Rats	Zemmiphobia
Reptiles	Herpetophobia
Snakes	Ophidiophobia
Spiders	Arachnophobia
Vomiting	Emetophobia
X-rays	Radiophobia

Treatment

- **Exposure therapy:** In this method, therapists desensitize patients by using a series of gradual, self-paced exposures to the phobic stimuli, and they teach patients various techniques to deal with anxiety, including relaxation, breathing control, and cognitive approaches.
- **Most effective therapy for Agarophobia**–Exposure based behavioural therapy
- **Cognitive behavior therapy**–Psychological treatment of choice for social phobia and Panic disorder

Behavioural Therapy–Systemic desensitization→Therapeutic graded exposure→ Flooding→ Participant Modeling

- **Others:** Psychodynamic insight oriented therapy, Hypnosis, Supportive psychotherapy, Family therapy, Anxiolytics, TCA, SSRI, MAO Inhibitors

> - *Drug of choice for Phobia–SSRI*
> - *Drug of choice among Benzodiazepines–Alprazolam*

Ref: Kaplan and Sadock Synopsis of Psychiatry 11th Edition Page 9.3, Oxford Handbook of Psychiatry 3rd Edition Page 364, Niraj Ahuja 5th Edition Page 97, CDTP 2nd Edition Page 362

Ans: (C) Nyctophobia

2. **Feeling of pervasive sadness without apparent reason is seen in:**
   A. Extreme depression
   B. Melancholia
   C. Delusion
   D. Major depressive disorder

Key:

Melancholia is a severe depressive disorder with psychomotor retardation
Derived from Greek melaina kole (black bile) reflecting "intensity of idea"

- Mood can be defined as a **pervasive and sustained emotion** or **feeling tone** that influences a person's behavior and colors his or her perception of being in world.
- *Depressed mood and loss of interest/pleasure are key symptoms of major depressive disorder.*
- For a patient, the depressed mood often has a distinct quality that differentiates it from the normal emotion of sadness or grief.
- Patients often describe symptom of depression as one of agonizing emotional pain and sometimes complain about being unable to cry, symptom that resolves as they improve.
- In MDD, Depression is the key symptom, although about 50 percent of patients deny depressive feelings and do not appear to be particularly depressed.

Melancholia

- Melancholia term is used to refer to a depression characterized by severe anhedonia, early morning awakening, weight loss, and profound feelings of guilt (often over trivial events).
- It is marked by severe agitation and Multiple somatic symptoms.

DSM–V Criteria

A. Either one of the following:
- Loss of interest or pleasure in all/almost all activities that are normally enjoyable
- Lack of emotional reactivity to normally pleasurable surroundings and events

B. More than or equal to 3 of 6 endogeneity symptoms:
- Waking up in the morning 2 hours or more before the usual time
- Depression worse in the morning (regularly)
- *Objective evidence of definite psychomotor retardation or agitation (remarked on or reported by other people).*

Contd.

Contd.

- Marked loss of appetite
- Weight loss (often defined as 5% or more of body weight in past month) and Marked loss of libido
- Excessive or inappropriate guilt

Presence of 4/more symptoms out of above 8 indicate melancholic depression

Melancholia is associated with changes in autonomic nervous system and in endocrine functions. For that reason, melancholia is sometimes referred to as *"endogenous depression"* or depression that arises in absence of external life stressors or precipitants.

Rule Out Other Options

- ***Classification based on Severity of depression:*** Mild, Moderate, Severe depression without psychosis, Severe depression with psychosis.
- There is no term called as extreme depression in classification system.
- ***Delusion is false, unshakable belief that is out of keeping with patient's social and cultural background.***

Melancholia (PM)	DSM-IV-TR Criteria for Major Depressive
Excessive sorrow for no reason and crying	Depressed mood
Despair, affinity towards seclusion, isolation	Markedly diminished interest or pleasure in all or almost all activities
Emaciation	Significant (> 5% body weight) weight loss or gain
Excessive appetite	Increase or decrease in appetite
Insomnia, hypersomnia in individuals of phlegmatic temperament	Insomnia or hypersomnia
Agitation and restlessness	Psychomotor agitation or retardation
Dullness, decrease in physical motility	Fatigue or loss of energy
Excessive morbid fantasies	Feelings of worthlessness or excessive or inappropriate guilt (which may be delusional)
Excessive thought, perpetual obsession	Diminished ability to think or concentrate
Preoccupation with death	Recurrent thoughts of death (not just fear of dying) recurrent suicidal ideation

- Treatment of severe depression with Psychotic symptoms/Suicidal symptoms–***ECT***
- Drug of choice for Severe depression–***TCA***
- Drug of choice for Refractory depression- ***Flouxetine+Olanzapine***
- Drug of choice for depression in Suicidal tendency patient–***SSRI***
- Drug of choice for depression in Nicotine dependence patient–***Bupropion***
- Drug of choice for depression in Peptic ulcer patient–***Doxepin***
- Drug of choice for Atypical depression–***MAO Inhibitors***
- Drug of choice for Psychotic depression–***Amoxapine***
- Mainstay of Postpartum depression disorder–***Antidepressant + Cognitive therapy***

Ref: Kaplan and Sadock Synopsis of Psychiatry 11th Edition Page 840, Oxford Handbook of Psychiatry 3rd Edition Page 394 , Niraj Ahuja 5th Edition Page 86, CDTP 2nd Edition Page 305

Ans: (B) Melancholia

3. **Premature ejaculation is a sexual disorder involving which phase of human sexual act?**

A. Orgasmic phase
B. Excitement
C. Plateau phase
D. Resolution

Key:

Premature ejaculation is a sexual disorder that involves Orgasmic sexual phase

Normal Sexual Cycle Has 5 Phases		
Phase	**Name of phase**	**Disorders Associated with Specific Phase**
1	*Desire phase*	• Male Hypoactive Sexual Desire Disorder • Female Sexual Interest/Aversion
2	*Excitement phase*	• Erectile Disorder • Female sexual arousal Disorder
3	*Plateau phase*	
4	*Orgasmic phase*	• Female Orgasmic Disorder • Delayed Ejaculation • Premature (Early) Ejaculation
5	*Resolution phase*	• Post coital dysphoria • Postcoital headache

PREMATURE EJACULATION

- In premature ejaculation, men persistently or recurrently achieve orgasm and ejaculation before they wish to.
- Diagnosis is made when a man regularly ejaculates before or within approximately 1 minute after penetration.

DSM-5 Defines the Disorder	
Intensity	**Ejaculation**
Mild	Occurs within approximately 30 sec to 1 min of vaginal penetration
Moderate	Occurs within approximately 15 to 30 seconds of vaginal penetration
Severe	Occurs at the start of sexual activity or within approximately 15 seconds of vaginal penetration

- Premature ejaculation is more commonly reported among college-educated men than among men with less education.
- Complaint is thought to be related to their concern for partner satisfaction.

PREMATURE EJACULATION

- *Physiologically predisposed to climax quickly because of shorter nerve latency time*
- *Psychogenic/Behaviourally conditioned cause*

Management	
Non-pharmacological	**Pharmacological Treatment**
A. With young, inexperienced men, who have problem, it may ***resolve in time.*** **B.** ***Behavioural management is of first line of therapy.*** Includes Sex education, clarifying myths, relaxation and correction of situational factors. **Sex therapy has been most successful in treatment of premature ejaculation.** **C.** ***Squeeze technique*** is used to raise threshold of penile excitability. In this exercise, man or woman stimulates erect penis until earliest sensations of impending ejaculation are felt. At this point, woman forcefully squeezes coronal ridge of glans, erection is diminished, and ejaculation is inhibited. **D.** Variant of the exercise is ***Stop-Start technique (Semans technique)*** developed by James H. Semans, in which woman stops all stimulation of penis when the man first senses an impending ejaculation. ***No squeeze is used.***	**A.** Persons who have premature ejaculation in spite of use of behavioural techniques, can be treated with ***clomipramine*** 25-50 mg/d, ***fluoxetine*** 5-20 mg/day, ***dapoxetine*** 30-60 mg 1-2 hours before intercourse and sertraline 25-200 mg/d. **B.** **Combination of SSRI and PDE 5 inhibitors** like sildenafil has better outcome than SSRI alone.

Research shows presence/absence of circumcision has no bearing on man's ejaculatory control.

Ref: Kaplan and Sadock Comprehensive Textbook of Psychiatry 9h Edition Page 2039, Kaplan and Sadock Synopsis of Psychiatry Page 586, Niraj Ahuja 5th Edition Page 141

Ans: (A) Orgasmic phase

4. Drug that is useful in smoking cessation:

A. Varenicline B. Acamprostate
C. Nifedipine D. Riluzole

Key:

Varenicline, Agonist at alpha 7 nicotinic Acetylcholine receptor and partial agonist on Alpha 4 Beta 2 receptor is approved for usage in smoking cessation/tobacco dependence

TOBACCO ABUSE

- 35% of adults in India use some form of tobacco.
- Smokeless tobacco use is more common than smoking (both in male and females).
- *Most common form of smoking–Beedi smoking.*
- *Active ingradient of tobacco that causes addiction–Nicotine.*
- Immediately following inhalation, smoking delivers a bolus of nicotine in cerebral arterial circulation.

- ***Use of smokeless tobacco produces slower delivery of nicotine.***
- **Nicotine** binds to brain cholinergic receptors and releases surge of dopamine, neurotransmitter in reward pathway, is responsible for its reinforcing effect.

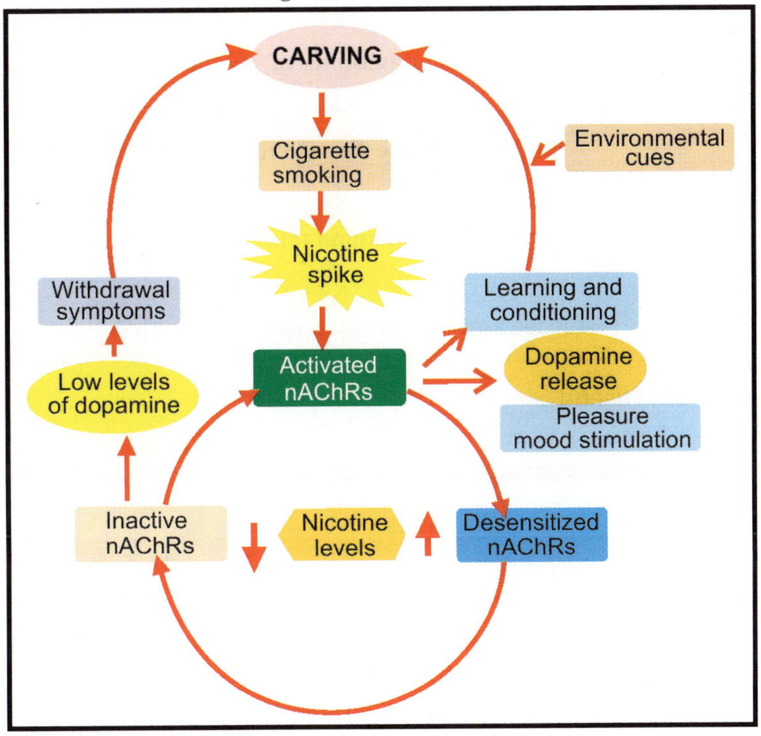

- *Nicotine and CO are responsible for Cardiovascular disorders.*

MANAGEMENT

NICOTINE DEPENDENCE

- **Non pharmacological**
  - Motivational interviewing, Counselling and motivational enhancement therapy
- **Pharmacological**
  - **Nicotine replacement therapy**
    Gum/Lozenges/Patch/Nasal spray/Inhaler
  - **Bupropion**
    (Acts on dopamine and NER receptor)
    150 mg tid for 3 days followed by 150 mg bd starting 1 week before quit date.
    Bupropion has not been significantly associated with increased tobacco abstinence
  - **Nortriptyline, Clonidine (2nd line)**
  - **Varenicline**

- ***90% of individuals who are nicotine dependent doesn't need pharmacotherapy.***

NICOTINE REPLACEMENT THERAPY

⇩

Smaller amounts of Nicotine

⇩

Bind to nicotinic Acetylcholine receptors

⇩

Dopamine release

⇩

Reduced cravings for cigarettes and other products

- Behavioural therapy is also useful

Varenicline

- ***Varenicline–Most effective agent for smoking cessation.***
- **Varenicline** is an alpha 4 beta 2 partial agonist at nicotinic acetylcholine receptors.
- FDA approved drug for use in treatment of nicotine addiction/dependence.
- One and half time more than bupropion and twice that of NRTs.

When administered with nicotine, reduces pleasurable effects of smoking and potentially reduces risk of relapse after temporary lapse.

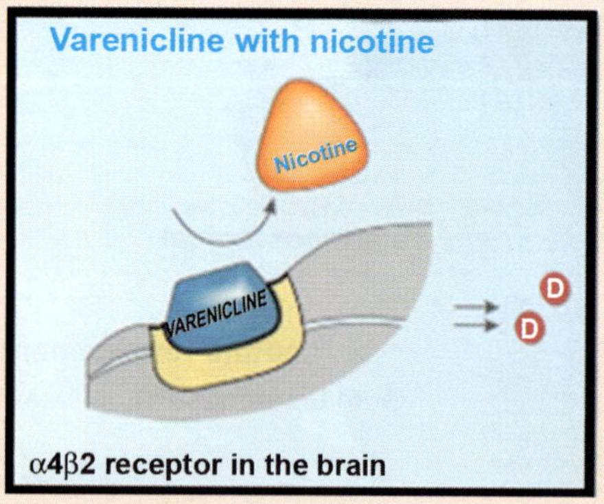

Relieves craving and withdrawal
Most effective agent for smoking cessation

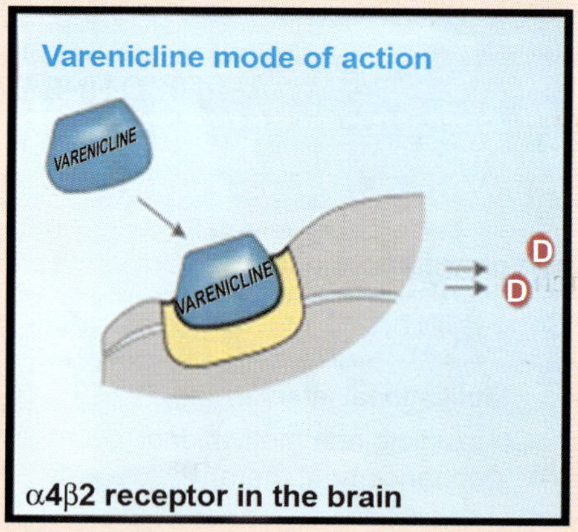

- Causes ***sustained but small amounts of dopamine release*** (less than with nicotine) and reduces nicotine withdrawal symptoms and the urge to smoke; increases abstinence.
- ***Unlike nicotine or bupropion, patient cannot "smoke over" varenicline since it will block effects of additional smoked nicotine if patient decides to smoke during treatment.***
- **Dosage:** 1-3 d 0.5 mg OD, 4-6 d 0.5 mg BD, 6 d-12 weeks 1 mg BD.

  Continue for another 12 weeks if it is effective.

  Start taking varenicline 1 week before quit date.
- **Side Effects:** Dose-dependent nausea, vomiting, constipation, flatulence, Insomnia, headache, abnormal dreams.
- Rare activation of agitation, depressed mood, suicidal ideation, suicidal behavior, seizures. Should be used with caution in patients with comorbid psychiatric illness.

Substance Abuse	Drug of Choice
Opoid overdose/Intoxication	**Naloxone IV**
Opoid Withdrawal symptoms	**Methadone** (Symptomatic relief)
Opoid detoxification	**Methadone, Buprenorphine, Clonidine** Accelerated detoxification–All above along with Naloxone
Opoid dependence	**Naloxone** (Maintenance treatment)
Alcohol detoxification	**Benzodiazepines (Chlordiazepoxide)**
Alcohol Abstinence/Maintenance	**Disulfiram, Naltrexone, Acamprosate, Baclofen, Topiramate, Fluoxetine**
Cannabis	**Short term–Benzodiapines** **Long term–Psychotherapeutic approach**

Ref: Kaplan and Sadock Synopsis of Psychiatry 11th Edition Page 632, Oxford 5th Edition Page 432, CDTP 2nd Edition Page 245, Niraj Ahuja 6th Edition Page 41

Ans: (A) Varenicline

5. **Confusion assessment method (CAM) is used to diagnose?**

A. Dementia
B. Alzhemeir disease
C. Delirium
D. Schizophrenia

Key:

Confusion assessment method (CAM) is used to diagnose Delerium

CONFUSION ASSESSMENT METHOD

- *CAM is a tool to aid in diagnosis of delirium.*
- Every older hospitalized patient should undergo brief but formal cognitive testing with use of instruments such as MMSE and CAM.
- *Administration time of CAM is approximately 2 minutes.*

1a. Acute Onset: Is there evidence of an acute change in mental status from the patient's baseline?

OR

1b. Fluctuating course: Did the (abnormal) behavior fluctuate during the day, that is tend to come and go or increase and decrease in severity?

AND

2. Inattention: Did the patients have difficulty focusing attention, for example being easily distractible, or having difficulty keeping track of what was being said?

AND

3. Disorganised thinking: Was the patient's thinking disorganized or incoherent, such as rambling or irrelevant conversation, unclear or illogical flow of ideas, or unpredictable switching from subject to subject?

OR

4. Altered level of consciousness: Overall, how would you rate this patient's level of consciousness? Any answer other than 'alert' indicates an abnormal level of consciousness.

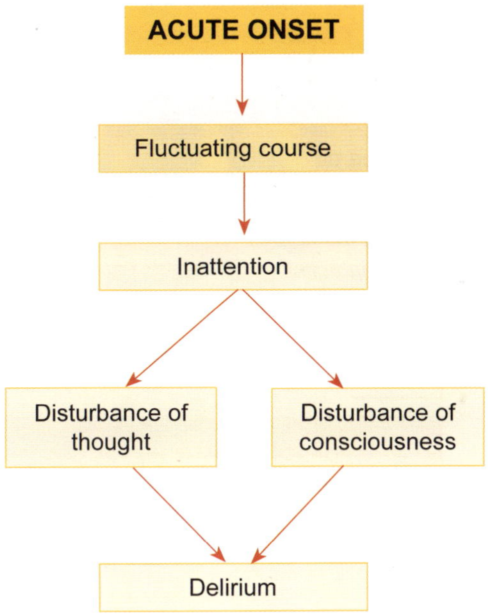

In order to diagnose delirium, first and second criteria must be present and either one of third/fourth criteria.

- CAM also looks for the ***evidence of disorientation, memory impairment, psychomotor changes, altered sleep-wake cycle changes, and perceptual disturbances.***
- CAM has been validated in number of settings, including ICU (CAM-ICU).

Delirium Scales

- NEECHAM Confusion scale
- Delirium Observation scale
- CAM (Confusion Assessment method)
- CAM-ICU (Confusion Assessment method for ICU)
- Delusion rating scale–Revised version (DRS-R 98)
- Memorial selirium assessment scale for diagnosis
- Delirium in Pediatric Age group
- Pediatric Anaesthesia Emergence Delirium scale
- Pediatric CAM-ICU

Ref: Kaplan and Sadock Comprehensive Textbook of Psychiatry 10th Edition Page 1159, Niraj Ahuja 7th Edition Page 38, CDTP 2nd Edition Page 190, Oxford 5th Edition Page 530

Ans: (C) Delirium

6. **Feeling of having experienced a current event in the past is known as:**

A. *déjà vu* B. *jamaisvous*
C. *déjà entendu* D. *déjà pense*

Key:

Déjà vu is not primarily memory disorder but a disturbance in which associated feeling of familiarity that normally occurs with previously experienced events occurs with a novel event, that is, when the event is experienced for the first time

Distortions of Recognition include

- *déjà vu*
- *jamaisvous*
- *déjà entendu*
- *déjà pense*

DÉJÀ VU

- ***Déjà vu*** is not primarily a memory disorder but a disturbance in which the associated feeling of familiarity that normally occurs with previously experienced events occurs with a novel event, that is, when the event is experienced for the first time.

Contd.

Contd.

- ***Déjà vu*** has been produced with brain stimulation.
- Penfeld and Kristiensen were able to reproduce a sensation of familiarity with stimulation of a brain electrode in epileptic patients.
- This stimulation clearly produced an abnormality of the feeling of familiarity, not an abnormality of memory. It was a disturbance of the feeling of recognition that accompanies recall in the process of memory.

Jamaisvous

- ***Jamaisvous*** is the knowledge that an event has been experienced before but is not presently associated with the appropriate feelings of familiarity.
- In *jamaisvous*, the patient may also have the feeling that some important memory is about to be recalled, although it does not actually arrive.

Déjà Entendu

- ***Déjà entendu***, the feeling of auditory recognition. Illusion that what one is hearing one has heard previously.

Déjà Pense

- Déjà pense, a new thought recognised as having previously occurred.

Déjà vu and jamais vu *are common, normal experiences but may also be signifcant symptoms of* ***temporal lobe epilepsy or cerebrovascular disorder.*** *Déjà vu and jamais vu are quite often described in* ***schizophrenia.***

Ref: Niraj Ahuja 5th Edition Page 253, Sims' Symptoms in the Mind 5th Edition 2015, Fish Clinical Psychopathology

Ans: (A) Déjà vu

7. **True about somnambulism are all except:**

A. Disorder of arousal of sleep
B. Consciousness of person is intact
C. Decreased motor skill is observed
D. Children are more affected

Key:

Somnambulism is defined as Arousal parasomnia that consists of series of complex behaviours resulting in large movements in bed or walking during sleep

- **Parasomnias:** Disorders of sleep arousal with dysfunctional events
- **Dyssomnias:** Abnormality in duration or quality of sleep

Parasomnia		
NREM sleep arousal disorders	**REM sleep arousal disorders**	**Other parasomnias**
Sleep walking Sleep eating Sex somnia Sleep related terror	REM sleep behavior disorder Nightmare disorder Recurrent isolated sleep paralysis	Enuresis Sleep related groaning Sleep related hallucinations

SOMNAMBULISM/SLEEP WALKING

- Parasomnia due to drug/substance use or a general medical condition.
- **Sleep walking** is a parasomnia and is ***disorder of partial arousal*** (NREM sleep arousal disorder).

- ***Common in children and has peak prevalence between ages 4 and 8 years.***
- After adolescence, it usually disappears spontaneously and is rarely seen in adults.
- Sleep walking in its classic form, is a condition in which an individual arises from bed and ambulates without fully awakening.
- It is sometimes called ***somnambulism,*** and ***individuals can engage in a variety of complex behaviors while unconscious.***
- Episodes may range from sitting up and attempting to walk to conducting an involved sequence of semi-purposeful actions ***(Can ambulate even though not fully awake).***
- An individual who is sleep walking is difficult to awaken.
- Sleep walker may ***interact with the environment inappropriately,*** which sometimes results in injury.
- Once awake, the sleep walker will ***usually appear confused.***
- In their confused state, sleep walkers may think they are being attacked and may react violently to defend themselves.
- It is best to gently attempt to lead sleep walkers back to bed rather than to attempt to awaken them by grabbing, shaking, or shouting.

Sleep related eating disorder: Syndrome involves an inability to get back to sleep after awakening unless individual has something to eat or drink. After eating/drinking, rest of sleep is normal.
Night terror (Sleep terror): Arousal in first one third of night. Invariably starts with piercing scream or cry with intense pain. No recall on waking up next day. More common in boys. No specific treatment required.
Nightmare: Vivid, anxiety producing dreams during REM sleep. Patient wakes up and is able to recall nightmare vividly. TCA, SSRI and Benzodiazepines are treatment.
Bruxism: Tooth grinding occurring during stage 2 NREM.
Somniloquy (Sleep talking): Occurs in all stages of sleep.
Sleep related head banging (Jactatio Capitis Nocturna): Rhythmic to and fro head rocking that occurs just before or during sleep.

Ref: Kaplan and Sadock Synopsis of Psychiatry 11th Edition Page 546, Niraj Ahuja 6th Edition Page 148, CDTP 2nd Edition Page 471, Oxford 5th Edition Page 371

Ans: (B) Consciousness of person is intact

8. Exposure and response prevention therapy has poor prognosis with which of the following components of OCD?

A. Pathological doubt
B. Contamination of dirt
C. Hoarding behaviour
D. Magical thinking

Key:

Hoarding behaviour has poor response to psychological therapy in OCD
Effective treatments for OCD have shown little benefit for patients with hoarding disorder

Poor Response to Exposure and Response Prevention in OCD

- Hoarding behaviour
- Increased OCD symptom severity and Increased anxiety
- OCD Subtypes like religious, sexual and contamination
- Unemployed
- Single/Unmarried

Magical Thinking

- Patient believes that mere thinking about an event in external worls can cause event to occur without intermediate physical action
- Most commonly seen in OCD and Schizophrenia
- **Example:** Patient believing that if he/she doesn't perform an act 3 times, great danger will befall him/her

Pathological Doubt

- *Obsession of doubt associated with compulsion of checking*
- **Example:** Repeated check of Locking of door

Dirt Contamination

- Most common presentation
- Repeated hand washing and avoidance of situations that provoke obsessive thoughts
- Frequently avoid public toilet usage

Hoarding Behaviour

- Disorder is characterized by acquiring and not discarding things that are deemed to be of little or no value, resulting in excessive clutter of living spaces.
- **Hoarding disorder now considered to be a separate diagnostic entity (Not a subtype of OCD)**
- Hoarding is associated with high rates of personality disorders like dependent, avoidant, schizotypal, and paranoid types in addition to OCD.
- *Effective treatments for OCD has little benefit for hoarding disorder patients.*
- Most effective treatment for the disorder is a cognitive behavioral model that includes training in decision making and categorizing; exposure and habituation to discarding; and cognitive restructuring.

Obsessive Compulsive Disorder

OBSESSIVE COMPULSIVE DISORDER

- **Obsession: Isolation of affect**
  - *Recurrent, persistent thoughts, impulses and images that are experienced as intrusive and inappropriate resulting in marked anxiety/distress*
- **Compulsion: Doing-Undoing**
  - *Repetitive Behaviour/Act performed repeatedly–Reduces distress caused by Obsession*

- ***Serotonin is major neurotransmitter involved in OCD***

Etiology

- Serotonin dysregulation–Linked to OCD symptomatology
- Regression to anal sadistic phase
- Group A beta hemolytic streptococcus–Neuroimmunological link
- **OCPD–**Obsessive compulsive personality disorder–Most patients don't have Pre morbid OCPD

Clinical Features

- **Contamination–Washing cycle (Washers)**
- **Pathological doubt (Checkers)**
- **Intrusive thoughts–**Pure obsessions but no compulsions→Repetitive sex thoughts
- **Symmetry–**Need for precision→ Need to keep books in order

Treatment

TREATMENT OF OCD

- **Pharmacotherapy**
- **Behaviour therapy**
- **Combination of pharmacotherapy and behaviour therapy (Most effective)**

Pharmacotherapy

- **Drug/Treatment of choice–**SSRI/Clomipramine
- Best SSRI for treatment of OCD–Fluvoxamine
- Best treatment for Resistant OCD–Clomipramine IV
- Lithium, Clonazepam, Buspirone, Risperidone, Venlafaxine can also be used

Behaviour Therapy

- ***Behaviour therapy is therapy of choice for OCD*** (Longer lasting benefits)
- Most common behaviour therapy used–Exposure and Response prevention
- **Others–**Thought stopping, Flooding and Systemic desensitization
- Electroconvulsive therapy and Psychosurgery–Other treatment options

Predictors of Prognosis–OCD

Poor prognosis	Good prognosis
Yielding compulsions	Sudden onset
Childhood onset	Episodic course

Contd.

Contd.

Bizarre compulsions Coexisting depression Presence of delusions Presence of personality disorders	Good socio-occupational functioning

Exposure and Response Prevention

- Aims to eliminate rituals and avoidance by teaching patients how to tolerate distress without engaging in counterproductive behaviours and providing ***"corrective information"*** that challenges people's existing fear response.

Current Guidelines Recommend ERP as First-line Treatment for OCD

- Only about half of patients who receive it will reach complete symptom remission.
- Approximately two-thirds of patients who received ERP experience improvement in symptoms and approximately 1/3rd of patients were considered to be recovered.
- Factors that are ***associated with poor response, including lack of adherence to treatment, poor insight, comorbid depression and OCD severity.***
- Individuals with contamination obsessions may be more resistant to treatment than those with other primary symptom presentations, as they did not fare as well as individuals with other types of symptoms.

Author's Note

Hoarding behavior is now not a part of OCD and more over it is resistant to treatment
If only OCD symptoms are given mark Contamination of Dirt as Poor prognostic for treatment

So final answer is Hoarding behavior/Pathology (No confusion)

Ref: Kaplan and Sadock Synopsis of Psychiatry 11th Edition Page 418, CDTP 2nd Edition Page 352, Niraj Ahuja 7th Edition Page 95, Oxford 5th Edition Page 199, Hezel DM, Simpson HB. Exposure and Response Prevention for Obsessive Compulsive Disorder: A Review and New Directions. Indian J Psychiatry 2019;61:S85-92

Ans: (C) Hoarding behaviour